CLINICAL
PHARMACOKINETICS
HANDBOOK

Notice

Medicine is an ever-changing science. As new research and clinical experience broaden our knowledge, changes in treatment and drug therapy are required. The authors and the publisher of this work have checked with sources believed to be reliable in their efforts to provide information that is complete and generally in accord with the standards accepted at the time of publication. However, in view of the possibility of human error or changes in medical sciences, neither the authors nor the publisher nor any other party who has been involved in the preparation or publication of this work warrants that the information contained herein is in every respect accurate or complete, and they disclaim all responsibility for any errors or omissions or for the results obtained from use of the information contained in this work. Readers are encouraged to confirm the information contained herein with other sources. For example and in particular, readers are advised to check the product information sheet included in the package of each drug they plan to administer to be certain that the information contained in this work is accurate and that changes have not been made in the recommended dose or in the contraindications for administration. This recommendation is of particular importance in connection with new or infrequently used drugs.

CLINICAL PHARMACOKINETICS HANDBOOK

Larry A. Bauer, Pharm.D.

Professor
Departments of Pharmacy and Laboratory Medicine
Schools of Pharmacy and Medicine
University of Washington
Seattle, Washington

McGraw-Hill
Medical Publishing Division

New York   Chicago   San Francisco   Lisbon   London   Madrid   Mexico City
Milan   New Delhi   San Juan   Seoul   Singapore   Sydney   Toronto

The *McGraw·Hill* Companies

Clinical Pharmacokinetics Handbook

1 2 3 4 5 6 7 8 9 0   DOC/DOC   0 9 8 7 6 5

ISBN: 0-07-142542-X

This book was set in Times Roman by International Typesetting and Composition.
The editors were Michael Brown and Karen Edmonson.
The production supervisor was Sherri Souffrance.
Project management was provided by International Typesetting and Composition.
The cover designer was Pehrsson Design.
RR Donnelley was printer and binder.

This book is printed on acid-free paper.

Cataloging-in-Publication data for this title is on file at the Library of Congress.

International Edition ISBN: 0-07-110492-5

Copyright © 2006. Exclusive rights by The McGraw-Hill Companies, Inc. for manufacture and export. This book cannot be re-exported from the country to which it is consigned by McGraw-Hill. The International Edition is not available in North America.

To my wife (S.P.B.)
for her unwavering, unlimited support and caring for over 25 years
and
to my daughters (L.A.B. & L.E.B.)
for their no-holds-barred, every-day-is-a-new-opportunity approach to
life—you both constantly teach me new things.

P.S. Dad, this one's for you.

Contents

PART V IMMUNOSUPPRESSANTS

PART VI OTHER DRUGS

About the Author

Larry A. Bauer, Pharm.D., is a Professor at the University of Washington School of Pharmacy and has been on the faculty since 1980. He also holds an adjunct appointment at the same rank in the Department of Laboratory Medicine, where he is a toxicology consultant. He received his Bachelor of Science in Pharmacy degree (1977) from the University of Washington, and his Doctor of Pharmacy degree (1980) from the University of Kentucky. He also completed an ASHP-accredited hospital pharmacy residency (1980), specializing in clinical pharmacokinetics, at A. B. Chandler Medical Center at the University of Kentucky, under the preceptorship of Dr. Paul Parker and under the guidance of Dr. Robert Blouin. Dr. Bauer is a fellow of the American College of Clinical Pharmacology and of the American College of Clinical Pharmacy.

Dr. Bauer's specialty area is in clinical pharmacokinetics, and he teaches courses and offers clinical clerkships in this area. His research interests include the pharmacokinetics and pharmacodynamics of drug interactions, the effects of liver disease and age on drug metabolism, the effects of renal disease and dialysis on drug elimination, and computer modeling of population pharmacokinetics. He has over 140 published research papers, abstracts, and book chapters. Also, he is author of the textbook entitled *Applied Clinical Pharmacokinetics* (McGraw-Hill, 2001). Dr. Bauer is a member of several clinical pharmacology and clinical pharmacy professional organizations. He is a reviewer for several scientific publications, was Consulting Editor of *Clinical Pharmacy* (1981–1990) and Field Editor of *ASHP Signal* (1981–1983), and is currently on the Editorial Boards of *Clinical Pharmacology and Therapeutics* and *Antimicrobial Agents and Chemotherapy*. Dr. Bauer has precepted three postdoctoral fellows in clinical pharmacokinetics who currently have faculty appointments in schools of pharmacy or positions in the pharmaceutical industry.

Preface

After writing *Applied Clinical Pharmacokinetics*, something unanticipated happened. While passing through the intensive care unit of our hospital, I encountered several advanced clerkship students who were carrying the textbook with them while on patient rounds. Later, on the same trip through the hospital, a couple of staff clinical pharmacists congratulated me on publishing the textbook, and one asked when a handbook with similar content would be available. I began considering ideas for such a handbook on that day.

My original concept was to write a handbook that focused solely on the dosing aspects of each drug, omitting other material that was included in the textbook. However, when I made a prototype for a couple of drugs that followed this plan and gave copies to a few clerkship students and clinical pharmacists, they all requested a handbook format that followed the one in the textbook. Clerkship students and beginning practitioners found the additional information for all drugs to be useful, while more advanced practitioners found the extra material helpful for drugs that they didn't use very often.

Based on this limited market research, *Clinical Pharmacokinetics Handbook* is an updated distillation of the information in *Applied Clinical Pharmacokinetics* that can easily be carried in a lab coat pocket in patient care areas. The handbook follows the same format as the textbook, it contains most of the same information (but in an outline form), and it uses many of the same patient examples for the various dosing techniques. As a result, previous users of the textbook will feel very comfortable with the format of the material. New users will find that each drug-specific chapter follows the same logical format, so that similar information about different medications can be easily found.

I remain convinced that the ideal approach to therapeutic drug monitoring is matching the best initial dosage and dosage adjustment techniques to the individual patient and the desired therapeutic goals. However, to provide some guidance in selecting methods that work well together, I have provided a new section entitled "Dosing Strategies." This section links together an initial dosing approach with a dose adjustment method that practitioners can consider during the treatment of patients. However, as long as the limitations for each dosing technique are adhered to, any of the initial dosing methods can be coupled with any of the dosing adjustment methods to achieve individualized drug dosage regimens.

From *Applied Clinical Pharmacokinetics*

Being a practitioner for over 20 years, I have had an opportunity to see the development of therapeutic drug monitoring almost from its inception. What began in the late 1960s and early 1970s as a way to optimize cardiac glycoside and aminoglycoside antibiotic treatment for patients has, in the 21st century, blossomed into an integral part of patient care for many drugs. On any given day, our clinical laboratory reports the results of over 200 patient drug concentration assays to clinicians.

My strong belief is that clinical pharmacokinetics cannot be practiced in a vacuum. Individuals interested in using these dosing techniques for their patients must also be excellent clinical practitioners. Although it is true that "kinetics = dose," clinicians must be able to select the best drug therapy among many choices and appropriately monitor patients for therapeutic response, adverse drug effects, potential drug interactions, disease states and conditions that alter drug dosage, and so on. Thus, it is not acceptable to simply suggest a dose and walk away from the patient, satisfied that the job has been done. It is my sincere hope that this book will help clinicians increase their knowledge in the area of therapeutic drug monitoring and improve care to their patients.

Larry A. Bauer, Pharm.D.

CLINICAL PHARMACOKINETICS HANDBOOK

1 | **BASIC CONCEPTS**

1 | Clinical Pharmacokinetic and Pharmacodynamic Concepts

Clinical pharmacokinetics is the discipline that applies pharmacokinetic concepts and principles in humans in order to design individualized dosage regimens that optimize the therapeutic response of a medication while minimizing the chance of an adverse drug reaction.

- Pharmacokinetics is the study of the *absorption, distribution, metabolism,* and *excretion* of drugs.[1]

  - When drugs are given extravascularly (e.g., orally, intramuscularly, applied to the skin via a transdermal patch, etc.), absorption must take place for the drug molecules to reach the systemic circulation.
  - *Distribution* occurs when drug molecules that have entered the vascular system pass from the bloodstream into various tissues and organs such as the muscle or heart.
  - *Metabolism* is the chemical conversion of the drug molecule, usually by an enzymatically mediated reaction, into another chemical entity referred to as a metabolite. The metabolite may have the same, or different, pharmacological effect as the parent drug, or even cause toxic side effects.
  - *Excretion* is the irreversible removal of drug from the body, and commonly occurs via the kidney or biliary tract.

- Pharmacodynamics is the relationship between drug concentration and pharmacological response (Figure 1-1).

LINEAR VERSUS NONLINEAR PHARMACOKINETICS

- When drugs are given on a constant basis, such as a continuous intravenous infusion or an oral medication given every 12 hours, serum drug concentrations increase until the rate of drug administration equals the rate of drug metabolism and excretion. At that point, serum drug concentrations become constant during a continuous intravenous infusion or exhibit a repeating pattern over each dosage interval for medications given at a scheduled time (Figure 1-2).
- Regardless of the mode of drug administration, when the rate of drug administration equals the rate of drug removal, the amount of drug contained in the body reaches a constant value. This equilibrium condition is known as *steady state* and is extremely important in clinical pharmacokinetics because steady-state serum or blood concentrations are often used to assess patient response and to compute new dosage regimens.
- If a patient is administered several different doses until steady state is established, and steady-state serum concentrations are obtained from the patient after each dosage level, it is possible to determine a pattern of drug accumulation (Figure 1-3). If a plot of steady-state concentration versus dose yields a straight line, the drug is said to follow *linear pharmacokinetics*. In this situation, steady-state serum concentrations increase or decrease proportionally with dose.

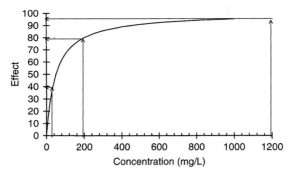

FIG. 1-1 The relationship between drug concentration and response is usually a hyperbolic function: Effect = $(E_{max} \cdot C)/(EC_{50} + C)$, where E_{max} is the maximum effect and EC_{50} is the drug concentration when the drug effect equals $E_{max}/2$. After a dosage change is made and drug concentrations increase, the drug effect does not change proportionally. Further, the increase in pharmacological effect is greater when the initial concentration is low compared to the change in drug effect observed when the initial concentration is high.

- If a patient has been taking a medication long enough for steady state to have been established, and it is determined that a dosage adjustment is necessary because of lack of drug effect or the presence of drug toxicity, steady-state drug concentrations will change in proportion to dose for drugs that follow linear pharmacokinetics.

- When steady-state concentrations change in a disproportionate fashion after the dose is altered, a plot of steady-state concentration versus dose is not a straight line and the drug is said to follow *nonlinear pharmacokinetics*.

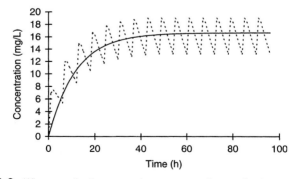

FIG. 1-2 When medications are given on a continuous basis, serum concentrations increase until the rate of drug administration equals the elimination rate. For the intravenous infusion, serum concentrations increase in a smooth pattern until steady state is achieved (solid line). During oral dosing of an equivalent amount, the serum concentrations oscillate around the intravenous profile, increasing during drug absorption and decreasing after absorption is complete and elimination takes place (dashed line).

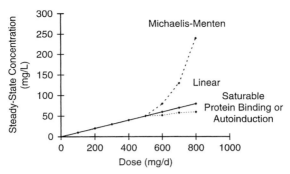

FIG. 1-3   When doses are increased for most drugs, steady-state concentrations increase in a proportional fashion, leading to linear pharmacokinetics (solid line). However, in some cases proportional increases in steady-state concentrations do not occur after a dosage increase. When steady-state concentrations increase more than expected after a dosage increase (upper dashed line), Michaelis-Menten pharmacokinetics may be taking place. If steady-state concentrations increase less than expected after a dosage increase (lower dashed line), saturable plasma protein binding or autoinduction are likely explanations.

- When steady-state concentrations increase more than expected after a dosage increase, the most likely explanation is that the processes removing the drug from the body have become saturated. This phenomenon is known as *saturable or Michaelis-Menten pharmacokinetics*. Phenytoin[2] follows Michaelis-Menten pharmacokinetics.
- When steady-state concentrations increase less than expected after a dosage increase, there are two typical explanations. Some drugs, such as valproic acid,[3] *saturate plasma protein binding sites* so that as the dosage is increased, steady-state serum concentrations increase less than expected. Other drugs, such as carbamazepine,[4] increase their own rate of metabolism from the body as dose is increased, so steady-state serum concentrations increase less than anticipated. This process is known as *autoinduction* of drug metabolism.

CLEARANCE

- Clearance (Cl) determines the maintenance dose (MD) that is required to obtain a given steady-state serum concentration (Css):

$$MD = Css \cdot Cl$$

- Target steady-state concentrations are usually chosen from previous studies in patients that have determined minimum effective concentrations and maximum concentrations that produce the desired pharmacological effect but avoid toxic side effects. This range of steady-state concentrations is known as the *therapeutic range* for the drug. The therapeutic range should be considered as an initial guideline for drug concentrations in a specific patient; drug dose and steady-state concentrations should then be titrated and individualized based on therapeutic response.

- The liver is most often the organ responsible for drug metabolism, while in most cases the kidney is responsible for drug elimination. The majority of drug metabolism is catalyzed by enzymes contained in the microsomes of hepatocytes known as the cytochrome P-450 enzyme system. The kidney eliminates drugs by glomerular filtration and tubular secretion in the nephron.
- Table 1-1 lists the cytochrome P-450 enzymes responsible for the majority of drug oxidative metabolism in humans, along with examples of known substrates, inhibitors, and inducers.[5] Also, some ethnic groups are deficient in certain enzyme families to a varying extent, and this information is included.
- P-glycoprotein (PGP) is a transport protein that is responsible for the active secretion of drugs into the bile, urine, and gastrointestinal tract. Table 1-2 lists PGP substrates, inhibitors, and inducers.
- The clearance for an organ, such as the liver or kidney, that metabolizes or eliminates drugs is determined by the blood flow to the organ and the ability of the organ to metabolize or eliminate the drug[6]. The drug clearance for an organ is equal to the product of the blood flow to the organ and the extraction ratio of the drug (Figure 1-4).

  - Liver blood flow (LBF) and renal blood flow (RBF) are each ~1– 1.5 L/min in adults with normal cardiovascular function. The ability of an organ to remove or extract the drug from the blood or serum is usually measured by determining the extraction ratio (ER), which is the fraction of drug removed by the organ, and is computed by measuring the concentrations of the drug entering (C_{in}) and leaving (C_{out}) the organ:

$$ER = \frac{(C_{in} - C_{out})}{C_{in}}$$

- Another way to think of hepatic clearance (Cl_H) is to recognize that its value is a function of the intrinsic ability of the enzyme to metabolize a drug (intrinsic clearance, Cl'_{int}); the fraction of drug present in the bloodstream that is not bound to cells or proteins, such as albumin, α_1-acid glycoprotein, or lipoproteins, but is present in the unbound, or "free," state (unbound fraction of drug, f_B); and liver blood flow (LBF):

$$Cl_H = \frac{LBF \cdot (f_B \cdot Cl_{int})}{LBF + (f_B \cdot Cl_{int})}$$

VOLUME OF DISTRIBUTION

- Volume of distribution (V) determines the loading dose (LD) that is required to achieve a particular steady-state drug concentration immediately after the dose is administered (Figure 1-5):

$$LD = Css \cdot V$$

  - It is rare to know the exact volume of distribution for a patient, because it is necessary to administer a dose on a previous occasion in order to have computed this parameter. Thus, usually an average volume of distribution measured in other patients with similar demographics (age, weight, gender, etc.) and medical conditions (renal failure, liver failure, heart failure, etc.) is used to estimate a loading dose (Figure 1-6). As a result, most patients will not actually attain steady state after a loading dose, but it can be hoped that serum drug concentrations will be high enough that the patient will experience the pharmacological effect of the drug.

TABLE 1-1 Cytochrome P-450 Enzymes, Substrates, Inhibitors, and Inducers[5]

Cytochrome P-450 enzyme	Substrates	Inhibitors	Inducers
CYP1A2	Acetaminophen Caffeine Clozapine Imipramine Ondansetron Phenacetin Ropinirole Tacrine Theophylline (R)-Warfarin Zileuton	Allopurinol Cimetidine Ciprofloxacin Enoxacin Erythromycin Fluvoxamine Isoniazid	Carbamazepine Charcoal-broiled meat Phenobarbital Primidone Rifampin Tobacco smoke
CYP2C9	Celecoxib Chlorpropamide Diclofenac Dronabinol Flurbiprofen Fluvastatin Glimepiride Glipizide Glyburide Ibuprofen Indomethacin Irbesartan Losartan Meloxicam Naproxen Nateglinide Phenytoin Piroxicam Ritonavir Rosiglitazone Tolbutamide Torsemide (S)-Warfarin Zafirlukast	Amiodarone Cimetidine Clopidogrel Cotrimoxazole Delavirdine Disulfiram Efavirenz Fluconazole Fluvastatin Fluvoxamine Gemfibrozil Imatinib Isoniazid Itraconazole Ketoconazole Metronidazole Sulfinpyrazole Zafirlukast	Barbiturates Carbamazepine Phenobarbital Phenytoin Primidone Rifampin
CYP2C19 PM: ~4% Caucasians ~20% Japanese & Chinese	Carisoprodol Desmethyldiazepam Diazepam Hexobarbital Imipramine Lansoprazole (S)-Mephenytoin Omeprazole Pantoprazole Pentamidine Phenytoin Propranolol Rabeprazole Selegiline Sertraline (R)-Warfarin	Cimetidine Delavirdine Efavirenz Felbamate Fluconazole Fluoxetine Fluvoxamine Omeprazole Ticlopidine	Artemisinin Barbiturates Phenytoin Rifampin

(Continued)

TABLE 1-1 Cytochrome P-450 Enzymes, Substrates, Inhibitors, and Inducers[5] (*Continued*)

Cytochrome P-450 enzyme	Substrates	Inhibitors	Inducers
CYP2D6 PM: ~8% Caucasians ~1% Japanese & Chinese	Alprenolol Amitriptyline Carvedilol Chlorpromazine Clomipramine Codeine Debrisoquin Desipramine Dextromethorphan Dihydrocodeine Encainide Fentanyl Flecainide Fluoxetine Fluvoxamine Fluphenazine Haloperidol Hydrocodone Imipramine Labetalol Maprotiline Methamphetamine Metoprolol Mexiletine Nortriptyline Oxycodone Paroxetine Perhexiline Perphenazine Promethazine Propafenone Propoxyphene Propranolol Risperidone Sertraline Sparteine Thioridazine Timolol Tolterodine Tramadol Trazodone Venlafaxine	Amiodarone Bupropion Chloroquine Cimetidine Citalopram Diphenhydramine Fluoxetine Imatinib Paroxetine Perphenazine Propafenone Propoxyphene Quinacrine Quinidine Quinine Ritonavir Sertraline Terbinafine Thioridazine	
CYP2E1	Acetaminophen Chlorzoxazone Enflurane Ethanol Halothane Isoflurane Isoniazid	Disulfiram	Ethanol Isoniazid
CYP3A4	Alfentanil Alprazolam Amiodarone Amlodipine	Clarithromycin Clotrimazole Danazol Delavirdine	Barbiturates Carbamazepine Dexamethasone Griseofulvin

(*Continued*)

TABLE 1-1 Cytochrome P-450 Enzymes, Substrates, Inhibitors, and Inducers[5] (*Continued*)

Cytochrome P-450 enzyme	Substrates	Inhibitors	Inducers
CYP3A4 (*Cont.*)	Amprenavir	Diltiazem	Nelfinavir
	Astemizole	Efavirenz	Oxcarbazine
	Atorvastatin	Erythromycin	Phenobarbital
	Bepridil	Ethinyl Estradiol	Phenytoin
	Bexarotene	Fluconazole	Primidone
	Bromocriptine	Fluvoxamine	Rifabutin
	Buspirone	Grapefruit Juice	Rifampin
	Carbamazepine	Indinavir	
	Cerivastatin	Isoniazid	
	Cilostazol	Itraconazole	
	Cisapride	Ketoconazole	
	Clarithromycin	Metronidazole	
	Cortisol	Mibefradil	
	Cyclosporine	Miconazole	
	Dapsone	Mifepristone	
	Delavirdine	Nefazodone	
	Dexamethasone	Nelfinavir	
	Diazepam	Ritonavir	
	Diltiazam	Saquinavir	
	Disopyramide	St. John's Wart	
	Donepezil	Troleandomycin	
	Doxorubicin	Verapamil	
	Ebastine	Zafirlukast	
	Efavirenz		
	Erythromycin		
	Ethinyl Estradiol		
	Etoposide		
	Felodipine		
	Fenofexadine		
	Fentanyl		
	Finasteride		
	Fluconazole		
	Galantamine		
	Hydrocortisone		
	Imipramine		
	Indinavir		
	Isradipine		
	Itraconazole		
	Ketoconazole		
	Lansoprazole		
	Lidocaine		
	Lopinavir		
	Loratadine		
	Losartan		
	Lovastatin		
	Methadone		
	Methylprednisolone		
	Mibefradil		
	Miconazole		
	Midazolam		
	Mifepristone		
	Nefazodone		
	Nelfinavir		

(*Continued*)

TABLE 1-1 Cytochrome P-450 Enzymes, Substrates, Inhibitors, and Inducers[5] (*Continued*)

Cytochrome P-450 enzyme	Substrates	Inhibitors	Inducers
CYP3A4 (*Cont.*)	Nicardipine		
	Nifedipine		
	Nimodipine		
	Nisoldipine		
	Nitrendipine		
	Paclitaxel		
	Pimozide		
	Pioglitazone		
	Progesterone		
	Prednisolone		
	Prednisone		
	Quetiapine		
	Quinidine		
	Quinine		
	Repaglinide		
	Rifabutin		
	Ritonavir		
	Saquinavir		
	Sertraline		
	Sildenafil		
	Simvastatin		
	Sirolimus		
	Sufentanil		
	Tacrolimus		
	Teniposide		
	Terfenadine		
	Testosterone		
	Triazolam		
	Troleandomycin		
	Verapamil		
	Vinblastine		
	Vincristine		
	Zaleplon		
	Ziprasidone		
	Zolpidem		
	Zonisamide		

TABLE 1-2 P-Glycoprotein Substrates, Inhibitors, and Inducers[5]

Substrates	Inhibitors	Inducers
Digoxin	Amiodarone	St. John's Wart
Diltiazem	Clarithromycin	Rifampin
Doxorubicin	Cyclosporine	
Erythromycin	Diltiazem	
Etoposide	Erythromycin	
Fexofenadine	Felodipine	
Loperamide	Itraconazole	
Rifampin	Ketoconazole	
Vinblastine	Nicardipine	
Vincristine	Quinidine	
	Tamoxifen	
	Testosterone	
	Verapamil	

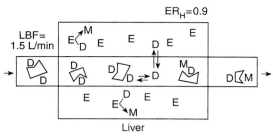

$$Cl_H = LBF \cdot ER_H = 1.5 \text{ L/min} \cdot 0.9 = 1.35 \text{ L/min}$$

FIG. 1-4   This schematic depicts the liver (large box) with the blood vessel supplying blood to it. When drug molecules (D) enter an organ (blood flows from left to right) that clears the drug, they may be bound to plasma proteins (trapezoid shapes) or exist in the unbound state. The unbound or "free" drug molecules are in equilibrium with the bound drug in the blood and unbound drug in the tissue. Drug–protein complexes are usually too big to diffuse across biological membranes into tissues. Drug molecules that have entered hepatic tissue may encounter an enzyme (E) that metabolizes the drug. When this occurs, the drug is chemically converted to a metabolite (M) which can diffuse back into the blood and leave the liver along with drug molecules that were not metabolized. The clearance of drug is equal to the blood flow to the organ (LBF) times the extraction ratio (ER_H) for the organ.

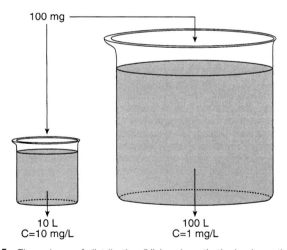

FIG. 1-5   The volume of distribution (V) is a hypothetical volume that is the proportionality constant which relates the concentration of drug in the blood or serum (C) and the amount of drug in the body (A_B): $A_B = C \cdot V$. It can be thought of as a beaker of fluid representing the entire space into which drug distributes. In this case, one beaker, representing a patient with a small volume of distribution, contains 10 L, while the other beaker, representing a patient with a large volume of distribution, contains 100 L. If 100 mg of drug are given to each patient, the resulting concentration will be 10 mg/L in the patient with the smaller volume of distribution, but 1 mg/L in the patient with the larger volume of distribution.

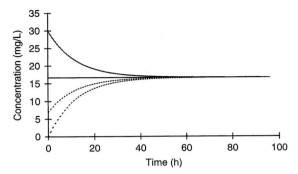

FIG. 1-6 If the volume of distribution (V) is known for a patient, it is possible to administer a loading dose (LD) that will attain a specified steady-state drug concentration (Css): LD = Css · V. This example depicts the ideal loading dose given as an intravenous bolus dose followed by a continuous intravenous infusion (solid line) so that steady state is achieved immediately and maintained. If a loading dose was not given and a continuous infusion started (bottom mixed dot and dashed line), it would take time to reach steady-state concentrations, and the patient may not experience an effect from the drug until a minimum effective concentration is achieved. This situation would not be acceptable for many clinical situations in which a quick onset of action is needed. Since the volume of distribution is not known for a patient before a dose is given, clinicians use an average volume of distribution previously measured in patients with similar demographics and disease states to compute loading doses. When this is done, the patient's volume of distribution may be smaller than average and result in higher-than-expected concentrations (top dashed line) or may be larger than average and result in lower-than-expected concentrations (middle dotted line). In these cases, it still takes 3–5 half-lives to reach steady state, but therapeutic drug concentrations are achieved much more quickly than when giving the drug by intravenous infusion only.

- The volume of distribution is a hypothetical volume that relates drug serum concentrations to the amount of drug in the body. At any given time after the drug has been absorbed from extravascular sites and the serum and tissue drug concentrations are in equilibrium, the serum concentration for a drug (C) is equal to the quotient of the amount of drug in the body (A_B) and the volume of distribution:

$$C = A_B/V$$

- The physiological determinates of volume of distribution are the actual volume of blood (V_B) and size (measured as a volume) of the various tissues and organs of the body (V_T). How the drug binds in the blood or serum (f_B, free fraction in the blood) compared to the binding in tissues (f_T, free fraction in the tissues) is also an important determinate of the volume of distribution for a drug. The equation that relates all of these physiological parameters to the volume of distribution is:[7]

$$V = V_B + (f_B/f_T)V_T$$

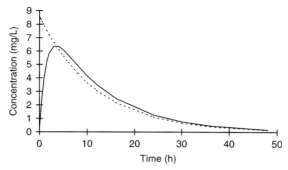

FIG. 1-7 Serum concentration–time profile for a patient receiving oral (solid line) and intravenous bolus (dashed line) doses of the same drug. When the drug is given orally, serum concentrations initially increase while the drug is being absorbed and decline after drug absorption is complete.

HALF-LIFE AND ELIMINATION RATE CONSTANT

- When drugs that follow linear pharmacokinetics are given to humans, serum concentrations decline in a curvilinear fashion (Figure 1-7). When the same data are plotted on a semilogarithmic axis, serum concentrations decrease in a linear fashion after drug absorption and distribution phases are complete (Figure 1-8). This part of the curve is known as the *elimination phase*. The time that it takes for serum concentrations to decrease by one-half in the elimination phase is a constant and is called the *half-life* ($t_{1/2}$).
- The half-life describes how quickly drug serum concentrations decrease in a patient after a medication is administered. Another common measurement used to denote how quickly drug serum concentrations decline in a patient

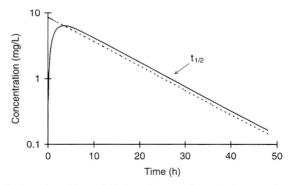

FIG. 1-8 Data from Figure 1-7 plotted on semilogarithmic axes. Serum concentrations decline in a straight line in both cases.

is the *elimination rate constant* (k_e). The half-life and elimination rate constant are related to each other by the following equation:

$$t_{1/2} = 0.693/k_e.$$

- The elimination rate constant can also be measured graphically by computing the slope of the log concentration versus time graph during the elimination phase. Using $\log_{10}$,

$$\frac{k_e}{2.303} = \frac{-(\log_{10} C_1 - \log_{10} C_2)}{(t_1 - t_2)}$$

or, using natural logarithms,

$$k_e = \frac{-(\ln C_1 - \ln C_2)}{(t_1 - t_2)}$$

- The half-life is important because it determines the time to steady state during the continuous dosing of a drug and the dosage interval for the medication.

  - The approach to steady-state serum concentrations is an exponential function. If a drug is administered on a continuous basis for 3 half-lives, serum concentrations are ~90% of steady-state values; on a continuous basis for 5 half-lives, serum concentrations equal ~95% of steady-state values; or on a continuous basis for 7 half-lives, serum concentrations achieve ~99% of steady-state values (Figure 1-9). Generally, drug serum concentrations used for pharmacokinetic monitoring can be safely measured after 3–5 estimated half-lives because most drug assays have 5–10% measurement error.
  - The dosage interval for a drug is also determined by the half-life of the medication. For example, if the therapeutic range of a drug is 10–20 mg/L, the ideal dosage interval would not let maximum serum concentrations exceed 20 mg/L or allow the minimum serum concentration to go

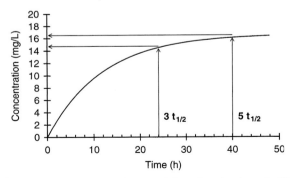

FIG. 1-9 Serum concentration–time graph for a drug that has a half-life equal to 8 hours. The arrows indicate concentrations at 3 half-lives (24 h, ~90% of Css) and at 5 half-lives (40 h, ~95% of Css). Since most drug assays have 5–10% measurement error, serum concentrations obtained between 3 and 5 half-lives after dosing commenced can be considered to be at steady state for clinical purposes and used to adjust drug doses.

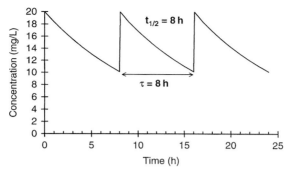

FIG. 1-10 The dosage interval for a drug is determined by the half-life of the agent. In this case, the half-life of the drug is 8 hours, and the therapeutic range of the drug is 10–20 mg/L. In order to ensure that maximum serum concentrations never go above and minimum serum concentrations never go below the therapeutic range, it is necessary to give the drug every 8 hours (τ = dosage interval).

below 10 mg/L (Figure 1-10). In this case, the dosage interval that would produce this steady-state concentration/time profile would be every half-life.

- The half-life and elimination rate constant are known as *dependent parameters* because their values depend on the clearance (Cl) and volume of distribution (V) of the agent:

$$t_{1/2} = \frac{0.693 \cdot V}{Cl} \qquad k_e = \frac{Cl}{V}$$

The half-life and elimination rate constant for a drug can change either because of a change in clearance or a change in the volume of distribution. Because the values for clearance and volume of distribution depend solely on physiological parameters and can vary independently of each other, they are known as *independent parameters*.

MICHAELIS-MENTEN OR SATURABLE PHARMACOKINETICS

- Michaelis-Menten or saturable pharmacokinetics is the type of nonlinear pharmacokinetics that occurs when the number of drug molecules saturates the enzymes' ability to metabolize the drug.[2,8] When this occurs, steady-state drug serum concentrations increase in a disproportionate manner after a dosage increase (Figure 1-3). In this case, the rate of drug removal is described by the classic Michaelis-Menten relationship that is used for all enzyme systems:

$$\text{Rate of metabolism} = \frac{V_{max} \cdot C}{Km + C}$$

where V_{max} is the maximum rate of metabolism, C is the substrate concentration, and Km is the substrate concentration when the rate of metabolism = $V_{max}/2$.
- The clinical implication of Michaelis-Menten pharmacokinetics is that the clearance of a drug is not a constant as it is with linear pharmacokinetics,

but is concentration- or dose-dependent. As the dose or concentration increases, the clearance rate (Cl) decreases as the enzyme approaches saturable conditions:

$$Cl = \frac{V_{max}}{Km + C}$$

This is the reason that concentrations increase disproportionately after a dosage increase.

- Since clearance is dose- or concentration-dependent, half-life also changes with dosage or concentration changes. As doses or concentrations increase for a drug that follows Michaelis-Menten pharmacokinetics, clearance decreases and half-life becomes longer for the drug: $\uparrow t_{1/2} = (0.693 \cdot V)/\downarrow Cl$. The clinical implication of this finding is that the time to steady state (3–5 $t_{1/2}$) is longer as the dose or concentration is increased for a drug that follows saturable pharmacokinetics.

- For a drug that is removed solely by metabolism via one enzyme system, the Michaelis-Menten equation can be used to compute the maintenance dose (MD) required to achieve a target steady-state serum concentration (Css):

$$MD = \frac{V_{max} \cdot Css}{Km + Css}$$

BIOAVAILABILITY

- When a drug is administered extravascularly, the entire dose may not enter the systemic circulation. The fraction of the administered dose that is delivered to the systemic circulation is known as the *bioavailability* for the drug and dosage form.

  - When medications are given by extravascular routes, the drug must be absorbed across several biological membranes before entering the vascular system. In these cases, drug serum concentrations rise while the drug is being absorbed into the bloodstream and reach a maximum concentration (C_{max}) when the rate of drug absorption equals the rate of drug elimination. The phase of the curve over which absorption takes place is known as the *absorption phase*, and the time that the maximum concentration occurs is called T_{max} (Figure 1-11).

- If a medication is given orally, drug molecules must pass through several organs before entering the systemic circulation. During absorption from the gastrointestinal tract, the drug molecules will encounter enzymes that may metabolize the agent (primarily CYP3A4 substrates, since ~90% of cytochrome P-450 contained in the gut wall is CYP3A4) or even pump the drug back into the lumen and prevent absorption from taking place (primarily P-glycoprotein substrates).

- If the drug is metabolized hepatically, part of the drug may be metabolized by the liver even though the majority of the drug was absorbed from the gastrointestinal tract. Drugs that are substrates for CYP3A4 and CYP2D6 are particularly susceptible to presystemic metabolism by the liver.

- The loss of drug from these combined processes is known as *presystemic metabolism* or the *first-pass effect*. Since the entire oral dose that was absorbed must take this route before entering the systemic vascular system, large amounts of drug can be lost via these processes.

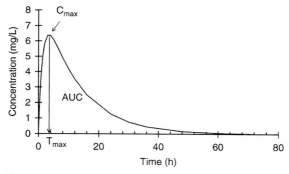

FIG. 1-11 Area under the serum concentration–time curve (AUC), the maximum concentration (C_{max}), and the time that the maximum concentration occurs (T_{max}) are considered primary bioavailability parameters. When the AUC, C_{max}, and T_{max} are the same within statistical limits for two dosage forms of the same drug, the dosage forms are considered to be bioequivalent.

- For drugs that follow linear pharmacokinetics, bioavailability is measured by comparing serum concentrations achieved after extravascular and intravenous doses in the same individual. Rather than compare drug concentrations at each time point, a composite of drug concentrations over time is derived by measuring the total area under the serum concentration–time curve (AUC) for each route of administration (Figure 1-11).

  - For an orally administered drug,

$$F = (AUC_{PO}/AUC_{IV})(D_{IV}/D_{PO})$$

where D_{IV} and AUC_{IV} are the intravenous dose and AUC, and D_{PO} and AUC_{PO} are the oral dose and AUC.

- Although it is not a requirement for generic drug products to be marketed by a pharmaceutical company, a desirable attribute of a generic drug dosage form is that it produces the same serum concentration–time profile as its brand-name counterpart. When it meets this requirement, the generic drug product is said to be *bioequivalent* to the brand-name drug.

  - In order to achieve the Food and Drug Administration's (FDA) definition of oral bioequivalence and be awarded an "AB" rating in the FDA publication, *Approved Drug Products with Therapeutic Equivalence Evaluations* (also known as the "Orange Book", http://www.fda.gov/cder/orange/default. htm), the pharmaceutical company producing a generic drug product must administer single doses or multiple doses of the drug until steady state is achieved of both the generic and brand-name drug dosage forms to a group of 18–24 humans and prove that the AUC (from time = 0 to infinity after a single dose, or over the dosage interval at steady state), C_{max}, and T_{max} values are statistically identical for the two dosage forms.

- Many states allow the substitution of generic drugs for brand-name drugs if the prescriber notes on the prescription order that generic substitution is acceptable, and the generic drug dosage form has an "AB" rating.

REFERENCES

1. Shargel L, Wu-Pong S, Yu ABC. Applied biopharmaceutics and pharmacokinetics. 5th ed. New York: McGraw-Hill, 2005.
2. Ludden TM, Allen JP, Valutsky WA, et al. Individualization of phenytoin dosage regimens. Clin Pharmacol Ther 1977;21(3):287–93.
3. Bowdle TA, Patel IH, Levy RH, Wilensky AJ. Valproic acid dosage and plasma protein binding and clearance. Clin Pharmacol Ther 1980;28(4):486–92.
4. Bertilsson L, Höjer B, Tybring G, Osterloh J, Rane A. Autoinduction of carbamazepine metabolism in children examined by a stable isotope technique. Clin Pharmacol Ther 1980;27(1):83–8.
5. Hansten PD, Horn JR. The top 100 drug interactions—a guide to patient management. Edmonds, WA: H&H Publications, 2005.
6. Rowland M, Benet LZ, Graham GG. Clearance concepts in pharmacokinetics. J Pharmacokinet Biopharm 1973;1:123–36.
7. Gibaldi M, McNamara PJ. Apparent volumes of distribution and drug binding to plasma proteins and tissues. Eur J Clin Pharmacol 1978;13:373–8.
8. Levy G. Pharmacokinetics of salicylate elimination in man. J Pharm Sci 1965;54(7):959–67.

2 | Clinical Pharmacokinetic Equations and Calculations

INTRODUCTION

Clinical pharmacokinetic dosage calculations are carried out using the easiest possible equations and methods. This is because there are usually only a few (sometimes as little as one or two) drug serum concentrations on which to base the calculations. Since the goal of therapeutic drug monitoring in patients is to individualize the drug dose and serum concentrations in order to produce the desired pharmacological effect and avoid adverse effects, it may not be possible, or even necessary, to compute pharmacokinetic parameters for every patient or clinical situation.

ONE-COMPARTMENT MODEL EQUATIONS FOR LINEAR PHARMACOKINETICS

- When medications are administered to humans, the body acts as if it were a series of compartments.[1] (Figure 2-1). In many cases, the drug distributes from the blood into the tissues quickly, and a pseudo-equilibrium of drug movement between blood and tissues is established rapidly. When this occurs, a one-compartment model can be used to describe the serum concentrations of a drug.[2,3]
- In some clinical situations, it is possible to use a one-compartment model to compute doses for a drug even if drug distribution takes time to complete.[4,5] In this case, drug serum concentrations are not obtained in a patient until after the distribution phase is over.

Intravenous Bolus Equation

- When a drug is given as an intravenous bolus and the drug distributes from the blood into the tissues quickly, the serum concentrations often decline in a straight line when plotted on semilogarithmic axes (Figure 2-2). In this case, a one-compartment model intravenous bolus equation can be used:

$$C = (D/V)e^{-k_e t}$$

where t is the time after the intravenous bolus was given (t = 0 at the time the dose was administered), C is the concentration at time t, V is the volume of distribution, and k_e is the elimination rate constant.

- Most drugs given intravenously cannot be given as an actual intravenous bolus because of side effects related to rapid injection. A short infusion of 5–30 minutes can avoid these types of adverse effects, and if the intravenous infusion time is very short compared to the half-life of the drug so that a large amount of drug is not eliminated during the infusion time, intravenous bolus equations can still be used.
- If drug distribution is not rapid, it is still possible to use a one-compartment model intravenous bolus equation if the duration of the distribution phase and infusion time is small compared to the half-life of the drug and only

19

One-compartment model

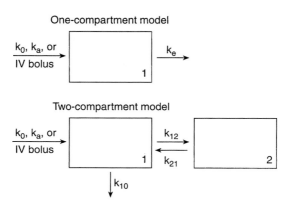

Two-compartment model

FIG. 2-1 Using compartment models, the body can be represented as a series of discrete sections. The simplest model is the one-compartment model, which depicts the body as one large container in which drug distribution between blood and tissues occurs instantaneously. Drug is introduced into the compartment, distributes immediately into a volume of distribution (V), and is removed from the body via metabolism and elimination via the elimination rate constant (k_e). The simplest multicompartment model is a two-compartment model which represents the body as a central compartment into which drug is administered and a peripheral compartment into which drug distributes. The central compartment (V_1) is composed of blood and tissues which equilibrate rapidly with blood. The peripheral compartment represents tissues that equilibrate slowly with blood. Rate constants represent the transfer between compartments (k_{1n}, k_{n1}) and elimination from the body (k_{10}).

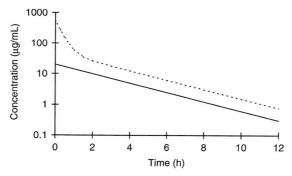

FIG. 2-2 The solid line shows the serum concentration-time graph for a drug that follows one-compartment model pharmacokinetics after intravenous bolus administration. Drug distribution occurs instantaneously, and serum concentrations decline in a straight line on semilogarithmic axes. The dashed line represents the serum concentration-time plot for a drug that follows two-compartment model pharmacokinetics after an intravenous bolus is given. Immediately after the dose is given, serum concentrations decline rapidly. This portion of the curve is known as the distribution phase. During the distribution phase, drug is distributing between blood and tissues and is removed from the body via hepatic metabolism and renal elimination. Later, serum concentrations decline more slowly during the elimination phase. During the elimination phase, drug is primarily being removed from the body.

a small amount of drug is eliminated during the infusion and distribution phases.[6] The strategy used in this situation is to infuse the medication and wait for the distribution phase to be over before obtaining serum concentrations in the patient.

- Pharmacokinetic parameters for patients can also be computed for use in the equations. If two or more serum concentrations are obtained after an intravenous bolus dose, the elimination rate constant, half-life, and volume of distribution can be calculated (Figures 2-3, 2-4). Alternatively, these parameters can be obtained by calculation without plotting the concentrations.

  - The elimination rate constant can be computed using the following equation:

$$k_e = \frac{-(\ln C_1 - \ln C_2)}{t_1 - t_2}$$

  where t_1 and C_1 are the first time/concentration pair and t_2 and C_2 are the second time/concentration pair.

  - The elimination rate constant can be converted into the half-life using the following equation:

$$t_{1/2} = 0.693/k_e$$

  - The volume of distribution can be calculated by dividing the dose by the serum concentration at time = 0:

$$V = D/C_0$$

  - The serum concentration at time = zero (C_0) can be computed using a variation of the intravenous bolus equation, $C_0 = C/e^{-k_e t}$, where t and C are a time/concentration pair that occur after the intravenous bolus dose.

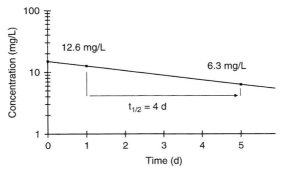

FIG. 2-3 Phenobarbital concentrations are plotted on semilogarithmic axes, and a straight line is drawn connecting the concentrations. Half-life ($t_{1/2}$) is determined by measuring the time needed for serum concentrations to decline by 1/2 (i.e., from 12.6 to 6.3 mg/L), and is converted to the elimination rate constant ($k_e = 0.693/t_{1/2} = 0.693/(4\ d) = 0.173\ d^{-1}$). The concentration-time line can be extrapolated to the concentration axis to derive the concentration at time zero ($C_0 = 15$ mg/L) and used to compute the volume of distribution ($V = D/C_0$).

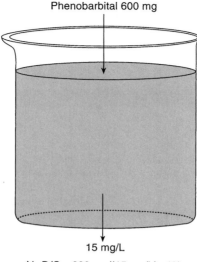

Phenobarbital 600 mg

15 mg/L

$V = D/C_0 = 600 \text{ mg}/(15 \text{ mg/L}) = 40\text{L}$

FIG. 2-4   For a one-compartment model, the body can be thought of as a beaker containing fluid. If 600 mg of phenobarbital is added to a beaker of unknown volume and the resulting concentration is 15 mg/L, the volume can be computed by taking the quotient of the amount placed into the beaker and the concentration: $V = D/C_0 = 600 \text{ mg}/(15 \text{ mg/L}) = 40$ L.

Continuous and Intermittent Intravenous Infusion Equations

• Some drugs are administered using a continuous intravenous infusion, and if the infusion is discontinued the serum concentration-time profile decreases in a straight line when graphed on a semilogarithmic axes (Figure 2-5). In this case, a one-compartment model intravenous infusion equation can be used to compute concentrations (C) while the infusion is running:

$$C = (k_0/Cl)(1 - e^{-k_e t}) = [k_0/(k_e V)](1 - e^{-k_e t})$$

where k_0 is the drug infusion rate (in amount per unit time, such as mg/h or μg/min), Cl is the drug clearance (since $Cl = k_e V$, this substitution was made in the second version of the equation), k_e is the elimination rate constant, and t is the time that the infusion has been running.

• If the infusion is stopped, postinfusion serum concentrations ($C_{postinfusion}$) can be computed by calculating the concentration when the infusion ended (C_{end}), using the appropriate equation above, and equation:

$$C_{postinfusion} = C_{end} e^{-k_e t_{postinfusion}}$$

where k_e is the elimination rate constant and $t_{postinfusion}$ is the postinfusion time ($t_{postinfusion} = 0$ at end of infusion and increases from that point).

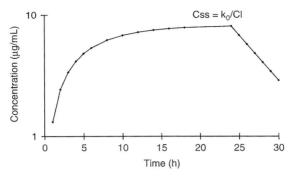

FIG. 2-5 If a drug is given as a continuous intravenous infusion, serum concentrations increase until a steady-state concentration (Css) is achieved in 5–7 half-lives. The steady-state concentration is determined by the quotient of the infusion rate (k_0) and drug clearance (Cl): Css = k_0/Cl. When the infusion is discontinued, serum concentrations decline in a straight line if the graph is plotted on semilogarithmic axes. When using $\log_{10}$ graph paper, the elimination rate constant (k_e) can be computed using the following formula: slope = $-k_e$/2.303.

- If the infusion is allowed to continue until steady state is achieved, the steady-state concentration (Css) can be calculated easily:

$$Css = k_0/Cl = k_0/(k_e V)$$

- Even if serum concentrations exhibit a distribution phase after the drug infusion has ended, it is still possible to use one-compartment model intravenous infusion equations for the drug without a large amount of error.[4,5] The strategy used in this instance is to infuse the medication and wait for the distribution phase to be over before measuring serum drug concentrations in the patient.
- Pharmacokinetic constants can also be calculated for use in the equations.

  - If a steady-state concentration is obtained after a continuous intravenous infusion has been running uninterrupted for 3–5 half-lives, the drug clearance (Cl) can be calculated by rearranging the steady-state infusion formula: Cl = k_0/Css.
  - If the infusion did not run until steady state was achieved, it is still possible to compute pharmacokinetic parameters from postinfusion concentrations.

    - By plotting the serum concentration-time information on semilogarithmic axes, the half-life can be determined by measuring the time it takes for serum concentrations to decline by one-half (Figure 2-6). The elimination rate constant (k_e) can be calculated using the following formula:

$$k_e = 0.693/t_{1/2}$$

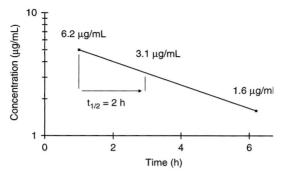

FIG. 2-6 Tobramycin concentrations are plotted on semilogarithmic axes, and a straight line is drawn connecting the concentrations. Half-life ($t_{1/2}$) is determined by measuring the time needed for serum concentrations to decline by 1/2 (i.e., from 6.2 to 3.1 mg/L), and is converted to the elimination rate constant ($k_e = 0.693/t_{1/2} = 0.693/2$ h $= 0.347$ h^{-1}). Volume of distribution is computed using the equation given in the text.

- Alternatively, the elimination rate constant can be calculated without plotting the concentrations using the following equation:

$$k_e = \frac{-(\ln C_1 - \ln C_2)}{t_1 - t_2}$$

where t_1 and C_1 are the first time/concentration pair and t_2 and C_2 are the second time/concentration pair.

- The volume of distribution (V) can be computed using the following equation:[4]

$$V = \frac{k_0(1 - e^{-k_e t'})}{k_e[C_{max} - (C_{predose}e^{-k_e t'})]}$$

where k_0 is the infusion rate, k_e is the elimination rate constant, t' = infusion time, C_{max} is the maximum concentration at the end of infusion, and $C_{predose}$ is the predose concentration.

Extravascular Equations

- When a drug is administered extravascularly [e.g., orally, intramuscularly, subcutaneously, transdermally, etc.), absorption into the systemic vascular system must take place (Figure 2-7)]. If serum concentrations decrease in a straight line when plotted on semilogarithmic axes after drug absorption is complete, a one-compartment model extravascular equation can be used to describe the serum concentration-time curve:

$$C = \{(Fk_aD)/[V(k_a - k_e)]\}(e^{-k_e t} - e^{-k_a t})$$

where t is the time after the extravascular dose was given (t = 0 at the time the dose was administered), C is the concentration at time = t, F is the bioavailability fraction, k_a is the absorption rate constant, D is the dose, V is the volume of distribution, and k_e is the elimination rate constant. The absorption rate constant describes how quickly the drug is absorbed, with

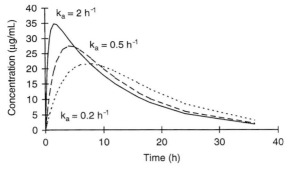

FIG. 2-7 Serum concentration-time curves for extravascular drug administration for agents following one-compartment pharmacokinetics. The absorption rate constant (k_a) controls how quickly the drug enters the body. A large absorption rate constant allows a drug to enter the body quickly, while a small elimination rate constant permits a drug to enter the body more slowly. The solid line shows the concentration-time curve on semilogarithmic axes for an elimination rate constant equal to 2 h^{-1}. The dashed and dotted lines depict serum concentration-time plots for elimination rate constants of 0.5 h^{-1} and 0.2 h^{-1}, respectively.

a large number indicating fast absorption and a small number indicating slow absorption.
- If the serum concentration-time curve displays a distribution phase, it is still possible to use one-compartment model equations after an extravascular dose is administered. In order to do this, serum concentrations are obtained only in the postdistribution phase. Since the absorption rate constant is also hard to measure in patients, it is also desirable to avoid drawing drug serum concentrations during the absorption phase in clinical situations.

  - When only postabsorption, postdistribution serum concentrations are obtained for a drug that is administered extravascularly, the equation simplifies to

$$C = [(FD)/V]e^{-k_e t}$$

  where C is the concentration at any postabsorption, postdistribution time; F is the bioavailability fraction; D is the dose; V is the volume of distribution; k_e is the elimination rate constant; and t is any postabsorption, postdistribution time.

- Pharmacokinetic constants can also be calculated and used in these equations. If two or more postabsorption, postdistribution serum concentrations are obtained after an extravascular dose, the volume of distribution, elimination rate constant, and half-life can be computed (Figure 2-8). An alternative approach is to calculate the parameters directly, without plotting the concentrations.

  - The elimination rate constant (k_e) is computed using the following relationship:

$$k_e = \frac{-(\ln C_1 - \ln C_2)}{t_1 - t_2}$$

  where C_1 is the first concentration at time = t_1, and C_2 is the second concentration at time = t_2.

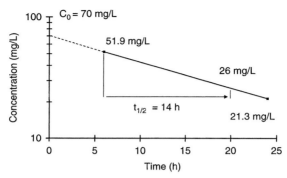

FIG. 2-8 Valproic acid concentrations are plotted on semilogarithmic axes, and a straight line is drawn connecting the concentrations. Half-life ($t_{1/2}$) is determined by measuring the time needed for serum concentrations to decline by 1/2 (i.e., from 51.9 to 26 mg/L), and is converted to the elimination rate constant ($k_e = 0.693/t_{1/2} = 0.693/(14\ h) = 0.0495\ h^{-1}$). The concentration-time line can be extrapolated to the concentration axis to derive the concentration at time zero ($C_0 = 70$ mg/L) and used to compute the hybrid constant volume of distribution/bioavailability fraction ($V/F = D/C_0$).

- The elimination rate constant can be translated into the half-life using the following equation:

$$t_{1/2} = 0.693/k_e$$

- The hybrid constant volume of distribution/bioavailability (V/F) is computed by taking the quotient of the dose and the extrapolated serum concentration at time = 0:

$$V/F = D/C_0$$

- The extrapolated serum concentration at time = zero (C_0) is calculated using a variation of the intravenous bolus equation: $C_0 = C/e^{-k_e t}$, where t and C are a time-concentration pair that occur after administration of the extravascular dose in the postabsorption and postdistribution phases.

Multiple-Dose and Steady-State Equations

- In most cases, medications are administered to patients as multiple doses, and drug serum concentrations for therapeutic drug monitoring are not obtained until steady state is achieved. For these reasons, multiple-dose equations that reflect steady-state conditions are usually more useful in clinical settings than single-dose equations. Whenever the multiple-dosing factor is used to change a single-dose equation to the multiple-dose or steady-state version, the time variable in the equation resets to zero at the beginning of each dosage interval.[7]
- In order to change a single-dose equation to the multiple-dose version, it is necessary to multiply each exponential term in the equation by the multiple-dosing factor:

$$(1 - e^{-nk_i\tau})/(1 - e^{-k_i\tau})$$

where n is the number of doses administered, k_i is the rate constant found in the exponential of the single-dose equation, and τ is the dosage interval.

- At steady state, the number of doses is large, the exponential term in the numerator of the multiple-dosing factor $(-nk_e\tau)$ becomes a large negative number, and the exponent approaches zero. Therefore, the steady-state version of the multiple-dosing factor becomes

$$1/(1 - e^{-k_e\tau})$$

where k_e is the elimination rate constant and τ is the dosage interval.
- Whenever the multiple-dosing factor is used to change a single-dose equation to the multiple-dose or steady-state version, the time variable in the equation resets to zero at the beginning of each dosage interval.
- Table 2-1 lists the one-compartment model equations for the different routes of administration under single-dose, multiple-dose, and steady-state conditions.
- Table 2-2 lists the methods to compute pharmacokinetic constants using a one-compartment model for different routes of administration under single dose, multiple dose, and steady-state conditions.

Average Steady-State Concentration Equations

- A very useful and easy equation can be used to compute the average steady-state concentration (Css) of a drug:

$$Css = [F(D/\tau)]/Cl$$

where F is the bioavailability fraction, D is the dose, τ is the dosage interval, and Cl is the drug clearance.[8] The average steady-state concentration equation is very useful when the half-life of the drug is long compared to the dosage interval or if a sustained-release dosage form is used.
- The steady-state concentration computed by this equation is the concentration that would have occurred if the dose, adjusted for bioavailability, was given as a continuous intravenous infusion. The equation works for any single- or multiple-compartment model, and because of this it is deemed a model-independent equation.
- If an average steady-state concentration (Css) is known for a drug, the hybrid pharmacokinetic constant clearance/bioavailability (Cl/F) can be computed:

$$Cl/F = (D/\tau)/Css$$

where D is dose and τ is the dosage interval.

Designing Individualized Dosage Regimens Using One-Compartment Model Equations

- The goal of therapeutic drug monitoring is to customize medication doses to provide optimal drug efficacy without adverse reactions. One-compartment model equations can be used to compute initial drug doses employing population pharmacokinetic parameters that estimate the constants for a patient.[4,5,9] To design initial doses, estimates of pharmacokinetic constants are obtained using patient characteristics such as weight, age, gender, renal and liver function, and other disease states and conditions that are known to affect the disposition and elimination of the drug. The patient's own, unique pharmacokinetic parameters can be computed once doses have been administered and drug serum concentrations measured. At that time, individualized dosage regimens at steady state can be designed for a patient. Table 2-3 lists the equations used to customize doses for the various routes of administration.

TABLE 2-1 Single-Dose, Multiple-Dose, and Steady-State One-Compartment Model Equations

Route of administration	Single-dose	Multiple-dose	Steady-state
Intravenous bolus	$C = (D/V)e^{-k_e t}$	$C = (D/V)e^{-k_e t}[(1 - e^{-nk_e\tau})/(1 - e^{-k_e\tau})]$	$C = (D/V)[e^{-k_e t}/(1 - e^{-k_e\tau})]$
Continuous intravenous infusion	$C = [k_0/(k_e V)](1 - e^{-k_e t})$	N/A	$Css = k_0/Cl = k_0/(k_e V)$
Intermittent intravenous infusion	$C = [k_0/(k_e V)](1 - e^{-k_e t'})$	$C = [k_0/(k_e V)](1 - e^{-k_e t'})$ $[(1 - e^{-nk_e\tau})/(1 - e^{-k_e\tau})]$	$C = [k_0/(k_e V)][(1 - e^{-k_e t'})/(1 - e^{-k_e\tau})]$
Extravascular (postabsorption, postdistribution)	$C = [(FD)/V]e^{-k_e t}$	$C = [(FD)/V]e^{-k_e t}[(1 - e^{-nk_e\tau})/(1 - e^{-k_e\tau})]$	$C = [(FD)/V][e^{-k_e t}/(1 - e^{-k_e\tau})]$
Average steady-state concentration (any route of administration)	N/A	N/A	$Css = [F(D/\tau)]/Cl$

Symbol key: C is drug serum concentration at time = t, D is dose, V is volume of distribution, k_e is the elimination rate constant, n is the number of administered doses, k_0 is the infusion rate, Cl is clearance, t' is the postinfusion time.

TABLE 2-2 Single-Dose, Multiple-Dose, and Steady-State Pharmacokinetic Constant Computations Utilizing a One-Compartment Model

Route of administration	Single-dose	Multiple-dose	Steady-state
Intravenous bolus	$k_e = -(\ln C_1 - \ln C_2)/(t_1 - t_2)$ $t_{1/2} = 0.693/k_e$ $V = D/C_0$ $Cl = k_e V$	$k_e = -(\ln C_1 - \ln C_2)/(t_1 - t_2)$ $t_{1/2} = 0.693/k_e$ $V = D/(C_0 - C_{predose})$ $Cl = k_e V$	$k_e = -(\ln C_1 - \ln C_2)/(t_1 - t_2)$ $t_{1/2} = 0.693/k_e$ $V = D/(C_0 - C_{predose})$ $Cl = k_e(V/F)$
Continuous intravenous infusion	N/A	N/A	$Cl = k_0/Css$
Intermittent intravenous infusion	$k_e = -(\ln C_1 - \ln C_2)/(t_1 - t_2)$ $t_{1/2} = 0.693/k_e$ $V = [k_0(1 - e^{-k_e t'})]/\{k_e[C_{max} - (C_{predose}\, e^{-k_e t'})]\}$ $Cl = k_e V$	$k_e = -(\ln C_1 - \ln C_2)/(t_1 - t_2)$ $t_{1/2} = 0.693/k_e$ $V = [k_0(1 - e^{-k_e t'})]/\{k_e[C_{max} - (C_{predose}\, e^{-k_e t'})]\}$ $Cl = k_e V$	$k_e = -(\ln C_1 - \ln C_2)/(t_1 - t_2)$ $t_{1/2} = 0.693/k_e$ $V = [k_0(1 - e^{-k_e t'})]/\{k_e[C_{max} - (C_{predose}\, e^{-k_e t'})]\}$ $Cl = k_e(V/F)$
Extravascular (postabsorption, postdistribution)	$k_e = -(\ln C_1 - \ln C_2)/(t_1 - t_2)$ $t_{1/2} = 0.693/k_e$ $V/F = D/C_0$ $Cl/F = k_e(V/F)$	$k_e = -(\ln C_1 - \ln C_2)/(t_1 - t_2)$ $t_{1/2} = 0.693/k_e$ $V/F = D/(C_0 - C_{predose})$ $Cl/F = k_e(V/F)$	$k_e = -(\ln C_1 - \ln C_2)/(t_1 - t_2)$ $t_{1/2} = 0.693/k_e$ $V/F = D/(C_0 - C_{predose})$ $Cl/F = k_e(V/F)$
Average steady-state concentration (any route of administration)	N/A	N/A	$Cl/F = (D/\tau)/Css$

Symbol key: C_1 is drug serum concentration at time = t_1, C_2 is drug serum concentration at time = t_2, k_e is the elimination rate constant, $t_{1/2}$ is the half-life, V is the volume of distribution, k_0 is the continuous infusion rate, t' is the infusion time, V/F is the hybrid constant volume of distribution/bioavailability fraction, D is dose, C_0 is the concentration at time = 0, Cl is drug clearance, Cl/F is the hybrid constant clearance/bioavailability fraction, $C_{predose}$ is the predose concentration, Css is the steady-state concentration.

TABLE 2-3 Equations Used to Compute Individualized Dosage Regimens for Various Routes of Administration

Route of administration	Dosage interval (τ), maintenance dose (D or k_0), and loading dose (LD) equations
Intravenous bolus	$\tau = (\ln Css_{max} - \ln Css_{min})/k_e$ $D = Css_{max} V(1 - e^{-k_e\tau})$ $LD = Css_{max} V$
Continuous intravenous infusion	$k_0 = Css\ Cl = Css\ k_e\ V$ $LD = Css\ V$
Intermittent intravenous infusion	$\tau = [(\ln Css_{max} - \ln Css_{min})/k_e] + t'$ $k_0 = Css_{max}\ k_e\ V[(1 - e^{-k_e\tau})/(1 - e^{-k_e t'})]$ $LD = k_0/(1 - e^{-k_e\tau})$
Extravascular (post-absorption, postdistribution)	$\tau = [(\ln Css_{max} - \ln Css_{min})/k_e] + T_{max}$ $D = [(Css_{max} V)/F][(1 - e^{-k_e\tau})/e^{-k_e T_{max}}]$ $LD = (Css_{max} V)/F$
Average steady-state concentration (any route of administration)	$D = (Css\ Cl\ \tau)/F = (Css\ k_e\ V\ \tau)/F$ $LD = (Css\ V)/F$

Symbol key: Css_{max} and Css_{min} are the maximum and minimum steady-state concentrations, k_e is the elimination rate constant, V is the volume of distribution, Css is the steady-state concentration, k_0 is the continuous infusion rate, t′ is the infusion time, T_{max} is the time at which Css_{max} occurs, F is the bioavailability fraction.

MULTICOMPARTMENT MODELS

• When serum concentrations decrease in a rapid fashion initially and then decline at a slower rate later (Figure 2-2), a multicompartment model can be used to describe the serum concentration-time curve [1] (Figure 2-1).

• The reason serum concentrations drop so rapidly after the dose is given is that all of the drug is in the bloodstream initially, and drug is leaving the vascular system by distribution to tissues and by hepatic metabolism and/or renal elimination. This portion of the curve is called the *distribution phase*. After this phase of the curve is finished, drug distribution is nearly complete and a pseudo-equilibrium is established between the blood and tissues. During the final part of the curve, serum concentrations drop more slowly since only metabolism and/or elimination are taking place. This portion of the curve is called the *elimination phase*, and the elimination half-life of the drug is measured in this part of the serum concentration-time graph.

• Digoxin, vancomycin, and lidocaine are examples of drugs that follow multicompartment pharmacokinetics.

• In order to obtain accurate values for the pharmacokinetic constants in multicompartment-model equations, 3–5 serum concentrations for each phase of the curve need to be obtained after a dose is given to a patient. Because of the cost and time involved in obtaining 6–10 serum concentrations after a dose, multicompartment models are rarely used in patient-care situations.

- If a drug follows multicompartment pharmacokinetics, serum concentrations are usually not drawn for clinical use until the distribution phase is over and the elimination phase has been established. In these cases, it is possible to use simpler one-compartment model equations to compute doses with an acceptable degree of accuracy.

MICHAELIS-MENTEN EQUATIONS FOR SATURABLE PHARMACOKINETICS

- The Michaelis-Menten expression describes the dose required to attain a given steady-state drug concentration:

$$MD = (V_{max} \cdot Css)/(Km + Css)$$

where MD is the maintenance dose, Css is the steady-state drug concentration, V_{max} is the maximum rate of drug metabolism, and Km is the concentration at which the rate of metabolism equals $V_{max}/2$. Phenytoin is an example of a drug that follows saturable pharmacokinetics.[10]
- Computing the Michaelis-Menten constants for a drug is not as straightforward as the calculation of pharmacokinetic parameters for a one-compartment linear pharmacokinetic model. The calculation of V_{max} and Km requires a graphical solution.[10]
- The Michaelis-Menten equation can be rearranged to the following formula:

$$D = V_{max} - [Km(D/Css)]$$

This version takes the form of the equation of a straight line:

$$y = \text{y-intercept} + [(\text{slope})x]$$

A plot of dose (D) versus dose divided by the steady-state concentration (D/Css) will yield a straight line with a slope equal to −Km and a y-intercept of V_{max} (Figure 2-9). Once V_{max} and Km are known, the Michaelis-Menten expression can be used to compute a dose to reach any steady-state concentration.

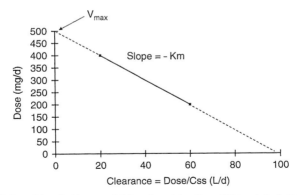

FIG. 2-9 Michaelis-Menten plot for phenytoin. Dose (D) is plotted versus the ratio of dose and steady-state concentration (D/Css) for two or more different doses, and a straight line is drawn connecting the points. The slope of the line is −Km , and the y-intercept is V_{max}. The Michaelis-Menten constants are then used to compute the dose needed to achieve a new desired steady-state concentration.

REFERENCES

1. Riegelman S, Loo JCK, Rowland M. Shortcomings in pharmacokinetic analysis by conceiving the body to exhibit properties of a single compartment. J Pharm Sci 1968;57:117–23.
2. Teorell T. Kinetics of distribution of substances administered to the body I. The extravascular modes of administration. Arch Int Pharmacodyn Ther 1937;57:205–25.
3. Teorell T. Kinetics of distribution of substances administered to the body II. The intravascular modes of administration. Arch Int Pharmacodyn Ther 1937;57:226–40.
4. Sawchuk RJ, Zaske DE, Cipolle RJ, Wargin WA, Strate RG. Kinetic model for gentamicin dosing with the use of individual patient parameters. Clin Pharmacol Ther 1977;21:362–5.
5. Matzke GR, McGory RW, Halstenson CE, Keane WF. Pharmacokinetics of vancomycin in patients with various degrees of renal function. Antimicrob Agents Chemother 1984;25:433–7.
6. Murphy JE, Winter ME. Clinical pharmacokinetics pearls: bolus versus infusion equations. Pharmacother 1996;16:698–700.
7. Benet LZ. General treatment of linear mammilary models with elimination from any compartment as used in pharmacokinetics. J Pharm Sci 1972;61:536–41.
8. Wagner JG, Northam JI, Alway CD, Carpenter OS. Blood levels of drug at the equilibrium state after multiple dosing. Nature 1965;207:1301–2.
9. Jusko WJ, Koup JR, Vance JW, Schentag JJ, Kuritzky P. Intravenous theophylline therapy: nomogram guidelines. Ann Intern Med 1977;86:400–4.
10. Ludden TM, Allen JP, Valutsky WA, et al. Individualization of phenytoin dosage regimens. Clin Pharmacol Ther 1977;21:287–93.

3 | Drug Dosing in Special Populations

Renal and Hepatic Disease, Dialysis, Heart Failure, Obesity, and Drug Interactions

INTRODUCTION

The dosing of most drugs may be altered by one or more of the important factors discussed in this chapter.

- Renal or hepatic disease may decrease the elimination or metabolism of the majority of drugs and change the clearance of the agent.
- Dialysis procedures, conducted using artificial kidneys in patients with renal failure, removes some medications from the body although the pharmacokinetics of other drugs are not changed.
- Heart failure results in low cardiac output, which decreases blood flow to eliminating organs, and the clearance rate of drugs with moderate to high extraction ratios are particularly sensitive to alterations in organ blood flow.
- Obesity adds excessive adipose tissue to the body, which may change the way that drugs distribute in the body and alter the volume of distribution for the medication.
- Drug interactions can inhibit or induce drug metabolism, alter drug protein binding, or change blood flow to organs that eliminate or metabolize the drug.

RENAL DISEASE

- Most water-soluble drugs are to some extent eliminated unchanged by the kidney. In addition, drug metabolites that have been made more water-soluble via oxidation or conjugation are typically removed by renal elimination (Figure 3-1).
- Unbound drug molecules that are relatively small are filtered at the glomerulus. Glomerular filtration is the primary elimination route for many medications.
- Drugs can be actively secreted into the urine, and this process usually takes place in the proximal tubules. Tubular secretion is an active process conducted by relatively specific carriers or pumps that move the drug from blood vessels in close proximity to the nephron into the proximal tubule.
- Some medications may be reabsorbed from the urine back into the blood by the kidney. Reabsorption is usually a passive process and requires a degree of lipid solubility for the drug molecule.
  - The equation that describes these various routes of renal elimination is

$$Cl_R = \left[(f_B \cdot GFR) + \frac{RBF \cdot (f_B Cl'_{sec})}{RBF + (f_B Cl'_{sec})} \right](1 - FR)$$

where f_B is the free fraction of drug in the blood, GFR is glomerular filtration rate, RBF is renal blood flow, Cl'_{sec} is the intrinsic clearance for tubular secretion of unbound drug, and FR is the fraction reabsorbed.[1]

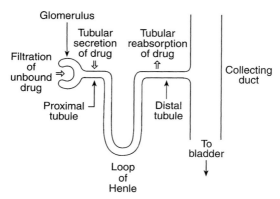

FIG. 3-1   The nephron is the functional unit of the kidney that is responsible for drug elimination. Unbound drug is filtered freely at the glomerulus (shown by arrow). Active tubular secretion of drug (denoted by arrow into nephron) usually occurs in the proximal tubule of the nephron. Passive tubular reabsorption (denoted by arrow out of nephron) usually occurs in the distal tubule of the nephron. Tubular reabsorption requires un-ionized drug molecules so that the molecules can pass through the lipid membranes of the nephron and surrounding capillaries.

MEASUREMENT AND ESTIMATION OF CREATININE CLEARANCE

- The most common method of estimating glomerular filtration for the purposes of drug dosing is to measure or estimate creatinine clearance (CrCl). Creatinine is a by-product of muscle metabolism that is eliminated primarily by glomerular filtration. Because of this property, it is used as a surrogate measurement of glomerular filtration rate (GFR).
- Creatinine clearance rates can be measured by collecting urine for a specified period and collecting a blood sample for determination of serum creatinine at the midpoint of the concurrent urine collection time:

$$\text{CrCl(in ml/min)} = \frac{U_{Cr} \cdot V_{urine}}{S_{Cr} \cdot T}$$

where U_{Cr} is the urine creatinine concentration in mg/dl, V_{urine} is the volume of urine collected in ml, S_{Cr} is the serum creatinine collected at the midpoint of the urine collection in mg/dl, and T is the time in minutes of the urine collection.

- Because creatinine renal secretion exhibits diurnal variation, most nephrologists use a 24-hour urine collection period for the determination of creatinine clearance. However, for the purpose of drug dosing, collection periods of 8–12 hours have been sufficient and provide a quicker turnaround time in emergency situations. Also, if renal function is stable, the blood sample for determination of serum creatinine may not need to be collected at the precise midpoint of the urine collection.
- Routine measurement of creatinine clearances in patients has been fraught with problems. Incomplete urine collections, serum creatinine concentrations obtained at incorrect times, and collection-time errors can produce

erroneous measured creatinine clearance values. This realization has prompted investigators to derive methods which estimate creatinine clearance from serum creatinine values and other patient characteristics in various populations. The most widely used of these formulas for adults aged 18 years and older is the method suggested by Cockcroft and Gault:[2]

$$CrCl_{est} = \frac{(140 - age)BW}{72 \cdot S_{Cr}} \quad \text{for males}$$

$$CrCl_{est} = \frac{0.85(140 - age)BW}{72 \cdot S_{Cr}} \quad \text{for females}$$

where $CrCl_{est}$ is estimated creatinine clearance in ml/min, age is in years, BW is body weight in kg, S_{Cr} is serum creatinine in mg/dl. The 0.85 correction factor for females is used because women have smaller muscle mass than men and therefore produce less creatinine per day.

- The Cockcroft-Gault method should be used only in patients ≥18 years old, of actual weight within 30% of their ideal body weight [IBW_{males} (in kg) = 50 + 2.3(Ht − 60) or $IBW_{females}$ (in kg) = 45 + 2.3(Ht − 60), where Ht is height in inches], and with stable serum creatinine concentrations.
- Some patients have decreased muscle mass due to disease states and conditions that affect muscles or prevent exercise. Patients with spinal cord injuries, cancer patients with muscle wasting, HIV-infected patients, cachectic patients, and patients with poor nutrition are examples of patients in whom muscle mass may be very small, resulting in low creatinine production. In these cases, serum creatinine concentrations are low because of the low creatinine production rate and not because of high renal clearance of creatinine.
  - Investigators have suggested that if serum creatinine values are <1.0 mg/dl for a patient with decreased muscle mass, an arbitrary value of 1 mg/dl be used in the Cockcroft-Gault formula to estimate creatinine clearance.[3–5] Although it appears that the resulting estimate of creatinine clearance is closer to the actual creatinine clearance in these patients, it can still result in misestimates. It may be necessary to measure creatinine clearance in patients with low muscle mass if an accurate reflection of glomerular filtration rate is needed.
- If serum creatinine values are not stable, but are increasing or decreasing in a patient, the Cockcroft-Gault equation cannot be used to estimate creatinine clearance. In this situation, an alternative method must be used, as suggested by Jelliffe and Jelliffe.[6]
  - The first step in this method is to estimate creatinine production. The formula for this is different for males and females because of gender-dependent differences in muscle mass:

$$Ess_{male} = IBW[29.3 - (0.203 \cdot age)] \quad \text{or}$$

$$Ess_{female} = IBW[25.1 - (0.175 \cdot age)]$$

where Ess is the excretion of creatinine, IBW is ideal body weight in kg, and age is in years.
  - The following equations correct creatinine production for renal function, and adjust the estimated creatinine clearance value according to whether

the renal function is getting better or worse:

$$Ess_{corrected} = Ess[1.035 - (0.0337 \cdot Scr_{ave})]$$

$$E = Ess_{corrected} - \frac{4IBW(Scr_2 - Scr_1)}{\Delta t}$$

$$CrCl \ (in \ ml/min/1.73m^2) = E/(14.4 \cdot Scr_{ave})$$

where Scr_{ave} is the average of the two serum creatinine determinations in mg/dl, Scr_1 is the first serum creatinine and Scr_2 is the second serum creatinine, both in mg/dl, and Δt is the time that expired between the measurement of Scr_1 and Scr_2 in minutes.

- If patients are not within 30% of their ideal body weight, other methods to estimate creatinine clearance should be used.[7] It has been suggested that use of ideal body weight instead of actual body weight in the Cockcroft-Gault equation gives an adequate estimate of creatinine clearance for obese individuals. However, a specific method suggested by Salazar and Corcoran[8] for estimating creatinine clearance for obese patients has been shown to be generally superior:

$$CrCl_{est(males)} = \frac{(137 - age)[(0.285 \cdot Wt) + (12.1 \cdot Ht^2)]}{51 \cdot S_{Cr}}$$

$$CrCl_{est(females)} = \frac{(146 - age)[(0.287 \cdot Wt) + (9.74 \cdot Ht^2)]}{60 \cdot S_{Cr}}$$

where age is in years, Wt is weight in kg, Ht is height in m, and S_{Cr} is serum creatinine in mg/dl.
- Methods to estimate creatinine clearance for children and young adults are also available according to their age:[9]

$$CrCl_{est} \ (in \ ml/min/1.73 \ m^2) = (0.45 \cdot Ht)/S_{Cr} \quad age \ 0-1 \ year$$

$$CrCl_{est} \ (in \ ml/min/1.73 \ m^2) = (0.55 \cdot Ht)/S_{Cr} \quad age \ 1-20 \ years$$

where Ht is in cm and S_{Cr} is in mg/dl.

- Note that for these formulas, estimated creatinine clearance is normalized to 1.73 m^2, which is the body surface area of an adult male with a height and weight of approximately 5′ 10″ and 70 kg, respectively.

ESTIMATION OF DRUG DOSING AND PHARMACOKINETIC PARAMETERS USING CREATININE CLEARANCE

- It is common practice to base initial doses of drugs that are eliminated renally on creatinine clearance. The rationale is that renal clearance of drug is smaller in patients with reduced glomerular filtration rate, and measured or estimated creatinine clearance is a surrogate marker for glomerular filtration rate.
- An implicit assumption used in this approach is that all drug-excreting processes of the kidney, including tubular section and reabsorption, decline in parallel with glomerular filtration. The basis of this assumption is the intact nephron theory. Although tubular secretion and reabsorption may not always decline in proportion to glomerular filtration, this approach approximates the

decline in tubular function and is useful for determining initial drug dosing in patients with renal dysfunction.

- Clinicians should bear in mind that the suggested doses for patients with renal impairment are an initial guideline only, and doses may need to be increased in patients who exhibit suboptimal drug response or decreased in patients who present adverse effects.
- Breakpoints at which to consider altering drug doses are useful for clinicians to keep in mind. Generally, one should consider a possible modest decrease in drug doses when creatinine clearance is <50–60 ml/min, a moderate decrease in drug doses when creatinine clearance is <25–30 ml/min, and a substantial decrease in drug doses when creatinine clearance is ≤15 ml/min.
- In modifying doses for patients with renal impairment, it is possible to decrease the drug dose and retain the usual dosage interval, retain the usual dose and increase the dosage interval, or both decrease the dosage and prolong the dosage interval. The approach used depends on the route of administration, the dosage forms available, and the pharmacodynamic response to the drug.

  - If the drug dose is reduced and the dosage interval is not altered in patients with decreased renal function, maximum drug concentrations are usually lower and minimum drug concentrations higher than those encountered in patients with normal renal function receiving the typical drug dose (Figure 3-2). If the dosage interval is prolonged and the drug dosage is kept the same, maximum and minimum drug concentrations are usually about the same as in patients with good renal function receiving the usual drug dose.

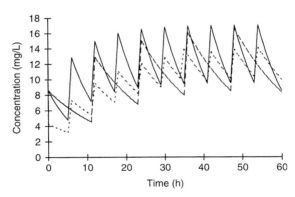

FIG. 3-2 Serum concentration/time profile for a patient with normal kidney function receiving a renally eliminated drug at the dose of 300 mg every 6 hours (solid line). In a patient with renal dysfunction, it is possible to give the same dose and prolong the dosage interval (300 mg every 12 hours, dashed line), or a reduced dose at the same dosage interval (150 mg every 6 hours, dotted line). Giving the same dose at a longer dosage interval in the patient with renal disease usually results in a concentration/time profile similar to that seen in a normal patient receiving the normal dose. However, giving a smaller dose and keeping the dosage interval the same usually produces a concentration/time profile with a lower peak steady-state concentration and a higher trough steady-state concentration. Note that since the total daily dose is the same for both renal disease dosage regimens (600 mg/d), the average steady-state concentration is identical for both dosage schemes. The same pattern occurs when hepatically metabolized drugs are administered to patients with liver disease.

- Since the mid-1980s, the Food and Drug Administration has required pharmacokinetic studies to be done for agents that are renally eliminated in patients with decreased creatinine clearance rates before they can receive agency approval. In these cases, the package insert for the drug probably contains reasonable initial dosage guidelines. Guidelines for changing drug doses for patients with decreased renal function are available for older drugs, as are updated guidelines for newer drugs that may not be included in the package insert.[10–15] Also, the primary literature should be consulted to ensure that the newest guidelines are used for all drugs. If no specific information is available for a medication, it is possible to calculate modified initial drug doses using the method described by Dettli.[16]
- For drugs with narrow therapeutic indexes, measured or estimated creatinine clearance may be used to estimate pharmacokinetic parameters for a patient based on prior studies conducted in other patients with renal dysfunction. Estimated pharmacokinetic parameters are then used in pharmacokinetic dosing equations to compute initial doses.

HEPATIC DISEASE

- Most lipid-soluble drugs are metabolized to some degree by the liver. Phase I-type reactions, such as oxidation, hydrolysis, and reduction, are often mediated by the cytochrome P-450 enzyme system (CYP), which is bound to the membrane of the endoplasmic reticulum inside hepatocytes. Phase II-type reactions, including conjugation to form glucuronides, acetates, or sulfates, may also be mediated in the liver by cytosolic enzymes contained in hepatocytes.
- The liver receives its blood supply via the hepatic artery, which contains oxygenated blood from the aorta via the superior mesenteric artery, and the portal vein, which drains the gastrointestinal tract (Figure 3-3). Liver blood flow averages 1–1.5 L/min in adults, with about one-third coming from the hepatic artery and about two-thirds coming from the portal vein.

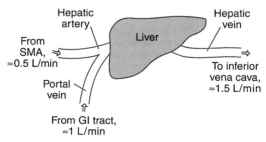

FIG. 3-3 Schematic representation of the liver. Liver blood flow to the organ is supplied by the hepatic artery and the portal vein. The hepatic artery branches off of the superior mesenteric artery and provides oxygenated blood to the liver at the rate of ~0.5 L/min. The portal vein drains blood from the gastrointestinal tract at the rate of ~1 L/min and passes its contents to the liver. Any chemicals, including orally administered drugs, must pass through the liver before it enters the systemic circulation. The hepatic vein drains the liver of blood and empties into the inferior vena cava.

- Orally administered medications must pass the systemic circulation, so if the drug is metab of the dose may be inactivated by the hepatic first-pa a chance to exert a pharmacological effect. In addition to lism, drugs can be eliminated unchanged by liver in the bile.
- The equation that describes hepatic drug metabolism is[17]

$$Cl_H = \frac{LBF \cdot (f_B \cdot Cl'_{int})}{LBF + (f_B \cdot Cl'_{int})}$$

where LBF is liver blood flow, f_B is the fraction of unbound drug in the blood, and Cl'_{int} is intrinsic clearance .
- There are two major types of liver disease: hepatitis and cirrhosis.

  - Patients with hepatitis experience an inflammation of the liver, and as a result, hepatocytes may experience decreased ability to function or die. Patients with acute hepatitis usually experience mild, transient decreases in drug metabolism that require no or minor changes in drug dosing.
  - If the patient develops chronic hepatitis, it is likely that irreversible hepatocyte damage will be more widespread, and drug dosage changes will be required at some point. With sufficient long-term hepatocyte damage, patients with chronic hepatitis can progress to hepatic cirrhosis.
  - In patients with hepatic cirrhosis, there is a permanent loss of functional hepatocytes. Drug dosage schedules usually need to be modified in patients with severe cirrhosis.

- When hepatocytes are damaged, they are no longer able to metabolize drugs efficiently and intrinsic clearance decreases, which reduces the hepatic clearance of the drug. If the drug has a hepatic first-pass effect, less drug will be lost by presystemic metabolism and bioavailability will increase. A simultaneous decrease in hepatic clearance and liver first-pass effect results in extremely large increases in steady-state concentrations for orally administered drugs.
- Liver blood flow also decreases in patients with cirrhosis because hepatocytes are replaced by nonfunctional connective tissue which increases intraorgan pressure, causing portal vein hypertension and shunting of blood flow around the liver. The decrease in liver blood flow results in less drug delivery to still-functioning hepatocytes and depresses hepatic drug clearance even further.
- The liver produces albumin and, probably, α-1-acid glycoprotein, the two major proteins that bind acidic and basic drugs, respectively, in the blood. In patients with cirrhosis, the production of these proteins declines. When this is the case, the free fraction of drugs in the blood increases because of a lack of binding proteins.
- High concentrations of endogenous substances in the blood that are normally eliminated by the liver, such as bilirubin, can displace drugs from plasma protein-binding sites. The increased free fraction in the blood will alter hepatic and renal drug clearance as well as the volume of distribution for drugs that are highly protein-bound.
- Since clearance typically decreases and volume of distribution usually increases or does not change appreciably for a drug in patients with liver disease, the half-life almost always increases in patients with decreased liver function.

| ...n Liver Disease[18] | |
Score 2 points	Score 3 points
2.0–3.0	>3.0
2.8–3.5	<2.8
4–6	>6
...ent Slight	Moderate
...ne Moderate	Severe

DETERM... ...LD-PUGH SCORES

- Unfortunately, th... ...single laboratory test that can be used to assess liver function in the same way that measured or estimated creatinine clearance is used to measure renal function. The most common way to estimate the ability of the liver to metabolize a drug is to determine the Child-Pugh score for a patient.[18]
- The Child-Pugh score consists of five laboratory tests or clinical symptoms. The five areas are serum albumin, total bilirubin, prothrombin time, ascites, and hepatic encephalopathy. Each of these areas is given a score of 1 (normal) to 3 (severely abnormal; Table 3-1), and the scores for the five areas are summed. The Child-Pugh score for a patient with normal liver function is 5, whereas the score for a patient with grossly abnormal serum albumin, total bilirubin, and prothrombin time values in addition to severe ascites and hepatic encephalopathy is 15.
- A Child-Pugh score of 8–9 is grounds for a moderate decrease (~25%) in initial daily drug dose for agents that are primarily (≥60%) metabolized hepatically, and a score of 10 or greater indicates that a significant decrease in initial daily dose (~50%) is required for drugs that are mostly liver-metabolized. As in any patient, with or without liver dysfunction, initial doses are meant as starting points for dosage titration based on patient response and avoidance of adverse effects.

ESTIMATION OF DRUG DOSING AND PHARMACOKINETIC PARAMETERS FOR DRUGS METABOLIZED BY THE LIVER

- When prescribing medications that are eliminated principally by the liver, in patients with liver dysfunction, it is possible to decrease the dose while retaining the normal dosage interval, retain the normal dose and prolong the dosage interval, or modify both the dose and the dosage interval.
- Compared to individuals with normal liver function receiving a drug at the usual dose and dosage interval, patients with hepatic disease who receive a normal dose but a prolonged dosage interval will have similar maximum and minimum steady-state serum concentrations (similar to renal drug dosing adjustments shown in Figure 3-2). However, if the dose is decreased but the dosage interval kept at the usual frequency, maximum steady-state concentrations will be lower and minimum steady-state concentrations will be higher for patients with liver disease than in patients with normal hepatic function.
- Table 3-2 gives values for theophylline clearance in a variety of patients, including patients with cirrhosis.[19] The theophylline dosage rates listed are designed to produce steady-state theophylline concentrations between 8 and 12 mg/L.

TABLE 3-2 Theophylline Clearance and Dosage Rates for Patients with Various Disease States and Conditions[19]

Disease state/ condition	Mean clearance (ml/min/kg)	Mean dose (mg/kg/h)
Children 1–9 years	1.4	0.8
Children 9–12 years or adult smokers	1.25	0.7
Adolescents 12–16 years or elderly smokers (>65 years)	0.9	0.5
Adult nonsmokers	0.7	0.4
Elderly nonsmokers (>65 years)	0.5	0.3
Decompensated CHF, cor pulmonale, cirrhosis	0.35	0.2

Mean volume of distribution = 0.5 L/kg.

IMPLICATIONS OF HEPATIC DISEASE FOR SERUM DRUG CONCENTRATION MONITORING AND DRUG EFFECTS

- The pharmacokinetic alterations that occur with hepatic disease result in complex changes in total and unbound steady-state concentrations and drug response. The changes that occur depend on whether the drug has a low or high hepatic extraction ratio.

  - For drugs with a low hepatic extraction ratio ($\leq 30\%$), hepatic clearance is equal to the product of free fraction in the blood (f_B) and the intrinsic clearance of the drug (Cl'_{int}):

$$Cl_H = f_B \cdot Cl'_{int}$$

  - For drugs with a high hepatic extraction ratio ($\geq 70\%$), hepatic clearance is equal to liver blood flow (LBF):

$$Cl_H = LBF$$

  - For drugs with intermediate hepatic extraction ratios, the entire liver clearance equation must be used and all three factors—liver blood flow, free fraction of drug in the blood and intrinsic clearance—are important parameters that must be taken into account:

$$Cl_H = \frac{LBF \cdot (f_B \cdot Cl'_{int})}{LBF + (f_B \cdot Cl'_{int})}$$

HEART FAILURE

- Heart failure is accompanied by a decrease in cardiac output which results in lower liver and renal blood flow. Changes in drug pharmacokinetics due to decreased renal blood flow are not widely reported. However, declines in hepatic clearance, especially for compounds with moderate to high hepatic extraction ratios, are reported for many drugs.
- Decreased drug bioavailability has been reported in patients with heart failure. The proposed mechanisms for decreased bioavailability are collection of edema fluid in the gastrointestinal tract, which makes absorption of drug molecules more difficult, and decreased blood flow to the gastrointestinal tract.

- The volume of distribution of some drugs decreases in patients with heart failure. Because clearance and volume of distribution may or may not change simultaneously, the alteration in half-life, if any, is difficult to predict in patients with heart failure.

DIALYSIS

- Dialysis is a process whereby substances move via a concentration gradient across a semipermeable membrane (Figure 3-4). Artificial kidneys (also known as dialysis coils or filters), which use a synthetic semipermeable membrane to remove waste products from the blood, are available for use in hemodialysis. Physiological membranes, such as those present in the peritoneal cavity in the lower abdomen, can be used with peritoneal dialysis as an endogenous semipermeable membrane.
- Substances that are small enough to pass through the pores in the semipermeable membrane will pass out of the blood into the dialysis fluid. Once in the dialysis fluid, waste products and other compounds can be removed from the body.
- In some cases, dialysis is used to remove drugs from the bodies of patients who have taken drug overdoses or who are experiencing severe adverse effects from the drug. However, in most cases drug molecules are removed from the blood coincidental to the removal of toxic waste products that would usually be eliminated by the kidney.
- Because drugs can be removed by dialysis, it is important to understand when drug dosing needs to be modified in renal failure patients undergoing the procedure. Often, dialysis removes enough drug from a patient's body that supplemental doses need to be given after dialysis has been completed (Figure 3-5)

Dialysis

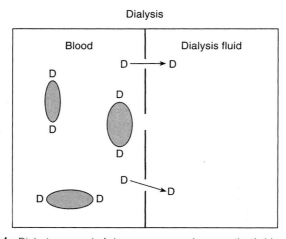

FIG. 3-4   Dialysis removal of drug can occur when a patient's blood comes in contact with a semipermeable membrane that has drug-free dialysis fluid on the other side. In this schematic, the semipermeable membrane has pores in it large enough for unbound drug to pass through (represented by D), but not for protein bound drug to pass through (denoted by D's attached to ovals representing plasma proteins).

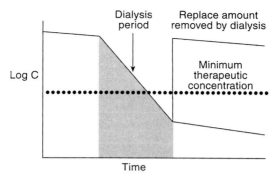

FIG. 3-5 Concentration/time graph for a drug removed by dialysis. The shaded area indicates the time period during which a dialysis procedure was conducted. Because extra drug was removed from the blood during dialysis, concentrations dropped much more quickly during that period. After dialysis is finished, the concentrations again drop at the predialysis rate. If drug concentrations drop below the minimum therapeutic concentration (shown by the dark, solid horizontal line), it may be necessary to give a supplemental dose to retain the pharmacological effect of the drug (indicated by increase in drug concentration after dialysis).

- In a renal failure patient, the only clearance mechanisms available to remove drugs from the body are nonrenal ($Cl = Cl_{NR}$, where Cl is total clearance and Cl_{NR} is nonrenal clearance). When the patient is receiving dialysis, clearance from both nonrenal routes and dialysis are present, which will accelerate drug removal from the body during the dialysis procedure if the compound is significantly removed by dialysis ($Cl = Cl_{NR} + Cl_D$, where Cl_D is dialysis clearance).
- In order to determine if dialysis clearance is significant, one should consider the absolute value of dialysis clearance and the relative contribution of dialysis clearance to total clearance. Additionally, if dialysis clearance is $\geq 30\%$ of total clearance or if the total amount of drug removed by the dialysis procedure is enough to warrant a postdialysis replacement dose, dialysis clearance is considered to be significant.

DRUG CHARACTERISTICS THAT AFFECT DIALYSIS REMOVAL

Molecular Size

- Molecular size relative to pore size in the semipermeable membrane is a factor that influences dialysis clearance of a compound. Most hemodialysis procedures are conducted using "low-flux" artificial kidneys which have relatively small pores in the semipermeable membranes.

  - For low-flux filters, small drug molecules (molecular weight <500 daltons) relative to the pore size of the semipermeable membrane tend to be readily eliminated by dialysis and have high extraction ratios for the artificial kidney. In this case, dialyzability of the drug is influenced by blood flow to the artificial kidney, dialysis fluid flow rate to the artificial kidney, and the surface area of the semipermeable membrane inside the artificial kidney.

- Increased blood flow delivers more drug to the dialysis coil, increased dialysis fluid flow rate removes drug that entered the dialysis fluid more quickly from the artificial kidney and increases the concentration gradient across the semipermeable membrane, and increased semipermeable membrane surface area increases the number of pores that a drug molecule will encounter, making it easier for drug molecules to pass from the blood into the dialysis fluid.
- Drug molecules with moderate molecular weights (molecular weight 500–1000 daltons) have a decreased ability to pass through the semipermeable membrane in low-flux filters. However, many drugs that fall into this intermediate category have sufficient dialysis clearances to require postdialysis replacement doses.
- Large drug molecules (molecular weight >1000 daltons) are not removed to a significant extent when low-flux filters are used for dialysis because pore sizes in these artificial kidneys are too small for the molecules to fit through.
- "High-flux" filters are now available and are widely used in some patients. The semipermeable membranes of these artificial kidneys have much larger pore sizes and larger surface areas, so large drug molecules that were previously considered not to be removable by hemodialysis can be cleared by high-flux filters. In some of these cases, supplemental postdialysis drug doses are needed to maintain therapeutic amounts of drug in the body.

Water/Lipid Solubility
- Drugs that have a high degree of water solubility tend to partition into the water-based dialysis fluid, while lipid-soluble drugs tend to remain in the blood.

Plasma Protein Binding
- Only unbound drug molecules are able to pass through the pores in the semipermeable membrane; drug–plasma protein complexes are too large to pass through the pores and gain access to the dialysis fluid side of the semipermeable membrane.

Volume of Distribution
- Medications with large volumes of distribution are located principally at tissue-binding sites and not in the blood, where dialysis can remove the drug. Compounds with small volumes of distribution (<1 L/kg) usually demonstrate high dialysis clearance rates. Drugs with moderate volumes of distribution (1–2 L/kg) have intermediate dialysis clearance values, while agents with large volumes of distribution (>2 L/kg) have poor dialysis characteristics.
  - When dialysis is completed, the blood and tissues have a chance to reequilibrate and serum concentrations increase, sometimes to their predialysis concentration. This "rebound" in serum concentration has been reported for several drugs.

HEMODIALYSIS

- Hemodialysis is a very efficient procedure to remove toxic waste from the blood of renal failure patients (Figure 3-6). Blood is pumped out of the patient at the rate of 300–400 ml/min and through one side of the semipermeable membrane of the artificial kidney by the hemodialysis machine. Cleansed blood is then pumped back into the vascular system of the patient.

- In acute situations, vascular access can be obtained through centrally placed catheters. For patients with chronic renal failure, vascular shunts made of synthetic materials can be placed surgically between a high-blood-flow artery and vein in the arm or other site for the purpose of conducting hemodialysis.

- Dialysis fluid is pumped through the artificial kidney at a rate of 400–600 ml/min on the other side of the semipermeable membrane, in the direction opposite to blood flow. This "countercurrent" flow is more efficient in removing waste products than running the blood and dialysis fluid in parallel to each other.

  - Dialysis fluid is electrolytically and osmotically balanced for the individual patient. It is possible to increase or decrease serum electrolytes by increasing or decreasing the concentration of the ion in the dialysis fluid compared to the concurrent serum value. By adding solutes to increase the osmolality of the dialysis fluid relative to the blood, it is possible to remove fluid from the patient's body by osmotic pressure across the semipermeable membrane of the artificial kidney. This process is known as ultrafiltration.

- Hemodialysis is usually performed for 3–4 hours 3 times a week using low-flux filters or for 1–1.5 hours 3 times a week using high-flux filters.

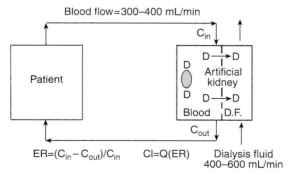

FIG. 3-6 Hemodialysis removes blood from the patient's body (indicated by arrows from patient to artificial kidney) and passes it through an artificial kidney that contains a semipermeable membrane. Inside the artificial kidney, waste products pass into the dialysis fluid and are eliminated from the body. If drug molecules can pass through the pores in the semipermeable membrane, they will also be eliminated from the body. The extraction ratio of the artificial kidney can be computed using the concentration into (C_{in}) and out of (C_{out}) the device. Dialysis clearance can be calculated by taking the product of the dialysis extraction ratio and blood flow to the dialysis machine.

- The Food and Drug Administration has required pharmacokinetic studies to be done for renally eliminated drugs in patients receiving chronic hemodialysis since the mid-1980s. Because of this, the package insert for the drug may include manufacturer-recommended doses to be administered to patients in the posthemodialysis period. Guidelines for the administration of posthemodialysis replacement doses are available for older drugs, as are updated guidelines for newer drugs that may not be included in the package insert.[10–15] Also, the primary literature should be consulted to ensure that the newest guidelines are used for all drugs.

  - When assessing the hemodialysis removal characteristics of a drug and the need for postdialysis replacement doses, it should be recognized that the majority of information available is for low-flux artificial kidneys. If a high-flux dialysis coil is used, the primary literature is probably the best source of information, but in many cases studies have not been conducted using this technology.

HEMOFILTRATION

- Hemofiltration comprises a family of techniques that have some similarities and some differences compared to hemodialysis.[20] The hemofilter used in hemofiltration is similar to the artificial kidney used in hemodialysis. The pore size in hemofilters is large, which allows drug molecules up to 20,000 daltons to cross its semipermeable membrane.

  - Continuous arteriovenous hemofiltration (CAVH) and continuous venovenous hemofiltration (CVVH) use an extracorporeal circuit that runs from an artery to a vein or from a vein to a vein, respectively. These processes do not use a dialysis fluid, so plasma water that passes through the hemofilter is collected and discarded.

  - Continuous arteriovenous hemodialysis with filtration (CAVHD) and continuous venovenous hemodialysis with filtration (CVVHD) are hybrids of conventional hemodialysis and CAVH or CVVH, respectively. The hemofilter has hemodialysis fluid on the other side of the semipermeable membrane containing the patient's blood.

  - For both CVVH and CVVHD, a mechanical pump is used to propel blood through the hemofilter. For CAVH and CAVHD, the patient's own blood pressure usually provides the propulsion of blood through the hemofilter.

- The sieving coefficient is the ratio of the drug concentration in the hemofiltrate to the drug concentration in the serum. Table 3-3 lists sieving coefficients for a variety of drugs.[21,22]

- The ultrafiltration rate (UFR) is the filtration provided by the specific hemofiltration technique. Typical ranges for UFR are 10–16 ml/min for procedures that do not use extracorporeal blood pumps, and 20–30 ml/min for procedures that use extracorporeal blood pumps. When hemofiltration procedures that incorporate dialysis fluid are used, an additional 15–20 ml/min is added to these values.[21,22]

- Several different methods of calculating additional doses during hemofiltration have been suggested.[21,22]

  - Based on the expected ultrafiltration rates noted above, hemofiltration is usually equivalent to a glomerular filtration rate (GFR) of 10–50 ml/min. In lieu of specific recommendations for a drug, clinicians can use this GFR rate with FDA or renal drug dosing guidelines to suggest an adjusted dose.[10–12]

TABLE 3-3 Hemofiltration Sieving Coefficients for Selected Drugs[21,22]

Drug	Sieving coefficient
Antibiotics	
Amikacin	0.95
Amphotericin B	0.35
Amphotericin B (liposomal)	0.10
Ampicillin	0.69
Cefepime	0.72
Cefoperazone	0.27
Cefotaxime	1.06
Cefoxitin	0.83
Ceftazidime	0.90
Ceftriaxone	0.20
Cephapirin	1.48
Cilastatin	0.75
Ciprofloxacin	0.58
Clavulanic acid	1.69
Clindamycin	0.49
Doxycycline	0.40
Erythromycin	0.37
Fluconazole	1.00
Flucytosine	0.80
Ganciclovir	0.84
Gentamicin	0.81
Imipenem	0.90
Meropenem	1.00
Metronidazole	0.84
Mezlocillin	0.71
Nafcillin	0.55
Netilmicin	0.93
Oxacillin	0.02
Perfloxacin	0.80
Penicillin	0.68
Piperacillin	0.82
Streptomycin	0.30
Sulfamethoxazole	0.30
Teichoplanin	0.05
Ticarcillin	0.83
Tobramycin	0.90
Vancomycin	0.80
Other drugs	
Amrinone	0.80
Chlordiazepoxide	0.05
Cisplatin	0.10
Clofibrate	0.06
Cyclosporine	0.58
Diazepam	0.02
Digoxin	0.70
Digitoxin	0.15
Famotidine	0.73
Glyburide	0.60
Glutethimide	0.02
Lidocaine	0.14
Lithium	0.90
Metamizole	0.40
N-acetylprocainamide	0.92

(Continued)

TABLE 3-3 Hemofiltration Sieving Coefficients for Selected
Drugs [21,22] (*Continued*)

Drug	Sieving coefficient
Nizatidine	0.59
Nitrazepam	0.08
Nomifensin	0.70
Oxazepam	0.10
Phenobarbital	0.80
Phenytoin	0.45
Procainamide	0.86
Ranitidine	0.78
Tacrolimus	0.26
Theophylline	0.80

- A supplemental dose (SD) can be estimated using a measured or estimated steady-state drug concentration (Css), unbound fraction in the serum (f_B), ultrafiltration rate (UFR), and drug dosing interval (τ):

$$SD = Css \cdot f_B \cdot UFR \cdot \tau$$

  Supplemental doses are given in addition to maintenance doses of the drug.
- A booster dose (BD) can be computed using an actual measured concentration (C_{actual}), a desired concentration ($C_{desired}$), and an estimated or actual volume of distribution (V):

$$BD = (C_{desired} - C_{actual})V$$

  Booster doses are given in addition to maintenance doses of the drug.

PERITONEAL DIALYSIS

- Peritoneal dialysis involves the surgical insertion of a catheter in the lower abdomen into the peritoneal cavity (Figure 3-7). The peritoneal membrane covering the internal organs is highly vascularized, so when dialysis fluid (1–3 L) is introduced into the peritoneal cavity using the catheter, waste products move from the blood vessels of the peritoneal membrane (a semipermeable membrane) into the dialysis fluid along a concentration gradient. The dialysis fluid is periodically removed (typically every 12–24 hours) from the peritoneal cavity and discarded. Outpatients undergoing chronic ambulatory peritoneal dialysis have dialysis fluid present in their peritoneal cavities all day or most hours of a day.
- Compared to hemodialysis, peritoneal dialysis removes drug much less efficiently. So, it is less likely that replacement drug doses will need to be given during intermittent peritoneal dialysis, and that drug dosages will need to be increased while patients receive chronic peritoneal dialysis. For patients undergoing peritoneal dialysis, clinicians should consult the manufacturer's package insert for drugs recently marketed (mid-1980s or later), reviews listing the peritoneal dialysis removal of older drugs and updated information on newer agents, and the primary literature for the newest guidelines for all compounds.

Peritoneal Dialysis

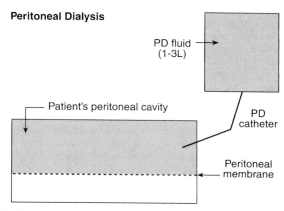

FIG. 3-7 Schematic of peritoneal dialysis procedure. A catheter (labeled PD catheter) is surgically inserted into the patient's peritoneal cavity and used to introduce 1–3 L of dialysis fluid (labeled PD fluid). The dialysis fluid comes into contact with capillaries in the peritoneal membrane, where waste products and drugs pass from the blood into the fluid. After the dwell time has concluded, the dialysis fluid is removed from the peritoneal cavity via the catheter and discarded.

- Drugs can also be added to peritoneal dialysis fluid. If the agent is absorbed from the dialysis fluid into the body, systemic effects due to the drug may occur. Because the development of peritonitis is a common problem in patients receiving peritoneal dialysis, antibiotics have been administered intraperitoneally for local treatment of the infection using dialysis fluid as the delivery vehicle. In most cases, antibiotics are absorbed into the body when given this way, but therapeutic serum concentrations may not be achieved for all agents, making systemically administered doses necessary.
- Clinicians should pay particular attention to whether studies measuring peritoneal dialysis removal or absorption of drugs were conducted in patients with peritonitis. Peritonitis involves inflammation of the peritoneal membrane and increases its permeability. Increased permeability allows for greater flux of drug across the membrane, which allows more drug removal during dialysis or more drug absorption if the drug is added to the peritoneal dialysis fluid.

OBESITY

- The presence of excessive adipose tissue can alter the pharmacokinetics of drugs by changing the volume of distribution. The general physiological equation for volume of distribution can be broken down into separate parameters for individual tissue types:

$$V = V_B + \frac{f_B}{f_A} V_T = V_B + \frac{f_B}{f_{heart}} V_{heart} + \frac{f_B}{f_{muscle}} V_{muscle} + \frac{f_B}{f_{fat}} V_{fat} + \cdots + \frac{f_B}{f_n} V_n$$

As a result, the sheer amount of adipose tissue will be a primary determinant of how much obesity will affect the volume of distribution of the drug.

- The magnitude of effect that adipose tissue has on the volume of distribution for a drug is also dependent on the binding of drug in the tissue itself. If the drug has a large affinity for adipose tissue and is highly bound there, the free fraction in adipose tissue will be small ($\downarrow f_{fat}$), and a large amount of drug will accumulate in that tissue.
- Medications that have high lipid solubility tend to partition into adipose tissue, and the volume of distribution in obese patients for these drugs can be dramatically larger than in normal-weight patients. However, hydrophilic drugs tend not to distribute into adipose tissue, so the volume of distribution for many water-soluble drugs is not significantly different in obese and normal-weight patients.
- Although the presence of excessive adipose tissue is the most obvious change that occurs in obese individuals, other physiological changes may also be present. While adipose cells contain >90% fat, there are additional supportive tissues, extracellular fluid, and blood present in adipose tissue. Also, some lean tissues hypertrophy in obese individuals. The net result of these changes is that hydrophilic drugs with small volumes of distribution may experience distribution alterations in obese patients. Another change that is found in obese individuals is increased glomerular filtration rates. This alteration primarily affects hydrophilic drug compounds that are eliminated renally and will increase the renal clearance of the agent.
- Obesity has variable effects on the metabolism of drugs. Clinicians should be aware of this variability and dose hepatically metabolized drugs cautiously in obese individuals in the absence of specific recommendations. Half-life changes vary according to the relative alterations in clearance (Cl) and volume of distribution (V):

$$t_{1/2} = (0.693 \cdot V)/Cl$$

where $t_{1/2}$ is half-life.

DRUG INTERACTIONS

- Pharmacokinetic drug interactions may occur between drugs when one agent changes the clearance or volume of distribution of another medication. There are several drug interaction mechanisms that result in altered drug clearance.

  - A drug can inhibit or induce the enzymes responsible for the metabolism of other drugs. Enzyme inhibition decreases intrinsic clearance, and enzyme induction increases intrinsic clearance.
  - Another type of drug interaction displaces a drug from plasma protein-binding sites because the two compounds share the same binding site, and the two compete for the same area on plasma proteins.
    - For a drug with a low hepatic extraction ratio, plasma protein-binding displacement drug interactions cause major pharmacokinetic alterations but are not clinically significant because the pharmacological effect of the drug does not change.
    - For drugs with high hepatic extraction ratios given intravenously, plasma protein-binding displacement drug interactions cause both major pharmacokinetic and pharmacodynamic changes.
    - Route of administration plays an important role in how important plasma protein-binding displacement drug interactions are for agents with high hepatic extraction ratios. If a drug with a high hepatic extraction ratio is given orally, a plasma protein-binding displacement drug interaction will

cause a simultaneous increase in the unbound fraction of drug in the blood ($\uparrow f_B$) and the hepatic presystemic metabolism of the drug.

- By virtue of its pharmacological effect, a drug may increase or decrease blood flow to an organ that eliminates or metabolizes another medication and thereby increase or decrease the clearance of the medication.
- Two drugs eliminated by the same active renal tubular secretion mechanism can compete for the pathway and decrease the renal clearance of one or both agents.

- Changes in plasma protein binding also cause alterations in volume of distribution. If two drugs share the same tissue-binding sites, it is possible for tissue-binding displacement drug interactions to occur and change the volume of distribution for one of the medications.
- Half-life may change as a result of drug interactions or, if clearance and volume of distribution alterations are about equal, half-life may remain constant even though a major drug interaction has occurred.

REFERENCES

1. Gibaldi M, Perrier D. Pharmacokinetics. 2nd ed. New York: Marcel Dekker; 1982.
2. Cockcroft DW, Gault MH. Prediction of creatinine clearance from serum creatinine. Nephron 1976;16:31–41.
3. Mohler JL, Barton SD, Blouin RA, Cowen DL, Flanigan RC. The evaluation of creatinine clearance in spinal cord injury patients. J Urol 1986;136(2):366–9.
4. Reichley RM, Ritchie DJ, Bailey TC. Analysis of various creatinine clearance formulas in prediciting gentamicin elimination in patients with low serum creatinine. Pharmacotherapy 1995;15(5):625–30.
5. Smythe M, Hoffman J, Kizy K, Dmuchowski C. Estimating creatinine clearance in elderly patients with low serum creatinine concentrations. Am J Hosp Pharm 1994;51(2):198–204.
6. Jelliffe RW, Jelliffe SM. A computer program for estimation of creatinine clearance from unstable serum creatinine levels, age, sex, and weight. Math Biosci 1972;14:17–24.
7. Dionne RE, Bauer LA, Gibson GA, Griffen WO, R.A. B. Estimating creatinine clearance in morbidly obese patients. Am J Hosp Pharm 1981;38:841–4.
8. Salazar DE, Corcoran GB. Predicting creatinine clearance and renal drug clearance in obese patients from estimated fat-free body mass. Am J Med 1988;84:1053–60.
9. Traub SL, Johnson CE. Comparison of methods of estimating creatinine clearance in children. Am J Hosp Pharm 1980;37:195–201.
10. Aronoff GR, Berns JS, Brier ME, et al. Drug prescribing in renal failure: dosing guidelines for adults. 4th ed. Philadelphia: American College of Physicians, 1999.
11. Bennett WM. Guide to drug dosage in renal failure. Clin Pharmacokinet 1988;15(5):326–54.
12. Aronoff GR, Berns JS, Brier ME, Golper TA, Morrison G, Singer I, Swan SK, Bennett WM. Drug prescribing in renal failure: dosing guidelines for adults. 3rd or 4th ed. Philadelphia: American College of Physicians, 1999.
13. Fillastre JP, Singlas E. Pharmacokinetics of newer drugs in patients with renal impairment (part I). Clin Pharmacokinet 1991;20(4):293–310.
14. Singlas E, Fillastre JP. Pharmacokinetics of newer drugs in patients with renal impairment (part II). Clin Pharmacokinet 1991;20(5):389–410.
15. Lam YW, Banerji S, Hatfield C, Talbert RL. Principles of drug administration in renal insufficiency. Clin Pharmacokinet 1997;32(1):30–57.
16. Dettli L. Drug dosage in renal disease. Clin Pharmacokinet 1976;1(2):126–34.
17. Wilkinson GR, Shand DG. A physiological approach to hepatic drug clearance. Clin Pharmacol Ther 1975;18(4):377–90.
18. Pugh RN, Murray-Lyon IM, Dawson JL, Pietroni MC, Williams R. Transection of the oesophagus for bleeding oesophageal varices. Br J Surg 1973;60(8):646–9.

19. Edwards DJ, Zarowitz BJ, Slaughter RL. Theophylline. In: Evans WE, Schentag JJ, Jusko WJ, eds. Applied pharmacokinetics: principles of therapeutic drug monitoring. 3rd ed. Vancouver, WA: Applied Therapeutics, 1992:557.
20. Forni LG, Hilton PJ. Continuous hemofiltration in the treatment of acute renal failure. N Engl J Med 1997;336(18):1303–9.
21. Golper TA, Marx MA. Drug dosing adjustments during continuous renal replacement therapies. Kidney Int Suppl 1998;66:S165–8.
22. Golper TA. Update on drug sieving coefficients and dosing adjustments during continuous renal replacement therapies. Contrib Nephrol 2001(132):349–53.

2 | ANTIBIOTICS

4 | Aminoglycoside Antibiotics

The aminoglycoside antibiotics are widely used for the treatment of severe gram-negative infections, often in combination with a β-lactam antibiotic. Aminoglycosides are also used for gram-positive infections in combination with penicillins when antibiotic synergy is required for optimal killing.

- Aminoglycoside antibiotics are bactericidal, and the drugs exhibit concentration-dependent bacterial killing.[1] Also, aminoglycosides have a concentration-dependent postantibiotic effect. The mechanisms of action of aminoglycosides are binding to the 30S ribosomal subunit, inhibiting protein synthesis and misreading of mRNA causing dysfunctional protein production.

THERAPEUTIC AND TOXIC CONCENTRATIONS

- The *conventional* method of dosing aminoglycoside antibiotics is to administer multiple daily doses (usually every 8 hours).[2] In order to take advantage of concentration-dependent bacterial killing and the postantibiotic effect, *extended-interval* (usually the total daily dose given once per day) aminoglycoside administration is also a dosing option.[3–5]
- Aminoglycoside antibiotics are given as short-term ($\frac{1}{2}$–1 hour) infusions. If a 1-hour infusion is used, maximum end-of-infusion concentrations are measured when the infusion is completed (Figure 4-1). If a $\frac{1}{2}$-hour infusion is used, serum concentrations exhibit a distribution phase so that drug in the blood and in the tissues are not yet in equilibrium. Because of this, before peak concentrations are measured, a $\frac{1}{2}$-hour waiting period is allowed for distribution to finish if a $\frac{1}{2}$-hour infusion is used.

Conventional Dosing

- Therapeutic steady-state peak concentrations for gentamicin, tobramycin, and netilmicin are generally 5–10 µg/ml for gram-negative infections. Therapeutic peak concentrations for amikacin are 15–30 µg/ml.

  - Infection sites with more susceptible bacteria, such as intra-abdominal infections, usually can be treated with steady-state peak concentrations at the lower end of this range (typically 5–7 µg/ml).
  - Infection sites that are difficult to penetrate and with bacteria that have higher minimum inhibitory concentration (MIC) values, such as pseudomonal pneumonia, usually require steady-state peak concentrations at the higher end of the range (typically 8–10 µg/ml).
  - When gentamicin, tobramycin, or netilmicin is used synergistically with penicillins or other antibiotics for the treatment of gram-positive infections, such as infective endocarditis, steady-state peak concentrations of 3–5 µg/ml are often adequate.

- Exceeding peak steady-state concentrations of 12–14 µg/ml for gentamicin, tobramycin, or netilmicin, or 35–40 µg/ml for amikacin, when using conventional dosing leads to an increased risk of ototoxicity.[6] The types of ototoxicity

55

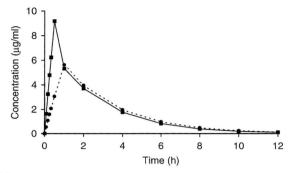

FIG. 4-1 Concentration/time plot for gentamicin 120 mg given as a $\frac{1}{2}$-hour infusion (squares with solid line) and as a 1-hour infusion (circles with dashed line). When given as a $\frac{1}{2}$-hour infusion, end-of-infusion concentrations are higher because the serum and tissues are not in equilibrium. A $\frac{1}{2}$-hour waiting time for aminoglycoside distribution to tissues is allowed before peak concentrations are measured. If aminoglycosides are given as 1-hour infusions, distribution has an opportunity to occur during the infusion time, and peak concentrations can be obtained immediately. In either case, concentrations 1 hour after the infusion was initiated are similar.

that aminoglycosides cause are auditory and vestibular, and the damage is permanent.

- Auditory ototoxicity usually is first noted at high frequencies (>4000 Hz) and is difficult to detect using clinical means. If aminoglycoside treatment is not discontinued in individuals with high-frequency auditory ototoxicity, hearing loss will progress to lower frequencies. As a result, aminoglycoside-induced hearing losses are not usually detected until the patient is unable to detect sounds in the conversational frequency zone (<4000 Hz).
- Often, the first sign of auditory ototoxicity is tinnitus. Vestibular ototoxicity results in the loss of balance. Besides loss of equilibrium, headache, ataxia, nausea, vomiting, nystagmus, and vertigo can all be signs of vestibular ototoxicity.

• Trough steady-state concentrations (predose or minimum concentrations, usually obtained within 30 minutes of the next dose) above 2–3 μg/ml for tobramycin, gentamicin, or netilmicin, or 10 μg/ml for amikacin, predispose patients to an increased risk of nephrotoxicity.[7,8]

- Nephrotoxicity due to aminoglycoside therapy is unlikely to occur before 3–5 days of therapy with proper dosing of the antibiotic. Because many patients receiving aminoglycosides are critically ill, other sources of nephrotoxicity, such as hypotension or other nephrotoxic drug therapy, should be ruled out before a diagnosis of aminoglycoside renal damage is made in a patient.
- Aminoglycoside-induced nephrotoxicity is usually reversible with little, if any, residual damage if the antibiotic is withdrawn soon after renal function tests change. With proper patient monitoring, mild renal dysfunction

resulting in serum creatinine increases of 0.5–2 mg/dl may be the only result of aminoglycoside nephrotoxicity.

- Keeping peak and trough concentrations within the suggested ranges does not completely avoid nephrotoxicity and ototoxicity in patients, but should decrease the likelihood that patients will experience these serious adverse effects.[9] Even though serum concentrations are controlled within the suggested ranges, duration of therapy exceeding 14 days, large total cumulative doses, and concurrent therapy with other nephrotoxic drugs such as vancomycin can predispose patients to these side effects of the aminoglycoside antibiotics.[10–13]

Extended-Interval Dosing

- Because aminoglycoside antibiotics exhibit concentration-dependent bacterial killing and the postantibiotic effect lasts longer with higher concentrations, investigators began studying the possibility of giving a higher dose of aminoglycoside once daily.[3–5] At the present time, there is not a consensus on how to approach concentration monitoring using this mode of administration.[14–20]
- Preliminary therapeutic concentrations for gentamicin, tobramycin, or netilmicin recommended by clinicians when using this mode of administration are steady-state peak concentrations of 20–30 μg/ml and trough concentrations <1 μg/ml.

CLINICAL MONITORING PARAMETERS

- Review current microbiological cultures and sensitivities to reaffirm correct antibiotic treatment.
- Confirm appropriate concurrent antibiotic therapy, such as β-lactam or anaerobic agents, when necessary to treat the infection.
- Measurement of serial white blood cell counts and body temperatures are useful to determine the efficacy of antibiotic therapy. A large number of neutrophils and immature neutrophils, known clinically as a "shift to the left," can also be observed in patients with severe bacterial infections.

  - Favorable response to antibiotic treatment is usually indicated by high white blood cell counts decreasing toward the normal range, the trend of body temperatures (plotted as body temperature versus time, also known as the "fever curve") approaching normal, and any specific infection-site tests or procedures resolving.
  - Clinicians should also be aware that immunocompromised patients with a bacterial infection may not be able to mount a fever or elevated white blood cell count.

- Aminoglycoside steady-state peak and trough serum concentrations should be measured after 3–5 estimated half-lives. Methods to estimate half-life are given in the initial-dose calculation portion of this chapter.

  - Since prolongation of the dosage interval is often used in patients with decreased elimination, a useful clinical rule when using conventional dosing is to measure serum concentrations after the third dose. Additionally, the third dose typically occurs 1–3 days after dosing has commenced, and this is a good time to assess clinical efficacy of the treatment as well.

- Steady-state serum concentrations, in conjunction with clinical response, are used to adjust the antibiotic dose, if necessary. Methods to adjust aminoglycoside doses using serum concentrations are discussed later in this chapter.
- If the dosage is adjusted, aminoglycoside elimination changes, or laboratory and clinical monitoring indicate that the infection is not resolving or worsening, clinicians should consider rechecking steady-state drug concentrations.

- When extended-interval aminoglycoside therapy is used, steady-state peak and trough concentrations can be measured and used to alter the dose and dosage interval, or an aminoglycoside serum concentration measured 6–14 hours after a dose and a dosage nomogram used to adjust the dosage interval (see dosing section later in the chapter for details).
- Serial monitoring of serum creatinine concentrations should be used to detect nephrotoxicity. Ideally, a baseline serum creatinine concentration is obtained before aminoglycoside therapy is initiated, and three times weekly or every other day during treatment. An increasing serum creatinine test on two or more consecutive measurement occasions indicates that more intensive monitoring of serum creatinine values, such as daily, is needed.

  - If serum creatinine measurements increase more than 0.5 mg/dl over the baseline value (or >25–30% over baseline for serum creatinine values >2 mg/dl) and other causes of declining renal function have been ruled out (other nephrotoxic drugs or agents, hypotension, etc.), alternatives to aminoglycoside therapy or, if that option is not possible, intensive aminoglycoside serum concentration monitoring should be initiated to ensure that excessive amounts of aminoglycoside do not accumulate in the patient.

- In the clinical setting, audiometry is rarely used to detect ototoxicity because it is difficult to accomplish in severely ill patients. Instead, clinical signs and symptoms of auditory (decreased hearing acuity in the conversational range, feeling of fullness or pressure in the ears, tinnitus) or vestibular (loss of equilibrium, headache, nausea, vomiting, vertigo, nystagmus, ataxia) ototoxicity are monitored at the same time intervals as serum creatinine determination.

BASIC CLINICAL PHARMACOKINETIC PARAMETERS

- The aminoglycosides are eliminated almost completely ($\geq$90%) unchanged in the urine, primarily by glomerular filtration (Table 4-1).[9,12,21]
- These antibiotics are usually given by short-term ($\frac{1}{2}$–1 hour) intermittent intravenous infusions, although they can be given intramuscularly. When aminoglycosides are given intramuscularly, they exhibit very good bioavailability of ~100% and are rapidly absorbed, with maximal concentrations occurring about 1 hour after injection.

  - Exceptions to this situation are patients who are hypotensive or obese. Intramuscularly administered drugs may be malabsorbed in hypotensive patients, such as those with gram-negative sepsis. Care must be taken when administering aminoglycoside antibiotics to obese individuals to use a long enough needle to penetrate subcutaneous fat and enter muscle tissue.

TABLE 4-1 Disease States and Conditions That Alter
Aminoglycoside Pharmacokinetics

Disease state/ condition	Half-life (h)	Volume of distribution (L/kg)	Comment
Adults, normal renal function	2 (range, 1.5–3)	0.26 (range, 0.2–0.3)	Usual doses 3–5 mg/kg/d for gentamicin, tobramycin, and netilmicin, or 15 mg/kg/d for amikacin
Adults, renal failure	50 (range, 36–72)	0.26	Renal failure patients commonly have fluid imbalances that may decrease (underhydration) or increase (overhydration) the volume of distribution and secondarily change half-life
Burn patients	1.5	0.26	Burn patients commonly have fluid imbalances that may decrease (underhydration) or increase (overhydration) the volume of distribution and secondarily change half-life
Penicillin therapy (patients with creatinine clearance <30 ml/min)	Variable	0.26	Some penicillins (penicillin G, ampicillin, nafcillin, carbenicillin, ticarcillin) can bind and inactivate aminoglycosides *in vivo*
Obese patients (>30% over IBW) with normal renal function	2–3	V (in L) = 0.26 [IBW + 0.4 (TBW − IBW)]	Aminoglycosides enter the extracellular fluid contained in adipose tissue requiring a correction factor to estimate volume of distribution
Cystic fibrosis patients	1.5	0.35	Larger volume of distribution and shorter half-life result in larger daily doses of 7.5–10 mg/kg/d (conventional therapy) for gentamicin, tobramycin, and netilmicin
Ascites/ overhydration patients	Variable	V (in L) = (0.26 · DBW) + (TBW − DBW)	Aminoglycosides distribute to excess extracellular fluid; correction equation assumes that weight gain is due to fluid accumulation; alterations in volume of distribution can cause secondary changes in half-life

(Continued)

TABLE 4-1 Disease States and Conditions That Alter
Aminoglycoside Pharmacokinetics (*Continued*)

Disease state/ condition	Half-life (h)	Volume of distribution (L/kg)	Comment
Hemodialysis patients	3–4	0.26	While receiving hemodialysis, aminoglycoside half-life will decrease from ~50 h to ~4 h. Renal failure patients commonly have fluid imbalances that may decrease (underhydration) or increase (overhydration) the volume of distribution and secondarily change half-life
Peritoneal dialysis patients	36	0.26	While receiving peritoneal dialysis, aminoglycoside half-life will decrease from ~50 h to ~36 h. Renal failure patients commonly have fluid imbalances that may decrease (underhydration) or increase (overhydration) the volume of distribution and secondarily change half-life

IBW = ideal body weight, TBW = total body weight, DBW = dry body weight.

- Oral bioavailability is poor (<10%), so systemic infections cannot be treated by this route of administration.
- Plasma protein binding is low (<10%).
- Manufacturer recommended doses for conventional dosing in patients with normal renal function are 3–5 mg/kg/d for gentamicin and tobramycin, 4–6 mg/kg/d for netilmicin, and 15 mg/kg/d for amikacin. These amounts are divided into three equal daily doses for gentamicin, tobramycin, or netilmicin, or two or three equal daily doses for amikacin.
- Extended-interval doses obtained from the literature for patients with normal renal function are 4–7 mg/kg/d for gentamicin, tobramycin, or netilmicin and 11–20 mg/kg/d for amikacin.[4,5,14–20,22–27]

EFFECTS OF DISEASE STATES AND CONDITIONS ON AMINOGLYCOSIDE PHARMACOKINETICS AND DOSING

- Nonobese adults with normal renal function (creatinine clearance >80 ml/min, Table 4-1) have an average aminoglycoside half-life of 2 hours (range: 1.5–3 hours), and the average aminoglycoside volume of distribution is 0.26 L/kg (range: 0.2–0.3 L/kg) in this population.[28–31] The volume of distribution is similar to extracellular fluid content of the body, and fluid balance will be an important factor when estimating the aminoglycoside volume of distribution for a patient. Patients who have been febrile due to their infections for 24 hours or more may be significantly dehydrated and have lower volumes of distribution until rehydrated.

Renal Dysfunction

• Because aminoglycosides are eliminated primarily by glomerular filtration, renal dysfunction is the most important disease state affecting aminoglycoside pharmacokinetics.[32,33] The elimination rate constant decreases in proportion to creatinine clearance because of the decline in drug clearance.[34, 35] Because the kidney is the organ responsible for maintaining fluid and electrolyte balance in the body, patients with renal failure are sometimes overhydrated.

Fluid Balance

• Body weight can be an effective way to detect overhydration in a patient. If the usual weight of the patient is 70 kg when he or she is in normal fluid balance—known as the patient's "dry weight"—and the patient is currently 75 kg with signs and symptoms of overhydration (pedal edema, extended neck veins, etc.), the additional 5 kg of weight could be considered extra fluid and added to the estimated volume of distribution for the patient.

  • Since a liter of water weights 1 kg, the estimated volume of distribution for this patient would be 18.2 L using the patient's dry weight (V = 0.26 L/kg · 70 kg = 18.2 L) plus 5 L to account for the additional 5 kg of extra fluid, yielding a total volume of distribution equal to 23.2 L (V = 18.2 L + 5 L = 23.2 L). Care would be needed to alter the estimated volume of distribution toward normal as the excess fluid was lost and the patient's weight returned to its usual value.

Burns

• A major body burn (>40% body surface area) can cause large changes in aminoglycoside pharmacokinetics.[36–38] Because basal metabolic rate increases 48–72 hours after a major burn, glomerular filtration rate increases, which increases aminoglycoside clearance. Because of the increase in drug clearance, the average half-life for aminoglycosides in burn patients is ~1.5 hour.

  • If the patient is in normal fluid balance, the average volume of distribution will be the same as in normal adults (0.26 L/kg). However, since the skin is the organ which prevents fluid evaporation from the body and the integrity of the skin has been violated by thermal injury, these patients can be dehydrated, especially if they have had a fever for more than 24 hours. The result is a lower volume of distribution for aminoglycosides. Alternatively, some burn patients may be overhydrated due to vigorous fluid therapy used to treat hypotension. This will result in a larger-than-expected aminoglycoside volume of distribution. Unfortunately, there is no precise way to correct for fluid balance in these patients. Frequent use of aminoglycoside serum concentrations is used to guide therapy in this population.

Penicillin Interaction

• Concurrent therapy with some penicillins can increase aminoglycoside clearance by chemically inactivating both the penicillin and aminoglycoside via formation of a covalent bond between the two antibiotic molecules.[39–43]

Penicillin G, ampicillin, nafcillin, carbenicillin, and ticarcillin are the penicillins most likely to cause this interaction. Piperacillin and mezlocillin, as well as cephalosporins, do not inactivate aminoglycosides to an appreciable extent.

- This *in vivo* interaction is most likely to occur in patients with poor renal function (creatinine clearance <30 ml/min). The addition of one of the interacting penicillins can decrease the aminoglycoside half-life from ~50 hours when given alone to ~12 hours when given in combination and result in a dosage increase for the aminoglycoside.

- This interaction is important to note when patients are receiving concurrent therapy with one of the interacting penicillins and an aminoglycoside antibiotic, and serum concentration monitoring of the aminoglycoside is planned. When a blood sample is obtained for measurement of the aminoglycoside serum concentration, penicillin contained in the blood collection tube can continue to inactivate aminoglycoside. This will lead to a spuriously low aminoglycoside concentration result, which can lead to dosing adjustment errors.

  - In order to prevent this *in vitro* inactivation interaction in patients receiving concurrent penicillin and aminoglycoside treatment when the drug assay will not be run for longer than 1–2 hours after specimen collection, the serum should be separated from the blood sample using centrifugation. The serum is removed and placed in a separate tube, then frozen to prevent chemical reaction from occurring. Alternatively, a small amount of β-lactamase (<5% of total blood volume to prevent sample dilution) can be added to break the β-lactam bond of the penicillin and avoid inactivation of the aminoglycoside antibiotic.

Obesity

- In patients who weigh more that 30% over their ideal body weight, the volume of distribution for aminoglycosides increases because of the additional extracellular fluid contained in adipose tissue (Figure 4-2).[44–46] To compensate for the increased extracellular fluid of adipose tissue and the greater volume of distribution found in obese patients (>30% over ideal body weight), the following formula can be used to estimate aminoglycoside volume of distribution (V in L) for initial dosing purposes:

$$V = 0.26 \cdot [IBW + 0.4(TBW - IBW)]$$

where IBW is ideal body weight and TBW is the patient's actual total body weight.

  - In morbidly obese (>90% above ideal body weight) patients with normal serum creatinine concentrations, the clearance of aminoglycoside antibiotics is also increased.[44–46] Because both volume of distribution and clearance change simultaneously in obese patients to about the same extent, the aminoglycoside half-life value is appropriate for the patient's renal function

$$(t_{1/2} = [0.693 \cdot V]/Cl).$$

Cystic Fibrosis

- Patients with cystic fibrosis have larger aminoglycoside volumes of distribution (0.35 L/kg).[22–25,47–50] These patients also have higher aminoglycoside clearance values due to increased glomerular filtration rates. Because clearance rates tend

140 kg Obese Patient with Ideal Body Weight of 70 kg

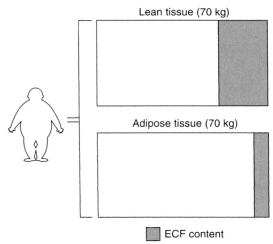

FIG. 4-2   Schematic of extracellular fluid content of lean and adipose tissue in a morbidly obese patient with an actual body weight of 140 kg and an ideal body weight of 70 kg. Lean tissue contains about 0.26 L/kg extracellular fluid, but adipose tissue has about 40% of the extracellular fluid content that lean tissue does. The equation that estimates volume of distribution for aminoglycosides in obese patients normalizes adipose tissue extracellular content into lean-tissue equivalents.

to increase more than volume-of-distribution values, the average aminoglycoside half-life is typically shorter in patients with cystic fibrosis ($t_{1/2} = 1.5$ h).

• Aminoglycosides can also be administered via inhalation at a dose of 300 mg twice daily in a cyclic fashion (4 weeks on, 4 weeks off) to patients with cystic fibrosis.[51]

Ascites/Overhydration

• Since aminoglycosides pass into ascitic fluid, the volume of distribution is increased in these patients. The approach to estimating an initial volume of distribution is similar to that used in renal failure patients who are fluid overloaded.

   • The weight of the patient when ascitic fluid is not present is known as the patient's dry weight. If this value is not known and the patient is not obese, ideal body weight can be used as an estimate of the dry weight. A reasonable value of the volume of distribution (V in L) for a patient with ascites, or who is overhydrated for other reasons, can be estimated using the following equation:

$$V = (0.26 \cdot DBW) + (TBW - DBW)$$

where DBW is the patient's dry body weight and TBW is the patient's actual total body weight.

- Because of the large variation in aminoglycoside volume of distribution for patients with ascites or overhydration, dosing should be guided by aminoglycoside serum concentrations. As excess fluid is lost, a decrease in the volume of distribution for these drugs should be anticipated.

Neonates/Infants/Children

- Premature infants (gestational age ≤34 weeks) have a larger aminoglycoside volume of distribution (0.5–0.6 L/kg) compared to adults.[26,52–54] Additionally, the kidneys are not completely developed so glomerular filtration and aminoglycoside clearance are decreased. A larger volume of distribution and lower clearance rate result in a prolonged average half-life equal to 6–10 hours.

  - Full-term neonates (gestational age ~40 weeks) also have a larger volume of distribution (mean $V = 0.4$–0.5 L/kg) and lower aminoglycoside clearance, resulting in longer half-life values ($t_{1/2} = 4$–5 h). By about 6 months, the mean volume of distribution is still large ($V = 0.3$–0.4 L/kg), but kidney development is complete, aminoglycoside clearance increases, and half-life is shorter ($t_{1/2} = 2$–3 h). These values remain relatively constant until about 2 years of age. At that time, aminoglycoside volume of distribution, clearance, and half-life gradually approach adult values at puberty (~12–14 years old).
- Doses for neonates are based on birth weight and age. Steady-state aminoglycoside serum concentrations are used to individualize doses:[55]

Drug	Route	Infants 0–4 wk old BW <1200 g	Infants <1 wk old BW ≤1200–2000 g	Infants <1 wk old BW >2000 g	Infants ≥1 wk old BW ≤1200–2000 g	Infants ≥1 wk old BW >2000 g
Amikacin	IV, IM	7.5 mg/kg every 18–24 h	7.5 mg/kg every 12 h	7.5–10 mg/kg every 12 h	7.5–10 mg/kg every 8 or 12 h	10 mg/kg every 8 h
Gentamicin or tobramycin	IV, IM	2.5 mg/kg every 18–24 h	2.5 mg/kg every 12 h	2.5 mg/kg every 12 h	2.5 mg/kg every 8 or 12 h	2.5 mg/kg every 8 h

- Doses for infants and children are: amikacin, 15–22.5 mg/kg/24 h IV or IM given every 8 hours; gentamicin or tobramycin, 6–7.5 mg/kg/24 h IV or IM given every 8 hours.[56] Steady-state aminoglycoside serum concentrations are used to individualize doses.

Dialysis

- Hemodialysis efficiently removes aminoglycoside antibiotics from the body.[57–61]

  - The average aminoglycoside half-life in a renal failure patient is 50 hours. During hemodialysis with a "low-flux" artificial kidney, half-life decreases to 4 hours and results in about 50% of the drug being removed during a typical dialysis period (3–4 h). Similarly, hemodialysis performed with a "high-flux" filter decreases aminoglycoside half-life to 2 hours.[62]
  - If the patient is properly hydrated, the volume of distribution for aminoglycosides is 0.26 L/kg. As discussed previously in the renal failure section in the above paragraphs, body weight is an effective way to assess

hydration status and can be used to adjust initial volume-of-distribution estimates.
- See the section on special dosing considerations at the end of this chapter for techniques used to individualize aminoglycoside dosing for patients undergoing hemodialysis.

- Peritoneal dialysis is much less efficient in removing aminoglycosides from the body.[63–65] Peritoneal dialysis will decrease the half-life of aminoglycosides in a renal failure patient from about 50 hours to about 36 hours during the dialysis procedure. If the patient is receiving peritoneal dialysis on a chronic, ongoing basis, such as continuous ambulatory peritoneal dialysis (CAPD), aminoglycoside half-life will be shorter all the time because of the additional dialysis clearance.

  - Patients receiving CAPD sometimes develop peritonitis, which can be treated by adding aminoglycoside (or other) antibiotics to the peritoneal dialysis fluid (typically, gentamicin, 8–10 mg/L of exchange fluid). While about one-half of the intraperitoneal aminoglycoside dose is absorbed systemically during a 5–6 hour dwell time, if a patient with peritonitis develops secondary bacteremia, it may be necessary to use parenteral antibiotics to cure the infection.[63–65] Peritonitis causes inflammation of the peritoneal membrane, which facilitates absorption of aminoglycoside administered via dialysis fluid and elimination of aminoglycoside present in the body.

- Continuous hemofiltration consists of a family of techniques that provides removal of toxic metabolic substances in patients with acute renal failure.[66] Considerable variability exists in aminoglycoside removal, depending on the type of hemofiltration used in a patient. Because continuous arteriovenous hemofiltration (CAVH) provides an average creatinine clearance of ~30 ml/min, this value is typically used to initiate therapy in patients, then aminoglycoside serum concentration monitoring is used early in therapy to individualize dosing.[67]

DRUG INTERACTIONS

- Most important drug interactions are pharmacodynamic, and not pharmacokinetic, in nature. Vancomycin,[10,13] amphotericin B,[13] cyclosporin,[68] and furosemide[12,13,69] enhance the nephrotoxicity potential of the aminoglycosides. Each of these agents can cause nephrotoxicity when administered alone. When these drugs are administered concurrently with an aminoglycoside, serum creatinine concentrations should be monitored on a daily basis. Additionally, serum concentrations of vancomycin or cyclosporin, as well as the aminoglycoside, should be measured.
- Loop diuretics,[70,71] including furosemide, bumetanide, and ethacrynic acid, can cause ototoxicity, and reports of an increased incidence of this adverse effect have been reported when aminoglycosides have been coadministered. If aminoglycoside antibiotics are administered with loop diuretics, clinical signs and symptoms of ototoxicity (auditory: decreased hearing acuity in the conversational range, feeling of fullness or pressure in the ears, tinnitus; vestibular: loss of equilibrium, headache, nausea, vomiting, nystagmus, vertigo, ataxia) should be monitored daily.
- Aminoglycosides have intrinsic nondepolarizing neuromuscular blocking activity and may prolong the effects of neuromuscular blocking agents such as succinylcholine.[72]

- Penicillins (primarily penicillin G, ampicillin, nafcillin, carbenicillin, ticarcillin) can inactivate aminoglycosides *in vivo* and in blood specimen tubes intended for the measurement of aminoglycoside serum concentrations.[39-43]

INITIAL DOSAGE DETERMINATION METHODS

- Several methods to initiate aminoglycoside therapy are available.

  - The *pharmacokinetic dosing method* is the most flexible of the techniques. It allows for individualized target serum concentrations to be chosen for a patient, so it can be used for both conventional and extended-interval dosing. Also, each pharmacokinetic parameter can be customized to reflect specific disease states and conditions present in the patient. However, it is computationally intensive.
  - The *Hull and Sarubbi nomogram* uses the dosing concepts in the pharmacokinetic dosing method. However, in order to simplify calculations, it makes simplifying assumptions: target concentration ranges consistent with conventional dosing only, fixed volume-of-distribution parameter in the normal range, limited dosage-interval selection (no longer than 24 hours). Thus, it should be used only in patients who have only renal dysfunction and/or obesity as complicating factors and only when conventional dosing is to be used.
  - The *Hartford nomogram* has similar strengths and weaknesses when compared to the Hull and Sarubbi nomogram, but is designed for use when extended-interval dosing is desired. This nomogram also incorporates a method to adjust aminoglycoside doses based on serum concentration feedback.

Pharmacokinetic Dosing Method

- The goal of initial dosing of aminoglycosides is to compute the best dose possible for the patient given his or her set of disease states and conditions that influence aminoglycoside pharmacokinetics and the site and severity of the infection. In order to do this, pharmacokinetic parameters for the patient are estimated using average parameters measured in other patients with similar disease state and condition profiles.

Elimination Rate Constant Estimate

- Aminoglycosides are eliminated almost totally unchanged in the urine, and there is a good relationship between creatinine clearance and aminoglycoside elimination rate constant. This relationship allows the estimation of the aminoglycoside elimination rate constant for a patient which can be used to compute an initial dose of the antibiotic:

$$k_e = 0.00293(CrCl) + 0.014$$

where k_e is the aminoglycoside elimination rate constant in h^{-1} and CrCl is creatinine clearance in ml/min.

Volume-of-Distribution Estimate

- The average volume of distribution is 0.26 L/kg. If a patient weights less than his or her ideal body weight, actual body weight is used to estimate volume of distribution. For patients whose weight is between their ideal body weight and 30% over ideal weight, actual body weight can be used to compute estimated volume of distribution, although some clinicians prefer to used ideal body weight for these individuals.

- In patients who are more than 30% above their ideal body weight, volume of distribution (V) is estimated using the following equation:

$$V = 0.26[IBW + 0.4(TBW - IBW)],$$

  where V is in L, IBW is ideal body weight in kg, and TBW is total body weight in kg.
- In patients who are overhydrated or with ascites, their dry body weight (weight without the extra fluid) can be used to provide an improved volume- of-distribution estimate (V in L) using the following formula:

$$V = (0.26 \cdot DBW) + (TBW - DBW),$$

  where DBW is the patient's dry body weight and TBW is the patient's actual total body weight.
- The average volume of distribution for cystic fibrosis patients is 0.35 L/kg.

Selection of Appropriate Pharmacokinetic Model and Equations

- A simple one-compartment model is widely used and allows accurate dosage calculation.[2,34,35,37,38,73] Generally, infusion equations should be used if the patient has a creatinine clearance greater than 30 ml/min. For creatinine clearances of 30 ml/min or less, very little aminoglycoside is eliminated during infusion and waiting-period times, and intravenous bolus or infusion equations accurately compute peak concentrations.[74]

  - Steady-state versions of one compartment model intermittent intravenous infusion ($C_{max,ss} = [k_0/(k_e V)][(1 - e^{-k_e t'})/(1 - e^{-k_e \tau})]$, $C_{min,ss} = C_{max,ss} e^{-[k_e(\tau - t')]}$, where k_0 is the infusion rate, k_e is the elimination rate constant, V is the volume of distribution, t' is the drug infusion time, and τ is the dosage interval) or intravenous bolus ($C_{max,ss} = (D/V)[e^{-k_e t}/(1 - e^{-k_e \tau})]$, $C_{min,ss} = C_{max,ss} e^{-k_e \tau}$, where D is the antibiotic dose, V is the volume of distribution, k_e is the elimination rate constant, t is time, and τ is the dosage interval) equations are chosen based on the patient's renal function to compute the required doses needed to achieve desired aminoglycoside concentrations.
  - Note that intermittent intravenous infusion equations will work well regardless of the patient's creatinine clearance. However, the intravenous bolus equations are easier to solve, save time, and are less likely to invoke a computational error.

Steady-State Concentration Selection

- Aminoglycoside peak steady-state concentrations are selected based on the site and severity of infection as well as the infecting organism.

  - Severe infections, such as gram-negative pneumonia or septicemia, or infections with organisms that have a high minimum inhibitory concentration (MIC) such as *Pseudomonas aeruginosa* (typical MIC ≈2 μg/ml for gentamicin, tobramycin, or netilmicin) generally require peak steady-state serum concentrations of 8–10 μg/ml for gentamicin, tobramycin, or netilmicin or 25–30 μg/ml for amikacin when using conventional dosing.
  - Moderate infections at sites that are easier to penetrate or with organisms that display lower MIC values, such as intra-abdominal infections, are usually

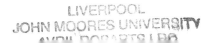

treated with peak gentamicin, tobramycin, or netilmicin steady-state serum concentrations equal to 5–7 µg/ml or with amikacin peak steady-state serum concentrations equal to 15–25 µg/ml.

- When treating urinary tract infections due to susceptible organisms or using aminoglycosides for synergy in combination with penicillins or other antibiotics for the treatment of gram-positive infections such as infective endocarditis, steady-state peak concentrations of 3–5 µg/ml are usually adequate for gentamicin, tobramycin, or netilmicin or 12–15 µg/ml for amikacin. Pyelonephritis is considered a soft-tissue infection, not a urinary tract infection, and requires higher peak steady-state concentrations to achieve a cure.

- Similar target peak steady-state concentrations for extended-interval aminoglycoside dosing are less established, although concentrations of 20–30 µg/ml for gentamicin, tobramycin, and netilmicin have been suggested for *Pseudomonas aeruginosa* and other serious infections.

- Desirable concentrations for steady-state trough concentrations are chosen based on avoidance of potential toxicity. For conventional dosing, steady-state trough concentrations should be maintained at <2 µg/ml for tobramycin, gentamicin, and netilmicin or <5–7 µg/ml for amikacin. Using extended-interval dosing, steady-state trough concentrations should be <1 µg/ml for gentamicin, tobramycin, and netilmicin.

Dosage Computation

- The equations given in Tables 4-2A through 4-2C are used to compute aminoglycoside doses (intermittent intravenous infusion for all patients, or, if desired, intravenous bolus for creatinine clearances ≤30 ml/min).

▶ ***Example 1***   JM is a 50-year-old, 70-kg (height = 5′10″) male with gram-negative pneumonia. His current serum creatinine is 0.9 mg/dl, and it has been stable over the 5 days since admission. Compute a gentamicin dose for this patient using conventional dosing.

1. *Estimate creatinine clearance.* This patient has a stable serum creatinine and is not obese. The Cockcroft-Gault equation can be used to estimate creatinine clearance:

$$CrCl_{est} = \frac{(140 - age)BW}{72 \cdot S_{Cr}} = \frac{(140 - 50y)70 \text{ kg}}{72 \cdot 0.9 \text{ mg/dl}}$$

$$CrCl_{est} = 97 \text{ ml/min}$$

TABLE 4-2A One-Compartment-Model Equations Used with Aminoglycoside Antibiotics

Route of administration	Single dose	Multiple dose	Steady state
Intravenous bolus	$C = (D/V)e^{-k_e t}$	$C = (D/V)e^{-k_e t}[(1 - e^{-nk_e \tau})/(1 - e^{-k_e \tau})]$	$C = (D/V)[e^{-k_e t}/(1 - e^{-k_e \tau})]$
Intermittent intravenous infusion	$C = [k_0/(k_e V)](1 - e^{-k_e t'})$	$C = [k_0/(k_e V)](1 - e^{-k_e t'})[(1 - e^{-nk_e \tau})/(1 - e^{-k_e \tau})]$	$C = [k_0/(k_e V)][(1 - e^{-k_e t'})/(1 - e^{-k_e \tau})]$

C is drug serum concentration at time = t, D is dose, V is volume of distribution, k_e is elimination rate constant, n is number of administered doses, τ is dosage interval, k_0 is infusion rate.

TABLE 4-2B Pharmacokinetic Constant Computations Utilizing a One-compartment Model Used with Aminoglycoside Antibiotics

Route of administration	Single dose	Multiple dose	Steady state
Intravenous bolus	$k_e = -(\ln C_1 - \ln C_2)/(t_1 - t_2)$	$k_e = -(\ln C_1 - \ln C_2)/(t_1 - t_2)$	$k_e = -(\ln C_1 - \ln C_2)/(t_1 - t_2)$
	$t_{1/2} = 0.693/k_e$	$t_{1/2} = 0.693/k_e$	$t_{1/2} = 0.693/k_e$
	$V = D/C_0$	$V = D/(C_0 - C_{predose})$	$V = D/(C_0 - C_{predose})$
	$Cl = k_e V$	$Cl = k_e V$	$Cl = k_e V$
Intermittent intravenous infusion	$k_e = -(\ln C_1 - \ln C_2)/(t_1 - t_2)$	$k_e = -(\ln C_1 - \ln C_2)/(t_1 - t_2)$	$k_e = -(\ln C_1 - \ln C_2)/(t_1 - t_2)$
	$t_{1/2} = 0.693/k_e$	$t_{1/2} = 0.693/k_e$	$t_{1/2} = 0.693/k_e$
	$V = [k_0(1 - e^{-k_e t'})]/ \{k_e[C_{max} - (C_{predose}e^{-k_e t'})]\}$	$V = [k_0(1 - e^{-k_e t'})]/ \{k_e[C_{max} - (C_{predose}e^{-k_e t'})]\}$	$V = [k_0(1 - e^{-k_e t'})]/ \{k_e[C_{max} - (C_{predose}e^{-k_e t'})]\}$
	$Cl = k_e V$	$Cl = k_e V$	$Cl = k_e V$

C_1 is drug serum concentration at time = t_1, C_2 is drug serum concentration at time = t_2, k_e is elimination rate constant, $t_{1/2}$ is half-life, V is volume of distribution, k_0 is continuous infusion rate, t' is infusion time, D is dose, C_0 is concentration at time = 0, Cl is drug clearance, $C_{predose}$ is predose concentration.

2. *Estimate elimination rate constant (k_e) and half-life ($t_{1/2}$).* The elimination rate constant-versus-creatinine clearance relationship is used to estimate the gentamicin elimination rate for this patient:

$$k_e = 0.00293(CrCl) + 0.014 = 0.00293(97 \text{ ml/min}) + 0.014 = 0.298 \text{ h}^{-1}$$

$$t_{1/2} = 0.693/k_e = 0.693/0.298 \text{ h}^{-1} = 2.3 \text{ h}$$

3. *Estimate volume of distribution (V).* The patient has no disease states or conditions that would alter the volume of distribution from the normal value of 0.26 L/kg:

$$V = 0.26 \text{ L/kg (70 kg)} = 18.2 \text{ L}$$

4. *Choose desired steady-state serum concentrations.* Gram-negative pneumonia patients treated with aminoglycoside antibiotics require steady-state

TABLE 4-2C Equations Used to Compute Individualized Dosage Regimens for Various Routes of Administration Used with Aminoglycoside Antibiotics

Route of administration	Dosage interval (t), maintenance dose (D or k_0), and loading dose (LD) equations
Intravenous bolus	$\tau = (\ln C_{max,ss} - \ln C_{min,ss})/k_e$
	$D = C_{max,ss} V(1 - e^{-k_e \tau})$
	$LD = C_{max,ss} V$
Intermittent intravenous infusion	$\tau = [(\ln C_{max,ss} - \ln C_{min,ss})/k_e] + t'$
	$k_0 = C_{max,ss} k_e V[(1 - e^{-k_e \tau})/(1 - e^{-k_e t'})]$
	$LD = k_0/(1 - e^{-k_e \tau})$

$C_{max,ss}$ and $C_{min,ss}$ are maximum and minimum steady-state concentrations, k_e is elimination rate constant, V is volume of distribution, k_0 is continuous infusion rate, t' is infusion time.

peak concentrations $(C_{max,ss})$ equal to 8–10 μg/ml; steady-state trough $(C_{min,ss})$ concentrations should be <2 μg/ml to avoid toxicity. Set $C_{max,ss}$ = 9 μg/ml and $C_{min,ss}$ = 1 μg/ml.

5. *Use intermittent intravenous infusion equations to compute dose* (*Table 4-2*). Calculate required dosage interval (τ) using a 1-hour infusion:

$$\tau = [(\ln C_{max,ss} - \ln C_{min,ss})/k_e] + t'$$
$$= [(\ln 9\ \mu g/ml - \ln 1\ \mu g/ml)/0.298\ h^{-1}] + 1\ h = 8.4\ h$$

Dosage intervals should be rounded to clinically acceptable intervals of 8, 12, 18, 24, 36, 48, 72 h, and multiples of 24 hours thereafter, whenever possible. In this case, the dosage interval would be rounded to 8 hours. Also, steady-state peak concentrations are similar if drawn immediately after a 1-hour infusion or $\frac{1}{2}$ hour after a $\frac{1}{2}$ hour infusion, so the dose could be administered either way.

$$k_0 = C_{max,ss} k_e V[(1 - e^{-k_e \tau})/(1 - e^{-k_e t'})]$$
$$k_0 = (9\ mg/L \cdot 0.298\ h^{-1} \cdot 18.2\ L)[(1 - e^{-(0.298\ h^{-1})(8\ h)})/$$
$$(1 - e^{-(0.298\ h^{-1})(1\ h)})] = 172\ mg$$

Aminoglycoside doses should be rounded to the nearest 5–10 mg. This dose would be rounded to 170 mg. (*Note:* μg/ml = mg/L, and this concentration unit was substituted for $C_{max,ss}$ so that unit conversion was not required.)

The prescribed maintenance dose would be 170 mg every 8 hours.

6. *Compute loading dose (LD), if needed.* Loading doses should be considered for patients with creatinine clearance values <60 ml/min. The administration of a loading dose in these patients will allow achievement of therapeutic peak concentrations more quickly than if maintenance doses alone are given. However, since the pharmacokinetic parameters used to compute these initial doses are only *estimated* values and not *actual* values, the patient's own parameters may be very different from the estimated constants and steady state will not be achieved until 3–5 half-lives have passed.

$$LD = k_0/(1 - e^{-k_e \tau}) = 170\ mg/(1 - e^{-(0.298\ h^{-1})(8\ h)}) = 187\ mg$$

As noted, this loading dose is only about 10% greater than the maintenance dose and would not be given to the patient. Since the expected half-life is 2.3 hour, the patient should be at steady state after the second dose is given.

▶ *Example 2*   Same patient profile as in Example 1, but serum creatinine is 3.5 mg/dl, indicating renal impairment.

1. *Estimate creatinine clearance.* This patient has a stable serum creatinine and is not obese. The Cockcroft-Gault equation can be used to estimate creatinine clearance:

$$CrCl_{est} = \frac{(140 - age)BW}{72 \cdot S_{Cr}} = \frac{(140 - 50\ y)70\ kg}{72 \cdot 3.5\ mg/dl}$$
$$CrCl_{est} = 25\ ml/min$$

2. *Estimate elimination rate constant (k_e) and half-life $(t_{1/2})$.* The elimination rate constant-versus-creatinine clearance relationship is used to estimate

the gentamicin elimination rate for this patient:

$$k_e = 0.00293(CrCl) + 0.014 = 0.00293(25 \text{ ml/min}) + 0.014$$
$$= 0.087 \text{ h}^{-1}$$
$$t_{1/2} = 0.693/k_e = 0.693/0.087 \text{ h}^{-1} = 8 \text{ h}$$

3. *Estimate volume of distribution* (*V*). The patient has no disease states or conditions that would alter the volume of distribution from the normal value of 0.26 L/kg:

$$V = 0.26 \text{ L/kg} (70 \text{ kg}) = 18.2 \text{ L}$$

4. *Choose desired steady-state serum concentrations.* Gram-negative pneumonia patients treated with aminoglycoside antibiotics require steady-state peak concentrations ($C_{max,ss}$) equal to 8–10 µg/ml; steady-state trough ($C_{min,ss}$) concentrations should be <2 µg/ml to avoid toxicity. Set $C_{max,ss} = 9$ µg/ml and $C_{min,ss} = 1$ µg/ml.

5. *Use intravenous bolus equations to compute dose* (*Table 4-2*). Calculate required dosage interval (τ):

$$\tau = \frac{(\ln C_{max,ss} - \ln C_{min,ss})}{k_e} = \frac{\ln 9 \text{ µg/ml} - \ln 1 \text{ µg/ml}}{0.087 \text{ h}^{-1}} = 25 \text{ h}$$

Dosage intervals should be rounded to clinically acceptable intervals of 8, 12, 18, 24, 36, 48, 72 h, and multiples of 24 hours thereafter, whenever possible. In this case, the dosage interval would be rounded to 24 hours. Also, steady-state peak concentrations are similar if drawn immediately after a 1-hour infusion or $\frac{1}{2}$-hour after a $\frac{1}{2}$-hour infusion, so the dose could be administered either way.

$$D = C_{max,ss} V(1 - e^{-k_e\tau})$$
$$D = 9 \text{ mg/L} \cdot 18.2 \text{ L}(1 - e^{-(0.087 \text{ h}^{-1})(24 \text{ h})}) = 143 \text{ mg}$$

Aminoglycoside doses should be rounded to the nearest 5–10 mg. This dose would be rounded to 145 mg. (*Note*: µg/ml = mg/L, and this concentration unit was substituted for $C_{max,ss}$ so that unit conversion was not required.)

The prescribed maintenance dose would be 145 mg every 24 hours.

Note: Although this dose is given once daily, it is not extended-interval dosing because desired serum concentrations are within the conventional range.

6. *Compute loading dose* (*LD*)*, if needed.* Loading doses should be considered for patients with creatinine clearance values <60 ml/min. The administration of a loading dose in these patients will allow achievement of therapeutic peak concentrations more quickly than if maintenance doses alone are given. However, since the pharmacokinetic parameters used to compute these initial doses are only *estimated* values and not *actual* values, the patient's own parameters may be very different from the estimated constants and steady state will not be achieved until 3–5 half-lives have passed.

$$LD = C_{max,ss} V = 9 \text{ mg/L} \cdot 18.2 \text{ L} = 164 \text{ mg}$$

Round the loading dose to 165 mg. It should be given as the first dose. The next dose should be a maintenance dose given a dosage interval away from the loading dose, in this case 24 hours later.

▶ *Example 3*   ZW is a 35-year-old, 150-kg (5'5'') female with an intra-abdominal infection. Her current serum creatinine is 1.1 mg/dl and is stable. Compute a tobramycin dose for this patient using conventional dosing.

1. *Estimate creatinine clearance.* This patient has a stable serum creatinine and is obese [$IBW_{females}$ (in kg) = 45 + 2.3(Ht − 60) = 45 + 2.3(65'' − 60) = 57 kg)]. The Salazar and Corcoran equation can be used to estimate creatinine clearance:

$$CrCl_{est(females)} = \frac{(146 - age)[(0.287 \cdot Wt) + (9.74 \cdot Ht^2)]}{60 \cdot S_{Cr}}$$

$$CrCl_{est(females)} = \frac{(146 - 35 \ y)\{(0.287 \cdot 150 \ kg) + [9.74 \cdot (1.65 \ m)^2]\}}{60 \cdot 1.1 \ mg/dl}$$

$$= 117 \ ml/min$$

   Note: Height is converted from inches to meters: Ht = (65 in · 2.54 cm/in)/(100 cm/m) = 1.65 m.

2. *Estimate elimination rate constant (k_e) and half-life ($t_{1/2}$).* The elimination rate constant-versus-creatinine clearance relationship is used to estimate the gentamicin elimination rate for this patient:

$$k_e = 0.00293(CrCl) + 0.014 = 0.00293(117 \ ml/min) + 0.014$$
$$= 0.357 \ h^{-1}$$

$$t_{1/2} = 0.693/k_e = 0.693/0.357 \ h^{-1} = 1.9 \ h$$

3. *Estimate volume of distribution (V).* The patient is obese, so the volume of distribution is estimated using the following formula:

$$V = 0.26[IBW + 0.4(TBW - IBW)]$$
$$= 0.26[57 \ kg + 0.4(150 \ kg - 57 \ kg)] = 24.5 \ L$$

4. *Choose desired steady-state serum concentrations.* Intra-abdominal infection patients treated with aminoglycoside antibiotics require steady-state peak concentrations ($C_{max,ss}$) equal to 5–7 µg/ml; steady-state trough ($C_{min,ss}$) concentrations should be <2 µg/ml to avoid toxicity. Set $C_{max,ss}$ = 6 µg/ml and $C_{min,ss}$ = 0.5 µg/ml.

5. *Use intermittent intravenous infusion equations to compute dose (Table 4-2).* Calculate required dosage interval (τ) using a 1-hour infusion:

$$\tau = [(\ln C_{max,ss} - \ln C_{min,ss})/k_e] + t'$$
$$= [(\ln 6 \ \mu g/ml - \ln 0.5 \ \mu g/ml)/0.357 \ h^{-1}] + 1 \ h = 8 \ h$$

   Dosage intervals should be rounded to clinically acceptable intervals of 8, 12, 18, 24, 36, 48, 72 h, and multiples of 24 hours thereafter, whenever possible. In this case, the dosage interval is 8 hours. Also, steady-state peak concentrations are similar if drawn immediately after a 1-hour infusion or $\frac{1}{2}$-hour after a $\frac{1}{2}$-hour infusion, so the dose could be administered either way.

$$k_0 = C_{max,ss}k_eV[(1 - e^{-k_e\tau})/(1 - e^{-k_et'})]$$
$$k_0 = (6 \ mg/L \cdot 0.357 \ h^{-1} \cdot 24.5 \ L)$$
$$[(1 - e^{-(0.357 \ h^{-1})(8 \ h)})/(1 - e^{-(0.357 \ h^{-1})(1 \ h)})]$$
$$= 165 \ mg$$

   Aminoglycoside doses should be rounded to the nearest 5–10 mg. This dose does not need to be rounded.

(*Note:* μg/ml = mg/L, and this concentration unit was substituted for $C_{max,ss}$ so that unit conversion was not required.)

The prescribed maintenance dose would be 165 mg every 8 hours.

5. *Compute loading dose (LD), if needed.* Loading doses should be considered for patients with creatinine clearance values <60 ml/min. The administration of a loading dose in these patients will allow achievement of therapeutic peak concentrations more quickly than if maintenance doses alone are given. However, since the pharmacokinetic parameters used to compute these initial doses are only *estimated* values and not *actual* values, the patient's own parameters may be very different from the estimated constants and steady-state will not be achieved until 3–5 half-lives have passed.

$$LD = k_0/(1 - e^{-k_e\tau}) = 165 \text{ mg}/(1 - e^{-(0.357 \text{ h}^{-1})(8 \text{ h})}) = 175 \text{ mg}$$

As noted, this loading dose is <10% greater than the maintenance dose and would not be given to the patient. Since the expected half-life is 1.9 hours, the patient should be at steady state after the second dose is given.

▶ *Example 4*   Same patient profile as in Example 2, but extended-interval dosing is used.

1. *Estimate creatinine clearance.* This patient has a stable serum creatinine and is not obese. The Cockcroft-Gault equation can be used to estimate creatinine clearance:

$$CrCl_{est} = \frac{(140 - age)BW}{72 \cdot S_{Cr}} = \frac{(140 - 50 \text{ y})70 \text{ kg}}{72 \cdot 3.5 \text{ mg/dl}}$$

$$CrCl_{est} = 25 \text{ ml/min}$$

2. *Estimate elimination rate constant (k_e) and half-life ($t_{1/2}$).* The elimination rate constant-versus-creatinine clearance relationship is used to estimate the gentamicin elimination rate for this patient:

$$k_e = 0.00293(CrCl) + 0.014$$
$$= 0.00293(25 \text{ ml/min}) + 0.014 = 0.087 \text{ h}^{-1}$$
$$t_{1/2} = 0.693/k_e = 0.693/0.087 \text{ h}^{-1} = 8 \text{ h}$$

3. *Estimate volume of distribution (V).* The patient has no disease states or conditions that would alter the volume of distribution from the normal value of 0.26 L/kg:

$$V = 0.26 \text{ L/kg } (70 \text{ kg}) = 18.2 \text{ L}$$

4. *Choose desired steady-state serum concentrations.* Gram-negative pneumonia patients treated with aminoglycoside antibiotics require steady-state peak concentrations ($C_{max,ss}$) >20 μg/ml; steady-state trough ($C_{min,ss}$) concentrations should be <1 μg/ml to avoid toxicity. Set $C_{max,ss}$ = 20 μg/ml and $C_{min,ss}$ = 0.5 μg/ml.

5. *Use intravenous bolus equations to compute dose (Table 4-2).* Calculate required dosage interval (τ):

$$\tau = [(\ln C_{max,ss} - \ln C_{min,ss})/k_e]$$
$$= (\ln 20 \text{ μg/ml} - \ln 0.5 \text{ μg/ml})/0.087 \text{ h}^{-1} = 42 \text{ h}$$

Dosage intervals should be rounded to clinically acceptable intervals of 24, 36, 48, 60, 72 h, and multiples of 12 hours thereafter, whenever possible. In this case, the dosage interval would be rounded to 48 hours. Also, steady-state peak concentrations are similar if drawn immediately after a 1-hour infusion or $\frac{1}{2}$ hour after a $\frac{1}{2}$-hour infusion, so the dose could be administered either way.

$$D = C_{max,ss} V(1 - e^{-k_e\tau})$$
$$D = 20 \text{ mg/L} \cdot 18.2 \text{ L}(1 - e^{-(0.087 \text{ h}^{-1})(48 \text{ h})}) = 358 \text{ mg}$$

Aminoglycoside doses should be rounded to the nearest 5–10 mg. This dose would be rounded to 360 mg.

(*Note:* μg/ml = mg/L, and this concentration unit was substituted for $C_{max,ss}$ so that unit conversion was not required.)

The prescribed maintenance dose would be 360 mg every 48 hours.

Hull and Sarubbi Nomogram Method

- For patients who do not have disease states or conditions that alter volume of distribution, the Hull and Sarubbi aminoglycoside dosing nomogram is a quick and efficient way to apply pharmacokinetic concepts for conventional dosing (Table 4-3).[34,35] Because cystic fibrosis requires a different volume of distribution (0.35 L/kg), this nomogram cannot be used for this patient population.
  - With a simple modification, it can also be used for obese patients. If the patient is ≥30% above ideal body weight, an adjusted body weight (ABW) can be calculated and used as the weight factor (ABW (in kg) = IBW + 0.4[TBW−IBW], where IBW is ideal body weight in kg and TBW is actual total body weight in kg).[44-46] Also, the Salazar and Corcoran method of estimating creatinine clearance in obese patients should be used to compute renal function in these individuals.[75,76]
- Steady-state peak concentrations are selected as discussed in the pharmacokinetic dosing method section and used to determine a loading dose from the nomogram (Table 4-3). Logically, lower loading doses produce lower expected peak concentrations, and higher loading doses result in higher expected peak concentrations.
- Once the loading dose is found, the patient's creatinine clearance is used to estimate the half-life, dosage interval, and maintenance dose (as a percent of the administered loading dose).
- To illustrate how the nomogram is used, the same patient examples utilized in the previous section will be repeated for this dosage approach. Since the nomogram uses slightly different estimates for volume of distribution and elimination rate constant, some minor differences in suggested doses are expected.

▶*Example 1*   JM is a 50-year-old, 70-kg (height = 5′10″) male with gram-negative pneumonia. His current serum creatinine is 0.9 mg/dl, and it has been stable over the 5 days since admission. Compute a gentamicin dose for this patient using conventional dosing.

1. *Estimate creatinine clearance.* This patient has a stable serum creatinine and is not obese. The Cockcroft-Gault equation can be used to estimate creatinine clearance:

$$CrCl_{est} = \frac{(140 - age)BW}{72 \cdot S_{Cr}} = \frac{(140 - 50 \text{ y})70 \text{ kg}}{72 \cdot 0.9 \text{ mg/dl}}$$
$$CrCl_{est} = 97 \text{ ml/min}$$

2. *Choose desired steady-state serum concentrations.* Gram-negative pneumonia patients treated with aminoglycoside antibiotics require steady-state peak concentrations ($C_{max,ss}$) equal to 8–10 μg/ml.

TABLE 4-3 Aminoglycoside Dosage Chart

1. Compute patient's creatinine clearance (CrCl) using Cockcroft-Gault method: CrCl = [(140 − age)BW]/(Scr × 72). Multiply by 0.85 for females.
2. Use patient's weight if within 30% of IBW, otherwise use adjusted body weight = IBW + [0.40(TBW − IBW)]
3. Select loading dose in mg/kg to provide peak serum concentrations in range listed below for the desired aminoglycoside antibiotic:

Aminoglycoside	Usual loading dose (mg/kg)	Expected peak serum concentrations (μg/ml)
Tobramycin Gentamicin Netilmicin	1.5–2.0	4–10
Amikacin Kanamycin	5.0–7.5	15–30

4. Select maintenance dose (as percentage of loading dose) to continue peak serum concentrations indicated above according to desired dosage interval and the patient's creatinine clearance. To maintain usual peak/trough ratio, use dosage intervals in clear areas.

CrCl (ml/min)	Est. half-life (h)	Percentage of loading dose required for dosage interval selected		
		8 h(%)	12 h(%)	24 h(%)
>90	2–3	90	—	—
90	3.1	84	—	—
80	3.4	80	91	—
70	3.9	76	88	—
60	4.5	71	84	—
50	5.3	65	79	—
40	6.5	57	72	92
30	8.4	48	63	86
25	9.9	43	57	81
20	11.9	37	50	75
17	13.6	33	46	70
15	15.1	31	42	67
12	17.9	27	37	61
10*	20.4	24	34	56
7*	25.9	19	28	47
5*	31.5	16	23	41
2*	46.8	11	16	30
0*	69.3	8	11	21

*Dosing for patients with CrCl ≤10 ml/min should be assisted by measuring serum concentrations. Adapted from Sarubbi and Hull.[34]

3. *Select loading dose* (Table 4-3). A loading dose (LD) of 2 mg/kg will provide a peak concentration of 8–10 μg/ml.

$$LD = 2 \text{ mg/kg (70 kg)} = 140 \text{ mg}$$

4. *Determine estimated half-life, maintenance dose, and dosage interval.* From the nomogram, the estimated half-life is 2–3 hours, the maintenance

dose (MD) is 90% of the loading dose [MD = 0.90(140 mg) = 126 mg], and the dosage interval is 8 hours.

Aminoglycoside doses should be rounded to the nearest 5–10 mg. Steady-state peak concentrations are similar if drawn immediately after a 1-hour infusion or $\frac{1}{2}$ hour after a $\frac{1}{2}$-hour infusion, so the dose could be administered either way.

The prescribed maintenance dose would be 125 mg every 8 hours.

▶*Example 2*   Same patient profile as in Example 1, but serum creatinine is 3.5 mg/dl, indicating renal impairment.

1. *Estimate creatinine clearance.* This patient has a stable serum creatinine and is not obese. The Cockcroft-Gault equation can be used to estimate creatinine clearance:

$$CrCl_{est} = \frac{(140 - age)BW}{72 \cdot S_{Cr}} = \frac{(140 - 50 \text{ y})70 \text{ kg}}{72 \cdot 3.5 \text{ mg/dl}}$$

$$CrCl_{est} = 25 \text{ ml/min}$$

2. *Choose desired steady-state serum concentrations.* Gram-negative pneumonia patients treated with aminoglycoside antibiotics require steady-state peak concentrations ($C_{max,ss}$) equal to 8–10 µg/ml.

3. *Select loading dose (Table 4-3).* A loading dose (LD) of 2 mg/kg will provide a peak concentration of 8–10 µg/ml.

$$LD = 2 \text{ mg/kg } (70 \text{ kg}) = 140 \text{ mg}$$

4. *Determine estimated half-life, maintenance dose, and dosage interval.* From the nomogram, the estimated half-life is 9.9 hours, the maintenance dose (MD) is 81% of the loading dose [MD = 0.81(140 mg) = 113 mg], and the dosage interval is 24 hours.

Aminoglycoside doses should be rounded to the nearest 5–10 mg. Steady-state peak concentrations are similar if drawn immediately after a 1-hour infusion or $\frac{1}{2}$ hour after a $\frac{1}{2}$-hour infusion, so the dose could be administered either way.

The prescribed maintenance dose would be 115 mg every 24 hours.

▶*Example 3*   ZW is a 35-year-old, 150-kg (5′5″) female with an intra-abdominal infection. Her current serum creatinine is 1.1 mg/dl and is stable. Compute a tobramycin dose for this patient using conventional dosing.

1. *Estimate creatinine clearance.* This patient has a stable serum creatinine and is obese [IBW$_{females}$ (in kg) = 45 + 2.3(Ht − 60) = 45 + 2.3(65″ − 60) = 57 kg]. The Salazar and Corcoran equation can be used to estimate creatinine clearance:

$$CrCl_{est(females)} = \frac{(146 - age)[(0.287 \cdot Wt) + (9.74 \cdot Ht^2)]}{60 \cdot S_{Cr}}$$

$$CrCl_{est(females)} = \frac{(146 - 35 \text{ y})\{(0.287 \cdot 150 \text{ kg}) + [9.74 \cdot (1.65 \text{ m})^2]\}}{60 \cdot 1.1 \text{ mg/dl}}$$

$$= 117 \text{ ml/min}$$

Note: Height is converted from inches to meters: Ht = (65 in · 2.54 cm/in)/(100 cm/m) = 1.65 m.

2. *Choose desired steady-state serum concentrations.* Intra-abdominal infection patients treated with aminoglycoside antibiotics require steady-state peak concentrations ($C_{max,ss}$) equal to 5–7 µg/ml.
3. *Select loading dose (Table 4-3).* A loading dose (LD) of 1.7 mg/kg will provide a peak concentration of 5–7 µg/ml.

   Because the patient is obese, adjusted body weight (ABW) will be used to compute the dose:

$$ABW = IBW + 0.4[TBW - IBW]$$
$$= 57 \text{ kg} + 0.4[150 \text{ kg} - 57 \text{ kg}] = 94 \text{ kg}$$

so

$$LD = 1.7 \text{ mg/kg} (94 \text{ kg}) = 160 \text{ mg}$$

4. *Determine estimated half-life, maintenance dose, and dosage interval.* From the nomogram, the estimated half-life is 2–3 hours, the maintenance dose (MD) is 90% of the loading dose [MD = 0.90(160 mg) = 144 mg], and the dosage interval is 8 hours.

   Aminoglycoside doses should be rounded to the nearest 5–10 mg. Steady-state peak concentrations are similar if drawn immediately after a 1 hour infusion or $\frac{1}{2}$ hour after a $\frac{1}{2}$-hour infusion, so the dose could be administered either way.

   The prescribed maintenance dose would be 145 mg every 8 hours.

Hartford Nomogram Method for Extended-Interval Dosing

- Extended-interval doses obtained from the literature for patients with normal renal function are 4–7 mg/kg/d for gentamicin, tobramycin, or netilmicin and 11–20 mg/kg/d for amikacin.[4,5,14–20,22–27]
- To date, the most widely used extended-interval aminoglycoside dosage approach for patients with renal dysfunction is the Hartford nomogram (Table 4-4).[4] The initial dose is 7 mg/kg of gentamicin or tobramycin (although it has not been tested with netilmicin, because of the pharmacokinetic similarity among the antibiotics it should be possible to use this aminoglycoside as well). The dosage interval is set according to the patient's creatinine clearance (Table 4-4).

  - The Hartford nomogram includes a method to adjust doses based on gentamicin or tobramycin serum concentrations. This portion of the nomogram contains average serum concentration/time lines in patients with creatinine clearances of 60, 40, and 20 ml/min. A gentamicin or tobramycin serum concentration is measured 6–14 hours after the first dose is given, and this concentration/time point is plotted on the graph (Table 4-4). The suggested dosage interval is indicated by which zone the serum concentration/time point falls in.
  - Assuming linear pharmacokinetics, clinicians have begun to use the Hartford nomogram for doses other than 7 mg/kg. Because this approach has not been formally evaluated, extreme care should be exercised when using it. For example, if the clinical situation warrants, a dose of 5 mg/kg could be administered to a patient, the initial dosage intervals suggested in the Hartford nomogram used, and a serum concentration measured to confirm the dosage interval. Assuming linear pharmacokinetics, the critical concentrations for changing dosage intervals on the Hartford nomogram graph would be decreased by 5/7 (the ratio of the 5-mg/kg dose administered to the 7-mg/kg dose suggested by the nomogram).

TABLE 4-4 Hartford Nomogram for Extended-Interval Aminoglycosides (Adapted from Nicolau, et al[4])

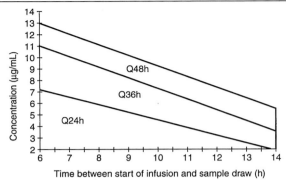

ODA nomogram for gentamicin and tobramycin at 7 mg/kg.

1. Administer 7 mg/kg gentamicin or tobramycin with initial dosage interval:

Estimated CrCl (ml/min)	Initial dosage interval
≥60	q24h
40–59	q36h
20–39	q48h
<20	Monitor serial conc. & administer next dose when <1 µg/ml

2. Obtain timed serum concentration, 6–14 hours after dose (ideally first dose).
3. Alter dosage interval to that indicated by the nomogram zone (above q48h zone, monitor serial concentrations and administer next dose when <1 µg/ml).

- Because cystic fibrosis requires a different volume of distribution (0.35 L/kg) and extended-interval dosing has not been adequately tested in patients with endocarditis, the Hartford nomogram should not be used in these situations.

▶*Example 1*　JM is a 50-year-old, 70-kg (height = 5'10") male with gram-negative pneumonia. His current serum creatinine is 0.9 mg/dl, and it has been stable over the 5 days since admission. Compute a gentamicin dose for this patient using extended-interval dosing.

1. *Estimate creatinine clearance.* This patient has a stable serum creatinine and is not obese. The Cockcroft-Gault equation can be used to estimate creatinine clearance:

$$CrCl_{est} = \frac{(140 - age)BW}{72 \cdot S_{Cr}} = \frac{(140 - 50 \text{ y})70 \text{ kg}}{72 \cdot 0.9 \text{ mg/dl}}$$

$$CrCl_{est} = 97 \text{ ml/min}$$

2. *Compute initial dose and dosage interval* (*Table 4-4*). A dose (D) of 7 mg/kg will provide a peak concentration >20 µg/ml.

$$D = 7 \text{ mg/kg} (70 \text{ kg}) = 490 \text{ mg}$$

Dosage interval would be 24 hours using the nomogram. Aminoglycoside doses should be rounded to the nearest 5–10 mg.

The prescribed maintenance dose would be 490 mg every 24 hours.

3. *Determine dosage interval using serum concentration monitoring.* A gentamicin serum concentration measured 10 hours after the dose equals 3 µg/ml. Based on the nomogram, a dosage interval of 24 hours is the correct value and does not need to be altered.

►*Example 2*   Same patient profile as in Example 1, but serum creatinine is 3.5 mg/dl, indicating renal impairment.

1. *Estimate creatinine clearance.* This patient has a stable serum creatinine and is not obese. The Cockcroft-Gault equation can be used to estimate creatinine clearance:

$$CrCl_{est} = \frac{(140 - age)BW}{72 \cdot S_{Cr}} = \frac{(140 - 50 \text{ y})70 \text{ kg}}{72 \cdot 3.5 \text{ mg/dl}}$$

$$CrCl_{est} = 25 \text{ ml/min}$$

2. *Compute initial dose and dosage interval (Table 4-4).* A dose (D) of 7 mg/kg will provide a peak concentration >20 µg/ml.

$$D = 7 \text{ mg/kg}(70 \text{ kg}) = 490 \text{ mg}$$

Dosage interval would be 48 hours using the nomogram. Aminoglycoside doses should be rounded to the nearest 5–10 mg.

The prescribed maintenance dose would be 490 mg every 48 hours.

3. *Determine dosage interval using serum concentration monitoring.* A gentamicin serum concentration measured 13 hours after the dose equals 9 µg/ml. Based on the nomogram, a dosage interval of 48 hours is too short and serial concentrations should be monitored. When the gentamicin serum concentration is <1 µg/ml, the next dose can be given. Based on the patient's estimated elimination rate constant [$k_e = 0.00293$(CrCl) + 0.014 = 0.00293 (25 ml/min) + 0.014 = 0.087 h^{-1}; $t_{1/2}$ = 0.693/k_e = 0.693/0.087 h^{-1} = 8 h], it will take approximately 3–4 half-lives or about an additional 24–32 hours after the gentamicin serum concentration for the value to drop below 1 µg/ml.

►*Example 3*   ZW is a 35-year-old, 150-kg (5′5″) female with an intra-abdominal infection. Her current serum creatinine is 1.1 mg/dl and is stable. Compute a tobramycin dose for this patient using conventional dosing.

1. *Estimate creatinine clearance.* This patient has a stable serum creatinine and is obese [IBW$_{females}$ (in kg) = 45 + 2.3(Ht − 60) = 45 + 2.3(65″ − 60) = 57 kg]. The Salazar and Corcoran equation can be used to estimate creatinine clearance:

$$CrCl_{est(females)} = \frac{(146 - age)[(0.287 \cdot Wt) + (9.74 \cdot Ht^2)]}{60 \cdot S_{Cr}}$$

$$CrCl_{est(females)} = \frac{(146 - 35 \text{ y})\{(0.287 \cdot 150 \text{ kg}) + [9.74 \cdot (1.65 \text{ m})^2]\}}{60 \cdot 1.1 \text{ mg/dl}}$$

$$= 117 \text{ ml/min}$$

Note: Height is converted from inches to meters: Ht = (65 in · 2.54 cm/in)/ (100 cm/m) = 1.65 m.

2. *Compute initial dose and dosage interval (Table 4-4).* A dose (D) of 7 mg/kg will provide a peak concentration >20 μg/ml. Because the patient is obese, adjusted body weight (ABW) will be used to compute the dose:

$$ABW = IBW + 0.4(TBW - IBW)$$

$$= 57 \text{ kg} + 0.4(150 \text{ kg} - 57 \text{ kg}) = 94 \text{ kg}$$

$$D = 7 \text{ mg/kg}(94 \text{ kg}) = 658 \text{ mg}$$

Dosage interval would be 24 hours using the nomogram. Aminoglycoside doses should be rounded to the nearest 5–10 mg.

The prescribed maintenance dose would be 660 mg every 24 hours.

3. *Determine dosage interval using serum concentration monitoring.* A gentamicin serum concentration measured 8 hours after the dose equals 4 μg/ml. Based on the nomogram, a dosage interval of 24 hours is the correct value and does not need to be altered.

USE OF AMINOGLYCOSIDE SERUM CONCENTRATIONS TO ALTER DOSAGES

- Because of pharmacokinetic variability among patients, it is likely that doses computed using patient population characteristics will not always produce aminoglycoside serum concentrations that are expected. Aminoglycoside serum concentrations are therefore measured in many patients to ensure that therapeutic, nontoxic levels are present.
- Not all patients require serum concentration monitoring. For example, if it is expected that only a limited number of doses will be administered, as is the case for surgical prophylaxis, or an appropriate dose for renal function and concurrent disease states of the patient is prescribed (e.g., 1 mg/kg every 8 hours for 3–5 days for a patient with a creatinine clearance of 80–120 ml/min for antibiotic synergy in the treatment of *Staphylococcus aureus* aortic or mitral valve endocarditis), aminoglycoside serum concentration monitoring may not be necessary.
- Whether or not aminoglycoside concentrations are measured, important patient parameters (fever curves, white blood cell counts, serum creatinine concentrations, etc.) should be followed to confirm that the patient is responding to treatment and not developing adverse drug reactions.
- When aminoglycoside serum concentrations are measured in patients and a dosage change is necessary, clinicians should seek to use the simplest, most straightforward method available to determine a dose that will provide safe and effective treatment.

  - In most cases, a simple dosage ratio can be used to adjust aminoglycoside doses, since these antibiotics follow *linear pharmacokinetics*.
  - Sometimes it is not possible simply to change the dose: the dosage interval must also be changed to achieve desired serum concentrations. In this case, it may be possible to use *pharmacokinetic concepts* to derive the aminoglycoside dose the patient needs.
  - In some situations it may be necessary to compute aminoglycoside pharmacokinetic parameters for the patient using the *Sawchuk-Zaske method* and utilize these to calculate the best drug dose. When steady-state concentrations are used, this method usually gives dosage adjustments similar to the pharmacokinetic concept method. While it is computationally

more difficult, many clinicians prefer the Sawchuk-Zaske method because pharmacokinetic parameters are calculated.

- Finally, computerized methods that incorporate expected population pharmacokinetic characteristics (*Bayesian pharmacokinetic computer programs*) can be used in difficult cases in which renal function is changing, serum concentrations are obtained at suboptimal times, or the patient was not at steady state when serum concentrations were measured.

Linear Pharmacokinetics Method

- Because aminoglycoside antibiotics follow linear, dose-proportional pharmacokinetics, steady-state serum concentrations change in proportion to dose according to the following equation:

$$D_{new}/C_{ss,new} = D_{old}/C_{ss,old} \qquad \text{or} \qquad D_{new} = (C_{ss,new}/C_{ss,old})D_{old}$$

where D is the dose, C_{ss} is the steady-state peak or trough concentration, old indicates the dose that produced the steady-state concentration that the patient is currently receiving, and new denotes the dose necessary to produce the desired steady-state concentration.

- The advantages of this method are that it is quick and simple. The disadvantages are that steady-state concentrations are required, and it may not be possible to attain desired serum concentrations by changing only the dose.

▶*Example 1*   JM is a 50-year-old, 70-kg (height = 5′10″) male with gramnegative pneumonia. His current serum creatinine is 0.9 mg/dl, and it has been stable over the 5 days since admission. A gentamicin dose of 170 mg every 8 hours was prescribed and expected to achieve steady-state peak and trough concentrations equal to 9 μg/ml and 1 μg/ml, respectively. After the third dose, steady-state peak and trough concentrations were measured and were 12 μg/ml and 1.4 μg/ml, respectively. Calculate a new gentamicin dose that would provide a steady-state peak of 9 μg/ml.

1. *Estimate creatinine clearance.* This patient has a stable serum creatinine and is not obese. The Cockcroft-Gault equation can be used to estimate creatinine clearance:

$$CrCl_{est} = \frac{(140 - age)BW}{72 \cdot S_{Cr}} = \frac{(140 - 50 \text{ y})70 \text{ kg}}{72 \cdot 0.9 \text{ mg/dl}}$$

$$CrCl_{est} = 97 \text{ ml/min}$$

2. *Estimate elimination rate constant* (k_e) *and half-life* ($t_{1/2}$). The elimination rate constant-versus-creatinine clearance relationship is used to estimate the gentamicin elimination rate for this patient:

$$k_e = 0.00293(CrCl) + 0.014 = 0.00293(97 \text{ ml/min}) + 0.014$$
$$= 0.298 \text{ h}^{-1}$$

$$t_{1/2} = 0.693/k_e = 0.693/0.298 \text{ h}^{-1} = 2.3 \text{ h}$$

Because the patient has been receiving gentamicin for more that 3–5 estimated half-lives, it is likely that the measured serum concentrations are steady-state values. *Note that these first two steps can be omitted if it is known that the patient is at steady-state.*

3. *Compute new dose to achieve desired serum concentration.* Using linear pharmacokinetics, the new dose to attain the desired concentration should be proportional to the old dose that produced the measured concentration:

$$D_{new} = (C_{ss,new}/C_{ss,old})D_{old} = (9 \ \mu g/ml \ /12 \ \mu g/ml) \ 170 \ mg$$
$$= 128 \ mg, \ round \ to \ 130 \ mg$$

The new suggested dose is 130 mg every 8 hours, to be started at the next scheduled dosing time.

4. *Check steady-state trough concentration for new dosage regimen.* Using linear pharmacokinetics, the new steady-state concentration can be estimated and should be proportional to the old dose that produced the measured concentration:

$$C_{ss,new} = (D_{new}/D_{old})C_{ss,old} = (130 \ mg/170 \ mg) \ 1.4 \ \mu g/ml = 1.1 \ \mu g/ml$$

This steady-state trough concentration should be safe and effective for the infection that is being treated.

Pharmacokinetic Concepts Method

- As implied by the name, the pharmacokinetics concepts technique derives alternative doses by estimating actual pharmacokinetic parameters or surrogates for pharmacokinetic parameters.[77] It is a very useful way to calculate drug doses when the linear pharmacokinetic method is not sufficient because a dosage change that will produce a proportional change in steady-state peak and trough concentrations is not appropriate. The only requirement is a steady-state peak and trough aminoglycoside serum concentration pair obtained before and after a dose (Figure 4-3). The following steps are used to compute new aminoglycoside doses:

  1. *Draw a rough sketch of the serum log concentration/time curve by hand, keeping track of the relative time between the serum concentrations (Figure 4-3).*

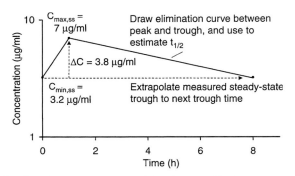

FIG. 4-3 Graphical representation of the pharmacokinetic concepts method, where a steady-state peak ($C_{max,ss}$) and trough ($C_{min,ss}$) concentration pair is used to individualize aminoglycoside therapy. Because the patient is at steady state, consecutive trough concentrations will be identical, so the trough concentration can be extrapolated to the next predose time. The change in concentration after a dose is given (ΔC) is a surrogate measure of the volume of distribution and is used to compute the new dose for the patient.

2. *Since the patient is at steady state, the trough concentration can be extrapolated to the next trough value time (Figure 4-3).*
3. *Draw the elimination curve between the steady-state peak concentration and the extrapolated trough concentration. Use this line to estimate half-life.* For example, a patient receives an gentamicin dose of 80 mg given every 8 hours that produces a steady-state peak equal to 7 μg/ml and a steady-state trough equal to 3.2 μg/ml, and the dose is infused over $\frac{1}{2}$ hour and the peak concentration is drawn $\frac{1}{2}$ hour later (Figure 4-3). The time between the measured steady-state peak and the extrapolated trough concentration is 7 hours (the 8-hour dosage interval minus the 1-hour combined infusion and waiting time). The definition of half-life is the time needed for serum concentrations to decrease by one-half. Because the serum concentration declined by approximately one-half from the peak concentration to the trough concentration, the aminoglycoside half-life for this patient is approximately 7 hours. This information will be used to set the new dosage interval for the patient.
4. *Determine the difference in concentration between the steady-state peak and trough concentrations. The difference in concentration will change proportionally with the dose size.* In the current example the patient is receiving a gentamicin dose equal to 80 mg every 8 hours, which produced steady-state peak and trough concentrations of 7 and 3.2 μg/ml, respectively. The difference between the peak and trough values is 3.8 μg/ml. The change in serum concentration is proportional to the dose, and this information is used to set a new dose for the patient.
5. *Choose new steady-state peak and trough concentrations.* For the purposes of this example, the desired steady-state peak and trough concentrations are approximately 7 and 1 μg/ml, respectively.
6. *Determine the new dosage interval for the desired concentrations.* In this example, the patient currently has the desired peak concentration of 7 μg/ml. In one half-life, the serum concentration will decline to 3.5 μg/ml, in an additional half-life the gentamicin concentration will decrease to 1.8 μg/ml, and in one more half-life the concentration will decline to 0.9 μg/ml (Figure 4-4). Since the approximate half-life is 7 hours

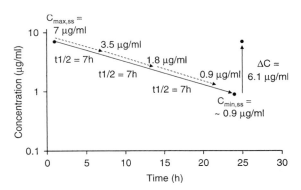

FIG. 4-4 The pharmacokinetic concepts method uses the estimated half-life to graphically compute the new dosage interval and the change in concentration to calculate the dose for a patient.

and 3 half-lives are required for serum concentrations to decrease from the desired peak concentration to the desired trough concentration, the dosage interval should be 21 hours (7 hours × 3 half-lives). This value will be rounded off to the clinically acceptable value of 24 hours, and the actual trough concentration can be expected to be slightly lower that 0.9 µg/ml.

7. *Determine the new dose for the desired concentrations.* The desired peak concentration is 7 µg/ml, and the expected trough concentration is 0.9 µg/ml. The change in concentration between these values is 6.1 µg/ml. It is known from measured serum concentrations that administration of 80 mg changes serum concentrations by 3.8 µg/ml and that the change in serum concentration between the peak and trough values is proportional to the size of the dose. Therefore, a simple ratio can be used to compute the required dose:

$$D_{new} = (\Delta C_{new}/\Delta C_{old})D_{old}$$

where D_{new} and D_{old} are the new and old doses, respectively; ΔC_{new} is the change in concentration between the peak and trough for the new dose; and ΔC_{old} is the change in concentration between the peak and trough for the old dose (*Note:* This relationship is appropriate because doses are given into a fixed, constant volume of distribution; it is not because the drug follows linear pharmacokinetics, so this method will work whether the agent follows nonlinear or linear pharmacokinetics). For this example,

$$D_{new} = (6.1 \ \mu g/ml/3.8 \ \mu g/ml) \ 80 \ mg = 128 \ mg$$

which can be rounded to 130 mg. Gentamicin, 130 mg every 24 hours, should be started 24 hours after the last dose of the previous dosage regimen.

- Once this method is mastered, it can be used without the need for a calculator. The following example uses the pharmacokinetic concepts method to change aminoglycoside doses.

▶*Example 1*   ZW is a 35-year-old, 150-kg (5′5″) female with an intra-abdominal infection. Her current serum creatinine is 1.1 mg/dl and is stable. A tobramycin dose of 165 mg every 8 hours was prescribed and expected to achieve steady-state peak and trough concentrations equal to 6 and 0.5 µg/ml, respectively. After the fifth dose, steady-state peak and trough concentrations were measured and were 5 and 2.6 µg/ml, respectively. Calculate a new tobramycin dose that would provide a steady-state peak of 6 µg/ml and a steady-state trough ≤1.

1. *Estimate creatinine clearance.* This patient has a stable serum creatinine and is obese [$IBW_{females}$ (in kg) = 45 + 2.3(Ht − 60) = 45 + 2.3(65″ − 60) = 57 kg]. The Salazar and Corcoran equation can be used to estimate creatinine clearance:

$$CrCl_{est(females)} = \frac{(146 - age)[(0.287 \cdot Wt) + (9.74 \cdot Ht^2)]}{60 \cdot S_{Cr}}$$

$$CrCl_{est(females)} = \frac{(146 - 35 \ y)\{(0.287 \cdot 150 \ kg) + [9.74 \cdot (1.65 \ m)^2]\}}{60 \cdot 1.1 \ mg/dl}$$

$$= 117 \ ml/min$$

Note: Height is converted from inches to meters: Ht = (65 in · 2.54 cm/in)/(100 cm/m) = 1.65 m.

2. *Estimate elimination rate constant (k_e) and half-life ($t_{1/2}$)* The elimination rate constant-versus-creatinine clearance relationship is used to estimate the tobramycin elimination rate for this patient:

$$k_e = 0.00293(CrCl) + 0.014 = 0.00293(117 \text{ ml/min}) + 0.014$$
$$= 0.357 \text{ h}^{-1}$$

$$t_{1/2} = 0.693/k_e = 0.693/0.357 \text{ h}^{-1} = 1.9 \text{ h}$$

Because the patient has been receiving tobramycin for more that 3–5 estimated half-lives, it is likely that the measured serum concentrations are steady-state values. *Note that these first two steps can be omitted if it is known that the patient is at steady state.*

3. *Use the pharmacokinetics concept method to compute a new dose.*

   a. *Draw a rough sketch of the serum log concentration/time curve by hand, keeping track of the relative time between the serum concentrations (Figure 4-5).*

   b. *Since the patient is at steady state, the trough concentration can be extrapolated to the next trough value time (Figure 4-5).*

   c. *Draw the elimination curve between the steady-state peak concentration and the extrapolated trough concentration. Use this line to estimate half-life.* The patient is receiving a tobramycin dose of 165 mg every 8 hours, which produces a steady-state peak equal to 5 µg/ml. and a steady-state trough equal to 2.6 µg/ml. The dose is infused over $\frac{1}{2}$ hour and the peak concentration is drawn $\frac{1}{2}$ hour later (Figure 4-5). The time between the measured steady-state peak and the extrapolated trough concentration is 7 hours (the 8-hour dosage interval minus the 1-hour combined infusion and waiting time). The definition of half-life is the time needed for serum concentrations to decrease by one-half. It will take 1 half-life for the peak serum concentration to decline from 5 to 2.5 µg/ml. The concentration of 2.6 µg/ml is very close to the extrapolated trough value of 2.5 µg/ml. Therefore, 1 half-life expired during the 7-hour time period between the peak concentration and extrapolated trough concentration,

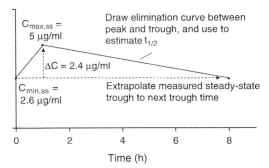

FIG. 4-5 Graphical representation of the pharmacokinetic concepts method, in which a steady state peak ($C_{max,ss}$) and trough ($C_{min,ss}$) concentration pair is used to individualize aminoglycoside therapy. Because the patient is at steady state, consecutive trough concentrations will be identical, so the trough concentration can be extrapolated to the next predose time. The change in concentration after a dose is given (ΔC) is a surrogate measure of the volume of distribution and is used to compute the new dose for the patient.

and the estimated half-life is 7 hours. This information will be used to set the new dosage interval for the patient.

d. *Determine the difference in concentration between the steady-state peak and trough concentrations. The difference in concentration will change proportionally with the dose size.* In the current example, the patient is receiving a tobramycin dose equal to 165 mg every 8 hours, which produced steady-state peak and trough concentrations of 5 and 2.6 μg/ml, respectively. The difference between the peak and trough values is 2.4 μg/ml. The change in serum concentration is proportional to the dose, and this information will be used to set a new dose for the patient.

e. *Choose new steady-state peak and trough concentrations.* For the purposes of this example, the desired steady-state peak and trough concentrations will be approximately 6 and ≤1 μg/ml, respectively.

f. *Determine the new dosage interval for the desired concentrations.* Using the desired concentrations, it will take one half-life for the peak concentration of 6 μg/ml to decrease to 3 μg/ml, one more half-life for the serum concentration to decrease to 1.5 μg/ml, and an additional half-life for serum concentrations to decline to 0.8 μg/ml. Therefore, the dosage interval will need to be approximately 3 half-lives or 21 hours (7 hours × 3 half-lives = 21 hours), which can be rounded to 24 hours.

g. *Determine the new dose for the desired concentrations.* The desired peak concentration is 6 μg/ml, and the expected trough concentration is 0.8 μg/ml. The change in concentration between these values is 5.2 μg/ml. It is known from measured serum concentrations that administration of 165 mg changes serum concentrations by 2.4 μg/ml and that the change in serum concentration between the peak and trough values is proportional to the size of the dose. In this case;

$$D_{new} = (\Delta C_{new}/\Delta C_{old})D_{old} = (5.2\ \mu g/ml/2.4\ \mu g/ml)165\ mg$$
$$= 358\ mg,\ rounded\ to\ 360\ mg.$$

Tobramycin 360 mg every 24 hours should be started 24 hours after the last dose of the previous dosage regimen.

Sawchuk-Zaske Method

- The Sawchuk-Zaske method of adjusting aminoglycoside doses was among the first techniques available to change doses using serum concentrations.[2,36–38,73] It allows the computation of an individual's, own, unique pharmacokinetic constants and uses those to calculate a dose to achieve desired aminoglycoside concentrations.

  - The standard Sawchuk-Zaske method conducts a small pharmacokinetic experiment using 3–4 aminoglycoside serum concentrations obtained during a dosage interval and does not require steady-state conditions.

  - The modified Sawchuk-Zaske method assumes that steady state has been achieved and requires only a steady-state peak and trough concentration pair obtained before and after a dose. The Sawchuk-Zaske method has also been used successfully to dose vancomycin and theophylline.

Standard Sawchuk-Zaske Method

- The standard version of the Sawchuk-Zaske method does not require steady-state concentrations. A trough aminoglycoside concentration is obtained before a dose, a peak aminoglycoside concentration is obtained after the dose is infused (immediately after a 1-hour infusion or $\frac{1}{2}$ hour after a $\frac{1}{2}$-hour infusion),

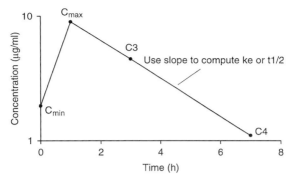

FIG. 4-6 The Sawchuk-Zaske method for individualization of aminoglycoside doses uses a trough (C_{min}), peak (C_{max}), and 1–2 additional postdose concentrations (C_3, C_4) to compute a patient's own, unique pharmacokinetic parameters. This version of the Sawchuk-Zaske method does not require steady-state conditions. The peak and trough concentrations are used to calculate the volume of distribution, and the postdose concentrations (C_{max}, C_3, C_4) are used to compute half-life. Once volume of distribution and half-life have been measured, they can be used to compute the exact dose needed to achieve desired aminoglycoside concentrations.

and 1–2 additional postdose serum aminoglycoside concentrations are obtained (Figure 4-6). Ideally, the 1–2 postdose concentrations should be obtained at least one estimated half-life from each other to minimize the influence of assay error.

- The postdose serum concentrations are used to calculate the aminoglycoside elimination rate constant and half-life (Figure 4-6). The half-life can be computed by graphing the postdose concentrations on semilogrithmic paper, drawing the best straight line through the data points, and determining the time needed for serum concentrations to decline by one-half. Once the half-life is known, the elimination rate constant (k_e) can be computed: $k_e = 0.693/t_{1/2}$.
- Alternatively, the elimination rate constant can be calculated directly using the postdose serum concentrations [$k_e = (\ln C_1 - \ln C_2)/\Delta t$, where C_1 and C_2 are postdose serum concentrations and Δt is the time that expired between the times at which C_1 and C_2 were obtained], and the half-life can be computed using the elimination rate constant ($t_{1/2} = 0.693/k_e$).
- The volume of distribution (V) is calculated using the following equation:

$$V = \frac{D/t'(1 - e^{-k_e t'})}{k_e[C_{max} - (C_{min}e^{-k_e t'})]}$$

where D is the aminoglycoside dose, t' is the infusion time, k_e is the elimination rate constant, C_{max} is the peak concentration, and C_{min} is the trough concentration.

- The elimination rate constant and volume of distribution measured in this fashion are the patient's own, unique aminoglycoside pharmacokinetic constants and can be used in one-compartment-model intravenous infusion equations to compute the required dose to achieve any desired serum concentration.

▶**Example 1** JH is a 24-year-old, 70-kg (height = 6'0") male with gram-negative pneumonia. His current serum creatinine is 1.0 mg/dl, and it has been stable over the 7 days since admission. An amikacin dose of 400 mg every 8 hours was prescribed. After the third dose, the following amikacin serum concentrations were obtained:

Time	Amikacin concentration (μg/ml)
0800 H	2.0
0800–0900 H	Amikacin 400 mg
0900 H	22.1
1100 H	11.9
1600 H	2.5

Medication administration sheets were checked, and the previous dose was given 2 hours early (2200 H the previous day). Because of this, it is known that the patient is not at steady state. Calculate a new amikacin dose that would provide a steady state peak of 28 μg/ml and a trough of 3 μg/ml.

Use the standard Sawchuk-Zaske method to compute a new dose.

1. *Plot serum concentration/time data (Figure 4-7). Because serum concentrations decrease in a straight line, use any two postdose concentrations to compute the patient's elimination rate constant and half-life.*

$$k_e = \frac{\ln C_{max,ss} - \ln C_{min,ss}}{\tau - t'} = \frac{\ln 22.1 \; \mu g/ml - \ln 2.5 \; \mu g/ml}{(16 \; H - 09 \; H)} = 0.311 \; h^{-1}$$

$$t_{1/2} = 0.693/k_e = 0.693/0.311 \; h^{-1} = 2.2 \; h$$

2. *Compute the patient's volume of distribution.*

$$V = \frac{D/t'(1 - e^{-k_e t'})}{k_e[C_{max,ss} - (C_{min,ss} e^{-k_e t'})]}$$

$$= \frac{(400 \; mg/l \; h)(1 - e^{-(0.311 \; h^{-1})(1 \; h)})}{0.311 \; h^{-1}[22.1 \; mg/L - (2.0 \; mg/L \; e^{-(0.311 \; h^{-1})(1 \; h)})]}$$

$$V = 16.7 \; L$$

3. *Choose new steady-state peak and trough concentrations.* For the purposes of this example, the desired steady-state peak and trough concentrations will be 28 and 3 μg/ml, respectively.

4. *Determine the new dosage interval for the desired concentrations.* As in the initial dosage section of this chapter, the dosage interval (τ) is computed using the following equation using a 1-hour infusion time (t'):

$$\tau = \left(\frac{\ln C_{max,ss} - \ln C_{min,ss}}{k_e}\right) + t' = \left(\frac{\ln 28 \; \mu g/ml - \ln 3 \; \mu g/ml}{0.311 \; h^{-1}}\right) + 1 \; h = 8 \; h$$

5. *Determine the new dose for the desired concentrations.* The dose is computed using the one-compartment-model intravenous infusion equation used in the initial dosing section of this chapter:

$$k_0 = C_{max,ss} k_e V[(1 - e^{-k_e \tau})/(1 - e^{-k_e t'})]$$

$$k_0 = (28 \; mg/L \cdot 0.311 \; h^{-1} \cdot 16.7 \; L)[(1 - e^{-(0.311 \; h^{-1})(8 \; h)})/(1 - e^{-(0.311 \; h^{-1})(1 \; h)})]$$

$$= 499 \; mg, \; rounded \; to \; 500 \; mg$$

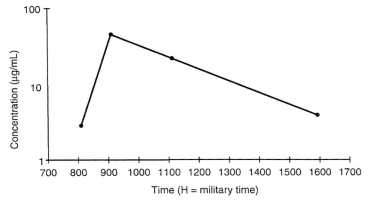

FIG. 4-7 Graph of amikacin serum concentrations used in Sawchuk-Zaske method example.

A dose of amikacin 500 mg every 8 hours should be prescribed to begin 8 hours after the last dose of the previous regimen.

Steady-State Sawchuk-Zaske Method

- If a steady-state peak and trough aminoglycoside concentration pair is available for a patient, the Sawchuk-Zaske method can be used to compute patient pharmacokinetic parameters and aminoglycoside doses (Figure 4-8).

  - Since the patient is at steady state, the measured trough concentration obtained before the dose was given can be extrapolated to the next dosage

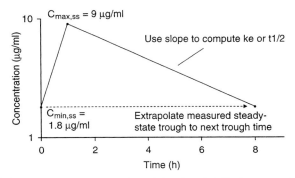

FIG. 4-8 The steady-state version of the Sawchuk-Zaske method uses a steady-state peak ($C_{max,ss}$) and trough ($C_{min,ss}$) concentration pair to individualize aminoglycoside therapy. Because the patient is at steady state, consecutive trough concentrations will be identical, so the trough concentration can be extrapolated to the next predose time. The steady-state peak and trough concentrations are used to calculate the volume of distribution and half-life. Once volume of distribution and half-life have been measured, they can be used to compute the exact dose needed to achieve desired aminoglycoside concentrations.

time and used to compute the aminoglycoside elimination rate constant ($k_e = [\ln C_{max,ss} - \ln C_{min,ss}]/\tau - t'$, where $C_{max,ss}$ and $C_{min,ss}$ are the steady-state peak and trough serum concentrations and t' and τ are the infusion time and dosage interval), and the half-life can be computed using the elimination rate constant ($t_{1/2} = 0.693/k_e$).

- The volume of distribution (V) is calculated using the following equation:

$$V = \frac{D/t'(1 - e^{-k_e t'})}{k_e[C_{max,ss} - (C_{min,ss}e^{-k_e t'})]}$$

where D is the aminoglycoside dose, t' is the infusion time, k_e is the elimination rate constant, $C_{max,ss}$ is the steady-state peak concentration, and $C_{min,ss}$ is the steady-state trough concentration.

- The elimination rate constant and volume of distribution measured in this way are the patient's own, unique aminoglycoside pharmacokinetic constants and can be used in one-compartment-model intravenous infusion equations to compute the required dose to achieve any desired serum concentration. The dosage calculations are similar to those done in the initial dosage section of this chapter, except that the patient's real pharmacokinetic parameters are used in the equations instead of population pharmacokinetic estimates.

▶**Example 1**   JM is a 50-year-old, 70-kg (height = 5'10") male with gram-negative pneumonia. His current serum creatinine is 3.5 mg/dl, and it has been stable over the 5 days since admission. A gentamicin dose of 115 mg every 24 hours was prescribed and expected to achieve steady-state peak and trough concentrations equal to 8–10 µg/ml and <2 µg/ml, respectively. After the third dose, steady-state peak and trough concentrations were measured and were 12 and 3.5 µg/ml, respectively. Calculate a new gentamicin dose that would provide a steady-state peak of 9 µg/ml and a trough <2 µg/ml.

1. *Estimate creatinine clearance.* This patient has a stable serum creatinine and is not obese. The Cockcroft-Gault equation can be used to estimate creatinine clearance:

$$CrCl_{est} = \frac{(140 - age)BW}{72 \cdot S_{Cr}} = \frac{(140 - 50 \text{ y})70 \text{ kg}}{72 \cdot 3.5 \text{mg/dl}}$$

$$CrCl_{est} = 25 \text{ ml/min}$$

2. *Estimate elimination rate constant (k_e) and half-life ($t_{1/2}$).* The elimination rate constant-versus-creatinine clearance relationship is used to estimate the gentamicin elimination rate for this patient:

$$k_e = 0.00293(CrCl) + 0.014$$
$$= 0.00293(25 \text{ ml/min}) + 0.014 = 0.087 \text{ h}^{-1}$$
$$t_{1/2} = 0.693/k_e = 0.693/0.087 \text{ h}^{-1} = 8 \text{ h}$$

Because the patient has been receiving gentamicin for more that 3–5 estimated half-lives, it is likely that the measured serum concentrations are steady-state values. *Note that these first two steps can be omitted if it is known that the patient is at steady state.*

3. *Compute the patient's elimination rate constant and half-life.* (*Note: For infusion times less than 1 hour, t′ is considered to be the sum of the infusion and waiting times*).

$$k_e = \frac{\ln C_{max,ss} - \ln C_{min,ss}}{\tau - t'} = \frac{\ln 12 \text{ μg/ml} - \ln 3.5 \text{ μg/ml}}{24 \text{ h} - 1 \text{ h}} = 0.054 \text{ h}^{-1}$$

$$t_{1/2} = 0.693/k_e = 0.693/0.054 \text{ h}^{-1} = 12.8 \text{ h}$$

4. *Compute the patient's volume of distribution.*

$$V = \frac{D/t'(1 - e^{-k_e t'})}{k_e[C_{max,ss} - (C_{min,ss} e^{-k_e t'})]}$$

$$= \frac{(115 \text{ mg/lh})(1 - e^{-(0.054 \text{ h}^{-1})(1 \text{ h})})}{0.054 \text{ h}^{-1}[12 \text{ mg/L} - (3.5 \text{ mg/L})(e^{-(0.054 \text{ h}^{-1})(1 \text{ h})})]}$$

$$V = 12.9 \text{ L}$$

5. *Choose new steady-state peak and trough concentrations.* For the purposes of this example, the desired steady-state peak and trough concentrations will be approximately 9 and 1.5 μg/ml, respectively.

6. *Determine the new dosage interval for the desired concentrations.* As in the initial dosage section of this chapter, the dosage interval (τ) is computed using the following equation using a 1-hour infusion time (t′):

$$\tau = \left(\frac{\ln C_{max,ss} - \ln C_{min,ss}}{k_e} \right) + t'$$

$$= \left(\frac{\ln 9 \text{ μg/ml} - \ln 1.5 \text{ μg/ml}}{0.054 \text{ h}^{-1}} \right) + 1 \text{ h}$$

$$= 34 \text{ h, rounded to 36 h}$$

7. *Determine the new dose for the desired concentrations.* The dose is computed using the one-compartment-model intravenous infusion equation used in the initial dosing section of this chapter:

$$k_0 = C_{max,ss} k_e V[(1 - e^{-k_e \tau})/(1 - e^{-k_e t'})]$$

$$k_0 = (9 \text{ mg/L} \cdot 0.054 \text{ h}^{-1} \cdot 12.9 \text{ L})[(1 - e^{-(0.054 \text{ h}^{-1})(36 \text{ h})})/(1 - e^{-(0.054 \text{ h}^{-1})(1 \text{ h})})]$$

$$= 102 \text{ mg, rounded to 100 mg}$$

A dose of gentamicin 100 mg every 36 hours should be prescribed to begin 36 hours after the last dose of the previous regimen.

Bayesian Pharmacokinetic Computer Programs

• Computer programs are available that can assist in the computation of pharmacokinetic parameters for patients.[78–82] The most reliable computer programs use a nonlinear regression algorithm that incorporates components of Bayes' theorem.

• An advantage of this approach is that consistent dosage recommendations can be made when several different practitioners are involved in therapeutic drug monitoring programs. However, since simpler dosing methods work just as well for patients with stable pharmacokinetic parameters and steady-state drug concentrations, many clinicians reserve the use of computer programs for more difficult situations. Those situations include serum concentrations that are not at steady state, serum concentrations not obtained at the specific times needed to employ simpler methods, and unstable pharmacokinetic parameters.

- Many Bayesian pharmacokinetic computer programs are available to users, and most should provide answers similar to the one used in the following example. The program used to solve problems in this book is DrugCalc, written by Dr. Dennis Mungall, and is available on his Internet web site (www.clinpharmacologist.bigstep.com/consumersurvey. html).[83]

▶**Example 1**   JM is a 50-year-old, 70-kg (height = 5′10″) male with gram-negative pneumonia. His current serum creatinine is 3.5 mg/dl, and it has been stable over the 5 days since admission. A gentamicin dose of 115 mg every 24 hours was prescribed and expected to achieve steady-state peak and trough concentrations equal to 8–10 μg/ml and <2 μg/ml, respectively. After the third dose, steady-state peak and trough concentrations were measured and were 12 and 3.5 μg/ml, respectively. Calculate a new gentamicin dose that will provide a steady-state peak of 9 μg/ml and a steady-state trough equal to 1.5 μg/ml.

1. *Enter patient demographic, drug dosing, and serum concentration/time data into the computer program.*

2. *Compute pharmacokinetic parameters for the patient using a Bayesian pharmacokinetic computer program.* The pharmacokinetic parameters computed by the program are a volume of distribution of 14.6 L, a half-life equal to 14.7 h, and an elimination rate constant of 0.047 h^{-1}. These values are slightly different than those computed using the steady-state Sawchuk-Zaske method (V = 12.9 L, $t_{1/2}$ = 12.8 h, k_e = 0.054 h^{-1}) because the patient probably was not at steady state when the serum concentrations were drawn.

3. *Compute dose required to achieve desired aminoglycoside serum concentrations.* The one-compartment-model intravenous infusion equations used by the program to compute doses indicates that a dose of 110 mg every 36 hours will produce a steady-state peak concentration of 9 μg/ml and a steady-state trough concentration of 1.7 μg/ml.

Dosing Strategies

- Initial dose and dosage adjustment techniques using serum concentrations can be used in any combination as long as the limitations of each method are observed.
- Some dosing approaches link together logically when considered according to their basic approaches or philosophies. Dosage strategies that follow similar pathways are given in Tables 4-5A and 4-5B.

TABLE 4-5A Conventional Dosing Schemes

Dosing approach/ philosophy	Initial dosing	Use of serum concentrations to alter doses
Pharmacokinetic parameters/equations	Pharmacokinetic dosing method	Sawchuk-Zaske method
Nomogram/ pharmacokinetic concepts	Hull & Sarubbi[34] nomogram	Pharmacokinetic concepts method
Computerized	Bayesian computer program	Bayesian computer program

TABLE 4-5B Extended-Interval Dosing Schemes

Dosing approach/ philosophy	Initial dosing	Use of serum concentrations to alter doses
Pharmacokinetic parameters/equations	Pharmacokinetic dosing method	Sawchuk-Zaske method
Nomogram/concepts	Hartford nomogram[4]	Hartford nomogram (1 concentration) or Pharmacokinetic concepts method (≥ 2 concentrations)
Computerized	Bayesian computer program	Bayesian computer program

SPECIAL DOSING CONSIDERATIONS

Hemodialysis Dosing

• Aminoglycoside antibiotics are eliminated by dialysis, so renal failure patients receiving hemodialysis must have aminoglycoside dosage regimens that take dialysis clearance into account.

▶*Example 1*   A 62-year-old, 5′8″ male, who weighs 65 kg, has chronic renal failure, and receives hemodialysis three times weekly with a low-flux dialysis filter. An initial dosage regimen for tobramycin needs to be computed for the patient to achieve peak concentrations of 6–7 mg/L and post-dialysis concentrations of 1–2 mg/L.

1. *Initial dosage determination.* Patients with renal failure are prone to having poor fluid balance because their kidneys are not able to provide this important function. Because of this, the patient should be assessed for overhydration (due to renal failure) or underhydration (due to renal failure and increased loss due to fever).

    • Weight is a good indication of fluid status, and this patient's weight is less than his ideal weight [IBW_{male} = 50 kg + 2.3(Ht − 60) = 50 kg + 2.3(68″ − 60) = 68 kg]. Other indications of state of hydration (skin turgor, etc.) indicate that the patient has normal fluid balance at this time. Because of this, the average volume of distribution for aminoglycoside antibiotics equal to 0.26 L/kg can be used.

    A loading dose of tobramycin would be appropriate for this patient because the expected half-life is long (~50 h); administration of maintenance doses only might not result in therapeutic maximum concentrations for a considerable time period while drug accumulation is occurring. The loading dose is to be given after hemodialysis ends at 1300 H on Monday (hemodialysis conducted on Monday, Wednesday, and Friday from 0900 to 1300 H).

    • Because the patient is expected to have a long half-life compared to the infusion time of the drug ($\frac{1}{2}$–1 h), little drug will be eliminated during the infusion period, and IV bolus one-compartment-model equations can be used. The loading dose for this patient should be based on the expected volume of distribution:

$$V = 0.26 \text{ L/kg} \cdot 65 \text{ kg} = 16.9 \text{ L}$$

$$LD = C_{max} \cdot V = 6 \text{ mg/L} \cdot 16.9 \text{ L} = 101 \text{ mg, rounded to } 100 \text{ mg}$$

where LD is loading dose and C_{max} is the maximum concentration after drug administration. This loading dose was given at 1400 H (Figure 4-9).

- Until the next dialysis period at 0900 H on Wednesday, tobramycin is cleared only by the patient's own body mechanisms. The expected elimination rate constant (k_e) for a patient with a creatinine clearance of approximately zero is

$$k_e \text{ (in h}^{-1}) = 0.00293 \cdot CrCl + 0.014$$

$$= 0.00293 (0 \text{ ml/min}) + 0.014 = 0.014 \text{ h}^{-1}$$

The expected concentration at 0900 H on Wednesday is

$$C = C_0 e^{-k_e t}$$

where C is the concentration at t hours after the initial concentration of C_0.

$$C = (6 \text{ mg/L})e^{-(0.014 \text{ h}^{-1})(43 \text{ h})} = 3.3 \text{ mg/L}$$

While the patient is receiving hemodialysis, tobramycin is eliminated by the patient's own mechanisms plus dialysis clearance. During hemodialysis

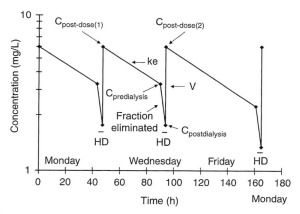

FIG. 4-9   Concentration/time graph for tobramycin in a hemodialysis patient using estimated, population pharmacokinetic parameters. The initial dose was given postdialysis at 1400 H on Monday (time = 0 h). Hemodialysis periods are shown by small horizontal bars labeled HD, and days are indicated on the time line. In order to compute patient-specific pharmacokinetic parameters, four serum concentrations are measured. The elimination rate constant (k_e) is computed using two concentrations after dosage administration ($C_{postdose(1)}$ and $C_{predialysis}$), the fraction eliminated by dialysis by two concentrations ($C_{predialysis}$ and $C_{postdialysis}$) before and after dialysis, and the volume of distribution using two concentrations ($C_{postdialysis}$ and $C_{postdose(2)}$) after another dosage administration.

with a low-flux filter, the average half-life for aminoglycosides is 4 hours. Because the patient is dialyzed for 4 hours, the tobramycin serum concentration should decrease by one-half, to 1.7 mg/L, or, using formal computations,

$$k_e = 0.693/(t_{1/2}) = 0.693/4 \text{ h} = 0.173 \text{ h}^{-1}$$

$$C = C_0 e^{-k_e t} = (3.3 \text{ mg/L}) e^{-(0.173 \text{ h}^{-1})(4 \text{ h})} = 1.7 \text{ mg/L}$$

- At this time, a postdialysis replacement dose could be given to increase the maximum concentration to its original value of 6 mg/L:

$$\text{Replacement dose} = (C_{max} - C_{baseline})V = (6 \text{ mg/L} - 1.7 \text{ mg/L})16.9 \text{ L}$$
$$= 73 \text{ mg, round to 75 mg}$$

where C_{max} is the maximum postdose concentration and $C_{baseline}$ is the predose concentration. The postdialysis replacement dose of 75 mg was administered at 1400 H on Wednesday. Because all time frames and pharmacokinetic parameters are the same for Monday–Wednesday and Wednesday–Friday, the postdialysis replacement dose on Friday at 1400 H should also be 75 mg.

- However, more time elapses from Friday after drug administration to Monday before dialysis (67 h), the next day for hemodialysis to be conducted in the patient, and this needs to be accounted for:

$$C = C_0 e^{-k_e t} = (6 \text{ mg/L}) e^{-(0.014 \text{ h}^{-1})(67 \text{ h})} = 2.3 \text{ mg/L}.$$

Again, a 4-hour hemodialysis period would decrease serum concentrations by one-half to 1.2 mg/L:

$$C = C_0 e^{-k_e t} = (2.3 \text{ mg/L}) e^{-(0.173 \text{ h}^{-1})(4 \text{ h})} = 1.2 \text{ mg/L}$$

At this time, a postdialysis replacement dose could be given to increase the maximum concentration to the original value of 6 mg/L:

$$\text{Replacement dose} = (C_{max} - C_{baseline})V = (6 \text{ mg/L} - 1.2 \text{ mg/L})16.9 \text{ L}$$
$$= 81 \text{ mg, round to 80 mg}$$

where C_{max} is the maximum postdose concentration and $C_{baseline}$ is the predose concentration. The postdialysis replacement dose of 80 mg was administered at 1400 H on Monday.
- Because all time frames and pharmacokinetic parameters will be the same in subsequent weeks, the following replacement doses should be prescribed postdialysis at 1400: Wednesday and Friday, 75 mg; Monday, 80 mg. In this particular example, recommended doses are within 5 mg of each other, and if the clinician wished, the same post-dialysis dose could be given on each day. However, this will not be true in every case.

2. *Use of aminoglycoside serum concentrations to alter dosages.* Since the initial dosage scheme outlined for this patient used average, estimated pharmacokinetic parameters, it is likely that the patient has different pharmacokinetic characteristics. It is possible to measure the patient's own unique pharmacokinetic parameters using four serum concentrations (Figure 4-9).

- The intradialysis elimination rate constant can be determined by obtaining postdose ($C_{postdose(1)}$) and predialysis ($C_{predialysis}$) concentrations [$k_e = (\ln C_{postdose} - \ln C_{predialysis})/\Delta t$, where Δt is the time between the two concentrations], the fraction of drug eliminated by dialysis can be computed using predialysis and postdialysis ($C_{postdialysis}$) concentrations (fraction eliminated = [$(C_{predialysis} - C_{postdialysis})/C_{predialysis}$], and the volume of distribution can be calculated using postdialysis and postdose concentrations [$V = D/(C_{postdose(2)} - C_{predialysis})$].
- Note that if the drug has a postdialysis "rebound" in drug concentrations, postdialysis serum samples should be obtained after blood and tissue have had the opportunity to reequilibrate. In the case of aminoglycosides, postdialysis samples should be collected no sooner that 3–4 hours after the end of dialysis.
- Once individualized pharmacokinetic parameters have been measured, they can be used in the same equations used to compute initial doses in the previous section in place of average, population pharmacokinetic parameters and used to calculate individualized doses for dialysis patients. It is also possible to use a mixture of measured and population-estimated pharmacokinetic parameters. For instance, a clinician may wish to measure the elimination rate constant or volume of distribution for a patient, but elect to use an average population estimate for fraction of drug removed by the artificial kidney.

REFERENCES

1. Chambers HF, Sande MA. Antimicrobial agents: the aminoglycosides. In: Hardman JG, Limbird LE, Molinoff PB, Ruddon RW, Gilman AG, eds. Goodman and Gilman's the pharmacological basis of therapeutics. 9th ed. New York: McGraw-Hill,1996:1103–22.
2. Zaske DE, Cipolle RJ, Rotschafer JC, Solem LD, Mosier NR, Strate RG. Gentamicin pharmacokinetics in 1,640 patients: method for control of serum concentrations. Antimicrob Agents Chemother 1982;21:407–11.
3. Prins JM, Buller HR, Kuijper EJ, Tange RA, Speelman P. Once versus thrice daily gentamicin in patients with serious infections [see comments]. Lancet 1993; 341(8841):335–9.
4. Nicolau DP, Freeman CD, Belliveau PP, Nightingale CH, Ross JW, Quintilliani R. Experience with a once-daily aminoglycoside program administered to 2,184 adult patients. Antimicrob Agent Chemother 1995;39:650–5.
5. Maller R, Ahrne H, Holmen C, Lausen I, Nilsson LE, Smedjegard J. Once- versus twice-daily amikacin regimen: efficacy and safety in systemic gram-negative infections. Scandinavian Amikacin Once Daily Study Group. J Antimicrob Chemother 1993;31(6):939–48.
6. Jackson GG, Arcieri G. Ototoxicity of gentamicin in man: a survey and controlled analysis of clinical experience in the United States. J Infect Dis 1971;124 (suppl): 130–7.
7. Smith CR, Maxwell RR, Edwards CQ, Rogers JF, Lietman PS. Nephrotoxicity induced by gentamicin and amikacin. Johns Hopkins Med J 1978;142(3):85–90.
8. Dahlgren JG, Anderson ET, Hewitt WL. Gentamicin blood levels: a guide to nephrotoxicity. Antimicrob Agents Chemother 1975;8:58–62.
9. Schentag JJ, Plaut ME, Cerra FB, Wels PB, Walczak P, Buckley RJ. Aminoglycoside nephrotoxicity in critically ill surgical patients. J Surg Res 1979;26:270–9.
10. Rybak MJ, Albrecht LM, Boike SC, Chandrasekar PH. Nephrotoxicity of vancomycin, alone and with an aminoglycoside. J Antimicrob Chemother 1990; 25(4):679–87.

11. Lane AZ, Wright GE, Blair DC. Ototoxicity and nephrotoxicity of amikacin: an overview of Phase II and Phase III experience in the United States. Am J Med 1977;62(6):911–8.
12. Schentag JJ, Cerra FB, Plaut ME. Clinical and pharmacokinetic characteristics of aminoglycoside nephrotoxicity in 201 critically ill patients. Antimicrob Agents Chemother 1982;21(5):721–6.
13. Bertino JS Jr, Booker LA, Franck PA, Jenkins PL, Franck KR, Nafziger AN. Incidence of and significant risk factors for aminoglycoside-associated nephrotoxicity in patients dosed by using individualized pharmacokinetic monitoring [see comments]. J Infect Dis 1993;167(1):173–9.
14. Barclay ML, Begg EJ, Hickling KG. What is the evidence for once-daily aminoglycoside therapy? Clin Pharmacokinet 1994;27(1):32–48.
15. Barclay ML, Duffull SB, Begg EJ, Buttimore RC. Experience of once-daily aminoglycoside dosing using a target area under the concentration-time curve. Austral N Z J Med 1995;25(3):230–5.
16. Barclay ML, Kirkpatrick CM, Begg EJ. Once daily aminoglycoside therapy. Is it less toxic than multiple daily doses and how should it be monitored? [In process citation]. Clin Pharmacokinet 1999;36(2):89–98.
17. Begg EJ, Barclay ML, Duffull SB. A suggested approach to once-daily aminoglycoside dosing. Br J Clin Pharmacol 1995;39(6):605–9.
18. Blaser J, Konig C, Simmen HP, Thurnheer U. Monitoring serum concentrations for once-daily netilmicin dosing regimens. J Antimicrob Chemother 1994;33(2):341–8.
19. Janknegt R. Aminoglycoside monitoring in the once- or twice-daily era. The Dutch situation considered. Pharm World Sci 1993;15(4):151–5.
20. Prins JM, Koopmans RP, Buller HR, Kuijper EJ, Speelman P. Easier monitoring of aminoglycoside therapy with once-daily dosing schedules. Eur J Clin Microbiol Infect Dis 1995;14(6):531–5.
21. Schentag JJ, Jusko WJ. Renal clearance and tissue accumulation of gentamicin. Clin Pharmacol Ther 1977;22:364–70.
22. Vic P, Ategbo S, Turck D, et al. Efficacy, tolerance, and pharmacokinetics of once daily tobramycin for pseudomonas exacerbations in cystic fibrosis. Arch Dis Child 1998;78(6):536–9.
23. Bragonier R, Brown NM. The pharmacokinetics and toxicity of once-daily tobramycin therapy in children with cystic fibrosis. J Antimicrob Chemother 1998;42(1):103–6.
24. Bates RD, Nahata MC, Jones JW, et al. Pharmacokinetics and safety of tobramycin after once-daily administration in patients with cystic fibrosis. Chest 1997;112(5):1208–13.
25. Bass KD, Larkin SE, Paap C, Haase GM. Pharmacokinetics of once-daily gentamicin dosing in pediatric patients. J Pediatr Surg 1998;33(7):1104–7.
26. Weber W, Kewitz G, Rost KL, Looby M, Nitz M, Harnisch L. Population kinetics of gentamicin in neonates. Eur J Clin Pharmacol 1993;44(suppl 1):S23–5.
27. Demczar DJ, Nafziger AN, Bertino JS Jr. Pharmacokinetics of gentamicin at traditional versus high doses: implications for once-daily aminoglycoside dosing. Antimicrob Agents Chemother 1997;41(5):1115–9.
28. Bauer LA, Blouin RA. Amikacin pharmacokinetics in young men with pneumonia. Clin Pharm 1982;1(4):353–5.
29. Bauer LA, Blouin RA. Influence of age on tobramycin pharmacokinetics in patients with normal renal function. Antimicrob Agents Chemother 1981;20(5):587–9.
30. Bauer LA, Blouin RA. Gentamicin pharmacokinetics: effect of aging in patients with normal renal function. J Am Geriatr Soc 1982;30(5):309–11.
31. Bauer LA, Blouin RA. Influence of age on amikacin pharmacokinetics in patients without renal disease. Comparison with gentamicin and tobramycin. Eur J Clin Pharmacol 1983;24(5):639–42.
32. Barza M, Brown RB, Shen D, Gibaldi M, Weinstein L. Predictability of blood levels of gentamicin in man. J Infect Dis 1975;132(2):165–74.

33. Kaye D, Levison ME, Labovitz ED. The unpredictability of serum concentrations of gentamicin: pharmacokinetics of gentamicin in patients with normal and abnormal renal function. J Infect Dis 1974;130(2):150–4.

34. Sarubbi FA Jr, Hull JH. Amikacin serum concentrations: prediction of levels and dosage guidelines. Ann Intern Med 1978;89(5 pt 1):612–8.

35. Hull JH, Sarubbi FA Jr. Gentamicin serum concentrations: pharmacokinetic predictions. Ann Intern Med 1976;85(2):183–9.

36. Bootman JL, Wertheimer AI, Zaske D, Rowland C. Individualizing gentamicin dosage regimens in burn patients with gram-negative septicemia: a cost–benefit analysis. J Pharm Sci 1979;68(3):267–72.

37. Zaske DE, Sawchuk RJ, Gerding DN, Strate RG. Increased dosage requirements of gentamicin in burn patients. J Trauma 1976;16(10):824–8.

38. Zaske DE, Sawchuk RJ, Strate RG. The necessity of increased doses of amikacin in burn patients. Surgery 1978;84(5):603–8.

39. Tindula RJ, Ambrose PJ, Harralson AF. Aminoglycoside inactivation by penicillins and cephalosporins and its impact on drug-level monitoring. Drug Intell Clin Pharm 1983;17(12):906–8.

40. Wallace SM, Chan LY. In vitro interaction of aminoglycosides with beta-lactam penicillins. Antimicrob Agents Chemother 1985;28(2):274–81.

41. Henderson JL, Polk RE, Kline BJ. In vitro inactivation of gentamicin, tobramycin, and netilmicin by carbenicillin, azlocillin, or mezlocillin. Am J Hosp Pharm 1981;38(8):1167–70.

42. Pickering LK, Rutherford I. Effect of concentration and time upon inactivation of tobramycin, gentamicin, netilmicin and amikacin by azlocillin, carbenicillin, mecillinam, mezlocillin and piperacillin. J Pharmacol Exp Ther 1981;217(2):345–9.

43. Hale DC, Jenkins R, Matsen JM. In-vitro inactivation of aminoglycoside antibiotics by piperacillin and carbenicillin. Am J Clin Pathol 1980;74(3):316–9.

44. Bauer LA, Blouin RA, Griffen WO Jr, Record KE, Bell RM. Amikacin pharmacokinetics in morbidly obese patients. Am J Hosp Pharm 1980;37(4):519–22.

45. Bauer LA, Edwards WA, Dellinger EP, Simonowitz DA. Influence of weight on aminoglycoside pharmacokinetics in normal weight and morbidly obese patients. Eur J Clin Pharmacol 1983;24(5):643–7.

46. Blouin RA, Mann HJ, Griffen WO Jr, Bauer LA, Record KE. Tobramycin pharmacokinetics in morbidly obese patients. Clin Pharmacol Ther 1979;26(4):508–12.

47. Bauer LA, Piecoro JJ Jr, Wilson HD, Blouin RA. Gentamicin and tobramycin pharmacokinetics in patients with cystic fibrosis. Clin Pharm 1983;2(3):262–4.

48. Bosso JA, Townsend PL, Herbst JJ, Matsen JM. Pharmacokinetics and dosage requirements of netilmicin in cystic fibrosis patients. Antimicrob Agents Chemother 1985;28(6):829–31.

49. Kearns GL, Hilman BC, Wilson JT. Dosing implications of altered gentamicin disposition in patients with cystic fibrosis. J Pediatr 1982;100(2):312–8.

50. Kelly HB, Menendez R, Fan L, Murphy S. Pharmacokinetics of tobramycin in cystic fibrosis. J Pediatr 1982;100(2):318–21.

51. Ramsey BW, Pepe MS, Quan JM, et al. Intermittent administration of inhaled tobramycin in patients with cystic fibrosis. Cystic Fibrosis Inhaled Tobramycin Study Group. N Engl J Med 1999;340(1):23–30.

52. Izquierdo M, Lanao JM, Cervero L, Jimenez NV, Dominguez-Gil A. Population pharmacokinetics of gentamicin in premature infants. Ther Drug Monit 1992;14(3):177–83.

53. Hindmarsh KW, Nation RL, Williams GL, John E, French JN. Pharmacokinetics of gentamicin in very low birth weight preterm infants. Eur J Clin Pharmacol 1983;24(5):649–53.

54. Rameis H, Popow C, Graninger W. Gentamicin monitoring in low-birth-weight newborns. Biol Res Pregnancy Perinatol 1983;4(3):123–6.

55. Diseases AAoPCoI. 2003 Red book: report of the committee on infectious diseases. 26th ed. Evanston, IL: American Academy of Pediatrics, 2003.

56. Gunn VL, Nechyba C, eds. The Harriet Lane handbook: a manual for pediatric house officers. 16th ed. Philadelphia: Mosby, 2002.

57. Madhavan T, Yaremchuk K, Levin N, et al. Effect of renal failure and dialysis on the serum concentration of the aminoglycoside amikacin. Antimicrob Agents Chemother 1976;10(3):464–6.

58. Armstrong DK, Hodgman T, Visconti JA, Reilley TE, Garner WL, Dasta JF. Hemodialysis of amikacin in critically ill patients. Crit Care Med 1988;16(5): 517–20.

59. Herrero A, Rius Alarco F, Garcia Diez JM, Mahiques E, Domingo JV. Pharmacokinetics of netilmicin in renal insufficiency and hemodialysis. Int J Clin Pharmacol Ther Toxicol 1988;26(2):84–7.

60. Halstenson CE, Berkseth RO, Mann HJ, Matzke GR. Aminoglycoside redistribution phenomenon after hemodialysis: netilmicin and tobramycin. Int J Clin Pharmacol Ther Toxicol 1987;25(1):50–5.

61. Matzke GR, Halstenson CE, Keane WF. Hemodialysis elimination rates and clearance of gentamicin and tobramycin. Antimicrob Agents Chemother 1984;25(1): 128–30.

62. Basile C, Di Maggio A, Curino E, Scatizzi A. Pharmacokinetics of netilmicin in hypertonic hemodiafiltration and standard hemodialysis. Clin Nephrol 1985;24(6):305–9.

63. Smeltzer BD, Schwartzman MS, Bertino JS, Jr. Amikacin pharmacokinetics during continuous ambulatory peritoneal dialysis. Antimicrob Agents Chemother 1988;32(2):236–40.

64. Pancorbo S, Comty C. Pharmacokinetics of gentamicin in patients undergoing continuous ambulatory peritoneal dialysis. Antimicrob Agents Chemother 1981;19(4): 605–7.

65. Bunke CM, Aronoff GR, Brier ME, Sloan RS, Luft FC. Tobramycin kinetics during continuous ambulatory peritoneal dialysis. Clin Pharmacol Ther 1983;34(1):110–6.

66. Forni LG, Hilton PJ. Continuous hemofiltration in the treatment of acute renal failure. N Engl J Med 1997;336(18):1303–9.

67. Gilbert DN, Moellering RC, Eliopoulos GM, Sande MA. The Sanford guide to antimicrobial therapy. 34th ed. Hyde Park, VT: Antimicrobial Therapy, 2004.

68. Chandrasekar PH, Cronin SM. Nephrotoxicity in bone marrow transplant recipients receiving aminoglycoside plus cyclosporine or aminoglycoside alone. J Antimicrob Chemother 1991;27(6):845–9.

69. Moore RD, Smith CR, Lipsky JJ, Mellits ED, Lietman PS. Risk factors for nephrotoxicity in patients treated with aminoglycosides. Ann Intern Med 1984;100(3): 352–7.

70. Harpur ES. The pharmacology of ototoxic drugs. Br J Audiol 1982;16(2):81–93.

71. Mathog RH, Klein WJ Jr. Ototoxicity of ethacrynic acid and aminoglycoside antibiotics in uremia. N Engl J Med 1969;280(22):1223–4.

72. Paradelis AG, Triantaphyllidis C, Giala MM. Neuromuscular blocking activity of aminoglycoside antibiotics. Methods Find Exp Clin Pharmacol 1980;2(1):45–51.

73. Sawchuk RJ, Zaske DE, Cipolle RJ, Wargin WA, Strate RG. Kinetic model for gentamicin dosing with the use of individual patient parameters. Clin Pharmacol Ther 1977;21(3):362–9.

74. Murphy JE, Winter ME. Clinical pharmacokinetic pearls: bolus versus infusion equations. Pharmacotherapy 1996;16(4):698–700.

75. Spinler SA, Nawarskas JJ, Boyce EG, Connors JE, Charland SL, Goldfarb S. Predictive performance of ten equations for estimating creatinine clearance in cardiac patients. Iohexol Cooperative Study Group. Ann Pharmacother 1998;32(12):1275–83.

76. Salazar DE, Corcoran GB. Predicting creatinine clearance and renal drug clearance in obese patients from estimated fat-free body mass. Am J Med 1988;84(6): 1053–60.

77. McCormack JP, Carleton B. A simpler approach to pharmacokinetic dosage adjustments. Pharmacotherapy 1997;17(6):1349–51.

78. Burton ME, Brater DC, Chen PS, Day RB, Huber PJ, Vasko MR. A Bayesian feedback method of aminoglycoside dosing. Clin Pharmacol Ther 1985;37(3):349–57.

79. Burton ME, Chow MS, Platt DR, Day RB, Brater DC, Vasko MR. Accuracy of Bayesian and Sawchuk-Zaske dosing methods for gentamicin. Clin Pharm 1986;5(2):143–9.

80. Rodvold KA, Blum RA. Predictive performance of Sawchuk-Zaske and Bayesian dosing methods for tobramycin. J Clin Pharmacol 1987;27(5):419–24.
81. Murray KM, Bauer LA, Koup JR. Predictive performance of computer dosing methods for tobramycin using two pharmacokinetic models and two weighting algorithms. Clin Pharm 1986;5(5):411–4.
82. Koup JR, Killen T, Bauer LA. Multiple-dose non-linear regression analysis program. Aminoglycoside dose prediction. Clin Pharmacokinet 1983;8(5):456–62.
83. Wandell M, Mungall D. Computer assisted drug interpretation and drug regimen optimization. Am Assoc Clin Chem 1984;6:1–11.

5 | Vancomycin

Vancomycin is a glycopeptide antibiotic used to treat severe gram-positive infections due to organisms that are resistant to other antibiotics. It is also used to treat infections caused by other sensitive gram-positive organisms in patients who are allergic to penicillins.

- Vancomycin is bactericidal and exhibits time-dependent or concentration-independent bacterial killing.[1] Many strains of enterococcus have high minimum inhibitory concentration (MIC) values for vancomycin, and for these bacteria vancomycin may demonstrate only bacteriostatic properties.
- The mechanism of action of vancomycin is inhibition of cell wall synthesis in susceptible bacteria by binding to the D-alanyl-D-alanine terminal end of cell wall precursor units.[2]

THERAPEUTIC AND TOXIC CONCENTRATIONS

- Vancomycin is administered as a short-term (1-hour) intravenous infusion. Infusion rate-related side effects have been noted when shorter infusion times (~30 minutes or less) have been used [urticarial or erythematous reactions, intense flushing (known as the "red-man" or "red-neck" syndrome), tachycardia, and hypotension].

  - For doses exceeding 1500 mg, longer infusion times (1.5–2 hours) may be necessary to avoid infusion rate-related adverse effects.

- The therapeutic range for steady-state peak concentrations is usually considered to be 20–40 μg/ml. Because vancomycin does not enter the central nervous system in appreciable amounts when given intravenously,[2] steady-state peak concentrations of 40–60 μg/ml or direct administration into the cerebral spinal fluid may be necessary to treat central nervous system infections.[3, 4]

  - Because vancomycin serum concentrations exhibit a postinfusion distribution phase, a $\frac{1}{2}$–1-hour waiting period is allowed for distribution to finish before maximum or "peak" concentrations are measured (Figure 5-1). Since vancomycin exhibits time-dependent killing, microbiological or clinical cure rates are not closely associated with peak serum concentrations.

- Vancomycin-associated ototoxicity has been reported when serum concentrations exceed 80 μg/ml[5,6] and is usually first noted by the appearance of tinnitus, dizziness, or high-frequency hearing loss (>4000 Hz).[4,6,7] Ototoxicity can be permanent if appropriate changes in vancomycin dosing are not made.[4, 6–8] In some reports of vancomycin-induced ototoxicity, it is unclear when vancomycin serum concentrations were obtained during the dosage interval, so the exact association between peak concentrations and ototoxicity is uncertain.

  - Since audiometry is difficult to conduct in seriously ill patients, it is rarely done in patients receiving ototoxic drugs. Thus, clinicians should monitor for signs and symptoms that may indicate ototoxicity is occurring in a patient (auditory: tinnitus, feeling of fullness or pressure in the ears, loss of hearing acuity in the conversational range; vestibular: loss of equilibrium, headache, nausea, vomiting, vertigo, dizziness, nystagmus, ataxia).

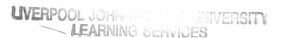

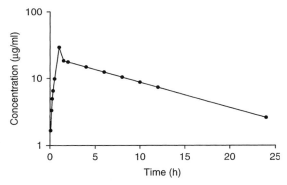

FIG. 5-1 Concentration/time plot for vancomycin 1000 mg given as a 1-hour infusion (circles with solid line). When given as a 1-hour infusion, end-of-infusion concentrations are higher because the serum and tissues are not in equilibrium. A $\frac{1}{2}$–1-hour waiting time for vancomycin distribution to tissues is allowed before peak concentrations are measured.

- Trough concentrations (predose or minimum concentrations, usually obtained within 30 minutes of the next dose) are usually related to therapeutic outcome for vancomycin because the antibiotic follows time-dependent bacterial killing.[1] Optimal bactericidal effects are found at concentrations 3–5 times the organism's MIC.[1,9] Because the average vancomycin MICs for *Staphylococcus aureus* and *S. epidermidis* are 1–2 µg/ml, minimum predose or trough steady-state concentrations equal to 5–10 µg/ml are usually adequate to resolve infections by susceptible organisms.

  - Trough vancomycin steady-state concentrations above 15 µg/ml are related to an increased incidence of nephrotoxicity.[10,11] Vancomycin-related nephrotoxicity is usually reversible with a low incidence of residual damage if the antibiotic is withdrawn or doses appropriately adjusted soon after renal function tests change. With adequate patient monitoring, the only result of vancomycin nephrotoxicity may be transient serum creatinine increases of 0.5–2.0 mg/dl.
  - Many patients receiving vancomycin are critically ill, so other sources of renal dysfunction, such as hypotension or other nephrotoxic drug therapy, should be ruled out before the diagnosis of vancomycin-induced renal damage is made in a patient. Compared to aminoglycoside antibiotics, vancomycin is usually considered to have less nephrotoxicity potential.[12]

- When using vancomycin, nephrotoxicity and ototoxicity cannot be completely avoided by keeping serum concentrations within the suggested ranges. However, by adjusting vancomycin dosage regimens so that potentially toxic serum concentrations are avoided, drug concentration-related adverse effects may be held to the absolute minimum.

CLINICAL MONITORING PARAMETERS

- Confirm that antibiotic therapy is appropriate for current microbiological cultures and sensitivities.

- Confirm appropriate concurrent antibiotic therapy, such as aminoglycosides or rifampin, when necessary to treat the infection.
- Measurements of serial white blood cell counts and body temperatures are useful to determine the efficacy of antibiotic therapy. A large number of neutrophils and immature neutrophils, known clinically as a "shift to the left," can also be observed in patients with severe bacterial infections.

  - Favorable response to antibiotic treatment is usually indicated by high white blood cell counts decreasing toward the normal range, the trend of body temperatures (plotted as body temperature versus time, also known as the "fever curve") approaching normal, and any specific infection-site tests or procedures resolving.
  - Clinicians should also be aware that immunocompromised patients with bacterial infections may not be able to mount a fever or elevated white blood cell count.

- Vancomycin steady-state serum concentrations should be measured after 3–5 estimated half-lives. Methods to estimate this parameter are given in the initial-dose calculation portion of this chapter.

  - Since the dosage interval is often prolonged in patients with decreased elimination, a useful clinical rule is to measure serum concentrations after the third dose. Additionally, the third dose typically occurs 1–3 days after dosing has commenced, and this is also a good time to assess clinical efficacy of the treatment.
  - Steady-state serum concentrations, in conjunction with clinical response, are used to adjust the antibiotic dose, if necessary. Methods for adjusting vancomycin doses using serum concentrations are discussed later in this chapter.
  - If the dosage is adjusted, vancomycin elimination changes, or laboratory and clinical monitoring indicate that the infection is not resolving or worsening, clinicians should consider rechecking steady-state drug concentrations.

- Some individuals advocate the measurement of only a steady-state trough concentration.[13]

  - The reasoning for trough-only monitoring is as follows. (1) Vancomycin follows time-dependent bacterial killing, and the efficacy of the drug should be most closely related to the minimum serum concentration encountered over the dosage interval. (2) Nephrotoxicity is related to high trough concentrations, so measurement of this value should ensure therapeutic, non-nephrotoxic drug concentrations. (3) If a patient has a therapeutic steady-state trough concentration (5–10 μg/ml) and the dose is in the usual range (500–1500 mg), it is difficult to produce a steady-state peak concentration that will be above the accepted toxic range (>80 μg/ml).[14]

- Serial monitoring of serum creatinine concentrations should be used to detect nephrotoxicity. Ideally, a baseline serum creatinine concentration is obtained before vancomycin therapy is initiated and three times weekly or every other day during treatment. An increasing serum creatinine test on two or more consecutive measurement occasions indicates that more intensive monitoring of serum creatinine values, such as daily, is needed.

  - If serum creatinine measurements increase more than 0.5 mg/dl over the baseline value (or >25–30% over baseline for serum creatinine values >2 mg/dl) and other causes of declining renal function have been ruled out (other nephrotoxic drugs or agents, hypotension, etc.), alternatives to vancomycin therapy or, if that option is not possible, intensive vancomycin serum concentration monitoring should be initiated to ensure that excessive amounts of vancomycin do not accumulate in the patient.

- In the clinical setting, audiometry is rarely used to detect ototoxicity because it is difficult to accomplish in severely ill patients. Instead, clinical signs and symptoms of auditory (decreased hearing acuity in the conversational range, feeling of fullness or pressure in the ears, tinnitus) or vestibular (loss of equilibrium, headache, nausea, vomiting, vertigo, nystagmus, ataxia) ototoxicity are monitored at the same time intervals as serum creatinine determination.
- Vancomycin can also cause allergic symptoms such as chills, fever, skin rashes, and anaphylactoid reactions.

BASIC CLINICAL PHARMACOKINETIC PARAMETERS

- Vancomycin is almost completely eliminated unchanged in the urine, primarily by glomerular filtration ($\geq 90\%$; Table 5-1).[15]
- This antibiotic is given by short-term (1-hour) intermittent intravenous infusion. Intramuscular administration is usually avoided because this route has been reported to cause tissue necrosis at the site of injection.
- Oral bioavailability is poor (<10%), so systemic infections cannot be treated by this route of administration.[5] However, patients with renal failure who

TABLE 5-1 Disease States and Conditions That Alter
Vancomycin Pharmacokinetics

Disease state/condition	Half-life (h)	Volume of distribution (L/kg)	Comment
Adults, normal renal function	8 (range; 7–9)	0.7 (range; 0.5–1.0)	Usual dose 30 mg/kg/d in two divided doses
Adults, renal failure	130 (range; 120–140)	0.7 (range; 0.5–1.0)	Under- or overhydration does not affect the volume of distribution as much as with aminoglycosides
Burn patients	4	0.7	Because of shorter half-life, some patients may need a 6–8-hour dosage interval to maintain therapeutic trough concentrations
Obese patients (>30% over IBW) with normal renal function	3–4	V = 0.7 IBW	Total daily doses are based on TBW, V estimates based on IBW; because of shorter half-life, some patients may require an 8-hour dosage interval to maintain therapeutic trough concentrations

IBW is ideal body weight, TBW is total body weight.

have been given oral vancomycin for the treatment of antibiotic-associated colitis have accumulated therapeutic concentrations because gut wall inflammation increased vancomycin bioavailability and renal dysfunction decreased drug clearance.[16–19]

- Plasma protein binding is ~55%.[20]
- The recommended dose for vancomycin in patients with normal renal function is 30 mg/kg/d given as two or four divided daily doses. In normal-weight adults, the dose is usually 2 gm/d given as 1000 mg every 12 hours.

EFFECTS OF DISEASE STATES AND CONDITIONS ON VANCOMYCIN PHARMACOKINETICS AND DOSING

- Nonobese adults with normal renal function (creatinine clearance > 80 ml/min, Table 5-1) have an average vancomycin half-life of 8 hours (range, 7–9 hours), and the average volume of distribution for vancomycin is 0.7 L/kg (range, 0.5–0.9 L/kg) in this population.[21,22] Because of the moderate size of volume of distribution, fluid balance (under- or overhydration) is less of an issue with vancomycin compared to the aminoglycoside antibiotics.

Renal Dysfunction

- Since vancomycin is eliminated principally by glomerular filtration, renal dysfunction is the most important disease state that influences vancomycin pharmacokinetics.[23–25] Vancomycin total clearance decreases proportionally to decreases in creatinine clearance.[23]

Burns

- Major body burns (>30–40% body surface area) can cause large changes in vancomycin pharmacokinetics.[26] Forty-eight to 72 hours after a major burn, glomerular filtration rate increases, which increases vancomycin clearance. Because of the increase in drug clearance, the average half-life for vancomycin in burn patients is 4 hours.

Obesity

- Obese individuals with normal serum creatinine concentrations have increased vancomycin clearance secondary to increased glomerular filtration rate and are best dosed with vancomycin using total body weight.[21, 22, 27, 28] Volume of distribution does not change significantly with obesity and is best estimated using ideal body weight (IBW) in patients who are more than 30% overweight (>30% over IBW, V = 0.7 L/kg IBW).[21,22,28] Because the primary pharmacokinetic change for vancomycin in obesity is increased drug clearance with a negligible change in volume of distribution, average half-life decreases to 3.3 hours ($t_{1/2} = [0.693 \cdot V]/Cl$).

  - While the average dose in morbidly obese and normal-weight patients with normal serum creatinine concentrations is ~30 mg/kg/d using total body weight in both populations, some morbidly obese patients require dosing every 8 hours to maintain vancomycin steady-state trough concentrations above 5 µg/ml.[21]

Neonates/Infants/Children

- Premature infants (gestational age <32 weeks) have a larger amount of body water compared to adults. However, vancomycin volume of distribution

(V = 0.7 L/kg) is not greatly affected by these larger amounts of body water as is the case with aminoglycoside antibiotics.[29] Kidneys are not completely developed at this early age, so glomerular filtration and vancomycin clearance (15 ml/min) are decreased.[29] A lower clearance rate with about the same volume of distribution as adults results in a longer average half-life for vancomycin in premature babies (10 hours).

- Full-term neonates (gestational age ~40 weeks) have similar volumes of distribution for vancomycin compared to premature infants, but their vancomycin clearance rate is twice that found in infants born prematurely (30 ml/min). The increase in drug clearance is due to additional renal development that occurred *in utero*. The vancomycin half-life in full-term babies is about 7 hours.
- At about 3 months of age, vancomycin clearance has nearly doubled again (50 ml/min), resulting in a half-life of approximately 4 hours. The increase in vancomycin clearance continues through 4–8 years of age, when clearance equals 130–160 ml/min while volume of distribution remains ~ 0.7 L/kg so that half-life is 2–3 hours. At that time, vancomycin clearance and half-life gradually approach adult values as children approach puberty (~12–14 years old).
- Intravenous doses for neonates are based on birthweight and age.[30] Steady-state vancomycin serum concentrations are used to individualize doses:

Weight	Postnatal age	
	<7 Days	≥7 Days
<1.2 kg	15 mg/kg every 24 h	15 mg/kg every 24 h
1.2–2 kg	10–15 mg/kg every 12–18 h	10–15 mg/kg every 8–12 h
>2 kg	10–15 mg/kg every 8–12 h	15–20 mg/kg every 8 h

- Intravenous doses for infants and children are 60 mg/kg/d given every 6 hours for central nervous system infections and 40 mg/kg/d given every 6–8 h for other infections, with a maximum of 1 g/dose.[30] Steady-state vancomycin serum concentrations are used to individualize doses.

Dialysis

- The effect of hemodialysis on vancomycin pharmacokinetics depends on the type of artificial kidney used for the procedure. Vancomycin is a relatively large molecule with a moderate-sized volume of distribution and intermediate protein binding. These characteristics lead to poor hemodialysis removal from the body. The mean vancomycin half-life for patients with renal failure is 120–140 hours.[25,31,32]

- Using traditional "low-flux" hemodialysis filters, an insignificant amount (<10%) of the total vancomycin body stores is removed during a 3–4-hour dialysis period.[24,33]
- Using a "high-flux" filter, vancomycin serum concentrations decrease by one-third during the dialysis period but then slowly increase or "rebound" for the next 10–12 hours, reaching nearly 90% of predialysis values.[34] To determine if supplemental doses of vancomycin are needed, postdialysis serum concentrations should be measured after the rebound period in patients receiving hemodialysis with a "high-flux" filter.

- Peritoneal dialysis removes only a negligible amount of vancomycin.[35–37]

  - Patients who develop peritonitis while receiving peritoneal dialysis can be treated by placing vancomycin into the dialysis fluid. Over a 6-hour dwell time, approximately 50% of a vancomycin dose (1000 mg in 2 L of dialysis fluid) is absorbed from the peritoneal cavity in renal failure patients without peritonitis.[35] Peritonitis causes inflammation of the peritoneal membrane, which facilitates absorption of vancomycin placed in the peritoneal dialysis fluid (up to 90% absorbed) and dialysis elimination of vancomycin from the body.[37]

- Hemofiltration removes vancomycin from the body. Recommended doses for critically ill patients with acute renal failure undergoing continuous venovenous hemofiltration (CVVH) are a loading dose of 15–20 mg/kg followed by 250–500 mg every 12 hours.[38] For patients undergoing continuous arteriovenous hemofiltration (CAVH), the recommended dose is 500 mg every 24–48 hours.[39] Because of pharmacokinetic variability, vancomycin concentrations should be measured in hemofiltration patients.

DRUG INTERACTIONS

- Most important drug interactions with vancomycin are pharmacodynamic, not pharmacokinetic, in nature. Coadministration of aminoglycoside antibiotics enhances the nephrotoxicity potential of vancomycin.[10,40,41] Aminoglycosides can cause nephrotoxicity when administered alone. When an aminoglycoside and vancomycin are administered concurrently, serum creatinine concentrations should be monitored on a daily basis. Additionally, serum concentrations of the aminoglycoside, as well as vancomycin, should be measured.

- When vancomycin is administered to patients stabilized on warfarin therapy, the hypoprothrombinemic effect of the anticoagulant may be augmented.[42] The mechanism of this interaction is unknown, but resulted in a mean 45% increase in prothrombin time over baseline values when warfarin was given alone. Patients receiving warfarin therapy who require vancomycin treatment should have a baseline prothrombin time ratio (INR) measured before the antibiotic is administered and daily INR tests until it is certain that anticoagulation status is stable.

INITIAL DOSAGE DETERMINATION METHODS

- Several methods to initiate vancomycin therapy are available.

  - The *pharmacokinetic dosing method* is the most flexible technique. It allows individualized target serum concentrations to be chosen for a patient, and each pharmacokinetic parameter can be customized to reflect specific disease states and conditions present in the patient. However, it is computationally intensive.

  - *Nomograms* use the dosing concepts in the pharmacokinetic dosing method. However, in order to simplify calculations, they make simplifying assumptions.

    - The *Moellering nomogram* is designed to achieve average steady-state concentrations equal to 15 µg/ml. Some clinicians find this approach confusing since target steady-state peak and trough concentrations are not stated by the nomogram. Since the computed dose provided by the nomogram is expressed in mg/kg/24 h, it can be difficult to determine the best dosage interval. However, once experience is gained with this approach, the Moellering nomogram computes doses similar, but not identical, to the pharmacokinetic dosing method.

- The *Matzke nomogram* is constructed to produce steady-state vancomycin peak and trough concentrations of 30 and 7.5 μg/ml, respectively. When these target concentrations are acceptable, the Matzke nomogram computes doses that are very similar to those calculated by the pharmacokinetic dosing method. However, since the expected peak and trough concentrations are in the middle of their respective therapeutic ranges, the Matzke nomogram computes relatively large doses for patients.

Pharmacokinetic Dosing Method

- The goal of initial dosing of vancomycin is to compute the best dose possible for the patient given the disease states and conditions that influence vancomycin pharmacokinetics and the site and severity of the infection. In order to do this, pharmacokinetic parameters for the patient are estimated using mean parameters measured in other individuals with similar disease state and condition profiles.

Clearance Estimate

- Vancomycin is eliminated by the kidney almost completely unchanged, and there is a good relationship between creatinine clearance and vancomycin clearance.[23] This relationship permits estimation of the vancomycin clearance for a patient, which can be used to calculate an initial dose of the drug: Cl = 0.695(CrCl) + 0.05, where Cl is vancomycin clearance in ml/min/kg and CrCl is creatinine clearance in ml/min/kg. The weight factor that is used for all individuals, including obese patients, is total body weight (TBW).[21,22,25,27,28]

Volume of Distribution Estimate

- The average volume of distribution of vancomycin is 0.7 L/kg.[21,22] The weight factor that is used to calculate vancomycin volume of distribution for obese patients (>30% overweight) is ideal body weight (IBW).[21,22,28]

Elimination Rate Constant and Half-Life Estimates

- The vancomycin elimination rate constant (k_e) is computed using the estimated clearance and volume of distribution values for the drug in the following equation: $k_e = Cl/V$. It is usually expressed using the unit of h^{-1}.

Selection of Appropriate Pharmacokinetic Model and Equations

- When given by intravenous infusion over an hour, vancomycin serum concentrations follow a two- or three-compartment pharmacokinetic model (Figure 5-1). While it is important to understand these models conceptually, they cannot easily be used clinically because of their mathematical complexity. Because of this, the simpler one-compartment model is widely used, which allows accurate dosage calculation when peak vancomycin serum concentrations are obtained after drug distribution is finished.[21,25]

  - Intravenously administered vancomycin is given over 1 hour as an intermittent continuous infusion. Since the drug has a long half-life relative to the infusion time (1 hour) and waiting time (0.5–1 hour) necessary to

TABLE 5-2A One Compartment-Model Equations Used with Vancomycin

Route of administration	Single dose	Multiple dose	Steady state
Intravenous bolus	$C = (D/V)e^{-k_e t}$	$C = (D/V)e^{-k_e t}[(1 - e^{-nk_e\tau})/(1 - e^{-k_e\tau})]$	$C = (D/V)[e^{-k_e t}/(1 - e^{-k_e\tau})]$

C is drug serum concentration at time = t, D is dose, V is volume of distribution, k_e is elimination rate constant, n is number of administered doses, τ is dosage interval.

allow for distribution to complete before peak concentrations are obtained, little of the drug is eliminated during this 1.5–2-hour time period. Intravenous-infusion pharmacokinetic equations that take into account the loss of drug during the infusion time are not generally needed because so little vancomycin is eliminated during the infusion and waiting-time periods.

• Although the antibiotic is given as an intravenous infusion, intravenous bolus equations accurately predict peak vancomycin concentrations and are mathematically simpler.[43] Steady-state versions of one-compartment-model intravenous bolus equations are as follows (Table 5-2):

$$C_{max,ss} = (D/V)/(1 - e^{-k_e\tau})$$
$$C_{min,ss} = C_{max,ss}\, e^{-k_e\tau}$$

where D is the antibiotic dose, V is the volume of distribution, k_e is the elimination rate constant, t is time, and τ is the dosage interval.

Steady-State Concentration Selection

• Vancomycin steady-state trough concentrations are selected based on site and severity of infection in addition to the infecting organism. A commonly used therapeutic range for this value is 5–10 µg/ml. Far less clinical data are available to aid in the selection of vancomycin serum concentrations compared to aminoglycoside serum concentrations. Severe, life-threatening infections should be treated with vancomycin trough steady-state concentrations in the upper end of this range (7.5–10 µg/ml).

TABLE 5-2B Pharmacokinetic Constants Computations Utilizing a One-Compartment Model for Vancomycin

Route of administration	Single dose	Multiple dose	Steady state
Intravenous bolus	$k_e = -(\ln C_1 - \ln C_2)/(t_1 - t_2)$	$k_e = -(\ln C_1 - \ln C_2)/(t_1 - t_2)$	$k_e = -(\ln C_1 - \ln C_2)/(t_1 - t_2)$
	$t_{1/2} = 0.693/k_e$	$t_{1/2} = 0.693/k_e$	$t_{1/2} = 0.693/k_e$
	$V = D/C_{max}$	$V = D/(C_{max} - C_{min})$	$V = D/(C_{max,ss} - C_{min,ss})$
	$Cl = k_e V$	$Cl = k_e V$	$Cl = k_e V$

C_1 is drug serum concentration at time = t_1, C_2 is drug serum concentration at time = t_2, k_e is elimination rate constant, $t_{1/2}$ is half-life, V is volume of distribution, D is dose, Cl is drug clearance, C_{min} is predose trough concentration, C_{max} is postdose peak concentration.

TABLE 5-2C Equations Used to Compute Individualized Dosage Regimens for Various Routes of Administration used with Vancomycin

Route of administration	Dosage interval (τ), maintenance dose (D), and loading dose (LD) equations
Intravenous bolus	$\tau = (\ln C_{max,ss} - \ln C_{min,ss})/k_e$ $D = C_{max,ss} V(1 - e^{-k_e\tau})$ $LD = C_{max,ss} V$

$C_{max,ss}$ and $C_{min,ss}$ are maximum and minimum steady-state concentrations, k_e is elimination rate constant, V is volume of distribution, k_0 is continuous infusion rate.

- Recent data suggest that steady-state trough concentrations as high as 15 μg/ml may pose no greater risk of vancomycin-induced nephrotoxicity than those within the traditional therapeutic range.[11]

  - If a patient does not respond adequately to vancomycin therapy that provides trough serum concentrations within the usual range, clinicians should consider prescribing an increased dose that produces a value as high as 15 μg/ml. In patients with sites of infection that are difficult to penetrate, such as the central nervous system or bone, it may be necessary to exceed this value with caution in order to eradicate the infecting organism. Whenever vancomycin doses are used that exceed steady-state trough concentrations of 10 μg/ml, serum creatinine concentrations should be monitored daily to detect early signs of nephrotoxicity.

- Steady-state peak vancomycin concentrations are chosen to provide adequate antibiotic penetration to the site of infection and to avoid adverse drug reactions. A commonly used therapeutic range for this value is 20–40 μg/ml.

  - In severe, life-threatening infections of the central nervous system, peak vancomycin serum concentrations as high as 60 mg/ml may be necessary to facilitate drug penetration. Whenever doses of vancomycin are used that exceed steady-state peak concentrations of 40 μg/ml, the patient should be monitored daily for early signs of ototoxicity (decreased hearing acuity in the conversational range, feeling of fullness or pressure in the ears, tinnitus, loss of equilibrium, headache, nausea, vomiting, vertigo, nystagmus, ataxia).

Dosage Computation

- The equations given in Table 5-2 are used to compute vancomycin doses.

▶ *Example 1* JM is a 50-year-old, 70-kg (height = 5′10″) male with a methicillin-resistant *Staphylococcus aureus* (MRSA) wound infection. His current serum creatinine is 0.9 mg/dl, and it has been stable over the 5 days since admission. Compute a vancomycin dose for this patient.

1. *Estimate creatinine clearance.* This patient has a stable serum creatinine and is not obese. The Cockcroft-Gault equation can be used to estimate creatinine clearance:

$$CrCl_{est} = \frac{(140 - age)BW}{72 \cdot S_{Cr}} = \frac{(140 - 50\ y)70\ kg}{72 \cdot 0.9\ mg/dl}$$

$$CrCl_{est} = 97\ ml/min$$

2. *Estimate vancomycin clearance.* The vancomycin clearance-versus-creatinine clearance relationship is used to estimate the vancomycin clearance for this patient:

$$Cl = 0.695(CrCl) + 0.05$$

$$= 0.695 \ [(97 \ \text{ml/min})/70 \ \text{kg}] + 0.05 = 1.013 \ \text{ml/min/kg}$$

3. *Estimate vancomycin volume of distribution.* The average volume of distribution for vancomycin is 0.7 L/kg:

$$V = 0.7 \ \text{L/kg} \cdot 70 \ \text{kg} = 49 \ \text{L}$$

4. *Estimate vancomycin elimination rate constant* (k_e) *and half-life* $(t_{1/2})$

$$k_e = Cl/V = (1.013 \ \text{ml/min/kg} \cdot 60 \ \text{min/h})/(0.7 \ \text{L/kg} \cdot 1000 \ \text{ml/L})$$

$$= 0.087 \ \text{h}^{-1}$$

$$t_{1/2} = 0.693/k_e = 0.693/0.087 \ \text{h}^{-1} = 8 \ \text{h}$$

5. *Choose desired steady-state serum concentrations.* Patients with *S. aureus* wound infections need to be carefully assessed. This patient did not appear to be in acute distress, with a normal temperature and slightly elevated white blood count. The wound was warm and red with a slight amount of purulent discharge. Because the infection was localized to the wound area, $C_{min,ss} = 7 \ \mu g/ml$ and $C_{max,ss} = 20 \ \mu g/ml$ were chosen.

6. *Use intravenous bolus equations to compute dose (Table 5-2).* Calculate required dosage interval (τ):

$$\tau = (\ln C_{max,ss} - \ln C_{min,ss})/k_e = (\ln 20 \ \mu g/ml - \ln 7 \ \mu g/ml)/0.087 \ \text{h}^{-1}$$

$$= 12.1 \ \text{h}$$

Dosage intervals should be rounded to clinically acceptable intervals of 12, 18, 24, 36, 48, 72 h, and multiples of 24 hours thereafter, whenever possible. In this case, the dosage interval would be rounded to 12 hours. Calculate required dose (D):

$$D = C_{max,ss} \ V(1 - e^{-k_e\tau}) = 20 \ \text{mg/L} \cdot 49 \ \text{L} \ (1 - e^{-(0.087 \ \text{h}^{-1})(12 \ \text{h})}) = 635 \ \text{mg}$$

Vancomycin doses should be rounded to the nearest 100–250 mg. This dose would be rounded to 750 mg. (*Note:* μg/ml = mg/L, and this concentration unit was substituted for $C_{max,ss}$ so that unit conversion was not required.)

The prescribed maintenance dose should be 750 mg every 12 hours.

7. *Compute loading dose (LD), if needed.* Loading doses should be considered for patients with creatinine clearance values below 60 ml/min. The administration of a loading dose in these patients will allow achievement of therapeutic concentrations more quickly than if maintenance doses alone are given. However, since the pharmacokinetic parameters used to compute these initial doses are only *estimated* values and not *actual* values, the patient's own parameters may be very different from the estimated constants, and steady state will not be achieved until 3–5 half-lives have passed.

$$LD = C_{max,ss} \ V = 20 \ \text{mg/L} \cdot 49 \ \text{L} = 980 \ \text{mg}$$

As noted, this patient has good renal function (CrCl ≥ 60 ml/min), so a loading dose would not be prescribed for this patient.

▶ **Example 2**   Same patient profile as in Example 1 except that serum creatinine is 3.5 mg/dl, indicating renal impairment.

1. *Estimate creatinine clearance.* This patient has a stable serum creatinine and is not obese. The Cockcroft-Gault equation can be used to estimate creatinine clearance:

$$CrCl_{est} = \frac{(140-age)BW}{72 \cdot S_{Cr}} = \frac{(140-50 \text{ y})70 \text{ kg}}{72 \cdot 3.5 \text{ mg/dl}}$$

$$CrCl_{est} = 25 \text{ ml/min}$$

2. *Estimate vancomycin clearance.* The vancomycin clearance-versus-creatinine clearance relationship is used to estimate the vancomycin clearance for this patient:

$$Cl = 0.695(CrCl) + 0.05 = 0.695[(25 \text{ ml/min})/70 \text{ kg}] + 0.05$$

$$= 0.298 \text{ ml/min/kg}$$

3. *Estimate vancomycin volume of distribution.* The average volume of distribution for vancomycin is 0.7 L/kg:

$$V = 0.7 \text{ L/kg} \cdot 70 \text{ kg} = 49 \text{ L}$$

4. *Estimate vancomycin elimination rate constant* (k_e) *and half-life* $(t_{1/2})$

$$k_e = Cl/V = (0.298 \text{ ml/min/kg} \cdot 60 \text{ min/h})/(0.7 \text{ L/kg} \cdot 1000 \text{ ml/L})$$

$$= 0.0256 \text{ h}^{-1}$$

$$t_{1/2} = 0.693/k_e = 0.693/0.0256 \text{ h}^{-1} = 27 \text{ h}$$

5. *Choose desired steady-state serum concentrations.* Patients with *S. aureus* wound infections need to be carefully assessed. This patient did not appear to be in acute distress, with a normal temperature and slightly elevated white blood counts. The wound was warm and red with a slight amount of purulent discharge. Because the infection was localized to the wound area, $C_{min,ss} = 7$ µg/ml and $C_{max,ss} = 20$ µg/ml were chosen.

6. *Use intravenous bolus equations to compute dose (Table 5-2).* Calculate required dosage interval (τ):

$$\tau = (\ln C_{max,ss} - \ln C_{min,ss})/k_e = (\ln 20 \text{ µg/ml} - \ln 7 \text{ µg/ml})/0.0256 \text{ h}^{-1}$$

$$= 41 \text{ h}$$

Dosage intervals should be rounded to clinically acceptable intervals of 12, 18, 24, 36, 48, 72 h, and multiples of 24 hours thereafter, whenever possible. In this case, the dosage interval would be rounded to 48 hours.

Calculate required dose (D):

$$D = C_{max,ss} V(1 - e^{-k_e\tau}) = 20 \text{ mg/L} \cdot 49 \text{ L } (1 - e^{-(0.0256 \text{ h}^{-1})(48 \text{ h})}) = 693 \text{ mg}$$

Vancomycin doses should be rounded to the nearest 100–250 mg. This dose would be rounded to 750 mg. (*Note:* µg/ml = mg/L, and this concentration unit was substituted for $C_{max,ss}$ so that unit conversion was not required.)

The prescribed maintenance dose should be 750 mg every 48 hours.

7. *Compute loading dose (LD), if needed.* Loading doses should be considered for patients with creatinine clearance values below 60 ml/min. The administration of a loading dose in these patients will allow achievement of therapeutic concentrations more quickly than if maintenance doses alone are given. However, since the pharmacokinetic parameters used to compute these initial doses are only *estimated* values and not *actual* values, the

patient's own parameters may be very different from the estimated constants, and steady state will not be achieved until 3–5 half-lives have passed.

$$LD = C_{max,ss} \cdot V = 20 \text{ mg/L} \cdot 49 \text{ L} = 980 \text{ mg}$$

As noted, this patient has poor renal function (CrCl <60 ml/min), so a loading dose would be prescribed for this patient and given as the first dose. Vancomycin doses should be rounded to the nearest 100–250 mg. This dose would be rounded to 1000 mg. (*Note:* μg/ml = mg/L, and this concentration unit was substituted for $C_{max,ss}$ so that unit conversion was not required.) The first maintenance dose would be given one dosage interval (48 hours) after the loading dose was administered.

▶ *Example 3*   ZW is a 35-year-old, 150-kg (5′5″) female with a *Staphylococcus epidermidis* infection of a prosthetic knee joint. Her current serum creatinine is 0.7 mg/dl and is stable. Compute a vancomycin dose for this patient.

1. *Estimate creatinine clearance.* This patient has a stable serum creatinine and is obese [$IBW_{females}$ (in kg) = 45 + 2.3(Ht − 60) = 45 + 2.3(65″ − 60) = 57 kg]. The Salazar-Corcoran equation can be used to estimate creatinine clearance:

$$CrCl_{est(females)} = \frac{(146 - age)[(0.287 \cdot Wt) + (9.74 \cdot Ht^2)]}{60 \cdot S_{Cr}}$$

$$CrCl_{est(females)} = \frac{(146 - 35 \text{ y})\{(0.287 \cdot 150 \text{ kg}) + [9.74 \cdot (1.65 \text{ m})^2]\}}{60 \cdot 0.7 \text{ mg/dl}}$$

$$= 184 \text{ ml/min}$$

Note: Height is converted from inches to meters: Ht = (65 in · 2.54 cm/in)/(100 cm/m) = 1.65 m.

2. *Estimate vancomycin clearance.* The vancomycin clearance-versus-creatinine clearance relationship is used to estimate the vancomycin clearance for this patient. Since maintenance doses are based on total body weight (TBW), this weight factor is used to compute clearance:

$$Cl = 0.695 (CrCl) + 0.05 = 0.695[(184 \text{ ml/min})/150 \text{ kg}] + 0.05$$
$$= 0.902 \text{ ml/min/kg TBW}$$

3. *Estimate vancomycin volume of distribution.* The average volume of distribution for vancomycin is 0.7 L/kg and is computed using the patient's ideal body weight because obesity does not significantly alter this parameter:

$$V = 0.7 \text{ L/kg} \cdot 57 \text{ kg} = 40 \text{ L}$$

4. *Estimate vancomycin elimination rate constant (k_e) and half-life ($t_{1/2}$).* Note that in the case of obese individuals, different weight factors are needed for vancomycin clearance and volume of distribution, so these weights are included in the equation for elimination rate constant:

$$k_e = \frac{Cl}{V}$$
$$= \frac{0.902 \text{ ml/min/kg TBW} \cdot 150 \text{ kg TBW} \cdot 60 \text{ min/h}}{0.7 \text{ L/kg IBW} \cdot 57 \text{ kg IBW} \cdot 1000 \text{ ml/L}} = 0.205 \text{ h}^{-1}$$
$$t_{1/2} = 0.693/k_e = 0.693/0.205 \text{ h}^{-1} = 3.4 \text{ h}$$

5. *Choose desired steady-state serum concentrations.* $C_{min,ss}$ = 7.5 μg/ml and $C_{max,ss}$ = 35 μg/ml were chosen for this patient with a *S. epidermidis* prosthetic joint infection.

6. *Use intravenous bolus equations to compute dose (Table 5-2).* Calculate required dosage interval (τ):

$$\tau = (\ln C_{max,ss} - \ln C_{min,ss})/k_e = (\ln 35 \text{ μg/ml} - \ln 7.5 \text{ μg/ml})/0.205 \text{ h}^{-1}$$
$$= 7.5 \text{ h}$$

Dosage intervals in obese individuals should be rounded to clinically acceptable intervals of 8, 12, 18, 24, 36, 48, 72 h, and multiples of 24 hours thereafter, whenever possible. In this case, the dosage interval would be rounded to 8 hours.

Calculate required dose (D):

$$D = C_{max,ss} V(1 - e^{-k_e\tau}) = 35 \text{ mg/L} \cdot 40 \text{ L} (1 - e^{-(0.205 \text{ h}^{-1})(8 \text{ h})})$$
$$= 1128 \text{ mg}$$

Vancomycin doses should be rounded to the nearest 100–250 mg. This dose would be rounded to 1250 mg. (*Note:* μg/ml = mg/L, this concentration unit was substituted for $C_{max,ss}$ so that unit conversion was not required.)

The prescribed maintenance dose should be 1250 mg every 8 hours.

7. *Compute loading dose (LD), if needed.* Loading doses should be considered for patients with creatinine clearance values below 60 ml/min. The administration of a loading dose in these patients will allow achievement of therapeutic concentrations more quickly than if maintenance doses alone are given. However, since the pharmacokinetic parameters used to compute these initial doses are only *estimated* values and not *actual* values, the patient's own parameters may be very different from the estimated constants, and steady state will not be achieved until 3–5 half-lives have passed.

$$LD = C_{max,ss} V = 35 \text{ mg/L} \cdot 40 \text{ L} = 1400 \text{ mg}$$

As noted, this patient has good renal function (CrCl ≥60 ml/min), so a loading dose would not be prescribed for this patient.

Moellering Nomogram Method

- The Moellering dosage nomogram was the first widely used approach that incorporated pharmacokinetic concepts to compute doses of vancomycin for patients with compromised renal function (Table 5-3).[23] The relationship between vancomycin clearance and creatinine clearance used in the pharmacokinetic dosing method is the one used to construct the Moellering nomogram. Hence, the dosage recommendations made by both these methods are generally similar although not identical, because vancomycin peak and trough concentrations cannot be specified using the nomogram.

- The goal of the nomogram is to provide average steady-state vancomycin concentrations equal to 15 μg/ml (or 15 mg/L). In order to use the nomogram, the patient's creatinine clearance is computed and divided by his or her body weight so that the units for creatinine clearance are ml/min/kg. This value is converted to a vancomycin maintenance dose in

TABLE 5-3 Moellering Nomogram Vancomycin Dosage Chart

1. Compute patient's creatinine clearance (CrCl) using Cockcroft-Gault method for normal weight or Salazar-Corcoran method for obese patients.
2. Divide CrCl by patient's weight.
3. Compute 24-hour maintenance dose for CrCl value.
4. Loading dose of 15 mg/kg should be given to patients with significant renal function impairment.

Creatinine clearance (ml/min/kg)*	Vancomycin dose (mg/kg/24 h)
2	30.9
1.9	29.3
1.8	27.8
1.7	26.3
1.6	24.7
1.5	23.2
1.4	21.6
1.3	20.1
1.2	18.5
1.1	17
1.0	15.4
0.9	13.9
0.8	12.4
0.7	10.8
0.6	9.3
0.5	7.7
0.4	6.2
0.3	4.6
0.2	3.1
0.1	1.5

*Dose for functionally anephric patients is 1.9 mg/kg/24 h.
Adapted from Moellering et al.[23]

terms of mg/kg/24 h. If the patient has renal impairment, a loading dose of 15 mg/kg is suggested. The nomogram does not provide a value for dosage interval.

- A modification of the vancomycin clearance/creatinine clearance equation can be made that provides a direct calculation of the vancomycin maintenance dose:[44] D (in mg/h/kg) = 0.626(CrCl in ml/min/kg) + 0.05.

- The use of this modification is straightforward. The patient's creatinine clearance is estimated using an appropriate technique [Cockcroft-Gault method[45] for normal-weight patients, Salazar-Corcoran method[46] for obese patients]. The vancomycin maintenance dose is computed directly using the dosing equation and then multiplied by the patient's weight to convert the answer into the units of mg/h. Guidance for the appropriate dosage interval (in hours) can be gained by dividing this dosage rate into a clinically acceptable dose, such as 1000 mg.

▶ **Example 1** JM is a 50-year-old, 70-kg (height = 5'10'') male with a methicillin-resistant *S. aureus* (MRSA) wound infection. His current serum creatinine is 0.9 mg/dl, and it has been stable over the 5 days since admission. Compute a vancomycin dose for this patient.

1. *Estimate creatinine clearance.* This patient has a stable serum creatinine and is not obese. The Cockcroft-Gault equation can be used to estimate creatinine clearance:

$$CrCl_{est} = \frac{(140 - age)BW}{72 \cdot S_{Cr}} = \frac{(140 - 50 \text{ y})70 \text{ kg}}{72 \cdot 0.9 \text{ mg/dl}}$$

$$CrCl_{est} = 97 \text{ ml/min}$$

2. *Determine dosage interval and maintenance dose.* The maintenance dose is calculated using the modified vancomycin dosing equation:

D (in mg/h/kg) = 0.626(CrCl in ml/min/kg) + 0.05

$$D = 0.626[(97 \text{ ml/min})/70 \text{ kg}] + 0.05 = 0.918 \text{ mg/h/kg}$$

$$D = 0.918 \text{ mg/h/kg} \cdot 70 \text{ kg} = 64.2 \text{ mg/h}$$

Because the patient has good renal function, the typical dosage interval of 12 hours will be used:

$$D = 64.2 \text{ mg/h} \cdot 12 \text{ h} = 770 \text{ mg}$$

Vancomycin doses should be rounded to the nearest 100–250 mg. This dose would be rounded to 750 mg. The prescribed maintenance dose should be 750 mg every 12 hours.

3. *Compute loading dose.* A loading dose (LD) of 15 mg/kg is suggested by the Moellering nomogram:

$$LD = 15 \text{ mg/kg}(70 \text{ kg}) = 1050 \text{ mg}$$

As noted, this patient has good renal function (CrCl ≥ 60 ml/min), so a loading dose could optionally be prescribed for this patient.

▶ ***Example 2*** Same patient profile as in Example 1 except that serum creatinine is 3.5 mg/dl, indicating renal impairment.

1. *Estimate creatinine clearance.* This patient has a stable serum creatinine and is not obese. The Cockcroft-Gault equation can be used to estimate creatinine clearance:

$$CrCl_{est} = \frac{(140 - age)BW}{72 \cdot S_{Cr}} = \frac{(140 - 50 \text{ y})70 \text{ kg}}{72 \cdot 3.5 \text{ mg/dl}}$$

$$CrCl_{est} = 25 \text{ ml/min}$$

2. *Determine dosage interval and maintenance dose.* The maintenance dose is calculated using the modified vancomycin dosing equation:

D (in mg/h/kg) = 0.626(CrCl in ml/min/kg) + 0.05

$$D = 0.626[(25 \text{ ml/min})/70 \text{ kg}] + 0.05 = 0.274 \text{ mg/h/kg}$$

$$D = 0.274 \text{ mg/h/kg} \cdot 70 \text{ kg} = 19.2 \text{ mg/h}$$

The standard dose of 1000 mg can be used to gain an approximation for an acceptable dosage interval (τ):

$$\tau = 1000 \text{ mg}/(19.2 \text{ mg/h}) = 52 \text{ h}$$

Dosage intervals should be rounded to clinically acceptable intervals of 12, 18, 24, 36, 48, 72 h, and multiples of 24 hours thereafter, whenever possible. In this case, the dosage interval would be rounded to 48 hours.

$$D = 19.2 \text{ mg/h} \cdot 48 \text{ h} = 922 \text{ mg}$$

Vancomycin doses should be rounded to the nearest 100–250 mg. This dose would be rounded to 1000 mg. The prescribed maintenance dose would be 1000 mg every 48 hours.

3. *Compute loading dose.* A loading dose (LD) of 15 mg/kg is suggested by the Moellering nomogram:

$$LD = 15 \text{ mg/kg}(70 \text{ kg}) = 1050 \text{ mg}$$

This patient has poor renal function (CrCl <60 ml/min), so a loading dose could be prescribed for this patient and given as the first dose. However, in this case the loading dose is nearly identical to the maintenance dose and would not be given.

▶ *Example 3*   ZW is a 35-year-old, 150-kg (5′5″) female with a *S. epidermidis* infection of a prosthetic knee joint. Her current serum creatinine is 0.7 mg/dl and is stable. Compute a vancomycin dose for this patient.

1. *Estimate creatinine clearance.* This patient has a stable serum creatinine and is obese [$IBW_{females}$ (in kg) = 45 + 2.3(Ht − 60) = 45 + 2.3(65″ − 60) = 57 kg]. The Salazar-Corcoran equation can be used to estimate creatinine clearance:

$$CrCl_{est(females)} = \frac{(146 - age)[(0.287 \cdot Wt) + (9.74 \cdot Ht^2)]}{60 \cdot S_{Cr}}$$

$$CrCl_{est(females)} = \frac{(146 - 35 \text{ y})\{(0.287 \cdot 150 \text{ kg}) + [9.74 \cdot (1.65 \text{ m})^2]\}}{60 \cdot 0.7 \text{ mg/dl}}$$

$$= 184 \text{ ml/min}$$

Note: Height is converted from inches to meters: Ht = (65 in · 2.54 cm/in)/(100 cm/m) = 1.65 m.

2. *Determine dosage interval and maintenance dose.* The maintenance dose is calculated using the modified vancomycin dosing equation:

$$D \text{ (in mg/h/kg)} = 0.626(CrCl \text{ in ml/min/kg}) + 0.05$$

$$D = 0.626[(184 \text{ ml/min})/150 \text{ kg}] + 0.05 = 0.818 \text{ mg/h/kg}$$

$$D = 0.818 \text{ mg/h/kg} \cdot 150 \text{ kg} = 122.7 \text{ mg/h}$$

Because the patient has excellent renal function and is obese, a dosage interval equal to 8 hours will be used:

$$D = 122.7 \text{ mg/h} \cdot 8 \text{ h} = 981 \text{ mg}$$

Vancomycin doses should be rounded to the nearest 100–250 mg. This dose would be rounded to 1000 mg. The prescribed maintenance dose would be 1000 mg every 8 hours.

3. *Compute loading dose.* A loading dose (LD) of 15 mg/kg is suggested by the Moellering nomogram. As noted, this patient has good renal function (CrCl ≥60 ml/min), so a loading dose would probably not be prescribed for this patient.

Matzke Nomogram Method

- The Matzke dosing nomogram is a quick and efficient way to apply pharmacokinetic dosing concepts without using complicated pharmacokinetic equations (Table 5-4).[25] The nomogram has not been tested in obese subjects (>30% over ideal body weight) and should not be employed in this patient population. Additionally, the authors suggest that the nomogram not be used in patients undergoing peritoneal dialysis.
- The nomogram is constructed to produce steady-state vancomycin peak and trough concentrations of 30 and 7.5 µg/ml, respectively. A loading dose of 25 mg/kg is given as the first dose, and subsequent maintenance doses of 19 mg/kg are given according to a dosage interval that varies according to the patient's creatinine clearance. While the Matzke nomogram has been shown to provide precise and unbiased dosage recommendations, it does supply relatively large doses because expected peak and trough concentrations are in the middle of their respective therapeutic ranges.

▶ ***Example 1*** JM is a 50-year-old, 70-kg (height = 5'10") male with a methicillin-resistant *S. aureus* (MRSA) wound infection. His current serum creatinine is 0.9 mg/dl, and it has been stable over the 5 days since admission. Compute a vancomycin dose for this patient.

1. *Estimate creatinine clearance.* This patient has a stable serum creatinine and is not obese. The Cockcroft-Gault equation can be used to estimate creatinine clearance:

$$CrCl_{est} = \frac{(140 - age)BW}{72 \cdot S_{Cr}} = \frac{(140 - 50 \text{ y})70 \text{ kg}}{72 \cdot 0.9 \text{ mg/dl}}$$

$$CrCl_{est} = 97 \text{ ml/min}$$

TABLE 5-4 Matzke Nomogram Vancomycin Dosage Chart

1. Compute patient's creatinine clearance (CrCl) using Cockcroft-Gault method: CrCl = [(140 − age)BW]/(Scr • 72). Multiply by 0.85 for females.
2. Nomogram not verified for obese individuals.
3. Dosage chart designed to achieve peak serum concentrations of 30 µg/ml and trough concentrations of 7.5 µg/ml.
4. Compute loading dose of 25 mg/kg.
5. Compute maintenance dose of 19 mg/kg given at the dosage interval listed in the following chart for the patient's CrCl:

CrCl (ml/min)	Dosage interval (d)
≥120	0.5
100	0.6
80	0.75
60	1.0
40	1.5
30	2.0
20	2.5
10	4.0
5	6.0
0	12.0

Adapted from Matzke et al.[25]

2. *Compute loading dose* (Table 5-4). A loading dose (LD) of 25 mg/kg will provide a peak concentration of 30 µg/ml.

$$LD = 25 \text{ mg/kg}(70 \text{ kg}) = 1750 \text{ mg}$$

3. *Determine dosage interval and maintenance dose.* From the nomogram, the dosage interval is 0.6 day, which would be rounded to every 12 hours. The maintenance dose would be 19 mg/kg · 70 kg = 1330 mg. Vancomycin doses should be rounded to the nearest 100–250 mg. This dose would be rounded to 1250 mg and given one dosage interval (12 hours) after the loading dose. The prescribed maintenance dose would be 1250 mg every 12 hours.

▶ ***Example 2*** Same patient profile as in Example 1 except that serum creatinine is 3.5 mg/dl, indicating renal impairment.

1. *Estimate creatinine clearance.* This patient has a stable serum creatinine and is not obese. The Cockcroft-Gault equation can be used to estimate creatinine clearance:

$$CrCl_{est} = \frac{(140 - \text{age})BW}{72 \cdot S_{Cr}} = \frac{(140 - 50 \text{ y})70 \text{ kg}}{72 \cdot 3.5 \text{ mg/dl}}$$
$$CrCl_{est} = 25 \text{ ml/min}$$

2. *Compute loading dose* (Table 5-4). A loading dose (LD) of 25 mg/kg will provide a peak concentration of 30 µg/ml.

$$LD = 25 \text{ mg/kg}(70 \text{ kg}) = 1750 \text{ mg}$$

3. *Determine dosage interval and maintenance dose.* After rounding creatinine clearance to 30 ml/min, the nomogram suggests a dosage interval of 2 days. The maintenance dose would be 19 mg/kg · 70 kg = 1330 mg. Vancomycin doses should be rounded to the nearest 100–250 mg. This dose would be rounded to 1250 mg and given one dosage interval (2 d × 24 h/d = 48 h) after the loading dose. The prescribed maintenance dose would be 1250 mg every 48 hours.

USE OF VANCOMYCIN SERUM CONCENTRATIONS TO ALTER DOSAGES

- Because of pharmacokinetic variability among patients, it is likely that doses calculated using patient population characteristics will not always produce vancomycin serum concentrations that are expected. Therefore, vancomycin serum concentrations are measured in many patients to ensure that therapeutic, nontoxic levels are present.
- Not all patients require serum concentration monitoring. For example, if it is expected that only a limited number of doses will be administered, as is the case for surgical prophylaxis, or an appropriate dose for the renal function and concurrent disease states of the patient is prescribed (e.g., 15 mg/kg every 12 hours for a patient with a creatinine clearance of 80–120 ml/min), vancomycin serum concentration monitoring may not be necessary.
- Whether or not vancomycin concentrations are measured, important patient parameters (fever curves, white blood cell counts, serum creatinine concentrations, etc.) should be followed to confirm that the patient is responding to treatment and not developing adverse drug reactions.
- When vancomycin serum concentrations are measured in patients and a dosage change is necessary, clinicians should seek to use the simplest, most

straightforward method available to determine a dose that will provide safe and effective treatment.

- In most cases, a simple dosage ratio can be used to adjust vancomycin doses, since these antibiotics follow *linear pharmacokinetics.*
- If only steady-state trough concentrations are being measured in a patient, a variant of linear pharmacokinetics can be used to perform *trough-only* dosage adjustments.
- Sometimes, it is not possible simply to change the dose, and the dosage interval must also be changed to achieve desired serum concentrations. In this case, it may be possible to use *pharmacokinetic concepts* to alter the vancomycin dose.
- In some situations, it may be necessary or desirable to compute the vancomycin pharmacokinetic parameters for the patient using the *one-compartment-model-parameter method* and utilize these to calculate the best drug dose.
- Finally, computerized methods that incorporate expected population pharmacokinetic characteristics (*Bayesian pharmacokinetic computer programs*) can be used in difficult cases in which renal function is changing, serum concentrations are obtained at suboptimal times, or the patient was not at steady state when serum concentrations were measured. If trough-only monitoring is being done for a patient, Bayesian computer programs can provide estimates for all vancomycin pharmacokinetic parameters even though only one serum concentration was measured.

Linear Pharmacokinetics Method

- Because vancomycin antibiotics follow linear, dose-proportional pharmacokinetics, steady-state serum concentrations change in proportion to dose according to the following equation:

$$D_{new}/C_{ss,new} = D_{old}/C_{ss,old} \qquad \text{or} \qquad D_{new} = (C_{ss,new}/C_{ss,old})D_{old}$$

where D is the dose, C_{ss} is the steady-state peak or trough concentration, old indicates the dose that produced the steady-state concentration that the patient is currently receiving, and new denotes the dose necessary to produce the desired steady-state concentration.

- The advantages of this method are that it is quick and simple. The disadvantages are that steady-state concentrations are required, and it may not be possible to attain desired serum concentrations by changing only the dose.

- ▸ *Example 1*   JM is a 50-year-old, 70-kg (height = 5′10″) male with a methicillin-resistant *S. aureus* (MRSA) pneumonia. His current serum creatinine is 0.9 mg/dl, and it has been stable over the 5 days since admission. A vancomycin dose of 1000 mg every 12 hours was prescribed and expected to achieve steady-state peak and trough concentrations equal to 25 and 7 μg/ml, respectively. After the third dose, steady-state peak and trough concentrations were measured and equaled 45 and 12 μg/ml, respectively. Calculate a new vancomycin dose that will provide a steady-state trough of 7 μg/ml.

1. *Estimate creatinine clearance.* This patient has a stable serum creatinine and is not obese. The Cockcroft-Gault equation can be used to estimate

creatinine clearance:

$$CrCl_{est} = \frac{(140 - age)BW}{72 \cdot S_{Cr}} = \frac{(140 - 50 \ y)70 \ kg}{72 \cdot 0.9 \ mg/dl}$$

$$CrCl_{est} = 97 \ ml/min$$

2. *Estimate elimination rate constant* (k_e) *and half-life* ($t_{1/2}$). The vancomycin clearance-versus-creatinine clearance relationship is used to estimate drug clearance for this patient:

$$Cl = 0.695(CrCl) + 0.05 = 0.695[(97 \ ml/min)/70 \ kg] + 0.05$$

$$= 1.013 \ ml/min/kg$$

The average volume of distribution for vancomycin is 0.7 L/kg:

$$V = 0.7 \ L/kg \cdot 70 \ kg = 49 \ L$$

$$k_e = Cl/V = (1.013 \ ml/min/kg \cdot 60 \ min/h)/(0.7 \ L/kg \cdot 1000 \ ml/L)$$

$$= 0.0868 \ h^{-1}$$

$$t_{1/2} = 0.693/k_e = 0.693/0.0868 \ h^{-1} = 8 \ h$$

Because the patient has been receiving vancomycin for ~3 estimated half-lives, it is likely that the measured serum concentrations are steady-state values. *Note that these first two steps can be omitted if it is known that the patient is at steady state.*

3. *Compute new dose to achieve desired serum concentration.* Using linear pharmacokinetics, the new dose to attain the desired concentration should be proportional to the old dose that produced the measured concentration:

$$D_{new} = (C_{ss,new}/C_{ss,old})D_{old} = (7 \ \mu g/ml/12 \ \mu g/ml) \ 1000 \ mg$$

$$= 583 \ mg, \ round \ to \ 500 \ mg$$

The new suggested dose would be 500 mg every 12 hours, to be started at the next scheduled dosing time.

4. *Check steady-state peak concentration for new dosage regimen.* Using linear pharmacokinetics, the new steady-state concentration can be estimated and should be proportional to the old dose that produced the measured concentration:

$$C_{ss,new} = (D_{new}/D_{old})C_{ss,old} = (500 \ mg/1000 \ mg) \ 45 \ \mu g/ml = 22.5 \ \mu g/ml$$

This steady-state peak concentration should be safe and effective for the infection that is being treated.

Trough-Only Method

- When clinicians choose to monitor only steady-state trough vancomycin concentrations, a modification of the linear pharmacokinetics method can be used to adjust doses. Usually, the linear pharmacokinetics method is used when only the dose, and not the dosage interval, needs to be changed. However, the same technique used to estimate a dosage interval for the Moellering nomogram can be utilized to calculate a new dosage interval for the trough-only method.

  - Because the dosage interval computation involves a simplification (e.g., steady-state concentrations vary according to the inverse of the dosage interval), the actual new steady-state trough concentration should be slightly higher than that calculated if a shorter dosage interval is used or slightly lower than that calculated if a longer dosage interval is used.

▶ **Example 1** ZW is a 35-year-old, 150-kg (height = 5′5″ = 65 in = 165 cm) female with enterococcal endocarditis. Her current serum creatinine is 1.1 mg/dl and is stable. A vancomycin dose of 1000 mg every 12 hours was prescribed and expected to achieve a steady-state trough concentration equal to 7 µg/ml. After the fifth dose, a steady-state concentration was measured and equaled 4 µg/ml. Calculate a new vancomycin dose that will provide a steady-state trough of 7 µg/ml.

1. *Estimate creatinine clearance.* This patient has a stable serum creatinine and is obese [$IBW_{females}$ (in kg) = 45 + 2.3(Ht − 60) = 45 + 2.3(65″ − 60) = 57 kg]. The Salazar-Corcoran equation can be used to estimate creatinine clearance:

$$CrCl_{est(females)} = \frac{(146 - age)[(0.287 \cdot Wt) + (9.74 \cdot Ht^2)]}{60 \cdot S_{Cr}}$$

$$CrCl_{est(females)} = \frac{(146 - 35\ y)\{(0.287 \cdot 150\ kg) + [9.74 \cdot (1.65\ m)^2]\}}{60 \cdot 1.1\ mg/dl}$$

$$= 117\ ml/min$$

Note: Height is converted from inches to meters: Ht = (65 in · 2.54 cm/in)/(100 cm/m) = 1.65 m.

2. *Estimate elimination rate constant* (k_e) *and half-life* ($t_{1/2}$). The vancomycin clearance-versus-creatinine clearance relationship is used to estimate drug clearance for this patient:

$$Cl = 0.695(CrCl) + 0.05 = 0.695[(117\ ml/min)/150\ kg] + 0.05$$

$$= 0.592\ ml/min/kg$$

The average volume of distribution for vancomycin is 0.7 L/kg IBW:

$$V = 0.7\ L/kg \cdot 57\ kg = 40\ L$$

$$k_e = Cl/V$$
$$= (0.592\ ml/min/kg \cdot 150\ kg \cdot 60\ min/h)/$$
$$(0.7\ L/kg \cdot 57\ kg \cdot 1000\ ml/L) = 0.134\ h^{-1}$$

$$t_{1/2} = 0.693/k_e = 0.693/0.134\ h^{-1} = 5.2\ h$$

Because the patient has been receiving vancomycin for more than 3–5 estimated half-lives, it is likely that the measured serum concentrations are steady-state values. *Note that these first two steps can be omitted if it is known that the patient is at steady state.*

3. *Compute new dose to achieve desired serum concentration.* Using linear pharmacokinetics, the new dose to attain the desired concentration should be proportional to the old dose that produced the measured concentration:

$$D_{new} = (C_{ss,new}/C_{ss,old})D_{old} = (7\ µg/ml/4\ µg/ml)\ 1000\ mg = 1750\ mg$$

The new suggested dose is 1750 mg every 12 hours. However, this dose is relatively large, and without a measured steady-state peak concentration, it is not possible to calculate a new steady-state peak concentration.

Since it is possible that the steady-state peak concentration from this dose might be too high, an alternative dosage interval and dose will be computed.

4. *Compute hourly dosage rate.* The dosage rate for the new dose is computed by dividing the dose (D) by the dosage interval (τ):

$$\text{Dosage rate (in mg/h)} = D/\tau$$
$$\text{Dosage rate} = 1750 \text{ mg}/(12 \text{ h}) = 146 \text{ mg/h}$$

5. *Set a standard dose empirically and compute the alternative dosage interval.* A standard dose of 1000 mg will be used to compute the alternative dosage interval.

$$\tau = 1000 \text{ mg}/(146 \text{ mg/h}) = 7 \text{ h}$$

Because the patient has excellent renal function and is obese, the dosage interval will be rounded to 8 hours. The prescribed maintenance dose would be 1000 mg every 8 hours. Because the calculation for the dosage interval involves an approximation, the actual steady-state concentration should be slightly different than 7 µg/ml.

Pharmacokinetic Concepts Method

- As implied by the name, the pharmacokinetics concepts technique derives alternative doses by estimating actual pharmacokinetic parameters or surrogates for pharmacokinetic parameters.[47] It is a very useful way to calculate drug doses when the linear pharmacokinetic method is not sufficient because a dosage change that will produce a proportional change in steady-state peak and trough concentrations is not appropriate. The only requirement is a steady-state peak and trough vancomycin serum concentration pair obtained before and after a dose (Figure 5-2). The following steps are used to compute new vancomycin doses.

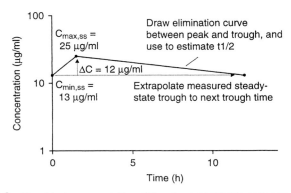

FIG. 5-2   Graphical representation of the pharmacokinetic concepts method in which a steady-state peak ($C_{max,ss}$) and trough ($C_{min,ss}$) concentration pair is used to individualize vancomycin therapy. Because the patient is at steady state, consecutive trough concentrations will be identical, so the trough concentration can be extrapolated to the next predose time. The change in concentration after a dose is given (ΔC) is a surrogate measure of the volume of distribution and will be used to compute the new dose for the patient.

1. *Draw a rough sketch of the serum log concentration/time curve by hand, keeping tract of the relative time between the serum concentrations (Figure 5-2).*
2. *Since the patient is at steady state, the trough concentration can be extrapolated to the next trough value time (Figure 5-2).*
3. *Draw the elimination curve between the steady-state peak concentration and the extrapolated trough concentration. Use this line to estimate half-life.* For example, a patient receives a vancomycin dose of 1000 mg given every 12 hours that produces a steady-state peak equal to 25 µg/ml and a steady-state trough equal to 13 µg/ml, and the dose is infused over 1 hour and the peak concentration is drawn $\frac{1}{2}$ hour later (Figure 5-2). The time between the measured steady-state peak and the extrapolated trough concentration is 10.5 hours (the 12-hour dosage interval minus the 1.5-hour combined infusion and waiting time). The definition of half-life is the time needed for serum concentrations to decrease by one-half. Because the serum concentration declined by approximately one-half from the peak concentration to the trough concentration, the vancomycin half-life for this patient is approximately 10.5 hours. This information will be used to set the new dosage interval for the patient.
4. *Determine the difference in concentration between the steady-state peak and trough concentrations. The difference in concentration will change proportionally with the dose size.* In the current example the patient is receiving a vancomycin dose equal to 1000 mg every 12 hours, which produced steady-state peak and trough concentrations of 25 and 13 µg/ml, respectively. The difference between the peak and trough values is 12 µg/ml. The change in serum concentration is proportional to the dose, and this information will be used to set a new dose for the patient.
5. *Choose new steady-state peak and trough concentrations.* For the purposes of this example, the desired steady-state peak and trough concentrations will be approximately 30 and 7 µg/ml, respectively.
6. *Determine the new dosage interval for the desired concentrations.* In this example, the patient has a desired peak concentration of 30 µg/ml. In one half-life, the serum concentration will decline to 15 µg/ml, and in an additional half-life the vancomycin concentration will decrease to 7.5 µg/ml (Figure 5-3). Since the approximate half-life is 10.5 hours and 2 half-lives are required for serum concentrations to decrease from the desired peak concentration to the desired trough concentration, the dosage interval should be 21 hours (10.5 hours × 2 half-lives). This value would be rounded off to the clinically acceptable value of 24 hours, and the actual trough concentration would be expected to be slightly lower than 7.5 µg/ml.
7. *Determine the new dose for the desired concentrations.* The desired peak concentration is 30 µg/ml, and the expected trough concentration is 7.5 µg/ml. The change in concentration between these values is 22.5 µg/ml. It is known from measured serum concentrations that administration of 1000 mg changes serum concentrations by 12 µg/ml and that the change in serum concentration between the peak and trough values is proportional to the size of the dose. Therefore, a simple ratio will be used to compute the required dose:

$$D_{new} = (\Delta C_{new}/\Delta C_{old})D_{old}$$

where D_{new} and D_{old} are the new and old doses, respectively; ΔC_{new} is the change in concentration between the peak and trough for the new dose;

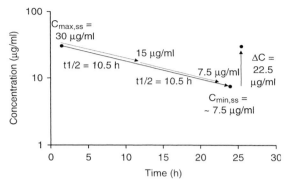

FIG. 5-3 The pharmacokinetic concepts method uses the estimated half-life to graphically compute the new dosage interval and the change in concentration to calculate the dose for a patient.

and ΔC_{old} is the change in concentration between the peak and trough for the old dose (*Note:* This relationship is appropriate because doses are given into a fixed, constant volume of distribution; it is not because the drug follows linear pharmacokinetics, so this method will work whether the agent follows nonlinear or linear pharmacokinetics). For this example,

$$D_{new} = (22.5 \ \mu g/ml/12 \ \mu g/ml) \ 1000 \ mg = 1875 \ mg$$

which would be rounded to 1750 mg. Vancomycin 1750 mg every 24 hours would be started 24 hours after the last dose of the previous dosage regimen.

- Once this method is mastered, it can be used without the need for a calculator. The following are examples that use the pharmacokinetic concepts method to change vancomycin doses.

▶ **Example 1** JM is a 50-year-old, 70-kg (height = 5'10") male with a methicillin-resistant *S. aureus* (MRSA) wound infection. His current serum creatinine is 3.5 mg/dl, and it has been stable over the 5 days since admission. A vancomycin dose of 800 mg every 24 hours was prescribed and expected to achieve steady-state peak and trough concentrations equal to 20 and 5 μg/ml, respectively. After the fourth dose, steady-state peak and trough concentrations were measured and equaled 25 and 12 μg/ml, respectively. Calculate a new vancomycin dose that will provide a steady-state peak of 20 μg/ml and a trough of 5 μg/ml.

1. *Estimate creatinine clearance.* This patient has a stable serum creatinine and is not obese. The Cockcroft-Gault equation can be used to estimate creatinine clearance:

$$CrCl_{est} = \frac{(140 - age)BW}{72 \cdot S_{Cr}} = \frac{(140 - 50 \ y)70 \ kg}{72 \cdot 3.5 \ mg/dl}$$

$$CrCl_{est} = 25 \ ml/min$$

2. *Estimate elimination rate constant* (k_e) *and half-life* $(t_{1/2})$. The vancomycin-clearance-versus-creatinine clearance relationship is used to estimate drug clearance for this patient:

$$Cl = 0.695(CrCl) + 0.05 = 0.695[(25 \text{ ml/min})/70 \text{ kg}] + 0.05$$
$$= 0.298 \text{ ml/min/kg}$$

The average volume of distribution for vancomycin is 0.7 L/kg:

$$V = 0.7 \text{ L/kg} \cdot 70 \text{ kg} = 49 \text{ L}$$

$$k_e = Cl/V = (0.298 \text{ ml/min/kg} \cdot 60 \text{ min/h})/(0.7 \text{ L/kg} \cdot 1000 \text{ ml/L})$$
$$= 0.0255 \text{ h}^{-1}$$

$$t_{1/2} = 0.693/k_e = 0.693/0.0255 \text{ h}^{-1} = 27 \text{ h}$$

Because the patient has been receiving vancomycin for ~3 estimated half-lives, it is likely that the measured serum concentrations are close to steady-state values. This steady-state concentration pair can be used to compute the patient's own unique pharmacokinetic parameters, which can be utilized to calculate individualized doses. *Note that these first two steps can be omitted if it is known that the patient is at steady state.*

3. *Use the Pharmacokinetic Concepts Method to compute a new dose.*

  a. *Draw a rough sketch of the serum log concentration/time curve by hand, keeping track of the relative time between the serum concentrations (Figure 5-4).*
  b. *Since the patient is at steady state, the trough concentration can be extrapolated to the next trough value time (Figure 5-4).*
  c. *Draw the elimination curve between the steady-state peak concentration and the extrapolated trough concentration. Use this line to estimate half-life.* The patient is receiving a vancomycin dose of 800 mg

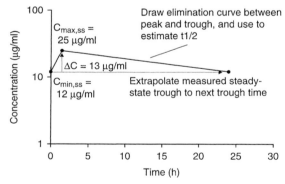

FIG. 5-4 Graphical representation of the pharmacokinetic concepts method in which a steady-state peak ($C_{max,ss}$) and trough ($C_{min,ss}$) concentration pair is used to individualize vancomycin therapy. Because the patient is at steady state, consecutive trough concentrations will be identical, so the trough concentration can be extrapolated to the next predose time. The change in concentration after a dose is given (ΔC) is a surrogate measure of the volume of distribution and will be used to compute the new dose for the patient.

given every 24 hours that produces a steady-state peak equal to 25 µg/ml and a steady-state trough equal to 12 µg/ml. The dose is infused over 1 hour and the peak concentration is drawn $\frac{1}{2}$ hour later (Figure 5-4). The time between the measured steady-state peak and the extrapolated trough concentration is 22.5 hours (the 24-hour dosage interval minus the 1.5-hour combined infusion and waiting time). The definition of half-life is the time needed for serum concentrations to decrease by one-half. It will take one half-life for the peak serum concentration to decline from 25 to 12.5 µg/ml. The concentration of 12 µg/ml is very close to the extrapolated trough value of 12.5 µg/ml. Therefore, 1 half-life expired during the 22.5-hour time period between the peak concentration and extrapolated trough concentration, and the estimated half-life is 22.5 hours. This information will be used to set the new dosage interval for the patient.

d. *Determine the difference in concentration between the steady-state peak and trough concentrations. The difference in concentration will change proportionally with the dose size.* In the current example the patient is receiving a vancomycin dose equal to 800 mg every 24 hours, which produced steady-state peak and trough concentrations of 25 and 12 µg/ml, respectively. The difference between the peak and trough values is 13 µg/ml. The change in serum concentration is proportional to the dose, and this information will be used to set a new dose for the patient.

e. *Choose new steady-state peak and trough concentrations.* For the purposes of this example, the desired steady-state peak and trough concentrations will be 20 and 5 µg/ml, respectively.

f. *Determine the new dosage interval for the desired concentrations* (Figure 5-5). Using the desired concentrations, it will take one half-life for the peak concentration of 20 µg/ml to decrease to 10 µg/ml, and an additional half-life for serum concentrations to decline from 10 µg/ml to 5 µg/ml. Therefore, the dosage interval will need to be approximately 2 half-lives or 45 hours (22.5 hours × 2 half-live = 45 hours). This dosage interval would be rounded off to 48 hours.

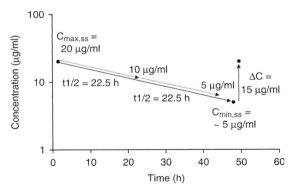

FIG. 5-5 The pharmacokinetic concepts method uses the estimated half-life to graphically compute the new dosage interval and the change in concentration to calculate the dose for a patient.

g. *Determine the new dose for the desired concentrations (Figure 5-5).* The desired peak concentration is 20 μg/ml, and the expected trough concentration is 5 μg/ml. The change in concentration between these values is 15 μg/ml. It is known from measured serum concentrations that administration of 800 mg changes serum concentrations by 13 μg/ml and that the change in serum concentration between the peak and trough values is proportional to the size of the dose. In this case,

$$D_{new} = (\Delta C_{new}/\Delta C_{old})D_{old} = (15 \text{ μg/ml}/13 \text{ μg/ml})800 \text{ mg}$$
$$= 923 \text{ mg, rounded to } 1000 \text{ mg.}$$

Vancomycin 1000 mg every 48 hours would be started 48 hours after the last dose of the previous dosage regimen.

One-Compartment-Model Parameter Method

- The one-compartment-model parameter method of adjusting drug doses was among the first techniques available to change doses using serum concentrations.[48] It allows the computation of an individual's own, unique pharmacokinetic constants and uses those to calculate a dose that achieves desired vancomycin concentrations.

  - The standard one-compartment-model parameter method conducts a small pharmacokinetic experiment using 3–4 vancomycin serum concentrations obtained during a dosage interval and does not require steady-state conditions.
  - The steady-state one-compartment-model parameter method assumes that steady-state has been achieved and requires only a steady-state peak and trough concentration pair obtained before and after a dose.

Standard One-Compartment-Model Parameter Method

- The standard version of the one-compartment-model parameter method does not require steady-state concentrations. A trough vancomycin concentration is obtained before a dose, a peak vancomycin concentration is obtained after the dose is infused ($\frac{1}{2}$–1 hour after a 1-hour infusion), and 1–2 additional postdose serum vancomycin concentrations are obtained (Figure 5-6). Ideally, the 1–2 postdose concentrations should be obtained at least 1 estimated half-life from each other to minimize the influence of assay error.

  - The postdose serum concentrations are used to calculate the vancomycin elimination rate constant and half-life (Figure 5-6). The half-life can be computed by graphing the postdose concentrations on semilogrithmic paper, drawing the best straight line through the data points, and determining the time needed for serum concentrations to decline by one-half. Once the half-life is known, the elimination rate constant (k_e) can be computed: $k_e = 0.693/t_{1/2}$.
  - Alternatively, the elimination rate constant can be calculated directly using the postdose serum concentrations [$k_e = (\ln C_1 - \ln C_2)/\Delta t$, where C_1 and C_2 are postdose serum concentrations and Δt is the time that expired between the times that C_1 and C_2 were obtained], and the half-life can be computed using the elimination rate constant ($t_{1/2} = 0.693/k_e$).
  - The volume of distribution (V) is calculated using the following equation:

  $$V = D/(C_{max} - C_{min})$$

  where D is the vancomycin dose, C_{max} is the peak concentration, and C_{min} is the trough concentration.

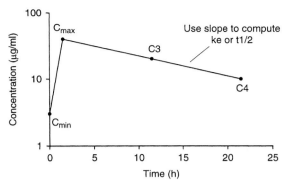

FIG. 5-6   The one-compartment-model parameter method for individualization of vancomycin doses uses a trough (C_{min}), peak (C_{max}), and 1–2 additional postdose concentrations (C_3, C_4) to compute a patient's own, unique pharmacokinetic parameters. This version of the one-compartment-model parameter method does not require steady-state conditions. The peak and trough concentrations are used to calculate the volume of distribution, and the postdose concentrations (C_{max}, C_3, C_4) are used to compute half-life. Once volume of distribution and half-life have been measured, they can be used to compute the exact dose needed to achieve desired vancomycin concentrations.

- The elimination rate constant and volume of distribution measured in this fashion are the patient's own, unique vancomycin pharmacokinetic constants and can be used in one-compartment-model intravenous bolus equations to compute the required dose to achieve any desired serum concentration.

▶ **Example 1**   JH is a 24-year-old, 70-kg (height = 6'0'') male with methicillin-resistant *S. aureus* endocarditis. His current serum creatinine is 1.0 mg/dl, and it has been stable over the 7 days since admission. A vancomycin dose of 1000 mg every 12 hours was prescribed. After the third dose, the following vancomycin serum concentrations were obtained:

Time	Vancomycin concentration (µg/ml)
0800 H	2.0
0800–0900 H	Vancomycin 1000 mg administered over 1 hour
1000 H	18.0
1500 H	10.1
2000 H	5.7

Medication administration sheets were checked, and the previous dose was given 2 hours early (1800 H the previous day). Because of this, it is known that the patient is not at steady state. Calculate a new vancomycin dose that will provide a steady-state peak of 30 µg/ml and a trough of 10 µg/ml.

Use the one-compartment-model parameter method to compute a new dose.

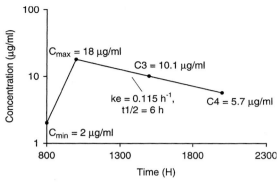

FIG. 5-7 Graph of vancomycin serum concentrations used in one-compartment-model parameter method example.

1. *Plot serum concentration/time data (Figure 5-7). Because serum concentrations decrease in a straight line, use any two postdose concentrations to compute the patient's elimination rate constant and half-life. Compute the patient's elimination rate constant and half-life.*

   $k_e = (\ln C_{max} - \ln C_{min})/\Delta t = (\ln 18 \, \mu g/ml - \ln 5.7 \, \mu g/ml)/(10 \, h)$
   $= 0.115 \, h^{-1}$

   $t_{1/2} = 0.693/k_e = 0.693/0.115 \, h^{-1} = 6 \, h$

2. *Compute the patient's volume of distribution:*

   $V = D/(C_{max} - C_{min}) = 1000 \, mg/(18 \, mg/L - 2.0 \, mg/L) = 62.5 \, L$

3. *Choose new steady-state peak and trough concentrations.* For the purposes of this example, the desired steady-state peak and trough concentrations will be 30 μg/ml and 10 μg/ml, respectively.

4. *Determine the new dosage interval for the desired concentrations.* As in the initial dosage section of this chapter, the dosage interval (τ) is computed using the following equation:

   $\tau = (\ln C_{max,ss} - \ln C_{min,ss})/k_e = (\ln 30 \, \mu g/ml - \ln 10 \, \mu g/ml)/0.115 \, h^{-1}$
   $= 10 \, h, \text{ rounded to } 12 \, h$

5. *Determine the new dose for the desired concentrations.* The dose is computed using the one-compartment-model intravenous bolus equation used in the initial dosing section of this chapter:

   $D = C_{max,ss} \, V(1 - e^{-k_e\tau}) = 30 \, mg/L \cdot 62.5 \, L \, (1 - e^{-(0.115 \, h^{-1})(12 \, h)})$
   $= 1403 \, mg, \text{ rounded to } 1500 \, mg$

A dose of vancomycin 1500 mg every 12 hours would be prescribed to begin 12 hours after the last dose of the previous regimen.

Steady-State One-Compartment-Model Parameter Method

- If a steady-state peak and trough vancomycin concentration pair is available for a patient, the one-compartment-model parameter method can be used to compute patient pharmacokinetic parameters and vancomycin doses (Figure 5-8).

  - Since the patient is at steady state, the measured trough concentration obtained before the dose was given can be extrapolated to the next dosage time and used to compute the vancomycin elimination rate constant ($k_e = (\ln C_{max,ss} - \ln C_{min,ss})/\tau - t'$, where $C_{max,ss}$ and $C_{min,ss}$ are the steady-state peak and trough serum concentrations and t' and τ are the infusion time and dosage interval), and the half-life can be computed using the elimination rate constant ($t_{1/2} = 0.693/k_e$).
  - The volume of distribution (V) is calculated using the following equation: $V = D/(C_{max,ss} - C_{min,ss})$, where D is the vancomycin dose, $C_{max,ss}$ is the steady-state peak concentration, and $C_{min,ss}$ is the steady-state trough concentration.
  - The elimination rate constant and volume of distribution measured in this way are the patient's own, unique vancomycin pharmacokinetic constants and can be used in one-compartment-model intravenous bolus equations to compute the required dose to achieve any desired serum concentration. The dosage calculations are similar to those done in the initial dosage section of this chapter, except that the patient's real pharmacokinetic parameters are used in the equations instead of population pharmacokinetic estimates.

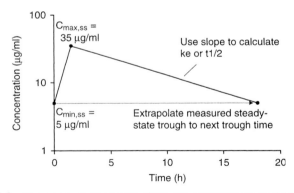

FIG. 5-8 The steady-state version of the one-compartment-model parameter method uses a steady-state peak ($C_{max,ss}$) and trough ($C_{min,ss}$) concentration pair to individualize vancomycin therapy. Because the patient is at steady state, consecutive trough concentrations will be identical, so the trough concentration can be extrapolated to the next predose time. The steady-state peak and trough concentrations are used to calculate the volume of distribution and half-life. Once volume of distribution and half-life have been measured, they can be used to compute the exact dose needed to achieve desired vancomycin concentrations.

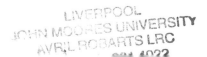

▶ *Example 1*   JM is a 50-year-old, 70-kg (height = 5′10″) male with a methicillin-resistant *S. aureus* (MRSA) wound infection. His current serum creatinine is 3.5 mg/dl, and it has been stable over the 5 days since admission. A vancomycin dose of 800 mg every 24 hours was prescribed and expected to achieve steady-state peak and trough concentrations equal to 20 and 5 µg/ml, respectively. After the fourth dose, steady-state peak and trough concentrations were measured and were 25 and 12 µg/ml, respectively. Calculate a new vancomycin dose that will provide a steady-state peak of 20 µg/ml and a trough of 5 µg/ml.

1. *Estimate creatinine clearance.* This patient has a stable serum creatinine and is not obese. The Cockcroft-Gault equation can be used to estimate creatinine clearance:

$$CrCl_{est} = \frac{(140 - age)BW}{72 \cdot S_{Cr}} = \frac{(140 - 50 \text{ y})70 \text{ kg}}{72 \cdot 3.5 \text{ mg/dl}}$$

$$CrCl_{est} = 25 \text{ ml/min}$$

2. *Estimate elimination rate constant (k_e) and half-life ($t_{1/2}$).* The vancomycin clearance versus creatinine clearance relationship is used to estimate drug clearance for this patient:

$$Cl = 0.695(CrCl) + 0.05 = 0.695[(25 \text{ ml/min})/70 \text{ kg}] + 0.05$$

$$= 0.298 \text{ ml/min/kg}$$

The average volume of distribution for vancomycin is 0.7 L/kg:

$$V = 0.7 \text{ L/kg} \cdot 70 \text{ kg} = 49 \text{ L}$$

$$k_e = Cl/V = (0.298 \text{ ml/min/kg} \cdot 60 \text{ min/h})/(0.7 \text{ L/kg} \cdot 1000 \text{ ml/L})$$

$$= 0.0255 \text{ h}^{-1}$$

$$t_{1/2} = 0.693/k_e = 0.693/0.0255 \text{ h}^{-1} = 27 \text{ h}$$

Because the patient has been receiving vancomycin for ~3 estimated half-lives, it is likely that the measured serum concentrations are close to steady-state values. This steady-state concentration pair can be used to compute the patient's own unique pharmacokinetic parameters, which can be utilized to calculate individualized doses. *Note that these first two steps can be omitted if it is known that the patient is at steady state.*

3. *Use the one-compartment-model parameter method to compute a new dose.*

   a. *Compute the patient's elimination rate constant and half-life (Note: t′= infusion time + waiting time of 1 hour and $\frac{1}{2}$ hour, respectively)*

$$k_e = (\ln C_{max,ss} - \ln C_{min,ss})/\tau - t'$$

$$= (\ln 25 \text{ µg/ml} - \ln 12 \text{ µg/ml})/(24 \text{ h} - 1.5 \text{ h})$$

$$= 0.0326 \text{ h}^{-1}$$

$$t_{1/2} = 0.693/k_e = 0.693/0.0326 \text{ h}^{-1} = 21.2 \text{ h}$$

   b. *Compute the patient's volume of distribution:*

$$V = D/(C_{max,ss} - C_{min,ss}) = 800 \text{ mg}/(25 \text{ mg/L} - 12 \text{ mg/L}) = 61.5 \text{ L}$$

   c. *Choose new steady-state peak and trough concentrations.* For the purposes of this example, the desired steady-state peak and trough concentrations will be 20 and 5 µg/ml, respectively.

d. *Determine the new dosage interval for the desired concentrations.* As in the initial dosage section of this chapter, the dosage interval (τ) is computed using the following equation:

$$\tau = (\ln C_{max,ss} - \ln C_{min,ss})/k_e$$
$$= (\ln 20\ \mu g/ml - \ln 5\ \mu g/ml)/0.0326\ h^{-1}$$
$$= 42\ h,\ \text{rounded to 48 hours}$$

e. *Determine the new dose for the desired concentrations.* The dose is computed using the one-compartment-model intravenous bolus equation utilized in the initial dosing section of this chapter:

$$D = C_{max,ss}\ V(1 - e^{-k_e\tau}) = 20\ mg/L \cdot 61.5\ L\ (1 - e^{-(0.0326\ h^{-1})(48\ h)})$$
$$= 974\ mg,\ \text{rounded to 1000 mg}$$

A dose of vancomycin 1000 mg every 48 hours would be prescribed to begin 48 hours after the last dose of the previous regimen.

BAYESIAN PHARMACOKINETIC COMPUTER PROGRAMS

- Computer programs are available that can assist in the computation of pharmacokinetic parameters for patients.[49–51] The most reliable computer programs use a nonlinear regression algorithm that incorporates components of Bayes' theorem.

  - An advantage of this approach is that consistent dosage recommendations can be made when several different practitioners are involved in therapeutic drug monitoring programs. However, since simpler dosing methods work just as well for patients with stable pharmacokinetic parameters and steady-state drug concentrations, many clinicians reserve the use of computer programs for more difficult situations. Those situations include serum concentrations that are not at steady state, serum concentrations not obtained at the specific times needed to employ simpler methods, and unstable pharmacokinetic parameters.
  - When trough-only monitoring is used during vancomycin therapy, Bayesian pharmacokinetic computer programs can be used to compute a complete patient pharmacokinetic profile that includes clearance, volume of distribution, and half-life.
  - Many Bayesian pharmacokinetic computer programs are available to users, and most should provide answers similar to the one used in the following example. The program used to solve problems in this book is DrugCalc, written by Dr. Dennis Mungall and is available on his Internet web site (www.clinpharmacologist.bigstep.com/consumersurvey.html).[52]

▶ *Example 1* JM is a 50-year-old, 70-kg (height = 5′10″) male with a methicillin-resistant *S. aureus* (MRSA) wound infection. His current serum creatinine is 3.5 mg/dl, and it has been stable over the 5 days since admission. A vancomycin dose of 800 mg every 24 hours was prescribed and expected to achieve steady-state peak and trough concentrations equal to 20 and 5 μg/ml, respectively. After the fourth dose, steady-state peak and trough concentrations were measured and were 25 and 12 μg/ml, respectively. Calculate a new vancomycin dose that will provide a steady-state peak of 20 μg/ml and a trough of 5 μg/ml.

TABLE 5-5 Dosing Schemes

Dosing approach/ philosophy	Initial dosing	Use of serum concentrations to alter doses
Pharmacokinetic parameters/ equations	Pharmacokinetic dosing method	One-compartment-model parameter method
Nomogram/ concepts	Moellering or Matzke nomogram	Trough-only method (1 concentration) or Pharmacokinetic concepts method (≥2 concentrations)
Computerized	Bayesian computer program	Bayesian computer program

1. *Enter patient demographic, drug dosing, and serum concentration/time data into the computer program.*
2. *Compute pharmacokinetic parameters for the patient using the Bayesian pharmacokinetic computer program.* The pharmacokinetic parameters computed by the program are a volume of distribution of 57.4 L, a half-life equal to 24.2 h, and an elimination rate constant of 0.0286 h^{-1}.
3. *Compute dose required to achieve desired vancomycin serum concentrations.* The one-compartment-model intravenous infusion equations used by the program to compute doses indicates that a dose of 1000 mg every 48 hours will produce a steady-state peak concentration of 23 μg/ml and a steady-state trough concentration of 6 μg/ml.

DOSING STRATEGIES

- Initial dose and dosage adjustment techniques using serum concentrations can be used in any combination as long as the limitations of each method are observed.
- Some dosing schemes link together logically when considered according to their basic approaches or philosophies. Dosage strategies that follow similar pathways are given in Table 5-5.

REFERENCES

1. Ackerman BH, Vannier AM, Eudy EB. Analysis of vancomycin time-kill studies with *Staphylococcus* species by using a curve stripping program to describe the relationship between concentration and pharmacodynamic response. Antimicrob Agents Chemother 1992;36(8):1766–9.
2. Kapusnik-Uner JE, Sande MA, Chambers HF. Antimicrobial agents: tetracyclines, chloramphenicol, erythromycin, and miscellaneous antibacterial agents. In: Hardman JG, Limbird LE, eds. Goodman & Gilman's the pharmacological basis of therapeutics. 9th ed. New York: McGraw-Hill, 1996:1123–54.
3. Young EJ, Ratner RE, Clarridge JE. Staphylococcal ventriculitis treated with vancomycin. South Med J 1981;74(8):1014–5.
4. Gump DW. Vancomycin for treatment of bacterial meningitis. Rev Infect Dis 1981;3 suppl:S289–92.
5. Geraci JE, Heilman FR, Nichols DR, Wellman WE, Ross GT. Some laboratory and clinical experience with a new antibiotic vancomycin. Antibiot Annu 1956–1957:90–106.

6. Kirby WMM, Perry DM, Bauer AW. Treatment of staphylococcal septicemia with vancomycin. N Engl J Med 1960;262:49–55.
7. Bailie GR, Neal D. Vancomycin ototoxicity and nephrotoxicity. A review. Med Toxicol Adverse Drug Exp 1988;3(5):376–86.
8. Mellor JA, Kingdom J, Cafferkey M, Keane C. Vancomycin ototoxicity in patients with normal renal function. Br J Audiol 1984;18(3):179–80.
9. Louria DB, Kaminski T, Buchman J. Vancomycin in severe staphylococcal infections. Arch Intern Med 1961;107:225–40.
10. Welty TE, Copa AK. Impact of vancomycin therapeutic drug monitoring on patient care. Ann Pharmacother 1994;28(12):1335–9.
11. Zimmermann AE, Katona BG, Plaisance KI. Association of vancomycin serum concentrations with outcomes in patients with gram-positive bacteremia. Pharmacotherapy 1995;15(1):85–91.
12. Cantu TG, Yamanaka-Yuen NA, Lietman PS. Serum vancomycin concentrations: reappraisal of their clinical value. Clin Infect Dis 1994;18(4):533–43.
13. Karam CM, McKinnon PS, Neuhauser MM, Rybak MJ. Outcome assessment of minimizing vancomycin monitoring and dosing adjustments. Pharmacotherapy 1999;19(3):257–66.
14. Saunders NJ. Why monitor peak vancomycin concentrations? Lancet 1994;344 (8939–8940):1748–50.
15. Kirby WMM, Divelbiss CL. Vancomycin: clinical and laboratory studies. Antibiot Annu 1956–1957:107–17.
16. Spitzer PG, Eliopoulos GM. Systemic absorption of enteral vancomycin in a patient with pseudomembranous colitis. Ann Intern Med 1984;100(4):533–4.
17. Dudley MN, Quintiliani R, Nightingale CH, Gontarz N. Absorption of vancomycin [letter]. Ann Intern Med 1984;101(1):144.
18. Thompson CM Jr, Long SS, Gilligan PH, Prebis JW. Absorption of oral vancomycin—possible associated toxicity. Int J Pediatr Nephrol 1983;4(1):1–4.
19. Matzke GR, Halstenson CE, Olson PL, Collins AJ, Abraham PA. Systemic absorption of oral vancomycin in patients with renal insufficiency and antibiotic-associated colitis. Am J Kidney Dis 1987;9(5):422–5.
20. Krogstad DJ, Moellering RC Jr, Greenblatt DJ. Single-dose kinetics of intravenous vancomycin. J Clin Pharmacol 1980;20(41):197–201.
21. Bauer LA, Black DJ, Lill JS. Vancomycin dosing in morbidly obese patients. Eur J Clin Pharmacol 1998;54(8):621–5.
22. Blouin RA, Bauer LA, Miller DD, Record KE, Griffen WO Jr. Vancomycin pharmacokinetics in normal and morbidly obese subjects. Antimicrob Agents Chemother 1982;21(4):575–80.
23. Moellering RC Jr, Krogstad DJ, Greenblatt DJ. Vancomycin therapy in patients with impaired renal function: a nomogram for dosage. Ann Intern Med 1981;94(3):343–6.
24. Matzke GR, Kovarik JM, Rybak MJ, Boike SC. Evaluation of the vancomycin-clearance:creatinine-clearance relationship for predicting vancomycin dosage. Clin Pharm 1985;4(3):311–5.
25. Matzke GR, McGory RW, Halstenson CE, Keane WF. Pharmacokinetics of vancomycin in patients with various degrees of renal function. Antimicrob Agents Chemother 1984;25(4):433–7.
26. Rybak MJ, Albrecht LM, Berman JR, Warbasse LH, Svensson CK. Vancomycin pharmacokinetics in burn patients and intravenous drug abusers. Antimicrob Agents Chemother 1990;34(5):792–5.
27. Vance-Bryan K, Guay DR, Gilliland SS, Rodvold KA, Rotschafer JC. Effect of obesity on vancomycin pharmacokinetic parameters as determined by using a Bayesian forecasting technique. Antimicrob Agents Chemother 1993;37(3):436–40.
28. Ducharme MP, Slaughter RL, Edwards DJ. Vancomycin pharmacokinetics in a patient population: effect of age, gender, and body weight. Ther Drug Monit 1994; 16(5):513–8.
29. Schaad UB, McCracken GH Jr, Nelson JD. Clinical pharmacology and efficacy of vancomycin in pediatric patients. J Pediatr 1980;96(1):119–26.

30. Gunn VL, Nechyba C, eds. The Harriet Lane handbook: a manual for pediatric house officers. 16th ed. Philadelphia: Mosby, 2002.

31. Rodvold KA, Blum RA, Fischer JH, et al. Vancomycin pharmacokinetics in patients with various degrees of renal function. Antimicrob Agents Chemother 1988;32(6):848–52.

32. Tan CC, Lee HS, Ti TY, Lee EJC. Pharmacokinetics of intravenous vancomycin in patients with end-stage renal disease. Ther Drug Monit 1990;12:29–34.

33. Salem NG, Blevin RB, Matzke GR. Clearance of vancomycin by hemodialysis (abstr). In: Thirtieth annual American Society for Artificial Internal Organs, 1984, Washington, DC, 1984: p. 54.

34. Pollard TA, Lampasona V, Akkerman S, et al. Vancomycin redistribution: dosing recommendations following high-flux hemodialysis. Kidney Int 1994;45(1):232–7.

35. Pancorbo S, Comty C. Peritoneal transport of vancomycin in 4 patients undergoing continuous ambulatory peritoneal dialysis. Nephron 1982;31(1):37–9.

36. Bunke CM, Aronoff GR, Brier ME, Sloan RS, Luft FC. Vancomycin kinetics during continuous ambulatory peritoneal dialysis. Clin Pharmacol Ther 1983; 34(5):631–7.

37. Morse GD, Nairn DK, Walshe JJ. Once weekly intraperitoneal therapy for gram-positive peritonitis. Am J Kidney Dis 1987;10(4):300–5.

38. Boereboom FT, Ververs FF, Blankestijn PJ, Savelkoul TJ, van Dijk A. Vancomycin clearance during continuous venovenous haemofiltration in critically ill patients. Intensive Care Med 1999;25(10):1100–4.

39. Gilbert DN, Moellering RC, Eliopoulos GM, Sande MA. The Sanford guide to antimicrobial therapy. 34th ed. Hyde Park, VT: Antimicrobial Therapy, 2004.

40. Rybak MJ, Albrecht LM, Boike SC, Chandrasekar PH. Nephrotoxicity of vancomycin, alone and with an aminoglycoside. J Antimicrob Chemother 1990;25(4): 679–87.

41. Farber BF, Moellering RC Jr. Retrospective study of the toxicity of preparations of vancomycin from 1974 to 1981. Antimicrob Agents Chemother 1983;23(1):138–41.

42. Angaran DM, Dias VC, Arom KV, et al. The comparative influence of prophylactic antibiotics on the prothrombin response to warfarin in the postoperative prosthetic cardiac valve patient. Cefamandole, cefazolin, vancomycin. Ann Surg 1987;206(2): 155–61.

43. Murphy JE, Winter ME. Clinical pharmacokinetic pearls: bolus versus infusion equations. Pharmacotherapy 1996;16(4):698–700.

44. Black DJ. Modification of Moellering vancomycin clearance/creatinine clearance relationship to allow direct calculation of vancomycin doses (personal communication). 1993.

45. Cockcroft DW, Gault MH. Prediction of creatinine clearance from serum creatinine. Nephron 1976;16:31–41.

46. Salazar DE, Corcoran GB. Predicting creatinine clearance and renal drug clearance in obese patients from estimated fat-free body mass. Am J Med 1988;84:1053–60.

47. McCormack JP, Carleton B. A simpler approach to pharmacokinetic dosage adjustments. Pharmacotherapy 1997;17(6):1349–51.

48. Shargel L, Yu ABC. Applied biopharmaceutics and pharmacokinetics. 4th ed. Stamford, CT: Appleton & Lange, 1999.

49. Pryka RD, Rodvold KA, Garrison M, Rotschafer JC. Individualizing vancomycin dosage regimens: one- versus two-compartment Bayesian models. Ther Drug Monit 1989;11(4):450–4.

50. Rodvold KA, Pryka RD, Garrison M, Rotschafer JC. Evaluation of a two-compartment Bayesian forecasting program for predicting vancomycin concentrations. Ther Drug Monit 1989;11(3):269–75.

51. Rodvold KA, Rotschafer JC, Gilliland SS, Guay DR, Vance-Bryan K. Bayesian forecasting of serum vancomycin concentrations with non-steady-state sampling strategies. Ther Drug Monit 1994;16(1):37–41.

52. Wandell M, Mungall D. Computer assisted drug interpretation and drug regimen optimization. Am Assoc Clin Chem 1984;6:1–11.

3 | CARDIOVASCULAR AGENTS

6 | Digoxin

Digoxin is the primary cardiac glycoside in clinical use. Digoxin is used for the treatment of congestive heart failure (CHF) because of its inotropic effects on the myocardium and for the treatment of atrial fibrillation because of its chronotropic effects on the electrophysiological system of the heart.

- The positive inotropic effect of digoxin is caused by binding to sodium- and potassium-activated adenosine triphosphatase, also known as Na,K-ATPase or the sodium pump.[1] The chronotropic effects of digoxin are mediated via increased parasympathetic activity and vagal tone.

THERAPEUTIC AND TOXIC CONCENTRATIONS

- When given as oral or intravenous doses, the serum digoxin concentration/time curve follows a two-compartment model and exhibits a long and large distribution phase of 8–12 hours (Figure 6-1).[2–4] During the distribution phase, digoxin in the serum is not in equilibrium with digoxin in the tissues, so digoxin serum concentrations should not be measured until the distribution phase is finished.
- When a digoxin serum concentration is very high but the patient is not exhibiting signs or symptoms of digitalis overdose, clinicians should consider the possibility that the blood sample for the determination of a digoxin serum concentration was obtained during the distribution phase.
- There is a great deal of inter- and intrapatient variability in the pharmacodynamic responses to digoxin. Because of pharmacodynamic variability, clinicians should consider these concentration ranges as initial guidelines and rely heavily on patient response to monitor digoxin therapy.

  - Clinically beneficial inotropic effects of digoxin are generally achieved at steady-state serum concentrations of 0.5–1 ng/ml.[5,6] Increasing steady-state serum concentrations to 1.2–1.5 ng/ml may provide some minor, additional inotropic effect.[5,6]
  - Chronotropic effects usually require higher digoxin steady-state serum concentrations of 0.8–1.5 ng/ml.[7,8] Additional chronotropic effects may be observed at digoxin steady-state serum concentrations as high as 2 ng/ml.

- Steady-state digoxin serum concentrations above 2 ng/ml are associated with an increased incidence of adverse drug reactions. At digoxin concentrations of 2.5 ng/ml or above, ~50% of all patients will exhibit some form of digoxin toxicity.[9] Most digoxin side effects involve the gastrointestinal tract, central nervous system, or cardiovascular system.[10]

  - Gastrointestinal-related adverse effects include anorexia, nausea, vomiting, diarrhea, abdominal pain, or constipation.
  - Central nervous system side effects are headache, fatigue, insomnia, confusion, or vertigo. Visual disturbances can also occur and are manifested as blurred vision and changes in color vision or colored halos around objects often times involving the yellow-green spectrum.
  - Cardiac side effects commonly include second- or third-degree atrioventricular block, atrioventricular dissociation, bradycardia, premature ventricular contractions, or ventricular tachycardia. Rarely, almost every cardiac arrhythmia

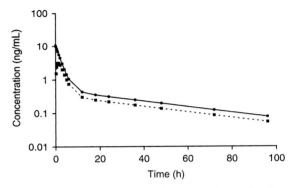

FIG. 6-1 Digoxin serum concentrations after 250-μg doses given intravenously (circles and solid line) and orally as a tablet (squares with dashed line). After an intravenous dose, digoxin serum concentrations are very high because all of the drug is initially in the blood. During the distribution phase, digoxin begins to move out of the vascular system into the tissues. It is also cleared from the body during this phase. Digoxin serum concentrations decline relatively rapidly over an 8–12-hour time period, until the blood and tissues are in pseudo-equilibrium with each other. During the elimination phase, digoxin serum concentrations in patients with good renal function (creatinine clearance >80 ml/min) decline with a half-life of about 36 hours. After oral tablet administration, about 70% of a digoxin dose is absorbed from the gastrointestinal tract. Maximum, or peak, concentrations occur about 1.5–2 hours after oral dosing with tablets, and the distribution phase still lasts 8–12 hours. During the elimination phase, intravenous and oral digoxin have the same terminal half-life.

has been reported to occur due to digoxin toxicity. If a patient develops a new arrhythmia while receiving digoxin treatment, consideration should be given to the possibility that it is digoxin-induced.

• In the case of life-threatening digoxin overdose, digoxin antigen-binding fragments or digoxin immune FAB (Digibind®) are portions of digoxin-specific antibodies that can be used to rapidly reverse the adverse symptoms (see Special Dosing Considerations at the end of the chapter).

CLINICAL MONITORING PARAMETERS

• In patients receiving digoxin for heart failure, the common signs and symptoms of CHF should be routinely monitored. A very useful functional classification for heart failure patients proposed by the New York Heart Association (NYHA) is given in Table 6-1.

  • Left-sided failure: dyspnea on exertion, paroxysmal nocturnal dyspnea, orthopnea, tachypnea, cough, hemoptysis, pulmonary rales/edema, S3 gallop, pleural effusion, Cheyne-Stokes respiration.
  • Right-sided failure: abdominal pain, anorexia, nausea, bloating, constipation, ascites, peripheral edema, jugular venous distention, hepatojugular reflux, hepatomegaly.
  • General symptoms: fatigue, weakness, nocturia, CNS symptoms, tachycardia, pallor, digital cyanosis, cardiomegaly.[11]

TABLE 6-1 New York Heart Association (NYHA) Functional Classification for Heart Failure[11]

NYHA heart failure class	Description
I	Patients with cardiac disease but without limitations of physical activity. Ordinary physical activity does not cause undue fatigue, dyspnea, or palpitation.
II	Patients with cardiac disease that results in slight limitations of physical activity. Ordinary physical activity results in fatigue, palpitation, dyspnea, or angina.
III	Patients with cardiac disease that results in marked limitations of physical activity. Although patients are comfortable at rest, less than ordinary activity will lead to symptoms.
IV	Patients with cardiac disease that results in an inability to carry on physical activity without discomfort. Symptoms of congestive heart failure are present even at rest. With any physical activity, increased discomfort is experienced.

- When used for the treatment of atrial fibrillation, digoxin will not stop the atrial arrhythmia but is used to decrease, or control, the ventricular rate to an acceptable value (usually <100 beats/min).[12] The patient's pulse or ventricular rate should be monitored, and an electrocardiogram can also be useful to clinicians able to interpret the output.
- Patients with severe heart disease such as coronary artery disease (angina, myocardial infarction) can have increased pharmacodynamic sensitivity to cardiac glycosides, and patients receiving these drugs should be monitored closely for adverse drug effects.[9,13]
- Augmented pharmacological responses to digitalis derivatives occur with serum electrolyte disturbances such as hypokalemia, hypomagnesemia, and hypercalcemia even though steady-state digoxin serum concentrations are in the therapeutic range.[1] Serum potassium concentrations should be routinely monitored in patients receiving digoxin and potassium-wasting diuretics.

  - Many patients receiving digoxin and diuretics will be receiving angiotensin I-converting enzyme (ACE) inhibitors, which can cause potassium retention. When receiving ACE inhibitors and diuretics, it can be difficult to reasonably ascertain what the patient's serum potassium status is without measuring it.

- As an adjunct to the patient's clinical response, postdistribution (8–12 hours postdose) steady-state digoxin serum concentrations can be measured 3–5 half-lives after a stable dose is initiated. Digoxin is primarily eliminated unchanged by the kidney (~75%), so its clearance is predominately influenced by renal function.[3,4]

  - Once stable, therapeutic steady-state digoxin serum concentrations and dosage levels have been established, serum creatinine measurements can be used to detect changes in renal function that may result in digoxin clearance and concentration alterations. Hospitalized patients with severe or acute heart failure may need to have serum creatinine determinations 2–3 times weekly to monitor renal function, while ambulatory patients with stable heart failure may need only yearly serum creatinine measurements.

BASIC CLINICAL PHARMACOKINETIC PARAMETERS

- The primary route of digoxin elimination from the body is by the kidney via glomerular filtration and active tubular secretion as unchanged drug (~75%).[3,4] The remainder of a digoxin dose (~25%) is removed by hepatic metabolism or biliary excretion. The primary transporter involved in active tubular secretion and biliary excretion is P-glycoprotein (PGP).
- Enterohepatic recirculation of digoxin occurs.[14]
- Digoxin is given as an intravenous injection or orally as a tablet, capsule, or elixir.

  - When given intravenously, doses should be infused over at least 5–10 minutes.
  - Average oral bioavailability constants (F) for the tablet, capsule, and elixir are 0.7, 0.9, and 0.8.[15–20]
  - Digoxin is available as tablets (125, 250 µg), capsules (50, 100, 200 µg), elixir (50 µg/ml), and intravenous injection (pediatric 100 µg/ml, adult 250 µg/ml).
  - Digoxin is not usually administered intramuscularly due to erratic absorption and severe pain at the injection site.

- Plasma protein binding is ~25% for digoxin.[21,22]
- Usual digoxin doses for adults are 250 µg/d (range 125–500 µg/d) in patients with good renal function (creatinine clearance ≥80 ml/min) and 125 µg every 2–3 days in patients with renal dysfunction (creatinine clearance ≤15 ml/min).

EFFECTS OF DISEASE STATES AND CONDITIONS ON DIGOXIN PHARMACOKINETICS AND DOSING

- Adults with normal renal function (creatinine clearance ≥80 ml/min, Table 6-2) have an average digoxin half-life of 36 hours (range 24–48 hours) and volume of distribution of 7 L/kg (range 5–9 L/kg).[23,24]
- Digoxin pharmacokinetics are not affected by obesity (>30% over ideal body weight), so volume of distribution and dosage estimates should be based on ideal body weight.[25,26]
- Renal dysfunction is the most important disease state that affects digoxin pharmacokinetics.[4]

  - The equation that estimates digoxin clearance from creatinine clearance is

$$Cl = 1.303(CrCl) + Cl_{NR}$$

  where Cl is digoxin clearance in ml/min, CrCl is creatinine clearance in ml/min, and Cl_{NR} is digoxin clearance by nonrenal routes of elimination, which equals 40 ml/min in patients with no or mild heart failure (NYHA CHF class I or II, Table 6-1).[4]
  - Digoxin volume of distribution, in addition to clearance, decreases with declining renal function.[2,27] The equation that estimates digoxin volume of distribution using creatinine clearance is

$$V = \left(226 + \frac{298 \cdot CrCl}{29.1 + CrCl}\right)(Wt/70)$$

  where V is digoxin volume of distribution in L, Wt is body weight in kg (use ideal body weight if >30% overweight) and CrCl is creatinine clearance in ml/min.[27]

TABLE 6-2 Disease States and Conditions That Alter Digoxin Pharmacokinetics

Disease state/condition	Half-life	Volume of distribution	Comment
Adult, normal renal function	36 h or 1.5 d (range 24–48 h)	7 L/kg (range 5–9 L/kg)	Usual dose 250 µg/d (range 125–500 µg/d), resulting in total body stores of 8–12 µg/kg for heart failure or 13–15 µg/kg for atrial fibrillation. Digoxin is eliminated ~75% unchanged renally/~25% nonrenally.
Adult, renal failure	120 h or 5 d	4.5 L/kg average $$V = \left(226 + \frac{298 \cdot CrCl}{29.1 + CrCl}\right)\left(\frac{Wt}{70}\right)$$ where V is digoxin volume of distribution in L, Wt is body weight in kg (use ideal body weight if >30% overweight), and CrCl is creatinine clearance in ml/min	Renal failure patients have decreased digoxin clearance and volume of distribution. As a result, half-life is not as long as might be expected $[t_{1/2} = (0.693V)/Cl]$. Digoxin total body stores decrease to 6–10 µg/kg because of reduced volume of distribution.
Moderate–severe heart failure	See comments	7 L/kg	Heart failure patients (NYHA III–IV) have decreased cardiac output, which causes decreased liver blood flow and digoxin hepatic clearance. In patients with good renal function (creatinine clearance >80 ml/min), the effect on digoxin total clearance is negligible. However in patients with poor renal function, (creatinine clearance <30 ml/min), nonrenal clearance is a primary elimination pathway.
Obesity (>30% over IBW) with normal renal function	36 h or 1.5 d	7 L/kg IBW	Digoxin does not distribute to adipose tissue, so volume of distribution calculations should be conducted with ideal body weight (IBW).
Hyperthyroidism with normal renal function	24 h or 1 d	7 L/kg	Hyperthyroid patients are hypermetabolic and have higher digoxin renal and nonrenal clearances.

- Because digoxin volume of distribution and clearance decrease simultaneously in patients with renal failure, the average half-life for digoxin of 5 days is shorter than what might be expected if clearance alone decreased $[t_{1/2} = (0.693 \cdot V)/Cl]$.
- Digoxin is not significantly eliminated by hemodialysis or peritoneal dialysis.[23,24]
- Hemofiltration does remove digoxin, with a typical sieving coefficient of 0.7.[28,29] In many cases, a sufficient amount of digoxin will not be removed to warrant an increased maintenance dose. However, because of pharmacokinetic variability, some patients may need a periodic booster dose to increase digoxin concentrations (see Special Dosing Consideration at the end of the chapter).[29]
- Heart failure decreases liver blood flow. Moderate–severe heart failure (NYHA CHF class III or IV, Table 6-1) decreases the hepatic clearance of digoxin by this mechanism.[4]

  - When estimating digoxin clearance for the purpose of computing initial drug doses, it is necessary to decrease the nonrenal clearance (Cl_{NR}) factor to 20 ml/min in the equation to compensate for decreased hepatic clearance:

    $$Cl = 1.303(CrCl) + 20$$

    where Cl is digoxin clearance in ml/min, CrCl is creatinine clearance in ml/min, and 20 is digoxin nonrenal clearance Cl_{NR} in ml/min.

- Patients who are hypothyroid have slower metabolic rates and eliminate digoxin more slowly that euthyroid patients (hypothyroid $t_{1/2}$ = 48 hours with normal renal function).[23,24,30–32] Hyperthyroid patients have faster metabolic rates and eliminate digoxin more quickly than euthyroid patients (hyperthyroid $t_{1/2}$ = 24 hours with normal renal function).[23,24,30–32] Hyperthyroid patients can present with atrial fibrillation which may be treated with digoxin. Generally, these patients require higher digoxin doses to control ventricular rate because of the increase in digoxin clearance.
- Digoxin clearance is lower in neonates and premature infants because renal and hepatic function are not completely developed.[33,34] Premature infants and neonates have average digoxin half-lives equal to 60 and 45 hours, respectively. In older babies and young children (6 months–8 years old), renal and hepatic function are fully developed and half-lives can be as short as 18 hours. Older children (≥12 years old) have mean digoxin half-lives ($t_{1/2}$ = 36 hours) that are similar to those found in adults. Also, volume of distribution is larger in infants and children compared to adults, as is found with many other drugs. Suggested doses are as follows.[35]

	Loading dose (μg/kg)		Maintenance dose (μg/kg/d)[a]	
Age	PO	IV/IM	PO	IV/IM
Premature	20	15	5	3–4
Full term	30	20	8–10	6–8
<2 years	40–50	30–40	10–12	7.5–9
2–10 years	30–40	20–30	8–10	6–8
>10 years and <100 kg	10–15	8–12	2.5–5	2–3

[a]Age <10 years, give as divided dose twice daily; age ≥10 years, give once daily.

- Malabsorption of oral digoxin has been reported in patients with severe diarrhea, radiation treatments to the abdomen, and gastrointestinal hypermotility.[30,36–40] In these cases, steady-state digoxin serum concentrations decrease due to poor bioavailability of the drug.

DRUG INTERACTIONS

- Digoxin has an extensive list of drug interactions with other agents. Therefore, only the most common and severe drug interactions will be discussed. Inhibition of P-glycoprotein, a drug efflux pump which is found in the kidney, liver, and intestine, appears to be involved in the majority of digoxin interactions.[41] Clinicians should consult a current drug interaction reference when other medications are prescribed to patients receiving digoxin therapy.

  - Quinidine decreases both the renal and nonrenal clearance of digoxin and also decreases the volume of distribution of digoxin.[42–47] The result of this complex interaction is that concurrent quinidine therapy increases the average steady-state digoxin concentration by 30–70%.
  - Verapamil, diltiazem, and bepridil inhibit digoxin clearance and increase mean digoxin steady-state concentrations by various degrees.[47–53] Of these calcium channel blockers, verapamil is the most potent inhibitor of digoxin clearance and increases digoxin steady-state serum concentrations up to 70%. Diltiazem and bepridil therapy each increase average digoxin steady-state serum concentrations by about 30%.
  - Amiodarone decreases digoxin clearance.[54–57] In addition to this drug interaction mechanism, amiodarone also simultaneously increases digoxin oral bioavailability. Digoxin steady-state serum concentrations increase 2–3 times over baseline values with concomitant amiodarone therapy. Because amiodarone has a very long half-life (~50 days), the onset of the drug interaction with digoxin can be very long.
  - Propafenone therapy decreases digoxin clearance and increases mean digoxin steady-state concentrations by 30–60% in a dose-dependent fashion, with propafenone doses of 450 mg/d causing digoxin concentration changes in the lower end of the range and propafenone doses of 900 mg/d causing digoxin concentration changes in the upper end of the range.[58–60]
  - Cyclosporine therapy has been reported to increase average steady-state digoxin concentrations up to 50%.[61]
  - About 10% of patients receiving digoxin therapy have significant amounts of *Eubacterium lentum* in their gastrointestinal tract that metabolizes orally administered digoxin before it can be absorbed.[62,63] Erythromycin, clarithromycin, and tetracycline are antibiotics that can kill these bacteria.[64–69] Digoxin steady-state serum concentrations increase an average of 30% in these select patients when one of these three antibiotics has been prescribed.

    - P-glycoprotein inhibition may be one of the mechanisms involved in this interaction with macrolide antibiotics.[69]

- The absorption of oral digoxin from the gastrointestinal tract is influenced by many different compounds.

  - Aluminum-containing antacids and kaolin-pectin physically adsorb digoxin, rending it unabsorbable.[70] These compounds should be administered no closer than 2 hours to an oral digoxin dose.

- Cholestyramine also reduces digoxin oral bioavailability by binding it in the gastrointestinal tract and should be given no closer than 8 hours to a digoxin oral dose.[71,72]
- Sulfasalazine and neomycin each decrease digoxin oral bioavailability by unknown mechanisms.[73,74]
- Propantheline increases oral digoxin bioavailability by prolonging gastrointestinal transit time, while metoclopramide and cisapride decreases oral digoxin bioavailability by decreasing gastrointestinal transit time.[72,75,76]

INITIAL DOSAGE DETERMINATION METHODS

- Several methods to initiate digoxin therapy are available:

  - The *pharmacokinetic dosing method* is the most flexible of the techniques. It allows individualized target serum concentrations to be chosen for a patient, and each pharmacokinetic parameter can be customized to reflect specific disease states and conditions present in the patient. However, it is computationally intensive.
  - The *Jelliffe method* is similar to the pharmacokinetic dosing method, except a target total body store is selected based on specific disease states and conditions present in the patient. It is also computationally intensive.
  - *Nomograms* use the dosing concepts of the Jelliffe dosing method. However, in order to make calculations easier, they make simplifying assumptions. The nomograms are for adults only, and separate versions are needed for intravenous injection (Table 6-3A), Tablets (Table 6-3B), and Capsules (Table 6-3C) because of bioavailability differences among the dosage forms.

TABLE 6-3A Jelliffe Nomogram for Intravenous Digoxin (in µg) in Adult Patients with Heart Failure to Provide Total Body Stores of 10 µg/kg[79]

Corrected CrCl (ml/min per 70 kg)[a]		Lean body weight						Number of days before steady state achieved[b]
	kg lb	50 110	60 132	70 154	80 176	90 198	100 220	
0		75[c]	75	100	100	125	150	22
10		75	100	100	125	150	150	19
20		100	100	125	150	150	175	16
30		100	125	150	150	175	200	14
40		100	125	150	175	200	225	13
50		125	150	175	200	225	250	12
60		125	150	175	200	225	250	11
70		150	175	200	225	250	275	10
80		150	175	200	250	275	300	9
90		150	200	225	250	300	325	8
100		175	200	250	275	300	350	7

[a]CrCl is creatinine clearance, corrected to 70-kg body weight or 1.73-m² body surface area. *For adults*, if only serum creatinine concentrations (Scr) are available, a CrCl (corrected to 70-kg body weight) may be estimated in men as (140 − Age)/Scr. For women, this result should be multiplied by 0.85. *Note: This equation cannot be used for estimating creatinine clearance in infants or children.*
[b]If no loading dose is administered.
[c]Daily maintenance doses have been rounded to the nearest 25-µg increment. 75 µg = 0.075 mg

TABLE 6-3B Jelliffe Nomogram for Oral Digoxin Tablets (in μg) in Adult Patients with Heart Failure to Provide Total Body Stores of 10 μg/kg[79]

Corrected CrCl (ml/min per 70 kg)[a]	kg lb	Lean body weight						Number of days before steady state achieved[b]
		50 110	60 132	70 154	80 176	90 198	100 220	
0		62.5[c]	125	125	125	187.5	187.5	22
10		125	125	125	187.5	187.5	187.5	19
20		125	125	187.5	187.5	187.5	250	16
30		125	187.5	187.5	187.5	250	250	14
40		125	187.5	187.5	250	250	250	13
50		187.5	187.5	250	250	250	250	12
60		187.5	187.5	250	250	250	375	11
70		187.5	250	250	250	250	375	10
80		187.5	250	250	250	375	375	9
90		187.5	250	250	250	375	500	8
100		250	250	250	375	375	500	7

[a]CrCl is creatinine clearance, corrected to 70-kg body weight or 1.73-m^2 body surface area. *For adults*, if only serum creatinine concentrations (Scr) are available, a CrCl (corrected to 70-kg body weight) may be estimated in men as (140 − Age)/Scr. For women, this result should be multiplied by 0.85. *Note:* This equation cannot be used for estimating creatinine clearance in infants or children.
[b]If no loading dose is administered.
[c]62.5 μg = 0.0625 mg

TABLE 6-3C Jelliffe Nomogram for Oral Digoxin Capsules (in μg) in Adult Patients with Heart Failure to Provide Total Body Stores of 10 μg/kg[79]

Corrected CrCl (ml/min per 70 kg)[a]	kg lb	Lean body weight						Number of days before steady state achieved[b]
		50 110	60 132	70 154	80 176	90 198	100 220	
0		50[c]	100	100	100	150	150	22
10		100	100	100	150	150	150	19
20		100	100	150	150	150	200	16
30		100	150	150	150	200	200	14
40		100	150	150	200	200	250	13
50		150	150	200	200	250	250	12
60		150	150	200	200	250	300	11
70		150	200	200	250	250	300	10
80		150	200	200	250	300	300	9
90		150	200	250	250	300	350	8
100		200	200	250	300	300	350	7

[a]CrCl is creatinine clearance, corrected to 70-kg body weight or 1.73-m^2 body surface area. *For adults*, if only serum creatinine concentrations (Scr) are available, a CrCl (corrected to 70-kg body weight) may be estimated in men as (140 − Age)/Scr. For women, this result should be multiplied by 0.85. *Note: This equation cannot be used for estimating creatinine clearance in infants or children.*
[b]If no loading dose is administered.
[c]50 μg = 0.05 mg

All three nomograms assume that digoxin total body stores of 10 μg/kg are adequate, so are limited to heart failure patients requiring this dose.

Pharmacokinetic Dosing Method

- The goal of initial dosing of digoxin is to compute the best dose possible for the patient given the set of disease states and conditions that influence digoxin pharmacokinetics and the cardiovascular disorder being treated. In order to do this, pharmacokinetic parameters for the patient are estimated using average parameters measured in other patients with similar disease state and condition profiles. This approach is also known as the Jusko-Koup method for digoxin dosing.[4,27]

Clearance Estimate

- Digoxin is predominately eliminated unchanged in the urine, and there is a good relationship between creatinine clearance and digoxin clearance. This relationship allows estimation of the digoxin clearance for a patient, which can be used to compute an initial dose of the cardiac glycoside:

$$Cl = 1.303(CrCl) + Cl_{NR}$$

where Cl is the digoxin clearance in ml/min, CrCl is creatinine clearance in ml/min, and Cl_{NR} is digoxin nonrenal clearance.[4]

  - A digoxin nonrenal clearance value of 40 ml/min is used for patients without heart failure or who have only mild signs and symptoms of heart failure (NYHA CHF class I or II). Patients with moderate or severe heart failure (NYHA CHF class III or IV) have significant decreases in cardiac output, which leads to a reduction in liver blood flow and digoxin hepatic clearance. In these cases, digoxin nonrenal clearance is set to 20 ml/min in the equation.

Volume of Distribution Estimate

- The average volume of distribution for patients without disease states and conditions that change this parameter is 7 L/kg.[23,24]

  - Because obesity does not change digoxin volume of distribution, the weight factor used in this calculation is ideal body weight (IBW) for patients who are significantly overweight (>30% over IBW).[25,26]

    - If a patient weighs less than his or her ideal body weight, actual body weight is used to estimate volume of distribution.
    - For patients whose weight is between their ideal body weight and 30% over ideal weight, actual body weight can be used to compute estimated volume of distribution, although some clinicians prefer to use ideal body weight for these individuals.

- For patients with renal dysfunction (creatinine clearance ≤30 ml/min), creatinine clearance should be used to provide an improved volume of distribution estimate (V in L) using the following formula:

$$V = \left(226 + \frac{298 \cdot CrCl}{29.1 + CrCl}\right)(Wt/70)$$

where CrCl is the patient's creatinine clearance in ml/min.[27] In patients who are more than 30% above their ideal body weight, volume of distribution

(V) estimates should be based on ideal body weight, so the weight factor used in the equation should be IBW.

Selection of Appropriate Pharmacokinetic Model and Equations

- When given by intravenous injection or orally, digoxin follows a two-compartment pharmacokinetic model (Figure 6-1). While this model is the most correct from a strict pharmacokinetic viewpoint, it cannot easily be used clinically because of its mathematical complexity.

  - A very simple pharmacokinetic equation that computes the average digoxin steady-state serum concentration (Css in ng/ml = μg/L) is widely used and allows maintenence dosage calculation:

$$Css = [F(D/\tau)]/Cl \qquad or \qquad D/\tau = (Css \cdot Cl)/F$$

    where F is the bioavailability fraction for the oral dosage form (F = 1 for intravenous digoxin), D is the digoxin dose in μg, τ is the dosage interval in days, and Cl is digoxin clearance in L/d.[4,27]

- The equation used to calculate loading dose (LD in μg) is based on a simple one-compartment model:

$$LD = (Css \cdot V)/F$$

  where Css is the desired digoxin steady-state concentration in μg/L (which is equivalent to ng/ml), V is the digoxin volume of distribution, and F is the bioavailability fraction for the oral dosage form (F = 1 for intravenous digoxin).

  - When digoxin loading doses are administered, they are usually given in divided doses separated by 4–6 hours (50% of dose at first, followed by two additional doses of 25%). A portion of the loading dose can be withheld if the patient is experiencing any adverse effects to digoxin, such as a low pulse rate. This technique is used to allow the assessment of clinical response before additional digoxin is given, in order to avoid accidental overdosage.
  - When rapid digitalization is indicated, loading doses can be administered as close as 2 hours apart, with intensive patient monitoring for effect and adverse drug reactions (American College of Cardiology, American Heart Association, European Society of Cardiology Joint Guidelines for Atrial Fibrillation).

Steady-State Concentration Selection

- Digoxin steady-state concentrations are selected based on the cardiovascular disease being treated.

  - For heart failure, steady-state serum concentrations of 0.5–1 ng/ml are usually effective.[5,6] For initial dosing purposes, a target digoxin concentration equal to 0.8 ng/ml is reasonable.
  - For patients with atrial fibrillation, steady-state serum concentrations of 0.8–1.5 ng/ml are usually needed to control the ventricular rate to 100 beats/min or less.[7,24] An initial target digoxin concentration of 1.2 ng/ml is reasonable for patients with this disease state.

▶ **Example 1**   MJ is a 50-year-old, 70-kg (height = 5′10″) male who has experienced atrial fibrillation for less than 24 hours. His current serum creatinine is 0.9 mg/dl, and it has been stable over the 5 days since admission. Compute an intravenous digoxin dose for this patient to control ventricular rate.

1. *Estimate creatinine clearance.* This patient has a stable serum creatinine and is not obese. The Cockcroft-Gault equation can be used to estimate creatinine clearance:

$$CrCl_{est} = \frac{(140 - age)BW}{72 \cdot S_{Cr}} = \frac{(140 - 50\,y)70\,kg}{72 \cdot 0.9\,mg/dl}$$

$$CrCl_{est} = 97\,ml/min$$

2. *Estimate clearance.* The drug clearance/creatinine clearance relationship is used to estimate the digoxin clearance for this patient ($Cl_{NR} = 40$ ml/min, since the patient does not have moderate–severe heart failure):

$$Cl = 1.303(CrCl) + Cl_{NR} = 1.303(97\,ml/min) + 40\,ml/min = 167\,ml/min$$

3. *Use average steady-state concentration equation to compute digoxin maintenance dose.* For a patient with atrial fibrillation, the desired digoxin concentration is 0.8–1.5 ng/ml. A serum concentration of 1.2 ng/ml is chosen for this patient, and intravenous digoxin will be used (F = 1). Note that for concentration units ng/ml = μg/L, and this conversion will be made before the equation is used. Also, conversion factors are needed to change ml units to L (1000 ml/L) and min units to days (1440 min/d).

$$D/\tau = (Css \cdot Cl)/F$$
$$= (1.2\ \mu g/L \cdot 167\ ml/min \cdot 1440\ min/d)/(1 \cdot 1000\ ml/L)$$
$$= 288\ \mu g/d,\ round\ to\ 250\ \mu g/d.$$

4. *Use loading dose equation to compute digoxin loading dose (if needed).* The patient has good renal function and is not obese. Therefore, a volume of distribution equal to 7 L/kg and actual body weight can be used to compute the digoxin loading dose. An intravenous loading dose (F = 1) could be used in this patient to achieve the desired pharmacological effect more quickly than would occur if maintenance doses alone were used and concentrations allowed to accumulate over 3–5 half-lives.

$$V = 7\ L/kg \cdot 70\ kg = 490\ L$$

$$LD = (Css \cdot V)/F = (1.2\ \mu g/L \cdot 490\ L)/1 = 588\ \mu g\ rounded\ to\ 500\ \mu g.$$

When digoxin loading doses are administered, they are usually given in divided doses separated by 4–6 hours (50% of dose at first, followed by two additional doses of 25%). In this case, an initial intravenous dose of 250 μg would be given initially, followed by two additional intravenous doses of 125 μg each. One of the loading doses could be withheld if pulse rate was less than 50–60 beats/min or other undesirable digoxin adverse effects were noted.

▶ *Example 2*   Same patient profile as in Example 1, but serum creatinine is 3.5 mg/dl, indicating renal impairment.

1. *Estimate creatinine clearance.* This patient has a stable serum creatinine and is not obese. The Cockcroft-Gault equation can be used to estimate creatinine clearance:

$$CrCl_{est} = \frac{(140 - age)BW}{72 \cdot S_{Cr}} = \frac{(140 - 50\,y)70\,kg}{72 \cdot 3.5\,mg/dl}$$

$$CrCl_{est} = 25\,ml/min$$

2. *Estimate clearance*. The drug clearance/creatinine clearance relationship is used to estimate the digoxin clearance for this patient (Cl_{NR} = 40 ml/min, since the patient does not have moderate–severe heart failure):

$$Cl = 1.303(CrCl) + Cl_{NR} = 1.303(25 \text{ ml/min}) + 40 \text{ ml/min} = 73 \text{ ml/min}$$

3. *Use average steady-state concentration equation to compute digoxin maintenance dose*. For a patient with atrial fibrillation, the desired digoxin concentration is 0.8–1.5 ng/ml. A serum concentration of 1.2 ng/ml is chosen for this patient, and intravenous digoxin will be used (F = 1). Note that for concentration units ng/ml = µg/L, and this conversion will be made before the equation is used. Also, conversion factors are needed to change ml units to L (1000 ml/L) and min units to days (1440 min/d).

$$D/\tau = (Css \cdot Cl)/F$$
$$= (1.2 \text{ µg/L} \cdot 73 \text{ ml/min} \cdot 1440 \text{ min/d})/(1 \cdot 1000 \text{ ml/L})$$
$$= 125 \text{ µg/d.}$$

4. *Use loading dose equation to compute digoxin loading dose (if needed)*. The patient has poor renal function and is not obese. Therefore, the volume of distribution equation that adjusts the parameter estimate for renal dysfunction can be used to compute the digoxin loading dose. An intravenous loading dose (F = 1) could be given in this patient to achieve the desired pharmacological effect more quickly than would occur if maintenance doses alone were used to allow concentrations to accumulate over 3–5 half-lives.

$$V = \left(226 + \frac{298 \cdot CrCl}{29.1 + CrCl} \right)(Wt/70)$$

$$= \left(226 + \frac{298 \cdot 25 \text{ ml/min}}{29.1 + 25 \text{ ml/min}} \right)(70 \text{ kg}/70) = 364 \text{ L}$$

$$LD = (Css \cdot V)/F = (1.2 \text{ µg/L} \cdot 364 \text{ L})/1 = 437 \text{ µg rounded to } 400 \text{ µg.}$$

When digoxin loading doses are administered, they are usually given in divided doses separated by 4–6 hours (50% of dose at first, followed by two additional doses of 25%). In this case, an initial intravenous dose of 200 µg would be given initially, followed by two additional intravenous doses of 100 µg each. One of the loading doses could be withheld if pulse rate was less than 50–60 beats/min or other undesirable digoxin adverse effects were noted.

▶ *Example 3*   Same patient profile as in Example 1, but serum creatinine is 3.5 mg/dl, indicating renal impairment. Additionally, the patient is being treated for NYHA class III moderate heart failure, not atrial fibrillation. Compute an oral digoxin tablet maintenance dose for this patient.

1. *Estimate creatinine clearance*. This patient has a stable serum creatinine and is not obese. The Cockcroft-Gault equation can be used to estimate creatinine clearance:

$$CrCl_{est} = \frac{(140 - age)BW}{72 \cdot S_{Cr}} = \frac{(140 - 50 \text{ y})70 \text{ kg}}{72 \cdot 3.5 \text{ mg/dl}}$$
$$CrCl_{est} = 25 \text{ ml/min}$$

2. *Estimate clearance.* The drug clearance/creatinine clearance relationship is used to estimate the digoxin clearance for this patient ($Cl_{NR} = 20$ ml/min, since the patient has moderate heart failure):

$$Cl = 1.303(CrCl) + Cl_{NR} = 1.303(25 \text{ ml/min}) + 20 \text{ ml/min} = 53 \text{ ml/min}$$

3. *Use average steady-state concentration equation to compute digoxin maintenance dose.* For a patient with heart failure, the desired digoxin concentration is 0.5–1 ng/ml. A serum concentration of 0.8 ng/ml is chosen for this patient, and oral digoxin will be used ($F = 0.7$). Note that for concentration units ng/ml = μg/L, and this conversion will be made before the equation is used. Also, conversion factors are needed to change ml units to L (1000 ml/L) and min units to days (1440 min/d).

$$D/\tau = (Css \cdot Cl)/F$$

$$= (0.8 \ \mu g/L \cdot 53 \text{ ml/min} \cdot 1440 \text{ min/d})/(0.7 \cdot 1000 \text{ ml/L}) = 87 \ \mu g/d$$

or 174 μg every 2 days (87 μg/d · 2 d = 174 μg every 2 days). This oral tablet dose would be rounded to 125 μg every other day.

▶ *Example 4* OI is a 65-year-old, 170-kg (height = 5′5″) female with NYHA class III moderate heart failure. Her current serum creatinine is 4.7 mg/dl and is stable. Compute an intravenous digoxin loading and maintenance dose for this patient.

1. *Estimate creatinine clearance.* This patient has a stable serum creatinine and is obese [$IBW_{females}$ (in kg) = 45 + 2.3(Ht − 60) = 45 + 2.3(65″ − 60) = 57 kg]. The Salazar and Corcoran equation can be used to estimate creatinine clearance:

$$CrCl_{est(females)} = \frac{(146 - age)[(0.287 \cdot Wt) + (9.74 \cdot Ht^2)]}{60 \cdot S_{Cr}}$$

$$CrCl_{est(females)} = \frac{(146 - 65 \text{ y})\{(0.287 \cdot 170 \text{ kg}) + [9.74 \cdot (1.65 \text{ m})^2]\}}{60 \cdot 4.7 \text{ mg/dl}}$$

$$= 22 \text{ ml/min}$$

Note: Height is converted from inches to meters: Ht = (65 in · 2.54 cm/in)/(100 cm/m) = 1.65 m.

2. *Estimate clearance.* The drug clearance/creatinine clearance relationship is used to estimate the digoxin clearance for this patient ($Cl_{NR} = 20$ ml/min, since the patient has moderate–severe heart failure):

$$Cl = 1.303(CrCl) + Cl_{NR} = 1.303(22 \text{ ml/min}) + 20 \text{ ml/min} = 48 \text{ ml/min}$$

3. *Use average steady-state concentration equation to compute digoxin maintenance dose.* For a patient with heart failure, the desired digoxin concentration is 0.5–1 ng/ml. A serum concentration of 0.8 ng/ml is chosen for this patient, and intravenous digoxin will be used ($F = 1$). Note that for concentration units ng/ml = μg/L, and this conversion will be made before the equation is used. Also, conversion factors are

needed to change ml units to L (1000 ml/L) and min units to days (1440 min/d).

$$D/\tau = (Css \cdot Cl)/F$$
$$= (0.8 \ \mu g/L \cdot 48 \ ml/min \cdot 1440 \ min/d)/(1 \cdot 1000 \ ml/L) = 55 \ \mu g/d$$

or 110 μg every 2 days (55 μg/d · 2 d = 110 μg every 2 days). This intravenous dose would be rounded to 125 μg every other day.

4. *Use loading dose equation to compute digoxin loading dose (if needed).* The patient has poor renal function and is obese. Therefore, the volume of distribution equation that adjusts the parameter estimate for renal dysfunction can be used to compute the digoxin loading dose, and ideal body weight will be used as the weight factor. An intravenous loading dose (F = 1) could be given in this patient to achieve the desired pharmacologic effect more quickly than would occur if maintenance doses alone were used to allow concentrations to accumulate over 3–5 half-lives.

$$V = \left(226 + \frac{298 \cdot CrCl}{29.1 + CrCl}\right)(Wt/70)$$
$$= \left(226 + \frac{298 \cdot 22 \ ml/min}{29.1 + 22 \ ml/min}\right)(57 \ kg/70) = 288 \ L$$

$$LD = (Css \cdot V)/F = (0.8 \ \mu g/L \cdot 288 \ L)/1 = 230 \ \mu g \ \text{rounded to} \ 250 \ \mu g.$$

When digoxin loading doses are administered, they are usually given in divided doses separated by 4–6 hours (50% of dose at first, followed by two additional doses of 25%). In this case, an initial intravenous dose of 125 μg would be given initially, followed by two additional intravenous doses of 62.5 μg each. One of the loading doses could be withheld if pulse rate was less than 50–60 beats/min or other undesirable digoxin adverse effects were noted.

Jelliffe Method

• Another approach to derive initial doses of digoxin is to compute an appropriate loading dose which provides an amount of the drug in the body that evokes the appropriate pharmacological response.[77,78] The amount of digoxin in the body that produces the desired effect is known as the total body store (TBS) of digoxin.

• Because the goal of therapy is to maintain total body stores of digoxin that cause the appropriate inotropic or chronotropic effect, the maintenance dose (D in μg/d) is the amount of digoxin eliminated on a daily basis:

$$D = \frac{TBS \cdot [14\% + 0.20(CrCl)]}{F \cdot 100}$$

where TBS is total body stores in μg/d, 14% is the percent of digoxin eliminated per day by nonrenal routes, CrCl is creatinine clearance in ml/min, F is the bioavailability factor for the dosage form, and 100 is a conversion factor to convert the percentage to a fraction.[78]

• For patients with creatinine clearance values over 30 ml/min, digoxin total body stores of 8–12 μg/kg are usually required to cause inotropic effects, while 13–15 μg/kg are generally needed to cause chronotropic effects.[79,80] Since renal disease (creatinine clearance <30 ml/min) decreases digoxin volume of distribution, initial digoxin total body stores of 6–10 μg/kg are recommended for patients with poor renal function.[79]

- If a loading dose is required, the total body store (TBS in µg) is calculated and used to compute the loading dose (LD in µg) after correction for dosage-form bioavailability (F):[77,78]

$$LD = TBS/F$$

- Because obesity does not change digoxin volume of distribution, the weight factor used in these calculations is ideal body weight (IBW) for patients who are significantly overweight (>30% over IBW).[25,26] If a patient weighs less than his or her ideal body weight, actual body weight is used to calculate total body stores. For patients whose weight is between their ideal body weight and 30% over ideal weight, actual body weight can be used to compute total body stores, although some clinicians prefer to use ideal body weight for these individuals.

- To contrast the Jelliffe dosage method with the Jusko-Koup dosage method, the same patient cases will be used as examples for this section.

▶ *Example 1*   MJ is a 50-year-old, 70-kg (height = 5′10″) male who has experienced atrial fibrillation for less than 24 hours. His current serum creatinine is 0.9 mg/dl, and it has been stable over the 5 days since admission. Compute an intravenous digoxin dose for this patient to control ventricular rate.

1. *Estimate creatinine clearance.* This patient has a stable serum creatinine and is not obese. The Cockcroft-Gault equation can be used to estimate creatinine clearance:

$$CrCl_{est} = \frac{(140 - age)BW}{72 \cdot S_{Cr}} = \frac{(140 - 50 \text{ y})70 \text{ kg}}{72 \cdot 0.9 \text{ mg/dl}}$$
$$CrCl_{est} = 97 \text{ ml/min}$$

2. *Estimate total body stores (TBS) and maintenance dose (D).* The patient has good renal function and is not obese. Digoxin total body stores of 13–15 µg/kg are effective in the treatment of atrial fibrillation. A digoxin dose of 14 µg/kg is chosen for this patient.

$$TBS = 14 \text{ µg/kg} \cdot 70 \text{ kg} = 980 \text{ µg}$$
$$D = \frac{TBS \cdot [14\% + 0.20(CrCl)]}{F \cdot 100} = \frac{980 \text{ µg} \cdot [14\% + 0.20(97 \text{ ml/min})]}{1 \cdot 100}$$
$$= 328 \text{ µg/d, rounded to 375 µg/d}$$

3. *Use loading dose equation to compute digoxin loading dose (if needed).* Digoxin total body store is used to calculate the loading dose after correcting for bioavailability:

$$LD = TBS/F = 980 \text{ µg}/1 = 980 \text{ µg, rounded to 1000 µg}$$

When digoxin loading doses are administered, they are usually given in divided doses separated by 4–6 hours (50% of dose at first, followed by two additional doses of 25%). In this case, an initial intravenous dose of 500 µg would be given initially, followed by two additional intravenous doses of 250 µg each. One of the loading doses could be withheld if pulse rate was less than 50–60 beats/min or other undesirable digoxin adverse effects were noted.

► *Example 2* Same patient profile as in Example 1, but serum creatinine is 3.5 mg/dl, indicating renal impairment.

1. *Estimate creatinine clearance.* This patient has a stable serum creatinine and is not obese. The Cockcroft-Gault equation can be used to estimate creatinine clearance:

$$CrCl_{est} = \frac{(140 - age)BW}{72 \cdot S_{Cr}} = \frac{(140 - 50 \text{ y})70 \text{ kg}}{72 \cdot 3.5 \text{ mg/dl}}$$

$$CrCl_{est} = 25 \text{ ml/min}$$

2. *Estimate total body stores* (*TBS*) *and maintenance dose* (*D*). The patient has poor renal function and is not obese. Digoxin total body stores of 6–10 µg/kg are recommended for patients with renal dysfunction. A digoxin dose of 8 µg/kg is chosen for this patient.

$$TBS = 8 \text{ µg/kg} \cdot 70 \text{ kg} = 560 \text{ µg}$$

$$D = \frac{TBS \cdot [14\% + 0.20(CrCl)]}{F \cdot 100} = \frac{560 \text{ µg} \cdot [14\% + 0.20(25 \text{ ml/min})]}{1 \cdot 100}$$

$$= 106 \text{ µg/d, rounded to } 125 \text{ µg/d}$$

3. *Use loading dose equation to compute digoxin loading dose* (*if needed*). Digoxin total body store is used to calculate the loading dose after correcting for bioavailability:

$$LD = TBS/F = 560 \text{ µg}/1 = 560 \text{ µg, rounded to } 500 \text{ µg}$$

When digoxin loading doses are administered, they are usually given in divided doses separated by 4–6 hours (50% of dose at first, followed by two additional doses of 25%). In this case, an initial intravenous dose of 250 µg would be given initially, followed by two additional intravenous doses of 125 µg each. One of the loading doses could be withheld if pulse rate was less than 50–60 beats/min or other undesirable digoxin adverse effects were noted.

► *Example 3* Same patient profile as in Example 1, but serum creatinine is 3.5 mg/dl, indicating renal impairment. Additionally, the patient is being treated for NYHA class III moderate heart failure, not atrial fibrillation. Compute an oral digoxin tablet maintenance dose for this patient.

1. *Estimate creatinine clearance.* This patient has a stable serum creatinine and is not obese. The Cockcroft-Gault equation can be used to estimate creatinine clearance:

$$CrCl_{est} = \frac{(140 - age)BW}{72 \cdot S_{Cr}} = \frac{(140 - 50 \text{ y})70 \text{ kg}}{72 \cdot 3.5 \text{ mg/dl}}$$

$$CrCl_{est} = 25 \text{ ml/min}$$

2. *Estimate total body stores* (*TBS*) *and maintenance dose* (*D*). The patient has poor renal function and is not obese. Digoxin total body stores of 6–10 µg/kg are recommended for patients with renal dysfunction. A digoxin dose of 8 µg/kg is chosen for this patient.

$$TBS = 8 \text{ µg/kg} \cdot 70 \text{ kg} = 560 \text{ µg}$$

$$D = \frac{TBS \cdot [14\% + 0.20(CrCl)]}{F \cdot 100} = \frac{560 \text{ µg} \cdot [14\% + 0.20(25 \text{ ml/min})]}{0.7 \cdot 100}$$

$$= 152 \text{ µg/d, rounded to } 125 \text{ µg/d}$$

▶ *Example 4*   OI is a 65-year-old, 170-kg (5′5″) female with NYHA class III moderate heart failure. Her current serum creatinine is 4.7 mg/dl and is stable. Compute an intravenous digoxin loading and maintenance dose for this patient.

1. *Estimate creatinine clearance.* This patient has a stable serum creatinine and is obese [$IBW_{females}$ (in kg) $= 45 + 2.3(Ht - 60) = 45 + 2.3(65″ - 60) = 57$ kg]. The Salazar and Corcoran equation can be used to estimate creatinine clearance:

$$CrCl_{est(females)} = \frac{(146 - age)[(0.287 \cdot Wt) + (9.74 \cdot Ht^2)]}{60 \cdot S_{Cr}}$$

$$CrCl_{est(females)} = \frac{(146 - 65 \text{ y})\{(0.287 \cdot 170 \text{ kg}) + [9.74 \cdot (1.65 \text{ m})^2]\}}{60 \cdot 4.7 \text{ mg/dl}}$$

$$= 22 \text{ ml/min}$$

Note: Height is converted from inches to meters: Ht $= (65 \text{ in} \cdot 2.54 \text{ cm/in})/(100 \text{ cm/m}) = 1.65$ m.

2. *Estimate total body stores* (TBS) *and maintenance dose* (D). The patient has poor renal function and is obese. Digoxin total body stores of 6–10 μg/kg are recommended for patients with renal dysfunction, and ideal body weight (IBW) should be used in the computation. A digoxin dose of 8 μg/kg is chosen for this patient.

$$TBS = 8 \text{ μg/kg} \cdot 57 \text{ kg} = 456 \text{ μg}$$

$$D = \frac{TBS \cdot [14\% + 0.20(CrCl)]}{F \cdot 100} = \frac{456 \text{ μg} \cdot [14\% + 0.20(22 \text{ ml/min})]}{1 \cdot 100}$$

$$= 84 \text{ μg/d}$$

or 168 μg every 2 days (84 μg/d · 2 days = 168 μg every 2 days). This intravenous dose would be rounded to 150 μg every other day.

3. *Use loading dose equation to compute digoxin loading dose* (if needed). Digoxin total body store is used to calculate the loading dose after correcting for bioavailability:

$$LD = TBS/F = 456 \text{ μg}/1 = 456 \text{ μg, rounded to } 500 \text{ μg}$$

When digoxin loading doses are administered, they are usually given in divided doses separated by 4–6 hours (50% of dose at first, followed by two additional doses of 25%). In this case, an initial intravenous dose of 250 μg would be given initially, followed by two additional intravenous doses of 125 μg each. One of the loading doses could be withheld if pulse rate was less than 50–60 beats/min or other undesirable digoxin adverse effects were noted.

USE OF DIGOXIN SERUM CONCENTRATIONS TO ALTER DOSAGES

• Because of pharmacokinetic variability among patients, it is likely that doses computed using patient population characteristics will not always produce digoxin serum concentrations that are expected. Because of this, digoxin serum concentrations are measured in many patients to ensure that therapeutic, nontoxic levels are present and to check for compliance to dosage regimens.

- Not all patients will require serum concentration monitoring. For example, if an appropriate dose for the renal function and concurrent disease states of the patient is prescribed (e.g., 250 μg/d in a patient with a creatinine clearance of 80–100 ml/min for heart failure) and the desired clinical effect is achieved without adverse effects, digoxin serum concentration monitoring may not be necessary.
- Whether or not digoxin concentrations are measured, important patient parameters (dyspnea, orthopnea, tachypnea, cough, pulmonary rales/edema, S3 gallop, etc.) should be followed to confirm that the patient is responding to treatment and not developing adverse drug reactions.
- When digoxin serum concentrations are measured in patients and a dosage change is necessary, clinicians should seek to use the simplest, most straightforward method available to determine a dose that will provide safe and effective treatment.

  - In most cases, a simple dosage ratio can be used to change digoxin doses, since digoxin follows *linear pharmacokinetics*. Sometimes it is not possible simply to change the dose because of the limited number of oral dosage strengths, and the dosage interval must also be changed. Available digoxin tablet strengths are 125 and 250 μg, while 50-, 100-, and 200-μg digoxin capsules are available.
  - In some situations it may be necessary or desirable to compute the digoxin *pharmacokinetic parameters* for the patient and utilize these to calculate the best drug dose.
  - Computerized methods that incorporate expected population pharmacokinetic characteristics (*Bayesian pharmacokinetic computer programs*) can be used in difficult cases in which renal function is changing, serum concentrations are obtained at suboptimal times, or the patient was not at steady state when serum concentrations were measured.

Linear Pharmacokinetics Method

- Because digoxin follows linear, dose-proportional pharmacokinetics, steady-state serum concentrations change in proportion to dose according to the following equation:

$$D_{new}/C_{ss,\,new} = D_{old}/C_{ss,old} \qquad \text{or} \qquad D_{new} = (C_{ss,new}/C_{ss,old})D_{old}$$

where D is the dose in μg, C_{ss} is the steady-state concentration in ng/ml, old indicates the dose that produced the steady-state concentration that the patient is currently receiving, and new denotes the dose necessary to produce the desired steady-state concentration.

  - The advantages of this method are that it is quick and simple. The main disadvantage is that steady-state concentrations are required. Also, because of a limited number of solid oral dosage strengths, it may not be possible to attain desired serum concentrations by changing only the dose. In these cases, dosage intervals are extended for patients receiving tablets so that doses can be given as multiples of 125 μg and for patients receiving capsules so that doses can be given in multiples of 50 μg.

- The estimated times to achieve steady-state concentrations on a stable digoxin dosage regimen vary according to renal function and are listed in Table 6-4.[79] An alternative to this way of estimating time to steady state is

TABLE 6-4   Estimated Time to Steady-State for Digoxin When a Stable Dosage Regimen is Administered.[79]

Creatinine clearance (ml/min/70 kg)	Number of days before steady-state achieved
0	22
10	19
20	16
30	14
40	13
50	12
60	11
70	10
80	9
90	8
100	7

to compute the expected digoxin half-life ($t_{1/2}$ in days) for a patient, using digoxin clearance (Cl in L/d) and volume of distribution (V in L), and allow 3–5 half lives to pass before obtaining digoxin serum concentrations:

$$t_{1/2} = (0.693 \cdot V)/Cl$$

▶ *Example 1*   MJ is a 50-year-old, 70-kg (height = 5′10″) male with moderate heart failure. His current serum creatinine is 0.9 mg/dl, and it has been stable over the last 6 months. A digoxin dose of 250 μg/d using oral tablets was prescribed and expected to achieve steady-state concentrations equal to 0.8 ng/ml. After a week of treatment, a steady-state digoxin concentration was measured and equalled 0.6 ng/ml. Calculate a new digoxin dose that will provide a steady-state concentration of 0.9 ng/ml.

1. *Estimate creatinine clearance.* This patient has a stable serum creatinine and is not obese. The Cockcroft-Gault equation can be used to estimate creatinine clearance:

$$CrCl_{est} = \frac{(140 - age)BW}{72 \cdot S_{Cr}} = \frac{(140 - 50 \text{ y})70 \text{ kg}}{72 \cdot 0.9 \text{ mg/dl}}$$
$$CrCl_{est} = 97 \text{ ml/min}$$

The patient has good renal function and can be expected to achieve steady-state after 7 days of treatment. *Note that this step can be omitted if it is known that the patient is at steady state.*

2. *Compute new dose to achieve desired serum concentration.* Using linear pharmacokinetics, the new dose to attain the desired concentration should be proportional to the old dose that produced the measured concentration:

$$D_{new} = (C_{ss,new}/C_{ss,old})D_{old} = (0.9 \text{ ng/ml}/0.6 \text{ ng/ml}) \, 250 \text{ μg/d} = 375 \text{ μg/d}$$

The new suggested dose is 375 μg/d given as digoxin tablets, to be started at the next scheduled dosing time.

▶ *Example 2* OI is a 65-year-old, 170-kg (5′5″) female with NYHA class III heart failure. Her current serum creatinine is 4.7 mg/dl and is stable. A digoxin dose of 125 μg/d given as tablets was prescribed and expected to achieve steady-state concentrations equal to 1 ng/ml. After 3 weeks of therapy, a steady-state digoxin concentration was measured and equalled 2.5 ng/ml. Calculate a new digoxin dose that will provide a steady-state concentration of 1.2 ng/ml.

1. *Estimate creatinine clearance.* This patient has a stable serum creatinine and is obese [$IBW_{females}$ (in kg) $= 45 + 2.3(Ht − 60) = 45 + 2.3(65″ − 60) = 57$ kg]. The Salazar and Corcoran equation can be used to estimate creatinine clearance:

$$CrCl_{est(females)} = \frac{(146 - age)[(0.287 \cdot Wt) + (9.74 \cdot Ht^2)]}{60 \cdot S_{Cr}}$$

$$CrCl_{est(females)} = \frac{(146 - 65 \text{ y})\{(0.287 \cdot 170 \text{ kg}) + [9.74 \cdot (1.65 \text{ m})^2]\}}{60 \cdot 4.7 \text{ mg/dl}}$$

$$= 22 \text{ ml/min}$$

Note: Height is converted from inches to meters: Ht = (65 in · 2.54 cm/in)/(100 cm/m) = 1.65 m.

This patient has poor renal function, but can be expected to be at steady-state with regard to digoxin serum concentrations after 3 weeks of treatment. *Note that this step can be omitted if it is known that the patient is at steady-state.*

2. *Compute new dose to achieve desired serum concentration.* Using linear pharmacokinetics, the new dose to attain the desired concentration should be proportional to the old dose that produced the measured concentration:

$$D_{new} = (C_{ss,new}/C_{ss,old})D_{old} = (1.2 \text{ ng/ml}/2.5 \text{ ng/ml}) \, 125 \text{ μg/d} = 60 \text{ μg/d}$$

or 120 μg every other day (60 μg/d · 2 days = 120 μg every 2 days). This would be rounded to digoxin tablets 125 μg every other day.

The new suggested dose would be 125 μg every other day given as digoxin tablets, to be started at the next scheduled dosing time. Since the dosage interval is being changed, a day should be skipped before the next dose is given.

Pharmacokinetic Parameter Method

- The pharmacokinetic parameter method calculates the patient-specific drug clearance, and uses it to design an improved dosage regimen.[23,24] Digoxin clearance can be measured using a single steady-state digoxin concentration (C_{ss}) and the following formula:

$$Cl = [F(D/\tau)]/C_{ss}$$

where Cl is digoxin clearance in L/d, F is the bioavailability factor for the dosage form used, τ is the dosage interval in days, and C_{ss} is the digoxin steady-state concentration in ng/ml, which also equals μg/L.

- Although this method does allow computation of digoxin clearance, it yields exactly the same digoxin dose as that supplied using linear pharmacokinetics. As a result, most clinicians prefer to calculate the new dose directly, using the simpler linear pharmacokinetics method. To illustrate this point, the patient cases used in the linear pharmacokinetics method will be used as examples for the pharmacokinetic parameter method.

▶ *Example 1* MJ is a 50-year-old, 70-kg (height = 5′10″) male with moderate heart failure. His current serum creatinine is 0.9 mg/dl, and it has been stable over the last 6 months. A digoxin dose of 250 μg/d using oral tablets was prescribed and expected to achieve steady-state concentrations equal to 0.8 ng/ml. After a week of treatment, a steady-state digoxin concentration was measured and equalled 0.6 ng/ml. Calculate a new digoxin dose that will provide a steady-state concentration of 0.9 ng/ml.

1. *Estimate creatinine clearance.* This patient has a stable serum creatinine and is not obese. The Cockcroft-Gault equation can be used to estimate creatinine clearance:

$$CrCl_{est} = \frac{(140 - age)BW}{72 \cdot S_{Cr}} = \frac{(140 - 50 \text{ y})70 \text{ kg}}{72 \cdot 0.9 \text{ mg/dl}}$$

$$CrCl_{est} = 97 \text{ ml/min}$$

The patient has good renal function and can be expected to have achieved steady-state after 7 days of treatment. *Note that this step can be omitted if it is known that the patient is at steady state.*

2. *Compute drug clearance.* Note that digoxin concentrations in ng/ml are the same as those for μg/L. This unit substitution will be made directly, to avoid conversion factors in the computation.

$$Cl = [F(D/\tau)]/C_{ss} = [0.7(250 \text{ μg/d})]/0.6 \text{ μg/L} = 292 \text{ L/d}$$

3. *Compute new dose to achieve desired serum concentration.* The average steady-state equation is used to compute the new digoxin dose.

$$D/\tau = (C_{ss} \cdot Cl)/F = (0.9 \text{ μg/L} \cdot 292 \text{ L/d})/0.7 = 375 \text{ μg/d}$$

The new suggested dose is 375 μg/d given as digoxin tablets, to be started at the next scheduled dosing time.

▶ *Example 2* OI is a 65-year-old, 170-kg (5′5″) female with NYHA class III heart failure. Her current serum creatinine is 4.7 mg/dl and is stable. A digoxin dose of 125 μg/d given as tablets was prescribed and expected to achieve steady-state concentrations equal to 1 ng/ml. After 3 weeks of therapy, a steady-state digoxin concentration was measured and equalled 2.5 ng/ml. Calculate a new digoxin dose that will provide a steady-state concentration of 1.2 ng/ml.

1. *Estimate creatinine clearance.* This patient has a stable serum creatinine and is obese [$IBW_{females}$ (in kg) = 45 + 2.3(Ht − 60) = 45 + 2.3(65″ − 60) = 57 kg]. The Salazar and Corcoran equation can be used to estimate creatinine clearance:

$$CrCl_{est(females)} = \frac{(146 - age)[(0.287 \cdot Wt) + (9.74 \cdot Ht^2)]}{60 \cdot S_{Cr}}$$

$$CrCl_{est(females)} = \frac{(146 - 65 \text{ y})\{(0.287 \cdot 170 \text{ kg}) + [9.74 \cdot (1.65 \text{ m})^2]\}}{60 \cdot 4.7 \text{ mg/dl}}$$

$$= 22 \text{ ml/min}$$

Note: Height is converted from inches to meters: Ht = (65 in · 2.54 cm/in)/(100 cm/m) = 1.65 m.

This patient has poor renal function, but can be expected to be at steady state with regard to digoxin serum concentrations after 3 weeks of treatment. *Note that this step can be omitted if it is known that the patient is at steady state.*

2. *Compute drug clearance.* Note that digoxin concentrations in ng/ml are the same as those for μg/L. This unit substitution will be made directly, to avoid conversion factors in the computation.

$$Cl = [F(D/\tau)]/C_{ss} = [0.7(125 \text{ μg/d})]/2.5 \text{ μg/L} = 35 \text{ L/d}$$

3. *Compute new dose to achieve desired serum concentration.* The average steady-state equation is used to compute the new digoxin dose.

$$D/\tau = (C_{ss} \cdot Cl)/F = (1.2 \text{ μg/L} \cdot 35 \text{ L/d})/0.7 = 60 \text{ μg/d}$$

or 120 μg every other day (60 μg/d · 2 days = 120 μg every 2 days). This would be rounded to digoxin tablets 125 μg every other day.

The new suggested dose is 125 μg every other day given as digoxin tablets, to be started at the next scheduled dosing time. Since the dosage interval is being changed, a day should be skipped before the next dose is given.

BAYESIAN PHARMACOKINETIC COMPUTER PROGRAMS

• Computer programs are available that can assist in the computation of pharmacokinetic parameters for patients.[81,82] The most reliable computer programs use a nonlinear regression algorithm that incorporates components of Bayes' theorem.

• An advantage of this approach is that consistent dosage recommendations are made when several different practitioners are involved in therapeutic drug monitoring programs. However, since simpler dosing methods work just as well for patients with stable pharmacokinetic parameters and steady-state drug concentrations, many clinicians reserve the use of computer programs for more difficult situations. Those situations include serum concentrations that are not at steady state, serum concentrations not obtained at the specific times needed to employ simpler methods, and unstable pharmacokinetic parameters.

• When only a limited number of digoxin concentrations are available, Bayesian pharmacokinetic computer programs can be used to compute a complete patient pharmacokinetic profile that includes clearance, volume of distribution, and half-life.

• Many Bayesian pharmacokinetic computer programs are available to users, and most should provide answers similar to the one used in the following examples. The program used to solve problems in this book is DrugCalc, written by Dr. Dennis Mungall and available at his Internet web site (www.clinpharmacologist.bigstep.com/consumersurvey.html).[83]

▶ *Example 1* MJ is a 50-year-old, 70-kg (height = 5′10″) male with moderate heart failure. His current serum creatinine is 0.9 mg/dl, and it has been stable over the last 6 months. A digoxin dose of 250 μg/d using oral tablets was prescribed and expected to achieve steady-state concentrations equal to 0.8 ng/ml. After a week of treatment, a steady-state digoxin concentration was measured and equalled 0.6 ng/ml. Calculate a new digoxin dose that will provide a steady-state concentration of 0.9 ng/ml.

1. *Enter patient demographic, drug dosing, and serum concentration/time data into a Bayesian pharmacokinetic computer program.*
2. *Compute pharmacokinetic parameters for the patient using the computer program.* The pharmacokinetic parameters computed by the program are a clearance of 8.8 L/h, a volume of distribution of 578 L, and a half-life of 46 h.
3. *Compute dose required to achieve desired digoxin serum concentration.* The one-compartment-model equations used by the program to compute doses indicates that a dose of 343 µg/d of digoxin tablets will produce a steady-state concentration of 0.9 ng/ml. This dose would be rounded off to 375 µg/d. Using the simpler linear pharmacokinetics method previously described in the chapter, the identical dose of 375 µg/d was computed.

▶ *Example 2*   OI is a 65-year-old, 170-kg (5'5″) female with NYHA class III heart failure. Her current serum creatinine is 4.7 mg/dl and is stable. A digoxin dose of 125 µg/d given as tablets was prescribed and expected to achieve steady-state concentrations equal to 1 ng/ml. After 3 weeks of therapy, a steady-state digoxin concentration was measured and equalled 2.5 ng/ml. Calculate a new digoxin dose that will provide a steady-state concentration of 1.2 ng/ml.

1. *Enter patient demographic, drug dosing, and serum concentration/time data into a Bayesian pharmacokinetic computer program.*
2. *Compute pharmacokinetic parameters for the patient using the computer program.* The pharmacokinetic parameters computed by the program are a clearance of 1.4 L/h, a volume of distribution of 516 L, and a half-life of 249 h. The clearance value is slightly different than that computed using the steady-state pharmacokinetic parameter method (35 L/d or 1.5 L/h) because the patient probably was not at steady state when the serum concentrations were drawn.
3. *Compute dose required to achieve desired digoxin serum concentration.* The one-compartment-model equations used by the program to compute doses indicates that a dose of 141 µg every 3 days will produce a steady-state concentration of 1.2 ng/ml. This would be rounded to 125 µg every 3 days. Using the steady-state pharmacokinetic parameter method previously described in the chapter, a similar dose of 125 µg every other day was computed.

▶ *Example 3*   JH is a 74-year-old, 85-kg (height = 5'8″) male with atrial fibrillation. His current serum creatinine is 1.9 mg/dl, and it has been stable over the 7 days since admission. An intravenous digoxin loading dose of 500 µg was prescribed (given as doses of 250, 125, and 125 µg every 4 hours at 0800, 1200, and 1600 H, respectively). An oral maintenance dose of digoxin tablets 125 µg was given the next morning at 0800 H. Because the patient still had a rapid ventricular rate, a digoxin concentration was obtained at 1600 H and equalled 0.9 ng/ml. Recommend a stat intravenous digoxin dose to be given at 2300 H that will achieve a digoxin serum concentration of 1.5 µg, and an oral maintenance dose that will provide a steady-state concentration of the same level.

1. *Enter patient demographic, drug dosing, and serum concentration/time data into a Bayesian pharmacokinetic computer program.*

2. *Compute pharmacokinetic parameters for the patient using the computer program.* The pharmacokinetic parameters computed by the program are a clearance of 4.8 L/h, a volume of distribution of 390 L, and a half-life of 57 h.

3. *Compute dose required to achieve desired digoxin serum concentration.* The stat intravenous digoxin dose is calculated using the volume of distribution supplied by the computer program. The booster dose (BD) that will change serum concentrations by the desired amount is BD = $[V(\Delta C)]/F$, where V is the volume of distribution in L, ΔC is the necessary change ($C_{desired} - C_{actual}$) in digoxin serum concentration in μg/L, and F is the bioavailability for the dosage form.

$$BD = [V(\Delta C)]/F = [390 \text{ L}(1.5 \text{ }\mu\text{g/L} - 0.9 \text{ }\mu\text{g/L})]/1$$

$$= 234 \text{ }\mu\text{g, round to } 250 \text{ }\mu\text{g IV stat}$$

The one-compartment-model equations used by the program to compute doses indicates that a digoxin tablet dose of 273 μg/d will produce a steady-state concentration of 1.5 ng/ml. This dose would be rounded to 250 μg/d of digoxin tablets and would be started at 0800 H the next morning.

DOSING STRATEGIES

- Initial dose and dosage adjustment techniques using serum concentrations can be used in any combination as long as the limitations of each method are observed.
- Some dosing schemes link together logically when considered according to their basic approaches or philosophies. Dosage strategies that follow similar pathways are given in Table 6-5.

SPECIAL DOSING CONSIDERATIONS

Use of Digoxin Immune FAB in Severe Digoxin Overdoses

- Digoxin immune FABs (Digibind®) are digoxin antibody molecule segments that bind and neutralize digoxin and that can be used in severe digoxin overdose situations.[84,85] Improvements in digoxin adverse effects can be seen within 30 minutes of digoxin immune FAB administration.
- Digoxin serum concentrations are not useful after digoxin immune FAB has been given to a patient, because pharmacologically inactive digoxin bound to the antibody segments will be measured and produce falsely high results.

TABLE 6-5 Dosing Strategies

Dosing approach/ philosophy	Initial dosing	Use of serum concentrations to alter doses
Pharmacokinetic parameters/ equations	Pharmacokinetic dosing or Jelliffe method	Pharmacokinetic parameter or linear pharmacokinetic method
Nomograms/ concepts	Nomograms	Linear pharmacokinetics method
Computerized	Bayesian computer program	Bayesian computer program

- The elimination half-life for digoxin immune FAB is 15–20 hours in patients with normal renal function, and it is eliminated by the kidney. The half-life of digoxin immune FAB is not known in patients with impaired renal function, but is assumed to be prolonged. In functionally anephric patients, the FAB fragment–digoxin complex may not be readily cleared from the body, so these patients should be closely monitored in the event digoxin dissociates from the FAB fragment and reintoxication occurs.
- Because digoxin immune FAB is a foreign protein, allergic reactions including anaphylactic shock can occur, so patient blood pressure and temperature should be closely monitored.

  - Intradermal skin testing may be helpful in high-risk individuals (known digoxin immune FAB allergy, previous treatment with digoxin immune FAB).[86]

- The electrocardiogram and serum potassium concentration should be closely followed in patients receiving this agent.

  - Initially, patients may be hyperkalemic due to digoxin-induced displacement of intracellular potassium. However, hypokalemia can occur rapidly as the FAB fragments bind digoxin. As a result, repeated measurements of serum potassium are necessary, especially after the first few hours of digoxin immune FAB.

- Because the pharmacological effects of digoxin will be lost, heart failure may worsen or a rapid ventricular rate may develop in patients treated for atrial fibrillation.
- Readministration of Digibind may be necessary if adverse effects to digoxin have not abated several hours after administration of the antibody fragments or if adverse effects recur.

  - When patients do not respond to Digibind, clinicians should consider the possibility that the patient is not digoxin-toxic and seek other etiologies for the patient's clinical symptomology.

- If a digoxin serum concentration or an estimate of the number of tablets ingested is not available, 20 vials of Digibind are usually adequate to treat most life-threatening acute overdoses in children and adults, while 6 vials are usually adequate to treat chronic digoxin overdoses in adults. One vial may be adequate for infants and small children weighing less than 20 kg.[86]
- If digoxin serum concentrations are available or a reasonable estimate of the number of digoxin tablets acutely ingested is available, the Digibind dose should be computed using one of the two approaches outlined below.[86] If it is possible to calculate a Digibind dose using both of the following methods, it is recommended that the higher dose be administered to the patient.

  - *Chronic overdose or acute overdose 8–12 hours after ingestion.* In these cases, a postabsorption, postdistribution digoxin concentration can be used to estimate the necessary dose of Digibind for a patient using the following formula:

$$\text{Digibind dose (in vials)} = (\text{digoxin concentration in ng/ml}) \times (\text{body weight in kg})/100$$

▶ *Example 1*   HY is a 72-year-old, 80-kg male (height = 5′7″) who has acci-
dently been taking twice his prescribed dose of digoxin tablets. The admit-
ting digoxin serum concentration is 4.1 ng/ml. Compute an appropriate dose
of Digibind for this patient.

$$\text{Digibind dose (in vials)} = \text{(digoxin concentration in ng/ml)}$$
$$\times \text{(body weight in kg)}/100$$
$$= (4.1 \text{ ng/ml} \cdot 80 \text{ kg})/100$$
$$= 3.3 \text{ vials, rounded to 4 vials}$$

- *Acute overdose when number of tablets is known or can be estimated.* In
this situation, digoxin total body stores are estimated using the number of
tablets ingested corrected for dosage-form bioavailability:

$$\text{TBS} = \text{F(\# dosage units)(dosage form strength)}$$

where TBS is digoxin total body stores in mg, F is the bioavailability for
the dosage form (*Note:* The suggested bioavailability constant for digoxin
in the Digibind package insert is 0.8 for tablets and 1 for capsules,
which allows for variability in the fraction of the dose that was absorbed.),
dosage units is the number of tablets or capsules, and dosage form
strength is in mg (*Note:* 250 μg = 0.25 mg).

  - Each vial of Digibind will inactivate approximately 0.5 mg of digoxin,
so the dose of Digibind (in vials) can be calculated using the following
equation:

$$\text{Digibind dose} = \text{TBS}/(0.5 \text{ mg/vial})$$

  where TBS is digoxin total body stores in mg.

▶ *Example 2*   DL is a 22-year-old, 85-kg male (height = 5′9″) who took
approximately 50 digoxin tablets of 0.25 mg strength about 4 hours ago.
Compute an appropriate dose of Digibind for this patient.

$$\text{TBS} = \text{F(\# dosage units)(dosage form strength)}$$
$$= 0.8 \text{ (50 tablets} \cdot 0.25 \text{ mg/tablet)} = 10 \text{ mg}$$

$$\text{Digibind dose} = \text{TBS}/(0.5 \text{ mg/vial}) = 10 \text{ mg}/(0.5 \text{ mg/vial}) = 20 \text{ vials}$$

Conversion of Patient Doses Between Dosage Forms

- When patients are switched between digoxin dosage forms, differences in
bioavailability should be accounted for within the limits of available oral
dosage forms using the following equation:

$$D_{IV} = D_{PO} \cdot F$$

where D_{IV} is the equivalent digoxin intravenous dose in μg, D_{PO} is the equivalent digoxin oral dose, and F is the bioavailability fraction appropriate for
the oral dosage form (F = 0.7 for tablets, 0.8 for elixir, 0.9 for capsules).

  - When possible, digoxin tablet doses should be rounded to the nearest 125 μg
to avoid the necessity of breaking tablets in half. Similarly, digoxin capsule
doses should be rounded to the nearest 50 μg, as that is the smallest
dosage size available.

666 **CARDIOVASCULAR AGENTS**

- It is best to avoid mixing tablet or capsule dosage strengths so that patients do not become confused with multiple prescription vials and take the wrong dose of medication. For example, if it were necessary to prescribe 375 µg/d of digoxin tablets, it would be preferable to have the patient take three 125-µg tablets daily or $1\frac{1}{2}$ 250-µg tablets daily rather than a 125-µg and a 250-µg tablet each day.

▶ *Example 1* YT is a 67-year-old, 60-kg male (height = 5′5″) with atrial fibrillation who is receiving 200 µg of intravenous digoxin daily, which produces a steady-state digoxin concentration of 1.3 ng/ml. Compute an oral tablet dose that will maintain steady-state digoxin concentrations at approximately the same level.

1. *Convert current digoxin dose to the equivalent amount for the new dosage form/route.*

   $D_{PO} = D_{IV}/F = 200$ µg/0.7 = 286 µg digoxin tablets, round to 250 µg

2. *Estimate change in digoxin steady-state concentration due to rounding of dose.* The oral tablet dose of 286 µg would produce a steady-state concentration similar to the intravenous dose of 200 µg. However, the dose had to be rounded to a dose that could be given as a tablet. The expected digoxin steady-state concentration from the rounded dose is proportional to the ratio of the rounded dose and the actual computed dose:

   $Css_{new} = Css_{old}(D_{rounded}/D_{computed}) = 1.3$ ng/ml(250 µg/286 µg) = 1.1 ng/ml

   where Css_{new} is the new expected digoxin steady-state concentration due to tablet administration in ng/ml, Css_{old} is the measured digoxin steady-state concentration due to intravenous administration in ng/ml, $D_{rounded}$ is the oral dose rounded to account for dosage form strengths in µg, and $D_{computed}$ is the exact oral dose computed during the intravenous to oral conversion calculation in µg. However, the steady-state digoxin concentration after the dosage-form change may not be exactly the value calculated, due to a variety of causes. Because of interindividual variations in digoxin bioavailability, the patient's actual bioavailability constant for oral tablets may be different than the average population bioavailability constant used to convert the dose. Also, there are day-to-day intrasubject variations in the rate and extent of digoxin absorption that will affect the actual steady-state digoxin concentration obtained while taking the drug orally. Finally, other oral drug therapy that did not influence digoxin pharmacokinetics when given intravenously may alter the expected digoxin concentration.

▶ *Example 2* KL is an 82-year-old, 45-kg female (height = 4′10″) with heart failure who is receiving 125 µg of oral digoxin daily as tablets, which produces a steady-state digoxin concentration of 1 ng/ml. Compute an intravenous dose that will maintain steady-state digoxin concentrations at approximately the same level.

1. *Convert current digoxin dose to the equivalent amount for the new dosage form/route.*

   $D_{IV} = D_{PO} \cdot F = 125$ µg · 0.7
   = 87.5 µg intravenous digoxin, round to 90 µg

2. *Estimate change in digoxin steady-state concentration due to rounding of dose*. The intravenous dose of 87.5 µg would produce a steady-state concentration similar to the oral tablet dose of 125 µg. However, the dose was rounded to an amount that could be reasonably measured in a syringe. The expected digoxin steady-state concentration from the rounded dose is proportional to the ratio of the rounded dose and the actual computed dose:

$$Css_{new} = Css_{old}(D_{rounded}/D_{computed}) = 1 \text{ ng/ml } (90 \text{ µg}/87.5 \text{ µg}) = 1 \text{ ng/ml}$$

where Css_{new} is the new expected digoxin steady-state concentration due to intravenous administration in ng/ml, Css_{old} is the measured digoxin steady-state concentration due to oral tablet administration in ng/ml, $D_{rounded}$ is the intravenous dose rounded to allow accurate dosage measurement in µg, and $D_{computed}$ is the exact intravenous dose computed during the intravenous-to-oral conversion calculation in µg. Since the rounded intravenous digoxin dose is so close to the exact dose needed, steady-state digoxin concentrations are not expected to change appreciably. However, the steady-state digoxin concentration after the dosage-form change may not be exactly the value calculated, due to a variety of causes. Because of interindividual variations in digoxin bioavailability, the patient's actual bioavailability constant for oral tablets may be different from the average population bioavailability constant used to convert the dose. Also, there are day-to-day intrasubject variations in the rate and extent of digoxin absorption that will affect the steady-state digoxin concentration obtained while taking the drug orally that will not be present when the drug is given intravenously. Finally, other oral drug therapy that influenced digoxin pharmacokinetics when given orally, but not intravenously, may alter the expected digoxin concentration.

Use of Digoxin Booster Doses to Immediately Increase Serum Concentrations

• If a patient has a subtherapeutic digoxin serum concentration in an acute situation, it may be desirable to increase the digoxin concentration as quickly as possible. A rational way to increase serum concentrations rapidly is to administer a booster dose of digoxin, a process also known as "reloading" the patient with digoxin, computed using pharmacokinetic techniques.

  • A modified loading dose equation is used to accomplish computation of the booster dose (BD) which takes into account the current digoxin concentration present in the patient:

$$BD = [(C_{desired} - C_{actual})V]/F$$

where $C_{desired}$ is the desired digoxin concentration, C_{actual} is the actual current digoxin concentration for the patient, F is the bioavailability fraction of the digoxin dosage form, and V is the volume of distribution for digoxin.
  • If the volume of distribution for digoxin is known for the patient, it can be used in the calculation. However, this value is not usually known and is assumed to equal the population average for the patient.

• Concurrent with the administration of the booster dose, the maintenance dose of digoxin is usually increased. Clinicians need to recognize that the administration of a booster dose does not alter the time required to achieve steady-state conditions when a new digoxin dosage rate is prescribed. It still requires a sufficient time period to attain steady state when the dosage rate is changed. Usually, however, the difference between the postbooster dose digoxin concentration and the ultimate steady-state concentration is reduced by giving the extra dose of drug.

▶ *Example 1* BN is a 52-year-old, 85-kg (height = 6′2″) male with atrial fibrillation who is receiving therapy with intravenous digoxin. He has normal liver and renal function. After receiving an initial loading dose of digoxin (1000 µg) and a maintenance dose of 250 µg/d of digoxin for 5 days, his digoxin concentration is measured at 0.6 ng/ml immediately after his pulse rate increased to 200 beats/min. Compute a booster dose of digoxin to achieve a digoxin concentration equal to 1.5 ng/ml.

1. *Estimate volume of distribution according to disease states and conditions present in the patient.* In the case of digoxin, the population average volume of distribution equals 7 L/kg, and this will be used to estimate the parameter for the patient. The patient is not obese, so his actual body weight will be used in the computation:

$$V = 7 \text{ L/kg} \cdot 85 \text{ kg} = 595 \text{ L}$$

2. *Compute booster dose.* The booster dose is computed using the following equation:

$$BD = [(C_{desired} - C_{actual})V]/F = [(1.5 \text{ µg/L} - 0.6 \text{ µg/L})595 \text{ L}]/1$$

$$= 536 \text{ µg, rounded to 500 µg}$$

(*Note*: ng/ml = µg/L, and this concentration unit was substituted for Css in the calculations so that unit conversion was not required.) This booster dose could be split into two equal doses given 4–6 hours apart with appropriate monitoring for adverse side effects. If the maintenance dose was also increased, it will take additional time for new steady-state conditions to be achieved. Digoxin serum concentrations should be measured at this time.

REFERENCES

1. Ooi H, Colucci W. Pharmacological treatment of heart failure. In: Hardman JG, Limbird LE, Gilman AG, eds. The pharmacologic basis of therapeutics. 10th ed. New York: McGraw-Hill; 2001:901–32.
2. Reuning RH, Sams RA, Notari RE. Role of pharmacokinetics in drug dosage adjustment. I. Pharmacologic effect kinetics and apparent volume of distribution of digoxin. J Clin Pharmacol New Drugs 1973;13(4):127–41.
3. Koup JR, Greenblatt DJ, Jusko WJ, Smith TW, Koch-Weser J. Pharmacokinetics of digoxin in normal subjects after intravenous bolus and infusion doses. J Pharmacokinet Biopharm 1975;3(3):181–92.
4. Koup JR, Jusko WJ, Elwood CM, Kohli RK. Digoxin pharmacokinetics: role of renal failure in dosage regimen design. Clin Pharmacol Ther 1975;18(1):9–21.
5. Slatton ML, Irani WN, Hall SA, et al. Does digoxin provide additional hemodynamic and autonomic benefit at higher doses in patients with mild to moderate heart failure and normal sinus rhythm? J Am Coll Cardiol 1997;29(6):1206–13.
6. Gheorghiade M, Hall VB, Jacobsen G, Alam M, Rosman H, Goldstein S. Effects of increasing maintenance dose of digoxin on left ventricular function and neurohormones in patients with chronic heart failure treated with diuretics and angiotensin-converting enzyme inhibitors. Circulation 1995;92(7):1801–7.

7. Beasley R, Smith DA, Mchaffie DJ. Exercise heart rates at different serum digoxin concentrations in patients with atrial fibrillation. Br Med J (Clin Res Ed) 1985;290(6461):9–11.
8. Aronson JK, Hardman M. ABC of monitoring drug therapy. Digoxin. Br Med J 1992;305(6862):1149–52.
9. Smith TW, Haber E. Digoxin intoxication: the relationship of clinical presentation to serum digoxin concentration. J Clin Invest 1970;49(12):2377–86.
10. Chung EK. Digitalis intoxication. Postgrad Med J 1972;48(557):163–79.
11. Johnson JA, Parker RB, Patterson JH. Heart failure. In: DiPiro JT, Talbert RL, Yee GC, Matzke GR, Wells BG, Posey LM, eds. Pharmacotherapy—a pathophysiologic approach. 5th ed. New York: McGraw-Hill; 2002:195–218.
12. Bauman JL, Schoen MD. Arrhythmias. In: DiPiro JT, Talbert RL, Yee GC, Matzke GR, Wells BG, Posey LM, eds. Pharmacotherapy—a pathophysiologic approach. 5th ed. New York: McGraw-Hill; 2002:273–304.
13. Beller GA, Smith TW, Abelmann WH, Haber E, Hood WB Jr. Digitalis intoxication. A prospective clinical study with serum level correlations. N Engl J Med 1971;284(18):989–97.
14. Norregaard-Hansen K, Klitgaard NA, Pedersen KE. The significance of the enterohepatic circulation on the metabolism of digoxin in patients with the ability of intestinal conversion of the drug. Acta Med Scand 1986;220(1):89–92.
15. Johnson BF, Smith G, French J. The comparability of dosage regimens of Lanoxin tablets and Lanoxicaps. Br J Clin Pharmacol 1977;4(2):209–11.
16. Johnson BF, Bye C, Jones G, Sabey GA. A completely absorbed oral preparation of digoxin. Clin Pharmacol Ther 1976;19(6):746–51.
17. Kramer WG, Reuning RH. Use of area under the curve to estimate absolute bioavailability of digoxin [letter]. J Pharm Sci 1978;67(1):141–2.
18. Beveridge T, Nuesch E, Ohnhaus EE. Absolute bioavailability of digoxin tablets. Arzneimittelforschung 1978;28(4):701–3.
19. Ohnhaus EE, Vozeh S, Nuesch E. Absolute bioavailability of digoxin in chronic renal failure. Clin Nephrol 1979;11(6):302–6.
20. Ohnhaus EE, Vozeh S, Nuesch E. Absorption of digoxin in severe right heart failure. Eur J Clin Pharmacol 1979;15(2):115–20.
21. Hinderling PH. Kinetics of partitioning and binding of digoxin and its analogues in the subcompartments of blood. J Pharm Sci 1984;73(8):1042–53.
22. Storstein L. Studies on digitalis. V. The influence of impaired renal function, hemodialysis, and drug interaction on serum protein binding of digitoxin and digoxin. Clin Pharmacol Ther 1976;20(1):6–14.
23. Iisalo E. Clinical pharmacokinetics of digoxin. Clin Pharmacokinet 1977;2:1–16.
24. Aronson JK. Clinical pharmacokinetics of digoxin 1980. Clin Pharmacokinet 1980;5(2):137–49.
25. Ewy GA, Groves BM, Ball MF, Nimmo L, Jackson B, Marcus F. Digoxin metabolism in obesity. Circulation 1971;44(5):810–4.
26. Abernethy DR, Greenblatt DJ, Smith TW. Digoxin disposition in obesity: clinical pharmacokinetic investigation. Am Heart J 1981;102(4):740–4.
27. Jusko WJ, Szefler SJ, Goldfarb AL. Pharmacokinetic design of digoxin dosage regimens in relation to renal function. J Clin Pharmacol 1974;14(10):525–35.
28. Golper TA, Marx MA. Drug dosing adjustments during continuous renal replacement therapies. Kidney Int Suppl 1998;66:S165–8.
29. Golper TA. Update on drug sieving coefficients and dosing adjustments during continuous renal replacement therapies. Contrib Nephrol 2001(132):349–53.
30. Ochs HR, Greenblatt DJ, Bodem G, Dengler HJ. Disease-related alterations in cardiac glycoside disposition. Clin Pharmacokinet 1982;7(5):434–51.
31. Bonelli J, Haydl H, Hruby K, Kaik G. The pharmacokinetics of digoxin in patients with manifest hyperthyroidism and after normalization of thyroid function. Int J Clin Pharmacol Biopharm 1978;16(7):302–6.
32. Koup JR. Distribution of digoxin in hyperthyroid patients. Int J Clin Pharmacol Ther Toxicol 1980;18(5):236.

33. Nyberg L, Wettrell G. Pharmacokinetics and dosage of digoxin in neonates and infants. Eur J Clin Pharmacol 1980;18(1):69–74.
34. Nyberg L, Wettrell G. Digoxin dosage schedules for neonates and infants based on pharmacokinetic considerations. Clin Pharmacokinet 1978;3(6):453–61.
35. Gunn VL, Nechyba C, eds. The Harriet Lane handbook: a manual for pediatric house officers. 16th ed. Philadelphia: Mosby; 2002.
36. Heizer WD, Pittman AW, Hammond JE, Fitch DD, Bustrack JA, Hull JH. Absorption of digoxin from tablets and capsules in subjects with malabsorption syndromes. Drug Intel Clin Pharm 1989;23(10):764–9.
37. Heizer WD, Smith TW, Goldfinger SE. Absorption of digoxin in patients with malabsorption syndromes. N Engl J Med 1971;285(5):257–9.
38. Kolibash AJ, Kramer WG, Reuning RH, Caldwell JH. Marked decline in serum digoxin concentration during an episode of severe diarrhea. Am Heart J 1977; 94(6):806–7.
39. Bjornsson TD, Huang AT, Roth P, Jacob DS, Christenson R. Effects of high-dose cancer chemotherapy on the absorption of digoxin in two different formulations. Clin Pharmacol Ther 1986;39(1):25–8.
40. Jusko WJ, Conti DR, Molson A, Kuritzky P, Giller J, Schultz R. Digoxin absorption from tablets and elixir. The effect of radiation-induced malabsorption. JAMA 1974;230(11):1554–5.
41. Fromm MF, Kim RB, Stein CM, Wilkinson GR, Roden DM. Inhibition of P-glycoprotein-mediated drug transport: a unifying mechanism to explain the interaction between digoxin and quinidine [see comments]. Circulation 1999;99(4): 552–7.
42. Ejvinsson G. Effect of quinidine on plasma concentrations of digoxin. Br Med J 1978;1(6108):279–80.
43. Leahey EB Jr, Reiffel JA, Drusin RE, Heissenbuttel RH, Lovejoy WP, Bigger JT Jr. Interaction between quinidine and digoxin. JAMA 1978;240(6):533–4.
44. Reiffel JA, Leahey EB Jr, Drusin RE, Heissenbuttel RH, Lovejoy W, Bigger JT Jr. A previously unrecognized drug interaction between quinidine and digoxin. Clin Cardiol 1979;2(1):40–2.
45. Hager WD, Fenster P, Mayersohn M, et al. Digoxin-quinidine interaction: pharmacokinetic evaluation. N Engl J Med 1979;300(22):1238–41.
46. Doering W. Quinidine-digoxin interaction: pharmacokinetics, underlying mechanism and clinical implications. N Engl J Med 1979;301(8):400–4.
47. Bauer LA, Horn JR, Pettit H. Mixed-effect modeling for detection and evaluation of drug interactions: digoxin-quinidine and digoxin-verapamil combinations. Ther Drug Monit 1996;18(1):46–52.
48. Pedersen KE, Dorph-Pedersen A, Hvidt S, Klitgaard NA, Nielsen-Kudsk F. Digoxin-verapamil interaction. Clin Pharmacol Ther 1981;30(3):311–6.
49. Klein HO, Lang R, Weiss E, et al. The influence of verapamil on serum digoxin concentration. Circulation 1982;65(5):998–1003.
50. Pedersen KE, Thayssen P, Klitgaard NA, Christiansen BD, Nielsen-Kudsk F. Influence of verapamil on the inotropism and pharmacokinetics of digoxin. Eur J Clin Pharmacol 1983;25(2):199–206.
51. Yoshida A, Fujita M, Kurosawa N, et al. Effects of diltiazem on plasma level and urinary excretion of digoxin in healthy subjects. Clin Pharmacol Ther 1984; 35(5):681–5.
52. Rameis H, Magometschnigg D, Ganzinger U. The diltiazem-digoxin interaction. Clin Pharmacol Ther 1984;36(2):183–9.
53. Belz GG, Wistuba S, Matthews JH. Digoxin and bepridil: pharmacokinetic and pharmacodynamic interactions. Clin Pharmacol Ther 1986;39(1):65–71.
54. Moysey JO, Jaggarao NS, Grundy EN, Chamberlain DA. Amiodarone increases plasma digoxin concentrations. Br Med J (Clin Res Ed) 1981;282(6260):272.
55. Maragno I, Santostasi G, Gaion RM, Paleari C. Influence of amiodarone on oral digoxin bioavailability in healthy volunteers. Int J Clin Pharmacol Res 1984;4(2):149–53.

56. Nademanee K, Kannan R, Hendrickson J, Ookhtens M, Kay I, Singh BN. Amiodarone-digoxin interaction: clinical significance, time course of development, potential pharmacokinetic mechanisms and therapeutic implications. J Am Coll Cardiol 1984;4(1):111–6.

57. Robinson K, Johnston A, Walker S, Mulrow JP, McKenna WJ, Holt DW. The digoxin-amiodarone interaction. Cardiovasc Drugs Ther 1989;3(1):25–8.

58. Nolan PE Jr, Marcus FI, Erstad BL, Hoyer GL, Furman C, Kirsten EB. Effects of coadministration of propafenone on the pharmacokinetics of digoxin in healthy volunteer subjects. J Clin Pharmacol 1989;29(1):46–52.

59. Bigot MC, Debruyne D, Bonnefoy L, Grollier G, Moulin M, Potier JC. Serum digoxin levels related to plasma propafenone levels during concomitant treatment. J Clin Pharmacol 1991;31(6):521–6.

60. Calvo MV, Martin-Suarez A, Martin Luengo C, Avila C, Cascon M, Dominguez-Gil Hurle A. Interaction between digoxin and propafenone. Ther Drug Monit 1989;11(1):10–5.

61. Dorian P, Strauss M, Cardella C, David T, East S, Ogilvie R. Digoxin-cyclosporine interaction: severe digitalis toxicity after cyclosporine treatment. Clin Invest Med 1988;11(2):108–12.

62. Dobkin JF, Saha JR, Butler VP Jr, Neu HC, Lindenbaum J. Inactivation of digoxin by *Eubacterium lentum,* an anaerobe of the human gut flora. Trans Assoc Am Physicians 1982;95:22–9.

63. Saha JR, Butler VP Jr, Neu HC, Lindenbaum J. Digoxin-inactivating bacteria: identification in human gut flora. Science 1983;220(4594):325–7.

64. Lindenbaum J, Rund DG, Butler VP Jr, Tse-Eng D, Saha JR. Inactivation of digoxin by the gut flora: reversal by antibiotic therapy. N Engl J Med 1981;305(14):789–94.

65. Morton MR, Cooper JW. Erythromycin-induced digoxin toxicity. Drug Intel Clin Pharm 1989;23(9):668–70.

66. Maxwell DL, Gilmour-White SK, Hall MR. Digoxin toxicity due to interaction of digoxin with erythromycin. Br Med J 1989;298(6673):572.

67. Brown BA, Wallace RJ Jr, Griffith DE, Warden R. Clarithromycin-associated digoxin toxicity in the elderly. Clin Infect Dis 1997;24(1):92–3.

68. Nawarskas JJ, McCarthy DM, Spinler SA. Digoxin toxicity secondary to clarithromycin therapy. Ann Pharmacother 1997;31(7-8):864–6.

69. Wakasugi H, Yano I, Ito T, et al. Effect of clarithromycin on renal excretion of digoxin: interaction with P-glycoprotein. Clin Pharmacol Ther 1998;64(1): 123–8.

70. Allen MD, Greenblatt DJ, Harmatz JS, Smith TW. Effect of magnesium–aluminum hydroxide and kaolin–pectin on absorption of digoxin from tablets and capsules. J Clin Pharmacol 1981;21(1):26–30.

71. Hall WH, Shappell SD, Doherty JE. Effect of cholestyramine on digoxin absorption and excretion in man. Am J Cardiol 1977;39(2):213–6.

72. Brown DD, Schmid J, Long RA, Hull JH. A steady-state evaluation of the effects of propantheline bromide and cholestyramine on the bioavailability of digoxin when administered as tablets or capsules. J Clin Pharmacol 1985;25(5): 360–4.

73. Juhl RP, Summers RW, Guillory JK, Blaug SM, Cheng FH, Brown DD. Effect of sulfasalazine on digoxin bioavailability. Clin Pharmacol Ther 1976;20(4): 387–94.

74. Lindenbaum J, Maulitz RM, Butler VP Jr. Inhibition of digoxin absorption by neomycin. Gastroenterology 1976;71(3):399–404.

75. Johnson BF, Bustrack JA, Urbach DR, Hull JH, Marwaha R. Effect of metoclopramide on digoxin absorption from tablets and capsules. Clin Pharmacol Ther 1984;36(6):724–30.

76. Kirch W, Janisch HD, Santos SR, Duhrsen U, Dylewicz P, Ohnhaus EE. Effect of cisapride and metoclopramide on digoxin bioavailability. Eur J Drug Metab Pharmacokinet 1986;11(4):249–50.

77. Jelliffe RW, Brooker G. A nomogram for digoxin therapy. Am J Med 1974;57(1):63–8.

78. Jelliffe RW. An improved method of digoxin therapy. Ann Intern Med 1968;69(4): 703–17.

79. GlaxoSmithKline Lanoxin web site, www.gsk.com/products/lanoxin_us.htm, 2005.

80. Mutnick AH. Digoxin. In: Schumacher GE, ed. Therapeutic drug monitoring. First ed. Stamford, CT: Appleton & Lange; 1995:469–91.

81. Sheiner LB, Halkin H, Peck C, Rosenberg B, Melmon KL. Improved computer-assisted digoxin therapy. A method using feedback of measured serum digoxin concentrations. Ann Intern Med 1975;82(5):619–27.

82. Peck CC, Sheiner LB, Martin CM, Combs DT, Melmon KL. Computer-assisted digoxin therapy. N Engl J Med 1973;289(9):441–6.

83. Wandell M, Mungall D. Computer assisted drug interpretation and drug regimen optimization. Am Assoc Clin Chem 1984;6:1–11.

84. Smith TW, Butler VP Jr, Haber E, et al. Treatment of life-threatening digitalis intoxication with digoxin-specific Fab antibody fragments: experience in 26 cases. N Engl J Med 1982;307(22):1357–62.

85. Smolarz A, Roesch E, Lenz E, Neubert H, Abshagen P. Digoxin specific antibody (Fab) fragments in 34 cases of severe digitalis intoxication. J Toxicol Clin Toxicol 1985;23(4-6):327–40.

86. GlaxoSmithKline Digibind web site, http://us.gsk.com/products/assets/us_digibind.pdf, 2005.

7 | Lidocaine

Lidocaine is a local anesthetic agent that also has antiarrhythmic effects. It is classified as a type IB antiarrhythmic agent and is used for the treatment of ventricular tachycardia or ventricular fibrillation.[1,2]

- Lidocaine inhibits transmembrane sodium influx into the His-Purkinje fiber conduction system, thereby decreasing conduction velocity.[2] It also decreases the duration of the action potential and as a result decreases the duration of the absolute refractory period in Purkinje fibers and the bundle of His. Automaticity is decreased during lidocaine therapy.

THERAPEUTIC AND TOXIC CONCENTRATIONS

- When lidocaine is given intravenously, the serum lidocaine concentration/ time curve follows a two-compartment model.[3,4] This is especially apparent when initial loading doses of lidocaine are given as rapid intravenous injections over 1–5 minutes (maximum rate 25–50 mg/min) and a distribution phase of 30–40 minutes is observed after drug administration (Figure 7-1).
- Unlike digoxin, the myocardium responds to the higher concentrations achieved during the distribution phase because lidocaine moves rapidly from the blood into the heart, and the onset of action for lidocaine after a loading dose is within a few minutes after completion of the intravenous injection.[1,2] Because of these factors, the heart is considered to be located in the central compartment of the two-compartment model for lidocaine.
- The generally accepted therapeutic range for lidocaine is 1.5–5 μg/ml. In the upper end of the therapeutic range (>3 μg/ml), some patients will experience minor side effects including drowsiness, dizziness, paresthesias, or euphoria.

  - Lidocaine serum concentrations above the therapeutic range can cause muscle twitching, confusion, agitation, dysarthria, psychosis, seizures, or coma.
  - Lidocaine-induced seizures are not as difficult to treat as theophylline-induced seizures and usually respond to traditional antiseizure medication therapy. Lidocaine metabolites (MEGX and GX; see Basic Clinical Pharmacokinetic Parameters) probably contribute to the central nervous system side effects attributed to lidocaine therapy.[5–7]
  - Cardiovascular adverse effects such as atrioventricular block, hypotension, and circulatory collapse have been reported at lidocaine concentrations above 6 μg/ml, but are not strongly correlated with specific serum levels.

- For dose-adjustment purposes, lidocaine serum concentrations are best measured at steady state after the patient has received a consistent dosage regimen for 3–5 drug half-lives. Lidocaine half-life varies from 1–1.5 hours in normal adults to 5 hours or more in adult patients with liver failure.
- If lidocaine is given as a continuous intravenous infusion, it can take a considerable amount of time (3–5 half-lives or 7.5–25 hours) for patients to achieve effective concentrations, so an intravenous loading dose is commonly administered to patients (Figure 7-2).

  - Since the patient's own, unique central volume of distribution will most likely be greater (resulting in too low a loading dose) or less (resulting in

173

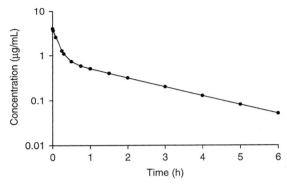

FIG. 7-1 Lidocaine serum concentrations initially drop rapidly after an intravenous bolus as drug distributes from blood into the tissues during the distribution phase. During the distribution phase, drug leaves the blood due to tissue distribution and elimination. After 0.5–1 hour, an equilibrium is established between the blood and tissues, and serum concentrations drop more slowly since elimination is the primary process removing drug from the blood. This type of serum concentration/time profile is described by a two-compartment model. The conduction system of the heart responds to the high concentrations of lidocaine present during the distribution phase, so lidocaine has a quick onset of action.

too large a loading dose) than the population average volume of distribution used to compute the loading dose, the desired steady-state lidocaine concentration will not be achieved. As a result, it will still take 3–5 half-lives for the patient to reach steady-state conditions while receiving a constant intravenous infusion rate (Figure 7-3).

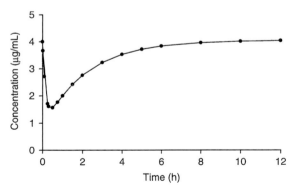

FIG. 7-2 To maintain therapeutic lidocaine concentrations, an intravenous bolus (over 2–8 minutes) of lidocaine is followed by a continuous intravenous infusion of the drug. Even though the infusion is started right after the loading dose is given, serum concentrations due to the infusion cannot increase rapidly enough to counter the large decrease in concentrations during the distribution phase from the bolus dose. The dip in serum lidocaine concentrations below therapeutic amounts can allow previously treated arrhythmias to recur.

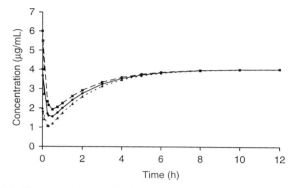

FIG. 7-3 Because the central volume of distribution is not known at the time an intravenous loading dose of lidocaine is administered, average population parameters must be assumed and almost always result in initial lidocaine serum concentrations that are higher (dashed line with squares) or lower (dotted line with triangles) than those that were expected (solid line with circles). So, the main clinical goal of administering loading doses of lidocaine is to achieve therapeutic concentrations as soon as possible, not to attain steady-state concentrations immediately after the loading dose is given.

- After a lidocaine loading dose is given, serum concentrations from this dose rapidly decline due to distribution from blood to tissues, and serum concentrations due to the infusion are not able to increase rapidly enough to avoid a temporary decline or dip in lidocaine concentrations (Figure 7-2). The decline may be severe enough that ventricular arrhythmias which were initially suppressed by lidocaine may recur as a result of subtherapeutic antiarrhythmic concentrations.

  - Because of this dip in concentrations due to distribution of drug after the intravenous loading dose, an additional dose (50% of original loading dose) can be given 20–30 minutes after the original loading dose, or several additional doses (33–50% of the original loading dose) can be given every 5–10 minutes to a total maximum of 3 mg/kg (Figure 7-4).[4]

CLINICAL MONITORING PARAMETERS

- In patients with ventricular tachycardia or fibrillation, the electrocardiogram (ECG or EKG) should be monitored to determine the response to lidocaine. The goal of therapy is suppression of ventricular arrhythmias and avoidance of adverse drug reactions.
- Because lidocaine is usually given for a short duration (<24 hours), it is often not necessary to obtain serum lidocaine concentrations in patients receiving appropriate doses who currently have no ventricular arrhythmia or adverse drug effects.

  - Lidocaine serum concentrations should be obtained in patients who have a recurrence of ventricular tachyarrhythmias, are experiencing possible lidocaine side effects, or are receiving lidocaine doses not consistent with disease states and conditions known to alter lidocaine pharmacokinetics (see Effects of Disease States and Conditions on Lidocaine Pharmacokinetics and Dosing).

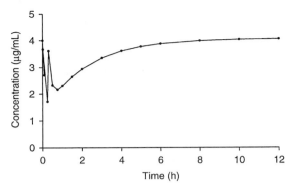

FIG. 7-4 Since the dip in serum lidocaine concentrations below therapeutic amounts can allow previously treated arrhythmias to recur, a supplemental loading or "booster" dose is typically given 20–30 minutes after the initial loading dose. This prevents lidocaine serum concentrations from declining too far during the distribution phase of the intravenous bolus dose and before serum concentrations from the intravenous infusion have had an opportunity to attain therapeutic concentrations.

- Patients receiving lidocaine infusions for longer than 24 hours are prone to unexpected accumulation of lidocaine concentrations in the serum and should be closely monitored for lidocaine side effects.[8–11]
- While they are receiving lidocaine, patients should be monitored for the following adverse drug effects: drowsiness, dizziness, paresthesias, euphoria, muscle twitching, confusion, agitation, dysarthria, psychosis, seizures, coma, atrioventricular block, or hypotension.

BASIC CLINICAL PHARMACOKINETIC PARAMETERS

- Lidocaine is almost completely eliminated by hepatic metabolism (>95%).[3,12] Hepatic metabolism is mainly via the CYP3A enzyme system.
- Monoethylglycinexylidide (MEGX) is the primary metabolite resulting from lidocaine metabolism.[5–7] While a portion of MEGX is eliminated renally, most of the metabolite is further converted hepatically to glycinexylidide (GX) and other, inactive metabolites. GX is eliminated primarily by the kidney.

  - MEGX and GX have some antiarrhythmic activity (MEGX ≈ 80% and GX ≈ 10%, relative to lidocaine), but have also been implicated as the cause of some adverse effects attributed to lidocaine therapy.[5–7] Because both metabolites are eliminated by the kidney, patients with renal failure should be monitored for adverse effects due to metabolite accumulation even though lidocaine serum concentrations are within the therapeutic range.

- The hepatic extraction ratio of lidocaine is about 70%, so lidocaine is typically classified as a high-extraction-ratio drug. As a result, it is expected that liver blood flow will be the predominant factor influencing the clearance of lidocaine (Cl ≈ LBF, where Cl is lidocaine clearance and LBF is liver blood flow, both in L/min), and many disease states and conditions that alter lidocaine clearance do so via changes in liver blood flow.

  - Because a hepatic extraction ratio greater than 70% is the definition of a high-extraction-ratio agent and the extraction ratio for lidocaine is at the margin of this range, it is very possible that changes in lidocaine intrinsic clearance or plasma protein binding will change lidocaine clearance.

- Lidocaine is usually given intravenously but may also be given intramuscularly.[13] After intramuscular injection, absorption is rapid and complete, with maximum concentrations occurring about 1 hour after administration and 100% bioavailability as long as the patient's peripheral circulation is not compromised because of hypotension or shock.

    - Intramuscular administration of medications can increase creatine kinase (CK) concentrations as a result of minor skeletal muscle trauma inflicted by the injection, and this enzyme is monitored in patients who may have had a myocardial infarction. Thus, the creatine kinase isozyme that is relatively specific to the heart (CK-MB) needs to be measured in myocardial infarction patients who have received intramuscular injections.

- Oral absorption of lidocaine is nearly 100%.[3] However, lidocaine is extensively metabolized by the CYP3A enzymes in the intestinal wall and liver, resulting in a large first-pass effect and low, variable oral bioavailability (F ≈ 30%). Because roughly 70% of an oral dose is converted to metabolites, MEGX and GX concentrations are high after oral administration of lidocaine and often result in a high incidence of adverse effects.
- Plasma protein binding in normal individuals is about 70%.[14–16] Of this value, approximately 30% is due to drug binding to albumin, while 70% is due to lidocaine bound to α_1-acid glycoprotein (AGP).[8,10,11]

    - AGP is classified as an acute-phase-reactant protein that is present in lower amounts in all individuals but is secreted in large amounts in response to certain stresses and disease states such as trauma, heart failure, and myocardial infarction. In patients with these disease states, lidocaine binding to AGP can be even larger, resulting in an unbound fraction as low as 10–15%.
    - AGP concentrations increase continuously during the first 12–72 hours after a myocardial infarction, and, as a result, the lidocaine unbound fraction decreases on average from about 30% to 20% during this time period. The continuous increase in protein binding due to AGP secretion causes a continuous decrease in lidocaine clearance in patients with myocardial infarction, and lidocaine concentrations can accumulate to unexpectedly high levels in patients who receive the drug for longer than 24 hours.

- Patients without myocardial infarction also experience accumulation of lidocaine concentrations during long-term (>24 hours) infusions, due to competition for hepatic metabolism between parent drug and metabolites.[9,17] Thus, monitoring for adverse reactions in patients receiving long-term lidocaine infusions is important, and lidocaine serum concentrations can be useful adjuncts to avoid lidocaine toxicity.

EFFECTS OF DISEASE STATES AND CONDITIONS ON LIDOCAINE PHARMACOKINETICS AND DOSING

- Normal adults without the disease states and conditions listed later in this section and who have normal liver function have an average lidocaine half-life of 1.5 hours (range 1–2 hours), a central volume of distribution of 0.5 L/kg (Vc = 0.4 − 0.6 L/kg) and the volume of distribution for the entire body of 1.5 L/kg (V_{area} = 1–2 L/kg; Table 7-1).[3,9,18]

TABLE 7-1 Disease States and Conditions That Alter Lidocaine Pharmacokinetics

Disease state/condition	Half-life (h)	Central volume of distribution, Vc (L/kg)	Volume of distribution for entire body, V_{area} (L/kg)	Comments
Adult, normal liver function	1.5 (range 1–2)	0.5 (range 0.4–0.6)	1.5 (range 1–2)	Lidocaine has a high hepatic extraction ratio of ~ 70%, so liver blood flow is the primary determinant of clearance rate. Accumulation of serum lidocaine concentrations can occur with long-term (>24-h) infusions.
Adult, hepatic disease (liver cirrhosis or acute hepatitis)	5	0.6	2.6	Lidocaine is metabolized >95% by hepatic microsomal enzymes (primarily CYP3A), so loss of functional liver tissue, as well as reduced liver blood flow, decreases lidocaine clearance. Pharmacokinetic parameters highly variable in liver disease patients. Volumes of distribution are larger due to decreased α_1-acid glycoprotein and albumin drug binding in the plasma.
Adult, heart failure	2	0.3	1	Decreased liver blood flow secondary to reduced cardiac output reduces lidocaine clearance. Volumes of distribution are smaller due to increased α_1-acid glycoprotein drug binding in the plasma. Heart failure results in large and variable reductions in lidocaine clearance.

178

Adult, post–myocardial infarction (<12 h)	4	0.5	1.5	Cardiac status must be monitored closely in heart failure patients, since lidocaine clearance changes with acute changes in cardiac output. Myocardial infarction reduces cardiac output, resulting in variable reductions in lidocaine clearance. These patients are especially prone to accumulation of serum lidocaine concentrations during long-term (>24-h) infusions, due to secretion of α_1-acid glycoprotein.
Adult, obese (>30% over IBW)	According to other disease states/conditions that affect lidocaine pharmacokinetics	According to other disease states/conditions that affect lidocaine pharmacokinetics	According to other disease states/conditions that affect lidocaine pharmacokinetics	For patients who weigh more that 30% above IBW, lidocaine doses should be based on ideal body weight.

- The volume of distribution for the central compartment of the two-compartment model is used to compute the loading dose because lidocaine distributes rapidly to the myocardium and the heart is considered to reside in the central compartment of the model.
- The elimination rate constant ($k = 0.693/t_{1/2}$, where $t_{1/2}$ is the half-life) and clearance ($Cl = kV_{area}$) can be computed from the aforementioned pharmacokinetic parameters.

Liver Dysfunction

- Patients who have liver cirrhosis or acute hepatitis have reduced lidocaine clearance, which results in a prolonged average lidocaine half-life of 5 hours.[12,19–22] The mechanism for depressed clearance in liver disease patients is destruction of liver parachymia where hepatic drug-metabolizing enzymes are present, and reduction of liver blood flow.
- The central volume of distribution and volume of distribution for the entire body are larger in patients with liver disease because albumin and α_1-acid glycoprotein (AGP) concentrations are lower in these patients and result in reduced lidocaine plasma protein binding (average $Vc = 0.6$ L/kg, average $V_{area} = 2.6$ L/kg).
- The effect that liver disease has on lidocaine pharmacokinetics is highly variable and difficult to predict accurately, especially in patients with acute hepatitis. It is possible for a patient with liver disease to have relatively normal or grossly abnormal lidocaine clearance, volumes of distribution, and half-life.
- An index of liver dysfunction can be gained by applying the Child-Pugh clinical classification system to the patient (Table 7-2).[23] Child-Pugh scores are discussed more fully in Chapter 3 (Drug Dosing in Special Populations: Renal and Hepatic Disease, Dialysis, Heart Failure, Obesity, and Drug Interactions).

  - The Child-Pugh score consists of five laboratory tests or clinical symptoms: serum albumin, total bilirubin, prothrombin time, ascites, and hepatic encephalopathy. Each of these areas is given a score of 1 (normal) to 3 (severely abnormal; Table 7-2), and the scores for the five areas are summed. The Child-Pugh score for a patient with normal liver function is 5, while the score for a patient with grossly abnormal serum albumin, total bilirubin, and prothrombin time values in addition to severe ascites and hepatic encephalopathy is 15.

TABLE 7-2 Child-Pugh Scores for Patients with Liver Disease[23]

Test/symptom	Score 1 point	Score 2 points	Score 3 points
Total bilirubin (mg/dl)	<2.0	2.0–3.0	>3.0
Serum albumin (g/dl)	>3.5	2.8–3.5	<2.8
Prothrombin time (seconds prolonged over control)	<4	4–6	>6
Ascites	Absent	Slight	Moderate
Hepatic Encephalopathy	None	Moderate	Severe

- A Child-Pugh score greater than 8 is grounds for a decrease in the initial daily drug dose for lidocaine ($t_{1/2}$ = 5 hours).
- As in any patient with or without liver dysfunction, initial doses are meant as starting points for dosage titration based on patient response and avoidance of adverse effects. Lidocaine serum concentrations and the presence of adverse drug effects should be monitored frequently in patients with liver cirrhosis.

Heart Failure

- Heart failure causes reduced lidocaine clearance because of decreased hepatic blood flow secondary to compromised cardiac output (Table 7-3).[5,12,21,24,25] Patients with cardiogenic shock experience extreme declines in lidocaine clearance due to severe decreases in cardiac output and liver blood flow.
- Central volume of distribution (Vc = 0.3 L/kg) and volume of distribution for the entire body (V_{area} = 1 L/kg) are decreased because heart failure patients have elevated AAG serum concentrations, which leads to increased lidocaine plasma protein binding and decreased lidocaine unbound fraction.
- Patients with heart failure have an average lidocaine half-life equal to 2 hours (range 1–24 hours). Half-life ($t_{1/2}$) does not change as much as expected from the change in clearance (Cl) because the volume of distribution decreases simultaneously [$t_{1/2} = (0.693 \cdot \downarrow V_{area})/\downarrow Cl$].
- The effect that heart failure has on lidocaine pharmacokinetics is highly variable and difficult to predict accurately. It is possible for a patient with heart failure to have relatively normal or grossly abnormal lidocaine clearance and half-life.
- For heart failure patients, initial doses are meant as starting points for dosage titration based on patient response and avoidance of adverse effects. Lidocaine serum concentrations and the presence of adverse drug effects should be monitored frequently in patients with heart failure.

TABLE 7-3 New York Heart Association (NYHA) Functional Classification for Heart Failure[36]

NYHA heart failure class	Description
I	Patients with cardiac disease but without limitations of physical activity. Ordinary physical activity does not cause undue fatigue, dyspnea, or palpitation.
II	Patients with cardiac disease that results in slight limitations of physical activity. Ordinary physical activity results in fatigue, palpitation, dyspnea, or angina.
III	Patients with cardiac disease that results in marked limitations of physical activity. Although patients are comfortable at rest, less than ordinary activity will lead to symptoms.
IV	Patients with cardiac disease that results in an inability to carry on physical activity without discomfort. Symptoms of congestive heart failure are present even at rest. With any physical activity, increased discomfort is experienced.

Myocardial Infarction

- Patients with myocardial infarction may develop serious ventricular arrhythmias that require therapy with lidocaine. After a myocardial infarction, serum AAG concentrations may increase up to 50% over a 12–72-hour time period.[8,10,11] As AAG serum concentrations increase, plasma protein binding of lidocaine decreases and the unbound fraction of lidocaine decreases from about 30% to about 20%.

  - Although lidocaine is considered a high-hepatic-extraction-ratio drug with liver blood flow having the major influence on lidocaine clearance, a decline in the unbound fraction of lidocaine in the plasma decreases lidocaine clearance. The reduction in lidocaine clearance is continuous as long as AAG concentrations continue to rise.
  - A result of this phenomenon is that lidocaine serum concentrations do not reach steady state during long-term (>24-hour) intravenous infusions of lidocaine in myocardial infarction patients, and results of pharmacokinetic studies in this patient population differ according to when the investigation took place in relation to the myocardial damage.
  - When similar myocardial infarction patients are studied after longer lidocaine infusions, the central volume of distribution and volume of distribution representing the entire body are smaller because AAG serum concentrations have had an opportunity to increase and change lidocaine plasma protein binding.[8,10,11]

- Patients studied within 12 hours of myocardial infarction had decreased lidocaine clearance due to decreased cardiac output and liver blood flow, relatively normal volumes of distribution (Vc = 0.5 L/kg, V_{area} = 1.5 L/kg), and a prolonged half-life of 4 hours.[25–27]

Obesity

- Although the volume of distribution representing the entire body (V_{area}) correlates most closely with total body weight, obese patients (>30% above ideal body weight or IBW) should have central volume of distribution and clearance estimates based on ideal body weight.[18]

Elderly

- For patients over the age of 65, studies indicate that lidocaine clearance is unchanged, the volumes of distribution are slightly larger, and half-life is longer (average half-life = 2.3 hours, range = 1.7–4.5 hours) compared to younger subjects.[24]

  - Most patients in all of the previously mentioned studies who had serious ventricular arrhythmias were older and the results include the influence of age. Thus, in most cases elderly patients are treated with lidocaine according to the other disease states or conditions present that influence lidocaine pharmacokinetics.

Pediatrics

- Pediatric doses are similar to those given to adults when adjusted for differences in body weight. Intravenous loading doses are 1 mg/kg, with up to two additional doses if needed (total dose not to exceed 3–5 mg/kg).

Continuous intravenous infusions doses are 20–50 µg/kg/min. For patients with shock, heart failure, or liver disease, initial doses should not exceed 20 µg/kg/min.[28]

Long-Term Infusions

• Lidocaine serum concentrations accumulate in patients receiving long-term (>24-hour) infusions even if the patient did not have a myocardial infarction.[9,17] Accumulation of lidocaine in these patients is due to competition for hepatic metabolism between parent drug and metabolites.

Renal Dysfunction

• Because MEGX and GX metabolites are eliminated to some extent by the kidney, patients with renal failure should be monitored for lidocaine adverse effects due to metabolite accumulation even though lidocaine serum concentrations are within the therapeutic range.

Dialysis and Hemofiltration

• Lidocaine is not appreciably removed by hemodialysis. Because lidocaine has a sieving coefficient of 0.14, continuous hemofiltration does not remove a significant amount of drug.[29,30]

DRUG INTERACTIONS

• Lidocaine has serious drug interactions with β-adrenergic receptor blockers and cimetidine, which decrease lidocaine clearance by 30% or more.[31]

  • Propranolol, metoprolol, and nadolol have been reported to reduce lidocaine clearance due to the decrease in cardiac output caused by β-blocker agents. Decreased cardiac output results in reduced liver blood flow, which explains the decline in lidocaine clearance caused by these drugs.
  • Cimetidine also decreases lidocaine clearance, but the mechanism of the interaction is different. Because cimetidine does not change liver blood flow, it is believed that cimetidine decreases lidocaine clearance by inhibiting hepatic microsomal enzymes.[32,33]

• Lidocaine clearance may be accelerated by concomitant use of phenobarbital or phenytoin.[31] Both of these agents are known to be hepatic drug-metabolizing enzyme inducers, and this is the probable mechanism of their drug interaction with lidocaine.

  • Phenytoin has antiarrhythmic effects and is also classified as a type IB antiarrhythmic agent. As a result, phenytoin and lidocaine may have additive pharmacological effects that could result in a pharmacodynamic drug interaction.

INITIAL DOSAGE DETERMINATION METHODS

• Several methods to initiate lidocaine therapy are available:

  • The *pharmacokinetic dosing method* is the most flexible of the techniques. It allows individualized target serum concentrations to be chosen for a patient, and each pharmacokinetic parameter can be customized to reflect specific disease states and conditions present in the patient.

- *Literature-based recommended dosing* is a very commonly used method for prescribing initial doses of lidocaine. Doses are based on those that commonly produce steady-state concentrations in the lower end of the therapeutic range, although there is a wide variation in the actual concentrations for a specific patient.

Pharmacokinetic Dosing Method

- The goal of initial dosing of lidocaine is to compute the best dose possible for the patient given his or her set of disease states and conditions that influence lidocaine pharmacokinetics and the arrhythmia being treated. In order to do this, pharmacokinetic parameters for the patient are estimated using average parameters measured in other patients with similar disease state and condition profiles.

Half-Life and Elimination Rate Constant Estimate

- Lidocaine is metabolized predominately by liver. Unfortunately, there is no good way to estimate the elimination characteristics of liver metabolized drugs using an endogenous marker of liver function in the same manner that serum creatinine and estimated creatinine clearance are used to estimate the elimination of agents that are renally eliminated.

  - A patient is categorized according to the disease states and conditions that are known to change lidocaine half-life, and the half-life previously measured in these studies is used as an estimate of the current patient's half-life (Table 7-1). Once the correct half-life is identified for the patient, it can be converted into the lidocaine elimination rate constant (k) using the following equation:

$$k = 0.693/t_{1/2}$$

  - To produce the most conservative lidocaine doses in patients with multiple concurrent disease states or conditions that affect lidocaine pharmacokinetics, the disease state or condition with the longest half-life should be used to compute doses. This approach will avoid accidental overdosage as much as is currently possible.

Volume of Distribution Estimate

- Lidocaine volume of distribution values are chosen according to the disease states and conditions that are present (Table 7-1). For obese patients (>30% above ideal body weight), ideal body weight is used to compute lidocaine volume of distribution.

  - The central volume of distribution (Vc) is used to compute loading doses because lidocaine has a rapid onset of action after administration, and the heart acts as if it is in the central compartment of the two-compartment model used to describe lidocaine pharmacokinetics.

    - The central volume of distribution is assumed to equal 0.6 L/kg for liver disease patients, 0.3 L/kg for heart failure and cardiogenic shock patients, and 0.5 L/kg for all other patients.

  - The volume of distribution for the entire body after distribution is complete (V_{area}) is used to help compute lidocaine clearance, and is assumed to equal 2.6 L/kg for liver disease patients, 1 L/kg for heart failure and cardiogenic shock patients, and 1.5 L/kg for all other patients.

Selection of Appropriate Pharmacokinetic Model and Equations

- When given by continuous intravenous infusion, lidocaine follows a two compartment pharmacokinetic model (Figures 7-1, 7-2, and 7-3).

  - A simple pharmacokinetic equation that computes the lidocaine steady-state serum concentration (Css in μg/ml = mg/L) is widely used and allows dosage calculation for a continuous infusion:

$$Css = k_0/Cl \qquad \text{or} \qquad k_0 = Css \cdot Cl$$

  where k_0 is the dose of lidocaine in mg and Cl is lidocaine clearance in L/h. Clearance is computed using estimates of lidocaine elimination rate constant (k) and volume of distribution for the entire body after distribution is complete (V_{area}):

$$Cl = kV_{area}$$

  - The equation used to calculate an intravenous loading dose (LD in mg) is based on a two-compartment model:

$$LD = (Css \cdot Vc)$$

  where Css is the desired lidocaine steady-state concentration in μg/ml (which is equivalent to mg/L), and Vc is the lidocaine central volume of distribution. Intravenous lidocaine loading doses should be given as an intravenous bolus no faster than 25–50 mg/min.

Steady-State Concentration Selection

- The generally accepted therapeutic range for lidocaine is 1.5–5 μg/ml. However, lidocaine therapy must be individualized for each patient in order to achieve optimal responses and minimal side effects.

▶ *Example 1*   LK is a 50-year-old, 75-kg (height 5′10″) male with ventricular tachycardia who requires therapy with intravenous lidocaine. He has normal liver and cardiac function. Suggest an initial intravenous lidocaine dosage regimen designed to achieve a steady-state lidocaine concentration equal to 3 μg/ml.

1. *Estimate half-life and elimination rate constant according to disease states and conditions present in the patient.* The expected lidocaine half-life ($t_{1/2}$) is 1.5 hours. The elimination rate constant is computed using the following formula:

$$k = 0.693/t_{1/2} = 0.693/1.5 \text{ h} = 0.462 \text{ h}^{-1}$$

2. *Estimate volume of distribution and clearance.* The patient is not obese, so the estimated lidocaine central volume of distribution and the volume of distribution for the entire body (V_{area}) can be based on actual body weight:

$$Vc = 0.5 \text{ L/kg} \cdot 75 \text{ kg} = 38 \text{ L}$$

$$V_{area} = 1.5 \text{ L/kg} \cdot 75 \text{ kg} = 113 \text{ L}$$

Estimated lidocaine clearance is computed by taking the product of V_{area} and the elimination rate constant:

$$Cl = kV_{area} = 0.462 \text{ h}^{-1} \cdot 113 \text{ L} = 52.2 \text{ L/h}$$

3. *Compute dosage regimen.* Therapy will be started by administering an intravenous loading dose of lidocaine to the patient (*Note:* μg/ml = mg/L, and this concentration unit was substituted for Css in the calculations so that unit conversion was not required):

$$LD = Css \cdot Vc = 3 \text{ mg/L} \cdot 38 \text{ L} = 114 \text{ mg}$$

rounded to 100 mg intravenously over 2–4 minutes. An additional dose equal to 50% of the loading dose can be given if arrhythmias recur within 20–30 minutes after the initial loading dose.

A continuous intravenous infusion of lidocaine will be started immediately after the loading dose has been administered. (*Note:* μg/ml = mg/L, and this concentration unit was substituted for Css in the calculations so unnecessary unit conversion was not required). The dosage equation for intravenous lidocaine is:

$$k_0 = Css \cdot Cl = (3 \text{ mg/L} \cdot 52.2 \text{ L/h})/(60 \text{ min/h})$$
$$= 2.6 \text{ mg/min, rounded to } 2.5 \text{ mg/min}$$

A steady-state lidocaine serum concentration can be measured after steady state is attained in 3–5 half- lives. Since the patient is expected to have a half-life equal to 1.5 hours, the lidocaine steady-state concentration could be obtained any time after the first 8 hours of dosing (5 half-lives = $5 \cdot 1.5$ h = 7.5 h). Lidocaine serum concentrations should also be measured if the patient experiences a return of ventricular arrhythmia, or if the patient develops potential signs or symptoms of lidocaine toxicity.

▶ *Example 2*   MN is a 64-year-old, 78-kg (height 5′9″) male with ventricular tachycardia who requires therapy with intravenous lidocaine. He has moderate heart failure [New York Heart Association (NYHA) CHF class III]. Suggest an initial intravenous lidocaine dosage regimen designed to achieve a steady-state lidocaine concentration of 3 μg/ml.

1. *Estimate half-life and elimination rate constant according to disease states and conditions present in the patient.* The expected lidocaine half-life ($t_{1/2}$) is 2 hours. The elimination rate constant is computed using the following formula:

$$k = 0.693/t_{1/2} = 0.693/2 \text{ h} = 0.347 \text{ h}^{-1}$$

2. *Estimate volume of distribution and clearance.* The patient is not obese, so the estimated lidocaine central volume of distribution and the volume of distribution for the entire body (V_{area}) can be based on actual body weight:

$$Vc = 0.3 \text{ L/kg} \cdot 78 \text{ kg} = 23 \text{ L}$$

$$V_{area} = 1 \text{ L/kg} \cdot 78 \text{ kg} = 78 \text{ L}$$

Estimated lidocaine clearance is computed by taking the product of V_{area} and the elimination rate constant:

$$Cl = kV_{area} = 0.347 \text{ h}^{-1} \cdot 78 \text{ L} = 27 \text{ L/h}$$

3. *Compute dosage regimen.* Therapy will be started by administering an intravenous loading dose of lidocaine to the patient (*Note:* μg/ml = mg/L,

and this concentration unit was substituted for Css in the calculations so that unit conversion was not required):

$$LD = Css \cdot Vc = 3 \text{ mg/L} \cdot 23 \text{ L} = 69 \text{ mg}$$

rounded to 75 mg intravenously over 2–3 minutes. An additional dose equal to 50% of the loading dose can be given if arrhythmias recur within 20–30 minutes after the initial loading dose.

A continuous intravenous infusion of lidocaine will be started immediately after the loading dose has been administered. (*Note:* μg/ml = mg/L, and this concentration unit was substituted for Css in the calculations so that unit conversion was not required). The dosage equation for intravenous lidocaine is:

$$k_0 = Css \cdot Cl = (3 \text{ mg/L} \cdot 27 \text{ L/h})/(60 \text{ min/h})$$
$$= 1.4 \text{ mg/min, rounded to } 1.5 \text{ mg/min}$$

A steady-state lidocaine serum concentration can be measured after steady state is attained in 3–5 half-lives. Since the patient is expected to have a half-life equal to 2 hours, the lidocaine steady-state concentration can be obtained any time after the first 10–12 hours of dosing (5 half-lives = 5 · 2 h = 10 h). Lidocaine serum concentrations should also be measured if the patient experiences a return of ventricular arrhythmia, or if the patient develops potential signs or symptoms of lidocaine toxicity.

Literature-Based Recommended Dosing

- Because of the large amount of variability in lidocaine pharmacokinetics, even when concurrent disease states and conditions are identified, many clinicians believe that the use of standard lidocaine doses for various situations is warranted.[34] The original computations of these doses were based on the pharmacokinetic dosing method described in the previous section, and the doses were subsequently modified based on clinical experience.
- In general, the lidocaine steady-state serum concentration expected from the lower end of the dosage range is 1.5–3 μg/ml and 3–5 μg/ml for the upper end of the dosage range. Suggested intravenous continuous-infusion lidocaine maintenance doses are 1–2 mg/min for patients with liver disease or heart failure and 3–4 mg/min for all other patients.
- When more than one disease state or condition is present in a patient, choosing the lowest infusion rate will result in the safest, most conservative dosage recommendation.
- With regard to loading doses, lidocaine is given intravenously at a dose of 1–1.5 mg/kg (not to exceed 25–50 mg/min) to all patients except those with heart failure. The suggested intravenous lidocaine loading dose for heart failure patients is 0.5–0.75 mg/kg (not to exceed 25–50 mg/min), although some clinicians advocate the administration of full loading doses of lidocaine in heart failure patients.
- Pediatric doses are similar to those given to adults when adjusted for differences in body weight. Intravenous loading doses are 1 mg/kg, with up to two additional doses if needed (total dose not to exceed 3–5 mg/kg). Continuous intravenous infusions doses are 20–50 μg/kg/min. For patients with shock, heart failure, or liver disease, initial doses should not exceed 20 μg/kg/min.[28]
- Ideal body weight is used to compute loading doses for obese patients (>30% over ideal body weight).

- To illustrate the similarities and differences between this method of dosage calculation and the pharmacokinetic dosing method, the same examples used in the previous section will be used.

▶ *Example 1*   LK is a 50-year-old, 75-kg (height 5′10″) male with ventricular tachycardia who requires therapy with intravenous lidocaine. He has normal liver and cardiac function. Suggest an initial intravenous lidocaine dosage regimen designed to achieve a steady-state lidocaine concentration of 3 μg/ml.

1. *Choose lidocaine dose based on disease states and conditions present in the patient.* A lidocaine loading dose of 1–1.5 mg/kg and maintenance infusion of 3–4 mg/min is suggested for a patient without heart failure or liver disease.

2. *Compute dosage regimen.* Because the desired concentration is near the lower end of the therapeutic range, a dose near the lower end of the suggested range will be used. A lidocaine loading dose of 1 mg/kg will be administered: LD = 1 mg/kg · 75 kg = 75 mg over 1.5–3 minutes. A lidocaine maintenance infusion equal to 3 mg/min will be administered after the loading dose is given. An additional dose equal to 50% of the loading dose can be given if arrhythmias recur within 20–30 minutes after the initial loading dose.

    Steady-state lidocaine serum concentration can be measured after steady state is attained in 3–5 half-lives. Since the patient is expected to have a half-life equal to 1.5 hours, the lidocaine steady-state concentration can be obtained any time after the first 8 hours of dosing (5 half-lives = 5 · 1.5 h = 7.5 h). Lidocaine serum concentrations should also be measured if the patient experiences a return of ventricular arrhythmia, or if the patient develops potential signs or symptoms of lidocaine toxicity.

▶ *Example 2*   MN is a 64-year-old, 78-kg (height 5′9″) male with ventricular tachycardia who requires therapy with intravenous lidocaine. He has moderate heart failure (NYHA CHF class III). Suggest an initial intravenous lidocaine dosage regimen designed to achieve a steady-state lidocaine concentration of 3 μg/ml.

1. *Choose lidocaine dose based on disease states and conditions present in the patient.* A lidocaine loading dose of 0.5–0.75 mg/kg and maintenance infusion of 1–2 mg/min is suggested for a patient with heart failure.

2. *Compute dosage regimen.* Because the desired concentration is near the lower end of the therapeutic range, a dose near the lower end of the suggested range will be used. A lidocaine loading dose of 0.5 mg/kg will be administered: LD = 0.5 mg/kg · 78 kg = 39 mg, rounded to 50 mg over 1–2 minutes. A lidocaine maintenance infusion of 1 mg/min will be administered after the loading dose is given. An additional dose equal to 50% of the loading dose can be given if arrhythmias recur within 20–30 minutes after the initial loading dose.

    Steady-state lidocaine serum concentration can be measured after steady state is attained in 3–5 half-lives. Since the patient is expected to have a half-life equal to 2 hours, the lidocaine steady-state concentration can be obtained any time after the first 10–12 hours of dosing (5 half-lives = 5 · 2 h = 10 h). Lidocaine serum concentrations should also be measured if the patient experiences a return of ventricular arrhythmia, or if the patient develops potential signs or symptoms of lidocaine toxicity.

USE OF LIDOCAINE SERUM CONCENTRATIONS TO ALTER DOSES

• Because of the extensive pharmacokinetic variability among patients, it is likely that doses computed using patient population characteristics will not always produce lidocaine serum concentrations that are expected or desirable. Because of this pharmacokinetic variability, the narrow therapeutic index of lidocaine, and the desire to avoid of lidocaine adverse side effects, measurement of lidocaine serum concentrations can be a useful adjunct for patients to ensure that therapeutic, nontoxic levels are present.

• Other important patient parameters (electrocardiogram, clinical signs and symptoms of the ventricular arrhythmia, potential lidocaine side effects, etc.) should be followed to confirm that the patient is responding to treatment and not developing adverse drug reactions.

• When lidocaine serum concentrations are measured in patients and a dosage change is necessary, clinicians should use the simplest, most straightforward method available to determine a dose that will provide safe and effective treatment.

  • In most cases, a simple dosage ratio can be used to change lidocaine doses, assuming the drug follows *linear pharmacokinetics.* Most clinicians use this straightforward method as their primary way to adjust lidocaine infusion rates.

    • Although it has been clearly demonstrated in research studies that lidocaine serum concentrations accumulate in patients during long-term (>24-hour) infusions, in the clinical setting most patients' steady-state serum concentrations change proportionally to lidocaine dose for shorter infusion times. Thus, assuming linear pharmacokinetics is adequate for dosage adjustments in most patients.

  • Sometimes, it is useful to compute lidocaine pharmacokinetic constants for a patient and base dosage adjustments on these. In this case, it may be possible to calculate and use *pharmacokinetic parameters* to alter the lidocaine dose. Since steady-state concentrations are used, this technique will give the same dosage as the linear pharmacokinetics method. However, since clearance is calculated, the value for the patient can be compared to the population average and previous measurements made in the patient.

  • In some situations, it may be necessary to compute lidocaine clearance for the patient during a continuous infusion before steady-state conditions occur, and then utilize this pharmacokinetic parameter to calculate the best drug dose. Computerized methods that incorporate expected population pharmacokinetic characteristics (*Bayesian pharmacokinetic computer programs*) can be used in difficult cases when serum concentrations are obtained at suboptimal times or the patient was not at steady state when serum concentrations were measured.

    • An additional benefit is that a complete pharmacokinetic workup (determination of clearance, volume of distribution, and half-life) can be done with one or more measured concentrations that do not have to be at steady state.

Linear Pharmacokinetics Method

• Because lidocaine follows linear, dose-proportional pharmacokinetics in most patients during short-term infusions (<24 hours), steady-state serum concentrations change in proportion to dose according to the following equation:

$$D_{new}/Css_{new} = D_{old}/Css_{old} \quad \text{or} \quad D_{new} = (Css_{new}/Css_{old})D_{old}$$

where D is the dose, Css is the steady-state concentration, old indicates the dose that produced the steady-state concentration that the patient is currently receiving, and new denotes the dose necessary to produce the desired steady-state concentration.

- The advantages of this method are that it is quick and simple. The disadvantages are that steady-state concentrations are required, and accumulation of serum lidocaine concentrations can occur with long-term (>24-hour) infusions.

  - When steady-state serum concentrations are higher than expected during long-term lidocaine infusions, lidocaine accumulation pharmacokinetics is a possible explanation for the observation. Therefore, suggested dosage increases greater than 75% using this method should be scrutinized by the prescribing clinician, and the risk versus benefit for the patient assessed before initiating large dosage increases (>75% over current dose).

▸ **Example 1**   OI is a 60-year-old, 85-kg (height 6'1") male with ventricular fibrillation who requires therapy with intravenous lidocaine. He has liver cirrhosis (Child-Pugh score = 11). The current steady-state lidocaine concentration is 6.4 µg/ml at a dose of 2 mg/min. Compute a lidocaine dose that will provide a steady-state concentration of 3 µg/ml.

1. *Compute new dose to achieve desired serum concentration.* The patient can be expected to achieve steady-state conditions after a day ($5t_{1/2} = 5 \cdot 5\ h = 25\ h$) of therapy.

   Using linear pharmacokinetics, the new dose to attain the desired concentration should be proportional to the old dose that produced the measured concentration:

   $$D_{new} = (Css_{new}/Css_{old})D_{old} = (3\ \mu g/ml/6.4\ \mu g/ml)\ 2\ mg/min$$
   $$= 0.9\ mg/min, \text{ rounded to } 1\ mg/min$$

The new suggested dose is 1 mg/min of intravenous lidocaine. If the patient is experiencing adverse drug effects, the infusion can be held for one estimated half-life (5 h) before the new dose is started.

A steady-state lidocaine serum concentration can be measured after steady state is attained in 3–5 half-lives. Since the patient is expected to have a half-life equal to 5 hours, the lidocaine steady-state concentration can be obtained any time after the first day of dosing (5 half-lives = $5 \cdot 5\ h = 25\ h$). Lidocaine serum concentrations should also be measured if the patient experiences a return of ventricular arrhythmia, or if the patient develops potential signs or symptoms of lidocaine toxicity.

Pharmacokinetic Parameter Method

- The pharmacokinetic parameter method of adjusting drug doses allows the computation of an individual's own, unique clearance and uses it to calculate a dose that achieves desired lidocaine concentrations. During a continuous intravenous infusion, the following equation is used to compute lidocaine clearance (Cl in L/min):

$$Cl = k_0/Css$$

where k_0 is the dose of lidocaine in mg/min and Css is the steady-state lidocaine concentration in mg/L or µg/ml.

- The clearance measured using this technique can be used in the intravenous continuous infusion equation to compute the required dose (k_0 in mg/min) to achieve any desired steady-state serum concentration (Css in mg/L or µg/ml):

$$k_0 = CssCl$$

where Cl is lidocaine clearance in L/min.

- Because this method also assumes linear pharmacokinetics, lidocaine doses computed using the pharmacokinetic parameter method and the linear pharmacokinetic method should be identical.

▶ **Example 1** OI is a 60-year-old, 85-kg (height 6′1″) male with ventricular fibrillation who requires therapy with intravenous lidocaine. He has liver cirrhosis (Child-Pugh score = 11). The current steady-state lidocaine concentration is 6.4 µg/ml at a dose of 2 mg/min. Compute a lidocaine dose that will provide a steady-state concentration of 3 µg/ml.

1. *Compute pharmacokinetic parameters.* The patient can be expected to achieve steady-state conditions after a day ($5t_{1/2} = 5 \cdot 5$ h = 25 h) of therapy.
    Lidocaine clearance can be computed using a steady-state lidocaine concentration:

$$Cl = k_0/Css = (2 \text{ mg/min})/(6.4 \text{ mg/L}) = 0.31 \text{ L/min}$$

(*Note:* µg/ml = mg/L, and this concentration unit was substituted for Css in the calculations so that unit conversion was not required.)
2. *Compute lidocaine dose.* Lidocaine clearance is used to compute the new lidocaine infusion rate:

$$k_0 = Css \cdot Cl = 3 \text{ mg/L} \cdot 0.31 \text{ L/min}$$
$$= 0.9 \text{ mg/min, rounded to 1 mg/min}$$

The new suggested dose is 1 mg/min of intravenous lidocaine. If the patient is experiencing adverse drug effects, the infusion can be held for one estimated half-life (5 h) before the new dose is started.
    A steady state lidocaine serum concentration can be measured after steady state is attained in 3–5 half-lives. Since the patient is expected to have a half-life equal to 5 hours, the lidocaine steady-state concentration can be obtained any time after the first day of dosing (5 half-lives = $5 \cdot 5$ h = 25 h). Lidocaine serum concentrations should also be measured if the patient experiences a return of ventricular arrhythmia, or if the patient develops potential signs or symptoms of lidocaine toxicity.

Bayesian Pharmacokinetic Computer Programs

- Computer programs are available that can assist in the computation of pharmacokinetic parameters for patients. The most reliable computer programs use a nonlinear regression algorithm that incorporates components of Bayes' theorem.

  - An advantage of this approach is that consistent dosage recommendations are made when several different practitioners are involved in therapeutic drug monitoring programs. However, since simpler dosing methods work just as well for patients with stable pharmacokinetic parameters and steady-state drug concentrations, many clinicians reserve the use of computer programs for more difficult situations. Those situations include

serum concentrations that are not at steady state, serum concentrations not obtained at the specific times needed to employ simpler methods, and unstable pharmacokinetic parameters.
- When only a limited number of lidocaine concentrations are available, Bayesian pharmacokinetic computer programs can be used to compute a complete patient pharmacokinetic profile that includes clearance, volume of distribution, and half life.

- Many Bayesian pharmacokinetic computer programs are available, and most should provide answers similar to the program used in the following examples. The program used to solve problems in this book is DrugCalc, written by Dr. Dennis Mungall and available at his Internet web site (www.clinpharmacologist.bigstep.com/consumersurvey.html).[35]

▶ *Example 1* SL is a 71-year-old, 82-kg (height 5′10″) male with ventricular fibrillation who requires therapy with intravenous lidocaine. He has liver cirrhosis (Child-Pugh score = 12, bilirubin = 3.2 mg/dl, albumin = 2.5 gm/dl) and normal cardiac function. He received a 150-mg loading dose of lidocaine at 1300 H, and a continuous intravenous infusion of lidocaine was started at 1305 H at the rate of 2 mg/min. The lidocaine serum concentration was 5.7 μg/ml at 2300 H. Compute a lidocaine infusion rate that will provide a steady-state concentration of 4 μg/ml.

1. *Enter patient demographic, drug dosing, and serum concentration/time data into a Bayesian pharmacokinetic computer program.* In this case it is unlikely that the patient is at steady state, so the linear pharmacokinetics method cannot be used. The DrugCalc program requires lidocaine infusion rates to be input in terms of mg/h. A 2-mg/min infusion rate is equivalent to 120 mg/h (k_0 = 2 mg/min · 60 min/h = 120 mg/h).
2. *Compute pharmacokinetic parameters for the patient using the computer program.* The pharmacokinetic parameters computed by the program are a volume of distribution for the entire body (V_{area}) of 142 L, a half-life of 6.5 h, and a clearance rate of 15 L/h.
3. *Compute dose required to achieve desired lidocaine serum concentrations.* The continuous intravenous infusion equation used by the program to compute doses indicates that a dose of 60 mg/h or 1 mg/min [k_0 = (60 mg/h)/(60 min/h) = 1 mg/min] will produce a steady-state lidocaine concentration of 4 μg/ml. This infusion rate can be started immediately, or if the patient is experiencing adverse drug effects, the infusion can be held for $\frac{1}{2}$–1 half-life to allow lidocaine serum concentrations to decline and then be restarted.

▶ *Example 2* TR is a 75-year-old, 85-kg (height 5′8″) male with ventricular tachycardia who requires therapy with intravenous lidocaine. He has moderate heart failure (NYHA CHF class III). He received a 75-mg loading dose of lidocaine at 0100 H, and a continuous intravenous infusion of lidocaine was started at 0115 H at the rate of 1 mg/min. The lidocaine serum concentration was 1.7 μg/ml at 0400 H. Compute a lidocaine infusion rate that will provide a steady-state concentration of 3 μg/ml.

1. *Enter patient demographic, drug dosing, and serum concentration/time data into a Bayesian pharmacokinetic computer program.* In this case it is unlikely that the patient is at steady state, so the linear pharmacokinetics method cannot be used. The DrugCalc program requires lidocaine

infusion rates be input in terms of mg/h. A 1-mg/min infusion rate is equivalent to 60 mg/h (k_0 = 1 mg/min · 60 min/h = 60 mg/h).

2. *Compute pharmacokinetic parameters for the patient using the computer program.* The pharmacokinetic parameters computed by the program are a volume of distribution for the entire body (V_{area}) of 74 L, a half-life of 1.8 h, and a clearance rate of 29 L/h.

3. *Compute dose required to achieve desired lidocaine serum concentrations.* The continuous intravenous infusion equation used by the program to compute doses indicates that a dose of 90 mg/h or 1.5 mg/min [k_0 = (90 mg/h)/(60 min/h) = 1.5 mg/min] will produce a steady-state lidocaine concentration of 3 μg/ml. This infusion rate would be started immediately.

DOSING STRATEGIES

• Initial dose and dosage adjustment techniques using serum concentrations can be used in any combination as long as the limitations of each method are observed.

• Some dosing schemes link together logically when considered according to their basic approaches or philosophies. Dosage strategies that follow similar pathways are given in Table 7-4.

USE OF LIDOCAINE BOOSTER DOSES TO IMMEDIATELY INCREASE SERUM CONCENTRATIONS

• If a patient has a subtherapeutic lidocaine serum concentration and is experiencing ventricular arrhythmias in an acute situation, it is desirable to increase the lidocaine concentration as quickly as possible. In this setting, it would not be acceptable simply to increase the maintenance dose and wait 3–5 half-lives for therapeutic serum concentrations to be established in the patient.

  • A rational way to increase the serum concentrations rapidly is to administer a booster dose (BD) of lidocaine, a process also known as "reloading" the patient with lidocaine, computed using pharmacokinetic techniques. A modified loading dose equation is used to accomplish computation of the booster dose which takes into account the current lidocaine

TABLE 7-4 Dosing Strategies

Dosing approach/ philosophy	Initial dosing	Use of serum concentrations to alter doses
Pharmacokinetic parameters/ equations	Pharmacokinetic dosing method	Pharmacokinetic parameter method
Literature-based/ concept	Literature-based recommended dosing	Linear pharmacokinetic method
Computerized	Bayesian computer program	Bayesian computer program

concentration in the patient:

$$BD = (C_{desired} - C_{actual})Vc$$

where $C_{desired}$ is the desired lidocaine concentration, C_{actual} is the actual current lidocaine concentration in the patient, and Vc is the central volume of distribution for lidocaine.

- If the central volume of distribution for lidocaine is known for the patient, it can be used in the calculation. However, this value is not usually known and is typically assumed to equal the population average appropriate for the disease states and conditions present in the patient (Table 7-1).

- Concurrent with the administration of the booster dose, the maintenance dose of lidocaine is usually increased. Clinicians need to recognize that the administration of a booster dose does not alter the time required to achieve steady-state conditions when a new lidocaine dosage rate is prescribed (Figure 7-3). It still requires 3–5 half-lives to attain steady state when the dosage rate is changed. However, usually the difference between the post-booster dose lidocaine concentration and the ultimate steady-state concentration is reduced by giving the extra dose of drug.

▶ **Example 1** BN is a 57-year-old, 50-kg (height 5′2″) female with ventricular tachycardia who is receiving therapy with intravenous lidocaine. She has normal liver function and does not have heart failure. After receiving an initial loading dose of lidocaine (75 mg) and a maintenance infusion of lidocaine of 2 mg/min for 2 hours, her arrhythmia reappears and a lidocaine concentration is measured at 1.2 mg/ml. Compute a booster dose of lidocaine to achieve a lidocaine concentration of 4 μg/ml.

1. *Estimate volume of distribution according to disease states and conditions present in the patient.* In the case of lidocaine, the population-average central volume of distribution equals 0.5 L/kg, and this will be used to estimate the parameter for the patient. The patient is not obese, so her actual body weight will be used in the computation:

$$V = 0.5 \text{ L/kg} \cdot 50 \text{ kg} = 25 \text{ L}$$

2. *Compute booster dose.* The booster dose is computed using the following equation:

$$BD = (C_{desired} - C_{actual})Vc = (4 \text{ mg/L} - 1.2 \text{ mg/L})25 \text{ L} = 70 \text{ mg}$$

rounded to 75 mg of lidocaine intravenously over 1.5–3 minutes. (*Note:* μg/ml = mg/L, and this concentration unit was substituted for C in the calculations so that unit conversion was not required.) If the maintenance dose is increased, it will take an additional 3–5 estimated half-lives for new steady-state conditions to be achieved. Lidocaine serum concentrations can be measured at this time. Lidocaine serum concentrations should also be measured if the patient experiences a return of ventricular arrhythmia, or if the patient develops potential signs or symptoms of lidocaine toxicity.

REFERENCES

1. Bauman JL, Schoen MD. Arrhythmias. In: DiPiro JT, Talbert RL, Yee GC, Matzke GR, Wells BG, Posey LM, eds. Pharmacotherapy. 5th ed. New York: McGraw-Hill, 2002:273–304.
2. Roden DM. Antiarrhythmic drugs. In: Hardman JG, Limbird LE, Gilman AG, eds. The pharmacological basis of therapeutics. 10th ed. New York: McGraw-Hill, 2001:933–70.

3. Boyes RN, Scott DB, Jebson PJ, Godman MJ, Julian DG. Pharmacokinetics of lidocaine in man. Clin Pharmacol Ther 1971;12(1):105–16.
4. Wyman MG, Lalka D, Hammersmith L, Cannom DS, Goldreyer BN. Multiple bolus technique for lidocaine administration during the first hours of an acute myocardial infarction. Am J Cardiol 1978;41(2):313–7.
5. Halkin H, Meffin P, Melmon KL, Rowland M. Influence of congestive heart failure on blood vessels of lidocaine and its active monodeethylated metabolite. Clin Pharmacol Ther 1975;17(6):669–76.
6. Strong JM, Mayfield DE, Atkinson AJ Jr, Burris BC, Raymon F, Webster LT Jr. Pharmacological activity, metabolism, and pharmacokinetics of glycinexylidide. Clin Pharmacol Ther 1975;17(2):184–94.
7. Narang PK, Crouthamel WG, Carliner NH, Fisher ML. Lidocaine and its active metabolites. Clin Pharmacol Ther 1978;24(6):654–62.
8. Barchowsky A, Shand DG, Stargel WW, Wagner GS, Routledge PA. On the role of alpha 1-acid glycoprotein in lignocaine accumulation following myocardial infarction. Br J Clin Pharmacol 1982;13(3):411–5.
9. Bauer LA, Brown T, Gibaldi M, et al. Influence of long-term infusions on lidocaine kinetics. Clin Pharmacol Ther 1982;31(4):433–7.
10. Routledge PA, Stargel WW, Wagner GS, Shand DG. Increased alpha-1-acid glycoprotein and lidocaine disposition in myocardial infarction. Ann Intern Med 1980;93(5):701–4.
11. Routledge PA, Shand DG, Barchowsky A, Wagner G, Stargel WW. Relationship between alpha 1-acid glycoprotein and lidocaine disposition in myocardial infarction. Clin Pharmacol Ther 1981;30(2):154–7.
12. Thomson PD, Rowland M, Melmon KL. The influence of heart failure, liver disease, and renal failure on the disposition of lidocaine in man. Am Heart J 1971;82(3):417–21.
13. Scott DB, Jebson PJ, Vellani CW, Julian DG. Plasma-lignocaine levels after intravenous and intramuscular injection. Lancet 1970;1(7636):41.
14. Routledge PA, Stargel WW, Kitchell BB, Barchowsky A, Shand DG. Sex-related differences in the plasma protein binding of lignocaine and diazepam. Br J Clin Pharmacol 1981;11(3):245–50.
15. Routledge PA, Barchowsky A, Bjornsson TD, Kitchell BB, Shand DG. Lidocaine plasma protein binding. Clin Pharmacol Ther 1980;27(3):347–51.
16. McNamara PJ, Slaughter RL, Pieper JA, Wyman MG, Lalka D. Factors influencing serum protein binding of lidocaine in humans. Anesth Analg 1981;60(6):395–400.
17. Suzuki T, Fujita S, Kawai R. Precursor-metabolite interaction in the metabolism of lidocaine. J Pharm Sci 1984;73(1):136–8.
18. Abernethy DR, Greenblatt DJ. Lidocaine disposition in obesity. Am J Cardiol 1984;53(8):1183–6.
19. Forrest JA, Finlayson ND, Adjepon-Yamoah KK, Prescott LF. Antipyrine, paracetamol, and lignocaine elimination in chronic liver disease. Br Med J 1977;1(6073): 1384–7.
20. Huet PM, Lelorier J. Effects of smoking and chronic hepatitis B on lidocaine and indocyanine green kinetics. Clin Pharmacol Ther 1980;28(2):208–15.
21. Thomson PD, Melmon KL, Richardson JA, et al. Lidocaine pharmacokinetics in advanced heart failure, liver disease, and renal failure in humans. Ann Intern Med 1973;78(4):499–508.
22. Williams RL, Blaschke TF, Meffin PJ, Melmon KL, Rowland M. Influence of viral hepatitis on the disposition of two compounds with high hepatic clearance: lidocaine and indocyanine green. Clin Pharmacol Ther 1976;20(3):290–9.
23. Pugh RN, Murray-Lyon IM, Dawson JL, Pietroni MC, Williams R. Transection of the oesophagus for bleeding oesophageal varices. Br J Surg 1973;60(8):646–9.
24. Nation RL, Triggs EJ, Selig M. Lignocaine kinetics in cardiac patients and aged subjects. Br J Clin Pharmacol 1977;4(4):439–48.
25. Prescott LF, Adjepon-Yamoah KK, Talbot RG. Impaired Lignocaine metabolism in patients with myocardial infarction and cardiac failure. Br Med J 1976;1(6015): 939–41.

26. Bax ND, Tucker GT, Woods HF. Lignocaine and indocyanine green kinetics in patients following myocardial infarction. Br J Clin Pharmacol 1980;10(4):353–61.
27. LeLorier J, Grenon D, Latour Y, et al. Pharmacokinetics of lidocaine after prolonged intravenous infusions in uncomplicated myocardial infarction. Ann Intern Med 1977;87(6):700–6.
28. Gunn VL, Nechyba C, eds. The Harriet Lane handbook: a manual for pediatric house officers. 16th ed. Philadelphia: Mosby, 2002.
29. Golper TA, Marx MA. Drug dosing adjustments during continuous renal replacement therapies. Kidney Int Suppl 1998;66:S165–8.
30. Golper TA. Update on drug sieving coefficients and dosing adjustments during continuous renal replacement therapies. Contrib Nephrol 2001(132):349–53.
31. Hansten PD, Horn JR. Drug interactions analysis and management. Vancouver, WA: Applied Therapeutics, 1998.
32. Bauer LA, Edwards WA, Randolph FP, Blouin RA. Cimetidine-induced decrease in lidocaine metabolism. Am Heart J 1984;108(2):413–5.
33. Bauer LA, McDonnell N, Horn JR, Zierler B, Opheim K, Strandness DE Jr. Single and multiple doses of oral cimetidine do not change liver blood flow in humans. Clin Pharmacol Ther 1990;48(2):195–200.
34. Mutnick AH, Burke TG. Antiarrhythmics. In: Schumacher GE, ed. Therapeutic Drug Monitoring. 1st ed. Stamford, CT: Appleton & Lange, 1995:684.
35. Wandell M, Mungall D. Computer assisted drug interpretation and drug regimen optimization. Am Assoc Clin Chem 1984;6:1–11.
36. Johnson JA, Parker RB, Geraci SA. Heart failure. In: DiPiro JT, Talbert RL, Yee GC, Matzke GR, Wells BG, Posey LM, eds. Pharmacotherapy—a pathophysiologic approach. 5th ed. New York: McGraw-Hill, 2002:185–218.

8 | Procainamide and N-Acetyl Procainamide

Procainamide is an effective antiarrhythmic agent that is used intravenously and orally. It is classified as a type IA antiarrhythmic agent and can be used for the treatment of supraventricular or ventricular arrhythmias.[1,2]

• Procainamide inhibits transmembrane sodium influx into the conduction system of the heart, thereby decreasing conduction velocity.[1,2] It also increases the duration of the action potential, increases threshold potential toward zero, and decreases the slope of phase 4 of the action potential. Automaticity is decreased during procainamide therapy. The net effect of these cellular changes is that procainamide causes increased refractoriness and decreased conduction in heart conduction tissue, which establishes a bidirectional block in reentrant pathways.

• N-acetyl procainamide (NAPA) is an active metabolite of procainamide that has type III antiarrhythmic effects.[1,2] A common characteristic of type III antiarrhythmic agents (bretylium, aminodarone, sotalol) is prolongation of the duration of the action potential, resulting in an increased absolute refractory period.

THERAPEUTIC AND TOXIC CONCENTRATIONS

• When given intravenously, the serum procainamide concentration/time curve follows a two-compartment model (Figure 8-1).[3] If an intravenous loading dose is followed by a continuous infusion, serum concentrations decline rapidly at first, due to distribution of the loading dose from blood to tissues (Figure 8-2).[3]

  • When oral dosage forms are given, absorption occurs more slowly than distribution, so a distribution phase is not seen (Figure 8-3).[4–8]

• The generally accepted therapeutic range for procainamide is 4–10 μg/ml. Serum concentrations near the upper end of the therapeutic range (≥8 μg/ml) may result in minor side effects such as gastrointestinal disturbances (anorexia, nausea, vomiting, diarrhea), weakness, malaise, decreased mean arterial pressure (less than 20%), and a 10–30% prolongation of electrocardiogram intervals (PR and QT intervals, QRS complex).

  • Procainamide serum concentrations above 12 μg/ml can cause increased PR interval, QT interval or QRS complex widening (>30%) on the electrocardiogram, heart block, ventricular conduction disturbances, new ventricular arrhythmias, or cardiac arrest.

• Procainamide therapy is also associated with torsades de pointes.[1,2] Torsades de pointes ("twisting of the points") is a form of polymorphic ventricular tachycardia preceded by QT interval prolongation.

  • It is characterized by polymorphic QRS complexes that change in amplitude and length, giving the appearance of oscillations around the electrocardiographic baseline. Torsade de pointes can develop into multiple episodes of nonsustained polymorphic ventricular tachycardia, syncope, ventricular fibrillation, or sudden cardiac death.

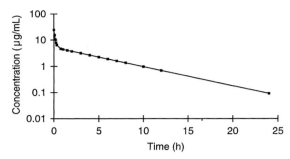

FIG. 8-1 Procainamide serum concentrations initially drop rapidly after an intravenous bolus as drug distributes from blood into the tissues during the distribution phase. During the distribution phase, drug leaves the blood due to tissue distribution and elimination. After 20–30 minutes, an equilibrium is established between the blood and tissues, and serum concentrations drop more slowly because elimination is the primary process removing drug from the blood. This type of serum concentration/time profile is described by a two-compartment model.

- Non–dose- or–concentration-related side effects to procainamide include rash, agranulocytosis, and a systemic lupus-like syndrome. Symptoms of the lupus-like syndrome include rash, photosensitivity, arthralgias, pleuritis or pericarditis, hemolytic anemia or leukopenia, and a positive antinuclear antibody (ANA) test.

  - Patients who metabolize the drug more rapidly via N-acetyltransferase, known as "rapid acetylators," appear to have a lower incidence of lupus or at least take more time and higher doses for it to appear.
  - While the lupus-like syndrome is usually not life-threatening, it does occur in 30–50% of patients taking procainamide for longer than 6–12 months

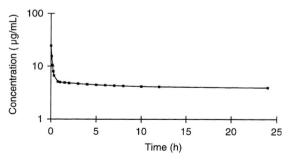

FIG. 8-2 To maintain therapeutic procainamide concentrations, an intravenous loading dose (over 25–30 minutes) of procainamide is followed by a continuous intravenous infusion of the drug. A distribution phase is still seen, due to the administration of the loading dose. Note that the administration of a loading dose may not establish steady-state conditions immediately, and the infusion needs to run 3–5 half-lives before steady-state concentrations are attained.

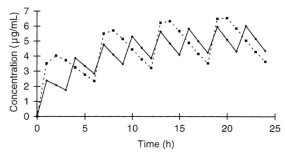

FIG. 8-3 Serum concentration/time profile for rapid-release procainamide (solid line, given every 3 hours) or sustained-release procainamide (dashed line, given every 6 hours) oral dosage forms after multiple doses until steady state is achieved. The curves shown are typical for an adult with normal renal and hepatic function.

and requires discontinuation of the drug. Most symptoms abate within several weeks to months, but some patients have required a year or more to recover completely.

- Intravenous procainamide doses must be given no faster than 25–50 mg/min, as faster injection can cause profound hypotension.
- An active procainamide metabolite, known as *N*-acetylprocainamide (NAPA) or acecainide, also possesses antiarrhythmic effects.[9–11] Based on limited clinical trials of NAPA, effective concentrations are 10–30 µg/ml.
- Concentration-dependent adverse effects for NAPA are similar to those given for procainamide. However, NAPA does not appear to cause a systemic lupus-like syndrome.

  - NAPA is not available commercially in the United States and has been given orphan drug status by the U.S. Food and Drug Administration with an indication for prevention of life-threatening ventricular arrhythmias in patients with documented procainamide-induced lupus.

- Some laboratories report the sum of procainamide and NAPA concentrations for a patient as the "total procainamide concentration," using the therapeutic range 10–30 µg/ml. However, because procainamide and NAPA have different antiarrhythmic potencies, serum concentrations for each agent should be considered individually.
- Many individuals feel that it is more important to maintain therapeutic procainamide concentrations in patients rather than NAPA or total procainamide levels in the suggested ranges.
- For dose-adjustment purposes, procainamide serum concentrations during oral administration are best measured as a predose or trough level at steady state after the patient has received a consistent dosage regimen for 3–5 drug half-lives.
- If the drug is given as a continuous intravenous infusion, procainamide serum concentrations can be measured at steady state after the patient has received a consistent infusion rate for 3–5 drug half-lives.
- Procainamide half-life varies from 2.5–5 hours in normal adults to 14 hours or more in adult patients with renal failure.

- Average NAPA half-lives are 6 hours for normal adults and 41 hours for adult patients with renal failure.
- If procainamide is given orally or intravenously on a stable schedule, steady-state serum concentrations for parent drug and metabolite will be achieved in about 1 day (5 · 5 h = 25 h for procainamide and 5 · 6 h = 30 h for NAPA). For a patient in renal failure, it will take 3 days for steady-state concentrations of procainamide to occur, and 9 days for steady-state conditions to be established for NAPA (5 · 14 h = 70 h or ~3 days for procainamide, 5 · 41 h = 205 h or ~9 days for NAPA).

CLINICAL MONITORING PARAMETERS

- The electrocardiogram (ECG or EKG) should be monitored to determine the response to procainamide. The goal of therapy is suppression of arrhythmias and avoidance of adverse drug reactions.
- Because many therapeutic and side effects of procainamide are not correlated with its serum concentration, it is often not necessary to obtain serum procainamide concentrations in patients receiving appropriate doses who currently have no arrhythmia or adverse drug effects.

  - Procainamide serum concentrations should be obtained in patients who have a recurrence of tachyarrhythmias, are experiencing possible procainamide side effects, or are receiving procainamide doses not consistent with disease states and conditions known to alter procainamide pharmacokinetics (see Effects of Disease States and Conditions on Procainamide Pharmacokinetics and Dosing).
  - Serum concentration monitoring can aid in the decision to increase or decrease the procainamide dose.

    - If an arrhythmia reappears and the procainamide serum concentration is <10 μg/ml, increasing the procainamide dose is a therapeutic option.
    - If the procainamide serum concentration is over 10–12 μg/ml, it is less likely that a dosage increase will be effective in suppressing the arrhythmia and there is an increased likelihood that drug side effects may occur. Some patients have responded to procainamide serum concentrations as high as 20 μg/ml without experiencing severe adverse effects.[12]

  - If a possible concentration-related procainamide adverse drug reaction is noted in a patient and the procainamide serum concentration is <4 μg/ml, it is possible that the observed problem may not be due to procainamide treatment and other sources can be investigated.

- While patients are receiving procainamide, they should be monitored for the following adverse drug effects: anorexia, nausea, vomiting, diarrhea, weakness, malaise, decreased blood pressure, electrocardiogram changes (increased PR interval, QT interval or QRS complex widening >30%), heart block, ventricular conduction disturbances, new ventricular arrhythmias, rash, agranulocytosis, and the systemic lupus-like syndrome.

BASIC CLINICAL PHARMACOKINETIC PARAMETERS

- Procainamide is eliminated by both hepatic metabolism (~50%) and renal elimination of unchanged drug (~50%).[9–11,13,14] Hepatic metabolism is mainly via *N*-acetyltransferase (NAT).[9–11]
- *N*-acetylprocainamide or NAPA is the primary active metabolite resulting from procainamide metabolism by *N*-acetyltransferase.

- *N*-acetyltransferase exhibits a bimodal genetic polymorphism that results in "slow acetylator" and "rapid acetylator" phenotypes. If the patient has normal renal function, acetylator status can be estimated using the ratio of NAPA and procainamide (PA) steady-state concentrations: acetylator ratio = NAPA/PA.[15,16]
  - If the NAPA/procainamide ratio is 1.2 or greater, it is likely the patient is a rapid acetylator. If the ratio is 0.8 or less, it is likely the patient is a slow acetylator.
- Ethnic background can play an important role in the procainamide dose required to achieve a therapeutic effect as well as the potential development of systemic lupus-like adverse effects.
  - The Caucasian and African-American populations appear to be about evenly split between slow and rapid acetylators. Up to 80–90% of the Japanese and Eskimo population are rapid acetylators, while only 20% or less of Egyptians and certain Jewish populations are of that phenotype.
- Metabolism of procainamide to other metabolites may be mediated by CYP2D6.[17]
- The ratio of procainamide renal clearance and creatinine clearance is 2–3, implying that net renal tubular secretion is taking place in the kidneys.[13,14] The renal secretion probably takes place in the proximal tubule.
- Although there have been some reports that procainamide follows nonlinear pharmacokinetics, for the purposes of clinical drug dosing in patients, linear pharmacokinetic concepts and equations can be used effectively to compute doses and estimate serum concentrations.[18,19]
- The average oral bioavailability of procainamide for both immediate-release and sustained-release dosage forms is 83%.[4–8] A lag time of 20–30 minutes occurs in some patients between oral dosage administration and the time procainamide first appears in the serum.
- Plasma protein binding of procainamide in normal individuals is only about 15%.

EFFECTS OF DISEASE STATES AND CONDITIONS ON PROCAINAMIDE PHARMACOKINETICS AND DOSING

Procainamide

- Normal adults without the disease states and conditions given later in this section and with normal liver and renal function have an average procainamide half-life of 3.3 hours (range 2.5–4.6 hours) and a volume of distribution for the entire body of 2.7 L/kg (V = 2–3.8 L/kg; Table 8-1).[20–22]
- *N*-acetyltransferase is the enzyme responsible for conversion of procainamide to *N*-acetylprocainamide (NAPA). The genetic polymorphism of *N*-acetyltransferase produces a bimodal frequency distribution for procainamide half-life and clearance that separates the population into rapid and slow acetylators (Figure 8-4).
  - The mean procainamide half-life for rapid acetylators is 2.7 hours, while for slow acetylators it is 5.2 hours.
  - Not all studies conducted with procainamide have separated results from rapid and slow acetylators when analyzing the pharmacokinetic data.

TABLE 8-1 Disease States and Conditions That Alter Procainamide Pharmacokinetics

Disease state/condition	Half-life (h)	Volume of distribution (L/kg)	Comments
Adult, normal renal and liver function	3.3 (range 2.6–4.6)	2.7 (range 2–3.8)	Procainamide is eliminated about 50% unchanged in the urine and about 50% metabolized. N-acetyltransferase converts procainamide to an active metabolite (N-acetylprocainamide or NAPA). Genetically, some individuals are "rapid acetylators" and convert more procainamide to NAPA than "slow acetylators." NAPA is 85% eliminated unchanged by the kidney.
Adult, renal failure (creatinine clearance ≤10 ml/min)	13.9	1.7	Because 50% of procainamide and 85% of NAPA are eliminated unchanged by the kidney, the clearance of both agents is reduced in renal failure.
Adult, liver cirrhosis	Not available	Not available	Procainamide is metabolized ~50% by hepatic enzymes (primarily N-acetyltransferase). Clearance of procainamide is decreased in liver cirrhosis patients, but NAPA clearance does not change substantially. Pharmacokinetic parameters are highly variable in liver disease patients.
Adult, uncompensated heart failure	5.5	1.6	Decreased liver blood flow secondary to reduced cardiac output reduces procainamide clearance. Heart failure results in variable reductions in procainamide clearance.
Adult, obese (>30% over ideal body weight)	According to other disease states/ conditions that affect procainamide pharmacokinetics	According to other disease states/ conditions that affect procainamide pharmacokinetics	Procainamide volume of distribution should be based on ideal body weight for patients who weigh more that 30% over IBW, but clearance should be based on total body weight or TBW (0.52 L/h/kg TBW for patients with normal renal function).

202

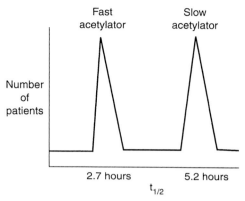

FIG. 8-4   *N*-acetyltransferase converts procainamide to its active metabolite, *N*-acetylprocainamide or NAPA. Patients can be phenotyped into two groups with regard to their ability to metabolize procainamide to NAPA via acetylation of the parent drug: Fast acetylators convert procainamide to NAPA rapidly and have a shorter procainamide half-life, whereas slow acetylators convert procainamide to NAPA more slowly and have a longer procainamide half-life. This leads to a bimodal distribution of procainamide half-life for adults with normal renal function.

- It is not practical to phenotype or genotype a patient as a slow or rapid metabolizer before administration of the drug, so an average population half-life and clearance is used for the purpose of initial dosage computation.
- Disease states and conditions that change procainamide pharmacokinetics and dosage requirements may alter clearance and the volume of distribution. The elimination rate constant ($k = 0.693/t_{1/2}$, where $t_{1/2}$ is the half-life) and clearance ($Cl = kV$) can be computed from the aforementioned pharmacokinetic parameters.

Renal Dysfunction

- Because about 50% of a procainamide dose is eliminated unchanged by the kidney, renal dysfunction is the most important disease state that affects procainamide pharmacokinetics.[23–25] Since the major route of renal clearance for procainamide is via proximal tubular secretion, creatinine clearance is not as reliable a parameter to aid in the estimation of procainamide clearance.

  - In patients with renal failure, the average procainamide half-life is 13.9 hours and the volume of distribution is 1.7 L/kg.

Heart Failure

- Uncompensated heart failure reduces procainamide clearance because of decreased hepatic blood flow secondary to compromised cardiac output (Table 8-2).[22,23] Volume of distribution (V = 1.6 L/kg) is decreased in uncompensated heart failure patients as well.

TABLE 8-2 New York Heart Association (NYHA) Functional Classification for Heart Failure[39]

NYHA heart failure class	Description
I	Patients with cardiac disease but without limitations of physical activity. Ordinary physical activity does not cause undue fatigue, dyspnea, or palpitation.
II	Patients with cardiac disease that results in slight limitations of physical activity. Ordinary physical activity results in fatigue, palpitation, dyspnea, or angina.
III	Patients with cardiac disease that results in marked limitations of physical activity. Although patients are comfortable at rest, less than ordinary activity will lead to symptoms.
IV	Patients with cardiac disease that results in an inability to carry on physical activity without discomfort. Symptoms of congestive heart failure are present even at rest. With any physical activity, increased discomfort is experienced.

- Because clearance and volume of distribution decrease simultaneously, the increase in half-life is not as dramatic as might be expected, and patients with uncompensated heart failure have an average procainamide half-life of 5.5 hours [$t_{1/2} = (0.693 \cdot \downarrow V)/\downarrow Cl$].
- The effect of uncompensated heart failure on procainamide pharmacokinetics is highly variable and difficult to predict accurately. It is possible for a patient with uncompensated heart failure to have relatively normal or grossly abnormal procainamide clearance and half-life.
- For uncompensated heart failure patients, initial doses are meant as starting points for dosage titration based on patient response and avoidance of adverse effects. Most clinicians reduce initial procainamide doses by 25–50% for patients with uncompensated heart failure (Table 8-3).
- Patients with compensated heart failure receiving appropriate treatment with good clinical response may have normal procainamide pharmacokinetics.[26]
- Procainamide serum concentrations and the presence of adverse drug effects should be monitored frequently in patients with heart failure.

Hepatic Dysfunction

- Patients with liver cirrhosis or hepatitis have not been adequately studied with regard to procainamide pharmacokinetics. However, the majority of *N*-acetyltransferase responsible for the conversion of procainamide to NAPA is thought to reside in the liver. Therefore, most clinicians recommend a decrease in initial doses for procainamide in patients with liver disease.[27]
- An index of liver dysfunction can be gained by applying the Child-Pugh clinical classification system to the patient (Table 8-4).[28] Child-Pugh scores are discussed more fully in Chapter 3 (Drug Dosing in Special Populations: Renal and Hepatic Disease, Dialysis, Heart Failure, Obesity, and Drug Interactions).

  - The Child-Pugh score consists of five laboratory tests or clinical symptoms: serum albumin, total bilirubin, prothrombin time, ascites, and

TABLE 8-3 Literature-Based Recommended Oral Procainamide Initial Dosage Ranges for Various Disease States and Conditions

Disease state/condition	Procainamide, oral tablets	Procainamide, continuous intravenous infusion
Adult, normal renal function (creatinine clearance >50 ml/min)	50 mg/kg/d	2–6 mg/min
Adult, renal dysfunction	Creatinine clearance = 10–50 ml/min: 25–50% dosage decrease Creatinine clearance <10 ml/min: 50–75% dosage decrease	Creatinine clearance = 10–50 ml/min: 25–50% dosage decrease Creatinine clearance <10 ml/min: 50–75% dosage decrease
Adult, uncompensated heart failure	NYHA CHF class II: 25% dosage decrease NYHA CHF class III or IV: 50% dosage decrease	NYHA CHF class II: 25% dosage decrease NYHA CHF class III or IV: 50% dosage decrease
Adult, liver disease	Child/Pugh score = 8–10: 25% dosage decrease Child-Pugh score >10: 50% dosage decrease	Child/Pugh score = 8–10: 25% dosage decrease Child-Pugh score >10: 50% dosage decrease
Adult, obese (>30% over ideal body weight)	Base dose on total body weight according to other disease states/conditions	Base dose on total body weight according to other disease states/conditions

hepatic encephalopathy. Each of these areas is given a score of 1 (normal) to 3 (severely abnormal; Table 8-4), and the scores for the five areas are summed. The Child-Pugh score for a patient with normal liver function is 5, while the score for a patient with grossly abnormal serum albumin, total bilirubin, and prothrombin time values in addition to severe ascites and hepatic encephalopathy is 15.

- A Child-Pugh score of 8 to 10 is grounds for a decrease of 25% in the initial daily drug dose for procainamide, while a score greater than 10 suggests a decrease of 50% (Table 8-3).

- As in any patient with or without liver dysfunction, initial doses are meant as starting points for dosage titration based on patient response and avoidance

TABLE 8-4 Child-Pugh Scores for Patients with Liver Disease[28]

Test/symptom	Score 1 point	Score 2 points	Score 3 points
Total bilirubin (mg/dl)	<2.0	2.0–3.0	>3.0
Serum albumin (g/dl)	>3.5	2.8–3.5	<2.8
Prothrombin time (seconds prolonged over control)	<4	4–6	>6
Ascites	Absent	Slight	Moderate
Hepatic Encephalopathy	None	Moderate	Severe

of adverse effects. Procainamide serum concentrations and the presence of adverse drug effects should be monitored frequently in patients with liver cirrhosis or hepatitis.

Obesity

• Studies investigating the impact of obesity (30% over ideal body weight) on procainamide pharmacokinetics have found that volume of distribution correlates best with ideal body weight, but clearance correlates best with total body weight.[29]

   • The volume of distribution for procainamide should be based on ideal body weight for obese individuals according to the other disease states and conditions present in the patient. Clearance should be based on total body weight (TBW) in obese individuals (0.52 L/h/kg TBW for normal renal failure).

Pediatrics

• Pediatric doses are similar to those given to adults when adjusted for differences in body weight.[30]

   • Intravenous loading doses can be administered in two different ways: (1) 15 mg/kg infused over 30–60 minutes or (2) 2–6 mg/kg over 5 minutes (maximum dose 100 mg), repeating as necessary every 5–10 minutes to a maximum dose of 15 mg/kg (no more than 500 mg should be given within a 30-minute time period).

   • Intravenous maintenance infusion rates equal 20–80 µg/kg/min (maximum dose 2 g/d).

   • Oral maintenance doses are 15–50 mg/kg/d. The dosage interval chosen should be appropriate for the dosage form administered.

Dialysis and Hemoperfusion

• Procainamide is significantly removed by hemodialysis but not by peritoneal dialysis.[31] Patients undergoing hemodialysis treatments may receive an additional dose of the usual amount taken after the procedure is finished.

   • Because procainamide has a sieving coefficient of 0.86, continuous hemoperfusion removes significant amounts of the drug.[32,33] Appropriate dosage increases should be determined using serum concentration measurements of both procainamide and NAPA.

N-Acetyl Procainamide

• NAPA is eliminated primarily unchanged in the urine via glomerular filtration and renal tubular secretion.[13,14,20,25,34] When NAPA is given orally, 85% of the administered dose is recovered in the urine as unchanged drug.

   • In patients with normal renal and liver function, NAPA has an average half-life of 6 hours and an an average volume of distribution of 1.4 L/kg.[10]

Renal Dysfunction

• NAPA half-life increases to 41 hours on average in patients with renal failure.[25,34]

   • In most patients with renal dysfunction, the ratio of NAPA to procainamide steady-state concentration exceeds 1, even if the patient is a slow acetylator.

The reason for this is that NAPA elimination is much more dependent on renal function, so NAPA concentrations accumulate more than procainamide concentrations do in patients with renal dysfunction. Thus, in patients with renal failure NAPA may be the predominate antiarrhythmic agent present in the serum.

Dialysis and Hemoperfusion

- NAPA is significantly removed by hemodialysis but not by peritoneal dialysis.[34] Because NAPA has a sieving coefficient of 0.92, continuous hemoperfusion removes significant amounts of the metabolite.[32,33]

DRUG INTERACTIONS

- Procainamide has serious drug interactions with other drugs that are capable of inhibiting its renal tubular secretion.[35,36]

  - Cimetidine, trimethoprim, ofloxacin, and levofloxacin are all drugs that compete for tubular secretion with procainamide and NAPA. When given with these other agents, procainamide renal clearance decreases by 30–50% and NAPA renal clearance decreases by 10–30%.

- Amiodarone increases the steady-state concentrations of procainamide and NAPA by 57% and 32%, respectively.

INITIAL DOSAGE DETERMINATION METHODS

- Several methods to initiate procainamide therapy are available:

  - The *pharmacokinetic dosing method* is the most flexible of the techniques. It allows individualized target serum concentrations to be chosen for a patient, and each pharmacokinetic parameter can be customized to reflect specific disease states and conditions present in the patient.
  - *Literature-based recommended dosing* is a very commonly used method for prescribing initial doses of procainamide. Doses are based on those that commonly produce steady-state concentrations near the lower end of the therapeutic range, although there is a wide variation in the actual concentrations for a specific patient.

Pharmacokinetic Dosing Method

- The goal of initial dosing of procainamide is to compute the best dose possible for the patient given the set of disease states and conditions that influence procainamide pharmacokinetics and the arrhythmia being treated. In order to do this, pharmacokinetic parameters for the patient are estimated using average parameters measured in other patients with similar disease state and condition profiles.

Half-Life and Elimination Rate Constant Estimate

- Depending on the acetylator status of the patient, procainamide is almost equally metabolized by the liver and eliminated unchanged by the kidney in patients with normal hepatic and renal function.

  - There is no good way to estimate the elimination characteristics of liver-metabolized drugs using an endogenous marker of liver function in the same manner that serum creatinine and estimated creatinine clearance are used to estimate the elimination of agents that are renally eliminated by glomerular filtration.

- To produce the most conservative procainamide doses in patients with multiple concurrent disease states or conditions that affect procainamide pharmacokinetics, the disease state or condition with the longest half-life should be used to compute doses. This approach will avoid accidental overdosage as much as is currently possible.
- Creatinine clearance does not accurately reflect the renal elimination of procainamide because the mechanism of elimination includes active tubular secretion.

  - A patient is categorized according to the disease states and conditions that are known to change procainamide half-life, and the half-life previously measured in these studies is used as an estimate of the current patient's half-life (Table 8-1). Once the correct half-life is identified for the patient, it can be converted into the procainamide elimination rate constant (k) using the following equation:

$$k = 0.693/t_{1/2}$$

Volume of Distribution Estimate

- Procainamide volume of distribution is chosen according to the disease states and conditions that are present (Table 8-1). For obese patients (>30% above ideal body weight), ideal body weight is used to compute procainamide volume of distribution.

Selection of Appropriate Pharmacokinetic Model and Equations

- When procainamide is given orally, it follows a one-compartment pharmacokinetic model (Figure 8-3).
- Because procainamide has such a short half-life, most patients receive oral procainamide therapy using sustained-release dosage forms. In the United States, two different sustained-release dosage forms have been approved that provide every-6-hour or every-12-hour dosing.

  - Procainamide sustained-release dosage forms provide good bioavailability (F = 0.83), supply a continuous release of procainamide into the gastrointestinal tract, and provide a smooth procainamide serum concentration/time curve that emulates an intravenous infusion when doses are given 2–4 times daily.
  - A very simple pharmacokinetic equation that computes the average procainamide steady-state serum concentration (Css in µg/ml = mg/L) is widely used and allows maintenance dosage calculation:

$$Css = \frac{F(D/\tau)}{Cl} \quad \text{or} \quad D = \frac{Css \cdot Cl \cdot \tau}{F}$$

where F is the bioavailability fraction for the oral dosage form (F = 0.83 for most oral procainamide sustained-release products), D is the dose of procainamide in mg, and τ is the dosage interval in hours.
  - Cl is procainamide clearance in L/h and is computed using estimates of procainamide elimination rate constant (k) and volume of distribution: Cl = kV.

- When intravenous therapy is required, the pharmacokinetic equation that computes the procainamide steady-state serum concentration (Css in µg/ml = mg/L) is widely used and allows dosage calculation for a continuous infusion:

$$Css = k_0/Cl \quad \text{or} \quad k_0 = Css \cdot Cl$$

where k_0 is the dose of procainamide in mg/min, Cl is procainamide clearance in L/min and is computed using estimates of procainamide elimination rate constant (k) and volume of distribution: Cl = kV.

- The equation used to calculate an intravenous loading dose (LD in mg) is based on a simple one-compartment model:

$$LD = Css \cdot V$$

where Css is the desired procainamide steady-state concentration in µg/ml (which is equivalent to mg/L), and V is the procainamide volume of distribution.

- Intravenous procainamide loading doses should be infusions no faster than 25–50 mg/min, to avoid severe hypotension.
- Two methods are used to administer procainamide loading doses to adults: (1) Administer 100 mg every 5 minutes to a maximum of 500 mg; a 10-minute waiting period to allow drug distribution to tissues is utilized if more than 500 mg is needed to abate the arrhythmia. (2) Administer the loading dose as a short-term infusion at a rate of 20 mg/min over 25–30 minutes, not to exceed a total dose of 500–600 mg.

Steady-State Concentration Selection

- The generally accepted therapeutic range for procainamide is 4–10 µg/ml. If procainamide + NAPA or "total procainamide" concentrations are used, the usual therapeutic range is 10–30 µg/ml, keeping in mind that procainamide and NAPA are not equipotent antiarrhythmics. However, procainamide therapy must be individualized for each patient in order to achieve optimal responses and minimal side effects.

▶ ***Example 1***   LK is a 50-year-old, 75-kg (height 5′10″) male with ventricular tachycardia who requires therapy with oral procainamide sustained-release tablets. He has normal liver and cardiac function. Suggest an initial oral procainamide dosage regimen designed to achieve a steady-state procainamide concentration of 4 µg/ml.

1. *Estimate half-life and elimination rate constant according to disease states and conditions present in the patient.* The expected procainamide half-life ($t_{1/2}$) for an individual with normal hepatic and renal function is 3.3 hours. The elimination rate constant is computed using the following formula:

$$k = 0.693/t_{1/2} = 0.693/3.3 \text{ h} = 0.210 \text{ h}^{-1}$$

2. *Estimate volume of distribution and clearance.* The patient is not obese, so the estimated procainamide volume of distribution is based on actual body weight:

$$V = 2.7 \text{ L/kg} \cdot 75 \text{ kg} = 203 \text{ L}$$

Estimated procainamide clearance is computed by taking the product of the volume of distribution and the elimination rate constant:

$$Cl = kV = 0.210 \text{ h}^{-1} \cdot 203 \text{ L} = 42.6 \text{ L/h}$$

3. *Compute dosage regimen.* Oral sustained-release procainamide tablets will be prescribed for this patient (F = 0.83). Because the patient has a rapid procainamide clearance and short half-life, the initial dosage interval (τ) will be set to 6 hours. (*Note:* µg/ml = mg/L, and this concentration unit was substituted for Css in the calculations

so that unit conversion was not required.) The dosage equation for oral procainamide is

$$D = \frac{Css \cdot Cl \cdot \tau}{F} = \frac{4 \text{ mg/L} \cdot 42.6 \text{ L/h} \cdot 6 \text{ h}}{0.83} = 1231 \text{ mg}$$

rounded to 1250 mg every 6 hours.

Steady-state procainamide and NAPA serum concentrations can be measured after steady-state is attained in 3–5 half-lives. Since the patient is expected to have a half-life of 3.3 hours for procainamide and 6 hours for NAPA, the steady-state concentrations can be obtained at any time after the first day of dosing (5 half-lives = $5 \cdot 3.3$ h = 16.5 h for procainamide, 5 half-lives = $5 \cdot 6$ h = 30 h for NAPA). Procainamide and NAPA serum concentrations should also be measured if the patient experiences a return of arrhythmia, or if the patient develops potential signs or symptoms of procainamide toxicity.

▶ **Example 2**   OI is a 60-year-old, 85-kg (height 6'1'') male with atrial fibrillation who requires therapy with intravenous procainamide. He has renal failure, with an estimated creatinine clearance of 9 ml/min. Suggest an initial intravenous procainamide dosage regimen designed to achieve a steady-state procainamide concentration of 4 μg/ml.

1. *Estimate half-life and elimination rate constant according to disease states and conditions present in the patient.* Patients with severe renal disease have highly variable procainamide pharmacokinetics and dosage requirements. Renal failure decreases procainamide renal clearance, and the expected procainamide half-life ($t_{1/2}$) is 13.9 hours. The elimination rate constant is computed using the following formula:

$$k = 0.693/t_{1/2} = 0.693/13.9 \text{ h} = 0.050 \text{ h}^{-1}$$

2. *Estimate volume of distribution and clearance.* The patient is not obese, so the estimated procainamide volume of distribution is based on actual body weight:

$$V = 1.7 \text{ L/kg} \cdot 85 \text{ kg} = 145 \text{ L}$$

Estimated procainamide clearance is computed by taking the product of the volume of distribution and the elimination rate constant:

$$Cl = kV = 0.050 \text{ h}^{-1} \cdot 145 \text{ L} = 7.25 \text{ L/h}$$

3. *Compute dosage regimen.* Therapy will be started by administering an intravenous loading dose of procainamide to the patient:

$$LD = Css \cdot V = 4 \text{ mg/L} \cdot 145 \text{ L} = 580 \text{ mg}$$

rounded to 600 mg intravenously over 25–30 minutes. (*Note:* μg/ml = mg/L, and this concentration unit was substituted for Css in the calculations so that unit conversion was not required.)

A continuous intravenous infusion of procainamide will be started immediately after the loading dose has been administered. (*Note:* μg/ml = mg/L, and this concentration unit was substituted for Css in the calculations so that unit conversion was not required.) The dosage equation for intravenous procainamide is:

$$k_0 = Css \cdot Cl = (4 \text{ mg/L} \cdot 7.25 \text{ L/h})/(60 \text{ min/h})$$
$$= 0.48 \text{ mg/min, rounded to 0.5 mg/min}$$

Steady-state procainamide and NAPA serum concentrations can be measured after steady-state is attained in 3–5 half-lives. Since the patient is expected to have a half-life of 13.9 hours for procainamide and 41 hours for NAPA, the steady-state concentrations can be obtained any time after 3–9 days of dosing (5 half-lives = 5 · 13.9 h = 69.5 h for procainamide, 5 half-lives = 5 · 41 h = 205 h for NAPA). Procainamide and NAPA serum concentrations should also be measured if the patient experiences a return of arrhythmia, or if the patient develops potential signs or symptoms of procainamide toxicity.

Literature-Based Recommended Dosing

- Because of the extensive variability in procainamide pharmacokinetics, even when concurrent disease states and conditions are identified, many clinicians believe that the use of standard procainamide doses for various situations are warranted. The original computations of these doses were based on the pharmacokinetic dosing method described in the previous section, and the doses were subsequently modified based on clinical experience.
- In general, the procainamide steady-state serum concentration expected from the lower end of the dosage range is 4–6 µg/ml and 6–10 µg/ml for the upper end of the dosage range. Suggested procainamide maintenance doses are given in Table 8-3.
- When a patient has more than one disease state or condition, choosing the lowest daily dose will result in the safest, most conservative dosage recommendation.
- Pediatric doses are similar to those given to adults when adjusted for differences in body weight.[30]

    - Intravenous loading doses can be administered in two different ways: (1) 15 mg/kg infused over 30–60 minutes or (2) 2–6 mg/kg infused over 5 minutes (maximum dose 100 mg), repeating as necessary every 5–10 minutes to a maximum dose of 15 mg/kg (no more than 500 mg should be given within a 30-minute time period).
    - Intravenous maintenance infusion rates equal 20–80 µg/kg/min (maximum dose 2 g/d).
    - Oral maintenance doses are 15–50 mg/kg/d. The dosage interval chosen should be appropriate for the dosage form administered.

- To illustrate the similarities and differences between this method of dosage calculation and the pharmacokinetic dosing method, the same examples used in the previous section will be used.

▶ **Example 1**   LK is a 50-year-old, 75-kg (height 5′10″) male with ventricular tachycardia who requires therapy with oral procainamide sustained-release tablets. He has normal liver and cardiac function. Suggest an initial oral procainamide dosage regimen designed to achieve a steady-state procainamide concentration of 4 µg/ml.

1. *Choose procainamide dose based on disease states and conditions present in the patient.* A procainamide maintenance dose of 50 mg/kg/d is suggested for a patient without heart failure or liver disease who requires a procainamide steady-state serum concentration near the lower end of the therapeutic range. The suggested initial dose is 3750 mg/d (50 mg/kg/d · 75 kg = 3750 mg/d), rounded to 4000 mg/d or 1000 mg every 6 hours.

    Steady-state procainamide and NAPA serum concentrations can be measured after steady state is attained in 3–5 half- lives. Since the patient is expected to have a half-life equal to 3.3 hours for procainamide and 6 hours for NAPA, the steady-state concentrations can be obtained at any time after the first day of dosing (5 half-lives = $5 \cdot 3.3$ h = 16.5 h for procainamide, 5 half-lives = $5 \cdot 6$ h = 30 h for NAPA). Procainamide and NAPA serum concentrations should also be measured if the patient experiences a return of arrhythmia, or if the patient develops potential signs or symptoms of procainamide toxicity.

▶ *Example 2*   OI is a 60-year-old, 85-kg (height 6′1″) male with atrial fibrillation who requires therapy with intravenous procainamide. He has renal failure, with an estimated creatinine clearance = 9 ml/min. Suggest an initial intravenous procainamide dosage regimen designed to achieve a steady-state procainamide concentration of 4 μg/ml.

1. *Choose procainamide dose based on disease states and conditions present in the patient.* A procainamide maintenance dose of 1–2 mg/min is suggested for a patient with renal failure who requires a procainamide steady-state serum concentration near the lower end of the therapeutic range. The suggested initial dose is 1 mg/min. If needed, a loading dose of 500 mg infused over 25–30 minutes can also be given.

   Steady-state procainamide and NAPA serum concentrations can be measured after steady-state is attained in 3–5 half-lives. Since the patient is expected to have a half-life of 13.9 hours for procainamide and 41 hours for NAPA, the steady-state concentrations can be obtained at any time after 3–9 days of dosing (5 half-lives = $5 \cdot 13.9$ h = 69.5 h for procainamide, 5 half-lives = $5 \cdot 41$ h = 205 h for NAPA). Procainamide and NAPA serum concentrations should also be measured if the patient experiences a return of arrhythmia, or if the patient develops potential signs or symptoms of procainamide toxicity.

USE OF PROCAINAMIDE AND *N*-ACETYLPROCAINAMIDE SERUM CONCENTRATIONS TO ALTER DOSES

- Because of the extensive pharmacokinetic variability among patients, it is likely that doses computed using patient population characteristics will not always produce procainamide or NAPA serum concentrations that are expected or desirable. Because of this pharmacokinetic variability, the narrow therapeutic index of procainamide, and the desire to avoid adverse side effects of procainamide, measurement of procainamide and NAPA serum concentrations can be a useful adjunct for patients to ensure that therapeutic, nontoxic levels are present.

  - Other important patient parameters (electrocardiogram, clinical signs and symptoms of the arrhythmia, potential procainamide side effects, etc.) should be followed to confirm that the patient is responding to treatment and not developing adverse drug reactions.

- When procainamide and NAPA serum concentrations are measured in patients and a dosage change is necessary, clinicians should use the simplest, most straightforward method available to determine a dose that will provide safe and effective treatment.

  - In most cases, a simple dosage ratio can be used to change procainamide doses, assuming the drug follows *linear pharmacokinetics*. Thus, assuming linear pharmacokinetics is adequate for dosage adjustments in most patients.

- Sometimes it is useful to compute procainamide pharmacokinetic constants for a patient and base dosage adjustments on these parameters. In this case it may be possible to calculate and use *pharmacokinetic parameters* to alter the procainamide dose.
- In some situations it may be necessary to compute procainamide pharmacokinetic parameters as soon as possible for the patient, before steady-state conditions occur, and then utilize these parameters to calculate the best drug dose.
  - The *Chiou method* allows clearance to be determined during a continuous intravenous infusion before steady state is achieved.
  - Computerized methods that incorporate expected population pharmacokinetic characteristics (*Bayesian pharmacokinetic computer programs*) can be used in difficult cases when serum concentrations are obtained at suboptimal times or the patient was not at steady state when serum concentrations were measured.
    - An additional benefit is that a complete pharmacokinetic workup (determination of clearance, volume of distribution, and half-life) can be done with one or more measured concentrations that do not have to be at steady state.

Linear Pharmacokinetics Method

- Because procainamide follows linear, dose-proportional pharmacokinetics in most patients, steady-state procainamide and NAPA serum concentrations change in proportion to dose according to the following equation:

$$D_{new}/Css_{new} = D_{old}/Css_{old} \qquad or \qquad D_{new} = (Css_{new}/Css_{old})D_{old}$$

where D is the dose, Css is the steady-state concentration, old indicates the dose that produced the steady-state concentration the patient currently has, and new denotes the dose necessary to produce the desired steady-state concentration.
- The advantages of this method are that it is quick and simple. The disadvantages are that steady-state concentrations are required.
- Because nonlinear pharmacokinetics for procainamide have been observed in some patients, suggested dosage increases greater than 75% using this method should be scrutinized by the prescribing clinician, and the risk versus benefit for the patient assessed before initiating large dosage increases (>75% over current dose).

▶ *Example 1*   LK is a 50-year-old, 75-kg (height 5′10″) male with ventricular tachycardia who requires therapy with procainamide sustained-release tablets. He has normal liver and cardiac function. The current steady-state procainamide and NAPA concentrations are 2.2 µg/ml and 1.5 µg/ml, respectively (total procainamide concentration = 3.7 µg/ml) at a dose of 1000 mg every 12 hours. Compute a procainamide dose that will provide a steady-state concentration of 4 µg/ml.

1. *Compute new dose to achieve desired serum concentration.* The patient can be expected to achieve steady-state conditions after the first day ($5t_{1/2} = 5 \cdot 3.3$ h = 17 h for procainamide, $5t_{1/2} = 5 \cdot 6$ h = 30 h for NAPA) of therapy.

    Using linear pharmacokinetics, the new dose to attain the desired concentration should be proportional to the old dose that produced the measured concentration (*Note:* Total daily dose = 1000 mg/dose · 2 dose/day = 2000 mg/d):

$$D_{new} = (Css_{new}/Css_{old})D_{old} = (4 \ \mu g/ml/2.2 \ \mu g/ml)(2000 \ mg/d)$$
$$= 3636 \ mg/d$$

rounded to 4000 mg/d or 2000 mg every 12 hours. The new suggested dose is 2000 mg every 12 hours of oral procainamide, to be started immediately.

The NAPA steady-state serum concentration should increase in proportion to the procainamide dosage increase:

$$Css_{new} = (D_{new}/D_{old}) \ Css_{old} = (4000 \ mg/d/2000 \ mg/d)(1.5 \ \mu g/ml)$$
$$= 3 \ \mu g/ml$$

Steady-state procainamide serum concentration can be measured after steady state is attained in 3–5 half-lives. Since the patient is expected to have a procainamide half-life of 3.3 hours and NAPA half-life of 6 hours, procainamide and NAPA steady-state concentrations can be obtained at any time after the first day of dosing (5 half-lives = 5 · 3.3 h = 17 h for procainamide, 5 half-lives = 5 · 6 h = 30 h for NAPA). Procainamide and NAPA serum concentrations should also be measured if the patient experiences a return of arrhythmia, or if the patient develops potential signs or symptoms of procainamide toxicity.

▶ *Example 2*   MN is a 64-year-old, 78-kg (height 5'9″) male with ventricular tachycardia who requires therapy with intravenous procainamide. He has moderate heart failure (NYHA CHF class III). The current steady-state procainamide and NAPA concentrations are 4.5 µg/ml and 7.9 µg/ml, respectively (total procainamide concentration = 12.4 µg/ml) at a dose of 1 mg/min. Compute a procainamide dose that will provide a steady-state concentration of 8 µg/ml.

1. *Compute new dose to achieve desired serum concentration.* The patient can be expected to achieve steady-state conditions after the second day ($5t_{1/2} = 5 \cdot 5.5 \ h = 28 \ h$ for procainamide, $5t_{1/2} = 5 \cdot 6 \ h = 30 \ h$, for NAPA assuming normal renal function) of therapy. Using linear pharmacokinetics, the new dose to attain the desired concentration should be proportional to the old dose that produced the measured concentration:

$$D_{new} = (Css_{new}/Css_{old})D_{old} = (8 \ \mu g/ml/4.5 \ \mu g/ml)(1 \ mg/min)$$
$$= 1.8 \ mg/min, \ rounded \ to \ 2 \ mg/min$$

The new suggested dose is 2 mg/min of intravenous procainamide, to be started immediately.

The NAPA steady-state serum concentration should increase in proportion to the procainamide dosage increase:

$$Css_{new} = (D_{new}/D_{old})Css_{old} = (2 \ mg/min/1 \ mg/min)(7.9 \ \mu g/ml)$$
$$= 15.8 \ \mu g/ml$$

Steady-state procainamide serum concentration can be measured after steady state is attained in 3–5 half-lives. Since the patient is expected to have a procainamide half-life of 5.5 hours and NAPA half-life of 6 hours, procainamide and NAPA steady-state concentrations can be obtained at any time after the second day of dosing (5 half-lives = 5 · 5.5 h = 28 h for procainamide, 5 half-lives = 5 · 6 h = 30 h for NAPA). Procainamide and NAPA serum concentrations should also be measured if the patient experiences a return of arrhythmia, or if the patient develops potential signs or symptoms of procainamide toxicity.

Pharmacokinetic Parameter Method

- The pharmacokinetic parameter method of adjusting drug doses allows the computation of an individual's own, unique pharmacokinetic constants and uses those to calculate a dose that achieves desired procainamide concentrations.

  - During a continuous intravenous infusion, the following equation is used to compute procainamide clearance (Cl):

  $$Cl = k_0/Css$$

  where k_0 is the dose of procainamide in mg/min.
  - For oral procainamide therapy, procainamide clearance (Cl) can be calculated using the following formula:

  $$Cl = \frac{F(D/\tau)}{Css}$$

  where F is the bioavailability fraction for the oral dosage form (F = 0.83 for most oral procainamide products), D is the dose of procainamide in mg, Css is the steady-state procainamide concentration, and τ is the dosage interval in hours.

- For both oral and intravenous procainamide routes of administration, the expected NAPA steady-state serum concentration will increase in proportion to the procainamide dosage increase:

$$Css_{new} = (D_{new}/D_{old})Css_{old}$$

where D is the dose, Css is the steady-state concentration, old indicates the dose that produced the steady-state concentration the patient is currently receiving, and new denotes the dose necessary to produce the desired steady-state concentration.

- Because this method also assumes linear pharmacokinetics, procainamide doses computed using the pharmacokinetic parameter method and the linear pharmacokinetic method should be identical.

▶ *Example 1*   LK is a 50-year-old, 75-kg (height 5′10″) male with ventricular tachycardia who requires therapy with procainamide sustained-release tablets. He has normal liver and cardiac function. The current steady-state procainamide and NAPA concentrations are 2.2 μg/ml and 1.5 μg/ml, respectively (total procainamide concentration = 3.7 μg/ml), at a dose of 1000 mg every 12 hours. Compute a procainamide dose that will provide a steady-state concentration of 4 μg/ml.

1. *Compute pharmacokinetic parameters.* The patient can be expected to achieve steady-state conditions after the first day ($5t_{1/2} = 5 \cdot 3.3$ h = 17 h for procainamide, $5t_{1/2} = 5 \cdot 6$ h = 30 h for NAPA) of therapy. Procainamide clearance can be computed using a steady-state procainamide concentration:

$$Cl = \frac{F(D/\tau)}{Css} = \frac{[0.83(1000 \text{ mg}/12 \text{ h})]}{2.2 \text{ mg/L}} = 31.4 \text{ L/h}$$

(*Note:* μg/ml = mg/L, and this concentration unit was substituted for Css in the calculations so that unit conversion was not required.)

2. *Compute procainamide dose.* Procainamide clearance is used to compute the new dose:

$$D = \frac{Css \cdot Cl \cdot \tau}{F} = \frac{4 \text{ mg/L} \cdot 31.4 \text{ L/h} \cdot 12 \text{ h}}{0.83} = 1816 \text{ mg}$$

which is rounded to 2000 mg every 12 hours.

The expected NAPA steady-state serum concentration will increase in proportion to the procainamide dosage increase:

$$Css_{new} = (D_{new}/D_{old})Css_{old} = [(4000 \text{ mg/d})/(2000 \text{ mg/d})](1.5 \text{ μg/ml})$$
$$= 3 \text{ μg/ml}$$

The new procainamide dose should be instituted immediately.

Steady-state procainamide serum concentration can be measured after steady state is attained in 3–5 half-lives. Since the patient is expected to have a procainamide half-life of 3.3 hours and NAPA half-life of 6 hours, procainamide and NAPA steady-state concentrations can be obtained at any time after the first day of dosing (5 half-lives = 5 · 3.3 h = 17 h for procainamide, 5 half-lives = 5 · 6 h = 30 h for NAPA). Procainamide and NAPA serum concentrations should also be measured if the patient experiences a return of arrhythmia, or if the patient develops potential signs or symptoms of procainamide toxicity.

▶ *Example 2* MN is a 64-year-old, 78-kg (height 5′9″) male with ventricular tachycardia who requires therapy with intravenous procainamide. He has moderate heart failure (NYHA CHF class III). The current steady-state procainamide and NAPA concentrations are 4.5 μg/ml and 7.9 μg/ml, respectively (total procainamide concentration = 12.4 μg/ml), at a dose of 1 mg/min. Compute a procainamide dose that will provide a steady-state concentration of 8 μg/ml.

1. *Compute pharmacokinetic parameters.* The patient can be expected to achieve steady-state conditions after the second day (5$t_{1/2}$ = 5 · 5.5 h = 28 h for procainamide, 5$t_{1/2}$ = 5 · 6 h = 30 h for NAPA, assuming normal renal function) of therapy. Procainamide clearance can be computed using a steady-state procainamide concentration:

$$Cl = k_0/Css = (1 \text{ mg/min})/(4.5 \text{ mg/L}) = 0.22 \text{ L/min}$$

(*Note:* μg/ml = mg/L, and this concentration unit was substituted for Css in the calculations so that unit conversion was not required.)

2. *Compute procainamide dose.* Procainamide clearance is used to compute the new dose:

$$k_0 = Css \ Cl = 8 \text{ mg/L} \cdot 0.22 \text{ L/min}$$
$$= 1.8 \text{ mg/min, rounded to 2 mg/min}$$

(*Note:* μg/ml = mg/L, and this concentration unit was substituted for Css in the calculations so that unit conversion was not required.)

The expected NAPA steady-state serum concentration will increase in proportion to the procainamide dosage increase:

$$Css_{new} = (D_{new}/D_{old})Css_{old} = (2 \text{ mg/min}/1 \text{ mg/min})(7.9 \text{ μg/ml})$$
$$= 15.8 \text{ μg/ml}$$

The new procainamide dose should be instituted immediately.

Steady-state procainamide serum concentration can be measured after steady state is attained in 3–5 half- lives. Since the patient is expected to have a procainamide half-life of 5.5 hours and NAPA half-life of 6 hours, procainamide and NAPA steady-state concentrations can be obtained any time after the second day of dosing (5 half-lives = 5 · 5.5 h = 28 h for procainamide, 5 half-lives = 5 · 6 h = 30 h for NAPA). Procainamide and NAPA serum concentrations should also be measured if the patient experiences a return of arrhythmia, or if the patient develops potential signs or symptoms of procainamide toxicity.

CHIOU METHOD

- For some patients it is desirable to individualize procainamide infusion rates as rapidly as possible, before steady state is achieved.[37] Examples of these cases include patients with renal dysfunction, heart failure, or hepatic cirrhosis who have variable procainamide pharmacokinetic parameters and long procainamide half-lives.

  - Two procainamide serum concentrations obtained at least 4–6 hours apart during a continuous infusion can be used to compute procainamide clearance and dosing rates. In addition, the only way procainamide can be entering the patient's body is via the intravenous infusion.
  - The last dose of sustained-release procainamide must have been administered no less than 12–16 hours before this technique is used, or some residual oral procainamide will still be absorbed from the gastrointestinal tract and cause computation errors.

- The following equation is used to compute procainamide clearance (Cl) using the procainamide concentrations:

$$Cl = \frac{2k_0}{C_1 + C_2} + \frac{2V(C_1 - C_2)}{(C_1 + C_2)(t_2 - t_1)}$$

where k_0 is the procainamide infusion rate, V is volume of distribution of procainamide (chosen according to disease states and conditions present in the patient, Table 8-1), C_1 and C_2 are the first and second procainamide serum concentrations, and t_1 and t_2 are the times at which C_1 and C_2 were obtained.

- Once procainamide clearance (Cl) is determined, it can be used to adjust the procainamide infusion rate (k_0) using the following relationship:

$$k_0 = Css \cdot Cl$$

▶ *Example 1*   JB is a 50-year-old, 60-kg (5′7″) male with heart failure (NYHA CHF class III) who was started on a 5-mg/min procainamide infusion after being administered an intravenous loading dose. The procainamide concentration was 10.6 µg/ml at 1000 H and 14.3 µg/ml at 1400 H. What procainamide infusion rate is needed to achieve Css = 8 µg/ml?

1. *Compute procainamide clearance and dose.*

$$Cl = \frac{2k_0}{C_1 + C_2} + \frac{2V(C_1 - C_2)}{(C_1 + C_2)(t_2 - t_1)}$$

$$Cl = \frac{2(5 \text{ mg/min})}{(10.6 \text{ mg/L}) + (14.3 \text{ mg/L})}$$

$$+ \frac{2(1.6 \text{ L/kg} \cdot 60 \text{ kg})(10.6 \text{ mg/L} - 14.3 \text{ mg/L})}{(10.6 \text{ mg/L} + 14.3 \text{ mg/L})240 \text{ min}} = 0.28 \text{ L/min}$$

(*Note:* μg/ml = mg/L, and this concentration unit was substituted for concentrations so that unit conversion was not required. In addition, the time difference between t_2 and t_1, in minutes, was determined and placed directly in the calculation.)

k_0 = Css · Cl = 8 mg/L · 0.28 L/h = 2.2 mg/min of procainamide

▶ ***Example 2*** YU is a 64-year-old, 80-kg (5′9″) male started on a 3 mg/min procainamide infusion after being administered an intravenous loading dose at 0900 H. The procainamide concentration was 10.3 μg/ml at 1000 H and 7.1 μg/ml at 1600 H. What procainamide infusion rate is needed to achieve Css = 10 μg/ml?

1. *Compute procainamide clearance and dose.*

$$Cl = \frac{2k_0}{C_1 + C_2} + \frac{2V(C_1 - C_2)}{(C_1 + C_2)(t_2 - t_1)}$$

$$Cl = \frac{2(3 \text{ mg/min})}{(10.3 \text{ mg/L}) + (7.1 \text{ mg/L})}$$

$$+ \frac{2(2.7 \text{ L/kg} \cdot 80 \text{ kg})(10.3 \text{ mg/L} - 7.1 \text{ mg/L})}{(10.3 \text{ mg/L} + 7.1 \text{ mg/L})360 \text{ min}} = 0.57 \text{ L/min}$$

(*Note:* μg/ml = mg/L, and this concentration unit was substituted for concentrations so that unit conversion was not required. In addition, the time difference between t_2 and t_1, in minutes, was determined and placed directly in the calculation).

k_0 = Css · Cl = 10 mg/L · 0.57 L/min = 5.7 mg/min of procainamide

BAYESIAN PHARMACOKINETIC COMPUTER PROGRAMS

- Computer programs are available that can assist in the computation of pharmacokinetic parameters for patients. The most reliable computer programs use a nonlinear regression algorithm that incorporates components of Bayes' theorem.

  - An advantage of this approach is that consistent dosage recommendations are made when several different practitioners are involved in therapeutic drug monitoring programs. However, since simpler dosing methods work just as well for patients with stable pharmacokinetic parameters and steady-state drug concentrations, many clinicians reserve the use of computer programs for more difficult situations. Those situations include serum concentrations that are not at steady state, serum concentrations not obtained at the specific times needed to employ simpler methods, and unstable pharmacokinetic parameters.
  - When only a limited number of procainamide concentrations are available, Bayesian pharmacokinetic computer programs can be used to compute a complete patient pharmacokinetic profile that includes clearance, volume of distribution, and half-life.

- Many Bayesian pharmacokinetic computer programs are available, and most should provide answers similar to the program used in the following examples. The program used to solve problems in this book is DrugCalc, written by Dr. Dennis Mungall and available at his Internet web site (www.clinpharmacologist.bigstep.com/consumersurvey.html).[38]

▶ *Example 1*   SL is a 71-year-old, 82-kg (height 5'10″) male with atrial fibrillation who requires therapy with oral procainamide. He has liver cirrhosis (Child-Pugh score = 12, bilirubin = 3.2 mg/dl, albumin = 2.5 gm/dl) and
normal cardiac function. He began procainamide sustained-release tablets
500 mg every 12 hours at 0700 H. On the second day of therapy, before the
morning dose was administered, the procainamide serum concentration was
4.5 µg/ml at 0700 H. Compute a procainamide dose that will provide a
steady-state concentration of 5 µg/ml.

1. *Enter patient demographic, drug dosing, and serum concentration/time
   data into a Bayesian pharmacokinetic computer program.* In this case it
   is unlikely that the patient is at steady state, so the linear pharmacokinetics method cannot be used.
2. *Compute pharmacokinetic parameters for the patient using the computer
   program.* The pharmacokinetic parameters computed by the program are
   a volume of distribution of 110 L, a half-life of 15.5 h, and a clearance of
   4.93 L/h.
3. *Compute dose required to achieve desired procainamide serum concentrations.* The oral one-compartment-model equation used by the program
   to compute doses indicates that 250 mg of procainamide sustained-
   release tablets every 8 hours will produce a steady-state trough concentration of 5.5 µg/ml. This dose should be started immediately.

DOSING STRATEGIES

• Initial dose and dosage adjustment techniques using serum concentrations
  can be used in any combination as long as the limitations of each method
  are observed.
• Some dosing schemes link together logically when considered according to
  their basic approaches or philosophies. Dosage strategies that follow similar pathways are given in Table 8-5.

USE OF PROCAINAMIDE BOOSTER DOSES TO IMMEDIATELY INCREASE SERUM CONCENTRATIONS

• If a patient has a subtherapeutic procainamide serum concentration in an acute
  situation, it may be desirable to increase the procainamide concentration as
  quickly as possible. A rational way to increase the serum concentration

TABLE 8-5 Dosing Strategies

Dosing approach/ philosophy	Initial dosing	Use of serum concentrations to alter doses
Pharmacokinetic parameters/ equations	Pharmacokinetic dosing method	Pharmacokinetic parameter method
Literature-based/ concept	Literature-based recommended dosing method	Linear pharmacokinetic method
Computerized	Bayesian computer program	Bayesian computer program

rapidly is to administer a booster dose of procainamide, a process also known as "reloading" the patient with procainamide, computed using pharmacokinetic techniques.

- A modified loading dose equation is used to accomplish computation of the booster dose (BD) which takes into account the current procainamide concentration present in the patient:

$$BD = (C_{desired} - C_{actual})V$$

where $C_{desired}$ is the desired procainamide concentration, C_{actual} is the actual current procainamide concentration for the patient, and V is the volume of distribution for procainamide.

- If the volume of distribution for procainamide is known for the patient, it can be used in the calculation. However, this value is not usually known and is assumed to equal the population average for the disease states and conditions present in the patient (Table 8-1).

- Concurrent with the administration of the booster dose, the maintenance dose of procainamide is usually increased. Clinicians need to recognize that the administration of a booster dose does not alter the time required to achieve steady-state conditions when a new procainamide dosage rate is prescribed. It still requires 3–5 half-lives to attain steady state when the dosage rate is changed. However, usually the difference between the post–booster dose procainamide concentration and the ultimate steady-state concentration is reduced by giving the extra dose of drug.

▸ *Example 1*   BN is a 42-year-old, 50-kg (height 5′2″) female with atrial flutter who is receiving therapy with intravenous procainamide. She has normal liver and cardiac function. After receiving an initial loading dose of procainamide (300 mg) and a maintenance infusion of procainamide of 4 mg/min for 16 hours, her procainamide concentration is measured at 2.1 μg/ml and her atrial rate continues to be rapid. Compute a booster dose of procainamide to achieve a procainamide concentration equal to 6 μg/ml.

1. *Estimate volume of distribution according to disease states and conditions present in the patient.* In the case of procainamide, the population average volume of distribution is 2.7 L/kg, and this is used to estimate the parameter for the patient. The patient is not obese, so her actual body weight will be used in the computation:

$$V = 2.7 \text{ L/kg} \cdot 50 \text{ kg} = 135 \text{ L}$$

2. *Compute booster dose.* The booster dose is computed using the following equation:

$$BD = (C_{desired} - C_{actual})V = (6 \text{ mg/L} - 2.1 \text{ mg/L})135 \text{ L} = 527 \text{ mg}$$

rounded to 500 mg of procainamide infused over 25–30 minutes. (*Note:* μg/ml = mg/L, and this concentration unit was substituted for Css in the calculations so that unit conversion was not required.) If the maintenance dose is increased, it will take an additional 3–5 estimated half-lives for new steady-state conditions to be achieved. Procainamide serum concentrations can be measured at this time.

CONVERSION OF PROCAINAMIDE DOSES FROM INTRAVENOUS TO ORAL ROUTE OF ADMINISTRATION

- Occasionally there is a need to convert a patient stabilized on procainamide therapy from the oral route of administration to an equivalent continuous infusion or vice versa. In general, oral procainamide dosage forms, including most sustained-release tablets and capsules, have a bioavailability of 0.83.
- Assuming that equal procainamide serum concentrations are desired, this makes conversion between the intravenous ($k_0 = Css \cdot Cl$) and oral [$D = (Css \cdot Cl \cdot \tau)/F$] routes of administration simple, since equivalent doses of drug (corrected for procainamide bioavailability) are prescribed:

$$k_0 = FD_{po}/(60 \text{ min/h} \cdot \tau) \qquad \text{or} \qquad D_{po} = (k_0 \cdot \tau \cdot 60 \text{ min/h})/F$$

where k_0 is the equivalent intravenous infusion rate for the procainamide in mg/min, D_{po} is the equivalent dose of oral procainamide in mg, τ is the dosage interval, and F is the bioavailability fraction for oral procainamide.

▶ ***Example 1***   JH is currently receiving oral sustained-release procainamide, 1000 mg every 6 hours. She is responding well to therapy, has no adverse drug effects, and has steady-state procainamide and NAPA concentrations of 8.3 and 14.7 μg/ml, respectively. Suggest an equivalent dose of procainamide to be given as an intravenous infusion to this patient.

1. *Calculate equivalent intravenous dose of procainamide.* The equivalent intravenous procainamide dose is

$$k_0 = FD_{po}/(60 \text{ min/h} \cdot \tau) = (0.83 \cdot 1000 \text{ mg})/(60 \text{ min/h} \cdot 6 \text{ h})$$

$$= 2.3 \text{ mg/min of procainamide as a continuous intravenous infusion}$$

▶ ***Example 2***   LK is currently receiving a continuous infusion of procainamide at the rate of 5 mg/min. He is responding well to therapy, has no adverse drug effects, and has steady-state procainamide and NAPA concentrations of 6.2 and 4.3 μg/ml, respectively. Suggest an equivalent dose of sustained-release oral procainamide for this patient.

1. *Calculate equivalent oral dose of procainamide.* The equivalent oral sustained-release procainamide dose using a 12-hour dosage interval is

$$D_{po} = (k_0 \cdot \tau \cdot 60 \text{ min/h})/F = (5 \text{ mg/min} \cdot 12 \text{ h} \cdot 60 \text{ min/h})/0.83$$

$$= 4337 \text{ mg, rounded to 4000 mg}$$

The patient should be prescribed procainamide sustained-release tablets 4000-mg orally every 12 hours.

REFERENCES

1. Bauman JL, Schoen MD. Arrhythmias. In: DiPiro JT, Talbert RL, Yee GC, Matzke GR, Wells BG, Posey LM, eds. Pharmacotherapy. 5th ed. New York: McGraw-Hill, 2002:273–304.
2. Roden DM. Antiarrhythmic drugs. In: Hardman JG, Limbird LE, Gilman AG, eds. The pharmacological basis of therapeutics. 10th ed. New York: McGraw-Hill, 2001:933–70.
3. Lima JJ, Conti DR, Goldfarb AL, Golden LH, Jusko WJ. Pharmacokinetic approach to intravenous procainamide therapy. Eur J Clin Pharmacol 1978;13(4):303–8.

4. Giardina EG, Fenster PE, Bigger JT Jr, Mayersohn M, Perrier D, Marcus FI. Efficacy, plasma concentrations and adverse effects of a new sustained release procainamide preparation. Am J Cardiol 1980;46(5):855–62.

5. Manion CV, Lalka D, Baer DT, Meyer MB. Absorption kinetics of procainamide in humans. J Pharm Sci 1977;66(7):981–4.

6. Graffner C, Johnsson G, Sjogren J. Pharmacokinetics of procainamide intravenously and orally as conventional and slow-release tablets. Clin Pharmacol Ther 1975;17(4):414–23.

7. Smith TC, Kinkel AW. Plasma levels of procainamide after administration of conventional and sustained-release preparations. Curr Ther Res 1980;27(2):217–28.

8. Koup JR, Abel RB, Smithers JA, Eldon MA, de Vries TM. Effect of age, gender, and race on steady state procainamide pharmacokinetics after administration of procanbid sustained-release tablets. Ther Drug Monit 1998;20(1):73–7.

9. Gibson TP, Matusik J, Matusik E, Nelson HA, Wilkinson J, Briggs WA. Acetylation of procainamide in man and its relationship to isonicotinic acid hydrazide acetylation phenotype. Clin Pharmacol Ther 1975;17(4):395–9.

10. Dutcher JS, Strong JM, Lucas SV, Lee WK, Atkinson AJ Jr. Procainamide and *N*-acetylprocainamide kinetics investigated simultaneously with stable isotope methodology. Clin Pharmacol Ther 1977;22(4):447–57.

11. Lima JJ, Conti DR, Goldfarb AL, Tilstone WJ, Golden LH, Jusko WJ. Clinical pharmacokinetics of procainamide infusions in relation to acetylator phenotype. J Pharmacokinet Biopharm 1979;7(1):69–85.

12. Myerburg RJ, Kessler KM, Kiem I, et al. Relationship between plasma levels of procainamide, suppression of premature ventricular complexes and prevention of recurrent ventricular tachycardia. Circulation 1981;64(2):280–90.

13. Galeazzi RL, Sheiner LB, Lockwood T, Benet LZ. The renal elimination of procainamide. Clin Pharmacol Ther 1976;19(1):55–62.

14. Reidenberg MM, Camacho M, Kluger J, Drayer DE. Aging and renal clearance of procainamide and acetylprocainamide. Clin Pharmacol Ther 1980;28(6):732–5.

15. Lima JJ, Jusko WJ. Determination of procainamide acetylator status. Clin Pharmacol Ther 1978;23(1):25–9.

16. Reidenberg MM, Drayer DE, Levy M, Warner H. Polymorphic acetylation procainamide in man. Clin Pharmacol Ther 1975;17(6):722–30.

17. Lessard E, Fortin A, Belanger PM, Beaune P, Hamelin BA, Turgeon J. Role of CYP2D6 in the N-hydroxylation of procainamide. Pharmacogenetics 1997;7(5):381–90.

18. Tilstone WJ, Lawson DH. Capacity-limited elimination of procainamide in man. Res Commun Chem Pathol Pharmacol 1978;21(2):343–6.

19. Coyle JD, Boudoulas H, Mackichan JJ, Lima JJ. Concentration-dependent clearance of procainamide in normal subjects. Biopharm Drug Dispos 1985;6(2):159–65.

20. Giardina EG, Dreyfuss J, Bigger JT Jr, Shaw JM, Schreiber EC. Metabolism of procainamide in normal and cardiac subjects. Clin Pharmacol Ther 1976;19(3):339–51.

21. Koch-Weser J. Pharmacokinetic of procainamide in man. Ann N Y Acad Sci 1971;179:370–82.

22. Koch-Weser J, Klein SW. Procainamide dosage schedules, plasma concentrations, and clinical effects. JAMA 1971;215(9):1454–60.

23. Bauer LA, Black D, Gensler A, Sprinkle J. Influence of age, renal function and heart failure on procainamide clearance and n-acetylprocainamide serum concentrations. Int J Clin Pharmacol Ther Toxicol 1989;27(5):213–6.

24. Gibson TP, Lowenthal DT, Nelson HA, Briggs WA. Elimination of procainamide in end stage renal failure. Clin Pharmacol Ther 1975;17(3):321–9.

25. Gibson TP, Atkinson AJ Jr, Matusik E, Nelson LD, Briggs WA. Kinetics of procainamide and N-acetylprocainamide in renal failure. Kidney Int 1977;12(6):422–9.

26. Tisdale JE, Rudis MI, Padhi ID, et al. Disposition of procainamide in patients with chronic congestive heart failure receiving medical therapy. J Clin Pharmacol 1996;36(1):35–41.

27. Mutnick AH, Burke TG. Antiarrhythmics. In: Schumacher GE, ed. Therapeutic Drug Monitoring. 1st ed. Stamford, CT: Appleton & Lange, 1995:684.
28. Pugh RN, Murray-Lyon IM, Dawson JL, Pietroni MC, Williams R. Transection of the oesophagus for bleeding oesophageal varices. Br J Surg 1973;60(8):646–9.
29. Christoff PB, Conti DR, Naylor C, Jusko WJ. Procainamide disposition in obesity. Drug Intell Clin Pharm 1983;17(7-8):516–22.
30. Gunn VL, Nechyba C, eds. The Harriet Lane handbook: a manual for pediatric house officers. 16th ed. Philadelphia: Mosby, 2002.
31. Atkinson AJ Jr, Krumlovsky FA, Huang CM, del Greco F. Hemodialysis for severe procainamide toxicity: clinical and pharmacokinetic observations. Clin Pharmacol Ther 1976;20(5):585–92.
32. Golper TA, Marx MA. Drug dosing adjustments during continuous renal replacement therapies. Kidney Int Suppl 1998;66:S165–8.
33. Golper TA. Update on drug sieving coefficients and dosing adjustments during continuous renal replacement therapies. Contrib Nephrol 2001(132):349–53.
34. Gibson TP, Matusik EJ, Briggs WA. N-Acetylprocainamide levels in patients with end-stage renal failure. Clin Pharmacol Ther 1976;19(2):206–12.
35. Hansten PD, Horn JR. Drug interactions analysis and management. Vancouver, WA: Applied Therapeutics, 1998.
36. Bauer LA, Black D, Gensler A. Procainamide-cimetidine drug interaction in elderly male patients. J Am Geriatr Soc 1990;38(4):467–9.
37. Chiou WL, Gadalla MA, Peng GW. Method for the rapid estimation of the total body drug clearance and adjustment of dosage regimens in patients during a constant-rate intravenous infusion. J Pharmacokinet Biopharm 1978;6(2):135–51.
38. Wandell M, Mungall D. Computer assisted drug interpretation and drug regimen optimization. Am Assoc Clin Chem 1984;6:1–11.
39. Johnson JA, Parker RB, Patterson JH. Heart failure. In: DiPiro JT, Talbert RL, Yee GC, Matzke GR, Wells BG, Posey LM, eds. Pharmacotherapy—a pathophysiologic approach. 5th ed. New York: McGraw-Hill, 2002:185–218.

9 | Quinidine

Quinidine was one of the first agents to be used for its antiarrhythmic effects. It is classified as a type IA antiarrhythmic agent and can be used for the treatment of supraventricular or ventricular arrhythmias.[1,2] Because of its side-effect profile, quinidine is considered by many clinicians to be a second-line antiarrhythmic choice.

- Quinidine inhibits transmembrane sodium influx into the conduction system of the heart, thereby decreasing conduction velocity.[1,2] It also increases the duration of the action potential, increases threshold potential toward zero, and decreases the slope of phase 4 of the action potential. Automaticity is decreased during quinidine therapy.
- The net effect of these cellular changes is that quinidine causes increased refractoriness and decreased conduction in heart conduction tissue, which establishes a bidirectional block in reentrant pathways.

THERAPEUTIC AND TOXIC CONCENTRATIONS

- When quinidine is given intravenously, the serum quinidine concentration/time curve follows a two-compartment model.[3–6]
- When oral quinidine is given as a rapidly absorbed dosage form such as quinidine sulfate tablets, a similar distribution phase is also observed, with a duration of 20–30 minutes.[3,4,7,8] If an extended-release oral dosage form is given, absorption occurs more slowly than distribution, so a distribution phase is not seen (Figure 9-1).[9–13]
- Because marked hypotension and tachycardia may occur in some patients given quinidine intravenously, the oral route of administration is far more common.
- The generally accepted therapeutic range for quinidine is 2–6 µg/ml. Quinidine serum concentrations above the therapeutic range can cause increased QT interval or QRS complex widening (>35–50%) on the electrocardiogram, cinchonism, hypotension, high-degree atrioventricular block, and ventricular arrhythmias.

  - Cinchonism is a collection of symptoms that includes tinnitus, blurred vision, lightheadedness, tremor, giddiness, and altered hearing, which decreases in severity with lower quinidine concentrations.
  - Adverse gastrointestinal effects such as anorexia, nausea, vomiting, and diarrhea are the most common side effects of quinidine therapy. Such side effects may occur after both oral and intravenous administration, but are not strongly correlated with specific serum levels.

- Quinidine therapy is also associated with syncope and torsades de pointes.

  - Quinidine syncope occurs when ventricular tachycardia, ventricular fibrillation, or a prolongation of QT intervals occurs in a non–dose-dependent manner.
  - Torsades de pointes ("twisting of the points") is a form of polymorphic ventricular tachycardia preceded by QT interval prolongation.

    - It is characterized by polymorphic QRS complexes that change in amplitude and length, giving the appearance of oscillations around the electrocardiographic baseline.

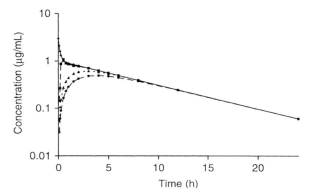

FIG. 9-1 Quinidine serum concentrations after an intravenous dose (diamonds with solid line) and three different oral tablets (doses normalized to provide 200 mg of quinidine base systemically). After an intravenous dose, quinidine serum concentrations decline according to a two-compartment model which demonstrates a distribution phase that lasts for 20–30 minutes postinjection. Immediate-release quinidine tablets (squares with dashed line) are rapidly absorbed and also show a distinct distribution phase. Extended-release quinidine gluconate (triangles with dotted line) and quinidine sulfate (circles with dashed line) have slower absorption profiles, so the drug has an opportunity to distribute to tissues while absorption is occurring. As a result, no distribution phase is observed for these dosage forms.

- Torsades de pointes can develop into multiple episodes of nonsustained polymorphic ventricular tachycardia, syncope, ventricular fibrillation, or sudden cardiac death.
- Hypersensitivity reactions to quinidine include rash, drug fever, thrombocytopenia, hemolytic anemia, asthma, respiratory depression, a systemic lupus-like syndrome, hepatitis, and anaphylactic shock.
- Quinidine metabolites (3-hydroxyquinidine, $2'$-quinidinone, quinidine-N-oxide, O-desmethylquinidine) all have antiarrhythmic effects in animal models.[14–17]
  - 3-Hydroxyquinidine is the most potent (60–80% compared to the parent drug) and achieves high enough serum concentrations in humans that its antiarrhythmic effects probably contribute to the clinical effects observed during quinidine treatment.
  - Dihydroquinidine is an impurity in commercially available quinidine products that also has antiarrhythmic effects.[18–20] Most products contain less than 10% of the labeled quinidine amount as dihydroquinidine.
- For dose-adjustment purposes, quinidine serum concentrations are best measured as a predose or trough level at steady state after the patient has received a consistent dosage regimen for 3–5 drug half-lives.
  - Quinidine half-life varies from 6–8 hours in normal adults to 9–10 hours or more in adult patients with liver failure. If quinidine is given orally or intravenously on a stable schedule, steady-state serum concentrations will be achieved in about 2 days (5 · 8 h = 40 h).

CLINICAL MONITORING PARAMETERS

- The electrocardiogram (ECG or EKG) should be monitored to determine the response to quinidine. The goal of therapy is suppression of arrhythmias and avoidance of adverse drug reactions.
- Because many therapeutic and side effects of quinidine are not correlated with its serum concentration, it is often not necessary to obtain serum quinidine concentrations in patients receiving appropriate doses who currently have no arrhythmia or adverse drug effects.
- Quinidine serum concentrations should be obtained in patients who have a recurrence of tachyarrhythmias, are experiencing possible quinidine side effects, or are receiving quinidine doses not consistent with disease states and conditions known to alter quinidine pharmacokinetics (see Effects of Disease States and Conditions on Quinidine Pharmacokinetics and Dosing).
- Serum concentration monitoring can aid in the decision to increase or decrease the quinidine dose.

  - If an arrhythmia reappears and the quinidine serum concentration is <6 μg/ml, increasing the quinidine dose is a therapeutic option.
  - If the quinidine serum concentration is over 6 μg/ml, it is unlikely that a dosage increase will be effective in suppressing the arrhythmia and there is an increased likelihood that drug side effects may occur.
  - If a possible concentration-related quinidine adverse drug reaction is noted in a patient and the quinidine serum concentration is <2 μg/ml, it is possible that the observed problem may not be due to quinidine treatment and other sources should be investigated.

- While patients are receiving quinidine, they should be monitored for the following adverse drug effects: anorexia, nausea, vomiting, diarrhea, cinchonism, syncope, increased QT interval or QRS complex widening (>35–50%) on the electrocardiogram, hypotension, high-degree atrioventricular block, ventricular arrhythmias, and hypersensitivity reactions (rash, drug fever, thrombocytopenia, hemolytic anemia, asthma, respiratory depression, a lupus-like syndrome, hepatitis, anaphylactic shock).

BASIC CLINICAL PHARMACOKINETIC PARAMETERS

- Quinidine is almost completely eliminated by hepatic metabolism (~80%).[4,7] Hepatic metabolism is mainly via the CYP3A enzyme system. Approximately 20% of a quinidine dose is eliminated unchanged in the urine.

  - 3-Hydroxyquinidine is the primary active metabolite resulting from quinidine metabolism, whereas dihydroquinidine is an active compound that is found as an impurity in most quinidine dosage forms.
  - The hepatic extraction ratio of quinidine is about 30%, so quinidine is typically classified as a intermediate-extraction-ratio drug. As a result, it is expected that liver blood flow, unbound fraction of drug in the blood, and intrinsic clearance will all be important factors influencing the clearance of quinidine.
  - After oral administration, quinidine is subject to moderate first-pass metabolism by CYP3A in the liver and intestinal wall.

- Although there have been some reports that quinidine follows nonlinear pharmacokinetics, for the purposes of clinical drug dosing in patients, linear pharmacokinetic concepts and equations can be used effectively to compute doses and estimate serum concentrations.[21]

- Three different salt forms of quinidine are available. Quinidine sulfate contains 83% quinidine base, quinidine gluconate contains 62% quinidine base, and quinidine polygalacturonate contains 60% quinidine base. The gluconate salt is available for both intravenous injection and oral use. Quinidine sulfate and polygalacturonate are available only for oral use.

- The oral bioavailability of all three quinidine-based drugs is moderate and generally equals 70%, reflecting first-pass metabolism in the intestinal wall and liver.[3,7]

- Although quinidine can be injected intramuscularly, this route of administration may lead to erratic absorption and serum concentrations.[6]

- Plasma protein binding of quinidine in normal individuals is about 80–90%.[22–24] The drug binds to both albumin and α_1-acid glycoprotein (AGP).

  - AGP is classified as an acute-phase reactant protein that is present in lower amounts in all individuals but is secreted in large amounts in response to certain stresses and disease states such as trauma, heart failure, and myocardial infarction. In patients with these disease states, quinidine binding to AGP can be even larger, resulting in an unbound fraction as low as 8%.

EFFECTS OF DISEASE STATES AND CONDITIONS ON QUINIDINE PHARMACOKINETICS AND DOSING

- Normal adults without the disease states and conditions discussed later in this section and who have normal liver function have an average quinidine half-life of 7 hours (range 6–8 hours) and a volume of distribution for the entire body of 2.4 L/kg (V = 2–3 L/kg; Table 9-1).[3–6,9,25–27] The elimination rate constant (k = 0.693/$t_{1/2}$, where $t_{1/2}$ is the half-life) and clearance (Cl = kV) can be computed from the aforementioned pharmacokinetic parameters.

Hepatic Dysfunction

- Patients with liver cirrhosis have increased quinidine clearance and volume of distribution, which results in a prolonged average quinidine half-life of 9 hours.[28,29] Clearance and volume of distribution are greater in patients with liver disease because albumin and α_1-acid glycoprotein (AAG) concentrations are lower in these patients and result in reduced quinidine plasma protein binding (average V = 3.8 L/kg).

  - The increased unbound fraction in the plasma allows more quinidine to enter the liver parenchyma, where hepatic drug-metabolizing enzymes are present, and leads to increased drug clearance. Decreased plasma protein binding also leads to higher unbound levels for a given total quinidine serum concentration.

  - The significance of this difference in unbound concentrations has not been assessed in cirrhosis patients, but clinicians should bear it in mind when monitoring quinidine levels, as only total serum concentrations are available from laboratories.

- The exact effect that liver disease has on quinidine pharmacokinetics is highly variable and difficult to predict accurately. It is possible for a patient with liver disease to have relatively normal or grossly abnormal quinidine clearance, volume of distribution, and half-life.

TABLE 9-1 Disease States and Conditions That Alter Quinidine Pharmacokinetics

Disease state/ condition	Half-life (h)	Volume of distribution (L/kg)	Comment
Adult, normal liver function	7 (range 6–8)	2.4 (range 2–3)	Quinidine has a moderate hepatic extraction ratio of ~30%, so liver blood flow, unbound fraction of drug in the blood, and intrinsic clearance are all important factors in clearance rate; ~20% of quinidine is eliminated unchanged in the urine.
Adult, liver cirrhosis	9	3.8	Quinidine is metabolized ~80% by hepatic microsomal enzymes (primarily CYP3A). Clearance of total drug is increased in cirrhosis patients, but intrinsic clearance is decreased. Pharmacokinetic parameters are highly variable in liver disease patients. Volume of distribution is larger, due to decreased α_1-acid glycoprotein and albumin production by the liver, which decreases drug binding in the plasma.
Adult, heart failure	7	1.7	Decreased liver blood flow secondary to reduced cardiac output reduces quinidine clearance. Volume of distribution is smaller due to increased α_1-acid glycoprotein drug binding in the plasma. Heart failure results in large and variable reductions in quinidine clearance. Cardiac status must be monitored closely in heart failure patients, since quinidine clearance changes with acute changes in cardiac output.
Adult, obese (>30% over ideal body weight, IBW)	According to other disease states/ conditions that affect quinidine pharmacokinetics	According to other disease states/ conditions that affect quinidine pharmacokinetics	Quinidine doses should be based on IBW for patients who weigh more that 30% over IBW.

TABLE 9-2 Child-Pugh Scores for Patients with Liver Disease[30]

Test/symptom	Score 1 point	Score 2 points	Score 3 points
Total bilirubin (mg/dl)	<2.0	2.0–3.0	>3.0
Serum albumin (g/dl)	>3.5	2.8–3.5	<2.8
Prothrombin time (seconds prolonged over control)	<4	4–6	>6
Ascites	Absent	Slight	Moderate
Hepatic Encephalopathy	None	Moderate	Severe

- An index of liver dysfunction can be gained by applying the Child-Pugh clinical classification system (Table 9-2).[30] Child-Pugh scores are discussed more fully in Chapter 3 (Drug Dosing in Special Populations: Renal and Hepatic Disease, Dialysis, Heart Failure, Obesity, and Drug Interactions).

- The Child-Pugh score consists of five laboratory tests or clinical symptoms: serum albumin, total bilirubin, prothrombin time, ascites, and hepatic encephalopathy. Each of these areas is given a score of 1 (normal) to 3 (severely abnormal; Table 9-2), and the scores for the five areas are summed. The Child-Pugh score for a patient with normal liver function is 5, while the score for a patient with grossly abnormal serum albumin, total bilirubin, and prothrombin time values in addition to severe ascites and hepatic encephalopathy is 15.

- A Child-Pugh score greater than 8 is grounds for a decrease of 25–50% in the initial daily drug dose of quinidine.

- As in any patient, with or without liver dysfunction, initial doses are meant as starting points for dosage titration based on patient response and avoidance of adverse effects. Quinidine serum concentrations and the presence of adverse drug effects should be monitored frequently in patients with liver cirrhosis.

Heart Failure

- Heart failure reduces quinidine clearance because of decreased hepatic blood flow secondary to compromised cardiac output (Table 9-3).[7,8,31,32] Volume of distribution (V = 1.7 L/kg) is decreased because heart failure patients have elevated AAG serum concentrations, which leads to increased quinidine plasma protein binding and decreased quinidine unbound fraction.

  - Because clearance and volume of distribution decrease simultaneously, patients with heart failure have an average quinidine half-life equal to 7 hours, which is similar to that in a normal individual ($t_{1/2} = [0.693 \cdot \downarrow V]/\downarrow Cl$).

  - Increased plasma protein binding also leads to lower unbound levels for a given total quinidine serum concentration.

  - The clinical significance of this difference in unbound concentrations has not been assessed in heart failure patients.

TABLE 9-3 New York Heart Association (NYHA) Functional Classification for Heart Failure[42]

NYHA heart failure class	Description
I	Patients with cardiac disease but without limitations of physical activity. Ordinary physical activity does not cause undue fatigue, dyspnea, or palpitation.
II	Patients with cardiac disease that results in slight limitations of physical activity. Ordinary physical activity results in fatigue, palpitation, dyspnea, or angina.
III	Patients with cardiac disease that results in marked limitations of physical activity. Although patients are comfortable at rest, less than ordinary activity will lead to symptoms.
IV	Patients with cardiac disease that results in an inability to carry on physical activity without discomfort. Symptoms of congestive heart failure are present even at rest. With any physical activity, increased discomfort is experienced.

- The effect of heart failure on quinidine pharmacokinetics is highly variable and difficult to predict accurately. It is possible for a patient with heart failure to have relatively normal or grossly abnormal quinidine clearance and half-life.
- For heart failure patients, initial doses are meant as starting points for dosage titration based on patient response and avoidance of adverse effects. Quinidine serum concentrations and the presence of adverse drug effects should be monitored frequently in patients with heart failure.

Myocardial Infarction

- After a myocardial infarction, serum AAG concentrations increase by up to 50% over a 12–72-hour time period. As AAG serum concentrations increase, plasma protein binding of quinidine increases and the unbound fraction of quinidine decreases. Because quinidine is considered a moderate-hepatic-extraction-ratio drug, a decline in the unbound fraction of quinidine in the plasma decreases quinidine clearance.

Elderly

- For patients over the age of 65, studies indicate that quinidine clearance is reduced, the volume of distribution is unchanged, and half-life is longer (average half-life = 10 hours) compared to younger subjects.[15,33]
- Most patients with serious arrhythmias studied in all of the previously mentioned investigations are older, and those results include any influence of age. Thus, in most cases elderly patients are treated with quinidine according to the other disease states or conditions present that influence quinidine pharmacokinetics.

Pediatrics

- The suggested dose of oral quinidine sulfate for children is 15–60 mg/kg/d given every 6 hours. For intravenous use, the dose of quinidine gluconate injection is 2–10 mg/kg/dose administered every 3–6 hours as needed. A 2- mg/kg test dose of oral quinidine sulfate or injectable quinidine gluconate (IM or IV) is recommended to determine if an idiosyncratic adverse effect will occur (maximum dose 200 mg).[34]

Obesity

• Because detailed studies have not been conducted in obese patients, ideal body weight should be used to compute initial doses of quinidine, to avoid accidental overdose in overweight individuals (>30% above ideal body weight or IBW).

Renal Dysfunction

• Since only 20% of a quinidine dose is eliminated unchanged by the kidney, dosage adjustments are usually not required for renal failure patients.[14,32]

Dialysis

• Quinidine is not appreciably removed by hemodialysis or peritoneal dialysis.[35,36]

DRUG INTERACTIONS

• Quinidine has serious drug interactions with other drugs that are capable of inhibiting the CYP3A enzyme system.[37] Because this isozyme is present in the intestinal wall and liver, quinidine serum concentrations may increase due to decreased clearance, decreased first-pass metabolism, or a combination of both.

  • Erythromycin, ketoconazole, and verapamil have been reported to increase quinidine serum concentrations or area under the concentration/time curve (AUC) by >30–50%.
  • Other macrolide antibiotics (such as clarithromycin) or azole antifungals (such as fluconazole, miconazole, and itraconazole) that inhibit CYP3A probably cause similar drug interactions with quinidine.
  • Cimetidine and aminodarone also have been reported to cause increases in quinidine concentrations or AUC of a similar magnitude.

• Drugs that induce CYP3A (phenytoin, phenobarbital, rifampin, rifabutin) decrease quinidine serum concentrations by increasing quinidine clearance and first-pass metabolism.

  • Phenytoin has antiarrhythmic effects and is also classified as a type IB antiarrhythmic agent. As a result, phenytoin and quinidine may have additive pharmacological effects that could result in a pharmacodynamic drug interaction.

• Although quinidine is not a substrate for CYP2D6, it is a potent inhibitor of that enzyme system.[37–40] As little as 50 mg of quinidine can effectively turn an "extensive metabolizer" into a "poor metabolizer" of this isozyme.

  • Because poor metabolizers of CYP2D6 substrates have little to none of this enzyme in their liver, the administration of quinidine does not result in a drug interaction in these individuals.
  • Quinidine can markedly decrease the clearance β-adrenergic receptor blockers eliminated via CYP2D6 by 30% or more. Propranolol, metoprolol, and timolol have decreased clearance due to quinidine coadministration.

- Tricyclic antidepressants (nortriptyline, imipramine, desipramine), haloperidol, and dextromethorphan also have increased serum concentrations when given with quinidine.
- Codeine is a prodrug with no analgesic effect that relies on conversion to morphine via the CYP2D6 enzyme system to decrease pain. When quinidine is given concomitantly with codeine, the conversion from codeine to morphine does not take place, and patients do not experience analgesia. A similar drug interaction may occur with dihydrocodeine and hydrocodone.
- Although it may not be reported in the literature for a specific compound, clinicians should consider that a drug interaction is possible between quinidine and any CYP2D6 substrate.

- Quinidine increases digoxin serum concentrations 30–50% by decreasing digoxin renal and nonrenal clearance as well as digoxin volume of distribution.[37] The probable mechanisms of this drug interaction are inhibition of digoxin renal and hepatic P-glycoprotein (PGP) elimination and tissue binding displacement of digoxin by quinidine.
- Antacids can increase urinary pH, leading to increased renal tubular reabsorption of un-ionized quinidine and decreased quinidine renal clearance.
- Kaolin–pectin administration results in physical adsorption of quinidine in the gastrointestinal tract and decreased quinidine oral absorption.
- The pharmacological effects of warfarin and neuromuscular blockers have been enhanced when given with quinidine.

INITIAL DOSAGE DETERMINATION METHODS

- Several methods to initiate quinidine therapy are available:

  - The *pharmacokinetic dosing method* is the most flexible of the techniques. It allows individualized target serum concentrations to be chosen for a patient, and each pharmacokinetic parameter can be customized to reflect specific disease states and conditions present in the patient.
  - *Literature-based recommended dosing* is a very commonly used method to prescribe initial doses of quinidine. Doses are based on those that commonly produce steady-state concentrations near the lower end of the therapeutic range, although there is a wide variation in the actual concentrations for a specific patient.

Pharmacokinetic Dosing Method

- The goal of initial dosing of quinidine is to compute the best dose possible for the patient given the set of disease states and conditions that influence quinidine pharmacokinetics and the arrhythmia being treated. In order to do this, pharmacokinetic parameters are estimated using average parameters measured in other patients with similar disease state and condition profiles.

Half-Life and Elimination Rate Constant Estimate

- Quinidine is metabolized predominantly by the liver. Unfortunately, there is no good way to estimate the elimination characteristics of liver-metabolized drugs using an endogenous marker of liver function in the same manner that serum creatinine and estimated creatinine clearance are used to estimate the elimination of agents that are eliminated renally.
- A patient is categorized according to the disease states and conditions that are known to change quinidine half-life, and the half-life previously measured in

these studies is used as an estimate of the current patient's half-life (Table 9-1). Once the correct half-life is identified for the patient, it can be converted into the quinidine elimination rate constant (k) using the following equation:

$$k = 0.693/t_{1/2}$$

- To produce the most conservative quinidine doses in patients with multiple concurrent disease states or conditions that affect quinidine pharmacokinetics, the disease state or condition with the longest half-life should be used to compute doses. This approach will avoid accidental overdosage as much as is currently possible.

Volume of Distribution Estimate

- The quinidine volume of distribution is chosen according to the disease states and conditions that are present (Table 9-1).

  - The volume of distribution is used to help compute quinidine clearance, and is assumed to equal 3.8 L/kg for liver disease patients, 1.7 L/kg for heart failure patients, and 2.4 L/kg for all other patients.
  - For obese patients (>30% above ideal body weight), ideal body weight is used to compute quinidine volume of distribution.

Selection of Appropriate Pharmacokinetic Model and Equations

- When quinidine is given orally, it follows a one- or two-compartment pharmacokinetic model (Figure 9-1).
- When oral therapy is required, most clinicians utilize a sustained-release dosage form that has good bioavailability (F = 0.7), supplies a continuous release of quinidine into the gastrointestinal tract, and provides a smooth quinidine serum concentration/time curve that emulates an intravenous infusion when given every 8–12 hours.
- A very simple pharmacokinetic equation that computes the average quinidine steady-state serum concentration (Css in μg/ml = mg/L) is widely used and allows maintenance dosage calculation:

$$Css = \frac{F \cdot S(D/\tau)}{Cl} \qquad or \qquad D = \frac{Css \cdot Cl \cdot \tau}{F \cdot S}$$

where F is the bioavailability fraction for the oral dosage form (F = 0.7 for most oral quinidine products), S is the fraction of the quinidine salt form that is active quinidine (S = 0.83 for sulfate, immediate-release tablets = 100, 200, 300 mg, extended-release tablets = 300 mg; S = 0.62 for gluconate, extended-release tablets = 324 mg; S = 0.60 for polygalacturonate, immediate-release tablets = 275 mg), D is the dose of quinidine salt in mg, and τ is the dosage interval in hours. Cl is quinidine clearance in L/h and is computed using estimates of quinidine elimination rate constant (k) and volume of distribution: Cl = kV.

Steady-State Concentration Selection

- The generally accepted therapeutic range for quinidine is 2–6 μg/ml. However, quinidine therapy must be individualized for each patient in order to achieve optimal response and minimize side effects.

▶ *Example 1*   LK is a 50-year-old, 75-kg (height 5′10″) male with ventricular tachycardia who requires therapy with oral quinidine gluconate. He has normal liver and cardiac function. Suggest an initial oral quinidine dosage regimen designed to achieve a steady-state quinidine concentration of 3 μg/ml.

1. *Estimate half-life and elimination rate constant according to disease states and conditions present in the patient.* The expected quinidine half-life ($t_{1/2}$) is 7 hours. The elimination rate constant is computed using the following formula:

$$k = 0.693/t_{1/2} = 0.693/7 \text{ h} = 0.099 \text{ h}^{-1}$$

2. *Estimate volume of distribution and clearance.* The patient is not obese, so the estimated quinidine volume of distribution is based on actual body weight:

$$V = 2.4 \text{ L/kg} \cdot 75 \text{ kg} = 180 \text{ L}$$

Estimated quinidine clearance is computed by taking the product of V and the elimination rate constant:

$$Cl = kV = 0.099 \text{ h}^{-1} \cdot 180 \text{ L} = 17.8 \text{ L/h}$$

3. *Compute dosage regimen.* Oral extended-release quinidine gluconate tablets will be prescribed for this patient (F = 0.7, S = 0.62). The initial dosage interval (τ) will be 8 hours. (*Note:* μg/ml = mg/L, and this concentration unit was substituted for Css in the calculations so that unit conversion was not required.) The dosage equation for oral quinidine is:

$$D = \frac{Css \cdot Cl \cdot \tau}{F \cdot S} = \frac{3 mg/L \cdot 17.8L/h \cdot 8h}{0.7 \cdot 0.62}$$
$$= 984 \text{ mg, rounded to 972 mg every 8h}$$

A steady-state quinidine serum concentration can be measured after steady state is attained in 3–5 half-lives. Since the patient is expected to have a drug half-life of 7 hours, the quinidine steady-state concentration can be obtained any time after the second day of dosing (5 half-lives = $5 \cdot 7$ h = 35 h). Quinidine serum concentrations should also be measured if the patient experiences a return of arrhythmia, or if the patient develops potential signs or symptoms of quinidine toxicity.

▶ *Example 2* OI is a 60-year-old, 85-kg (height 6′1″) male with atrial fibrillation who requires therapy with oral quinidine sulfate. He has liver cirrhosis (Child-Pugh score = 11). Suggest an initial extended-release quinidine sulfate dosage regimen designed to achieve a steady-state quinidine concentration of 2 μg/ml.

1. *Estimate half-life and elimination rate constant according to disease states and conditions present in the patient.* The expected quinidine half-life ($t_{1/2}$) is 9 hours. The elimination rate constant is computed using the following formula:

$$k = 0.693/t_{1/2} = 0.693/9 \text{ h} = 0.077 \text{ h}^{-1}$$

2. *Estimate volume of distribution and clearance.* The patient is not obese, so the estimated quinidine volume of distribution is based on actual body weight:

$$V = 3.8 \text{ L/kg} \cdot 85 \text{ kg} = 323 \text{ L}$$

Estimated quinidine clearance is computed by taking the product of V and the elimination rate constant:

$$Cl = kV = 0.077 \text{ h}^{-1} \cdot 323 \text{ L} = 24.9 \text{ L/h}$$

3. *Compute dosage regimen.* Oral extended-release quinidine sulfate tablets will be prescribed for this patient (F = 0.7, S = 0.83). The initial dosage interval (τ) will be 8 hours. (Note: μg/ml = mg/L, and this concentration unit was substituted for Css in the calculations so that unit conversion was not required.) The dosage equation for oral quinidine is:

$$D = \frac{Css \cdot Cl \cdot \tau}{F \cdot S} = \frac{2mg/L \cdot 24.9L/h \cdot 8h}{0.7 \cdot 0.83}$$

$$= 686 \text{ mg, rounded to } 600 \text{ mg every } 8h$$

A steady-state quinidine serum concentration can be measured after steady state is attained in 3–5 half-lives. Since the patient is expected to have a drug half-life of 9 hours, quinidine steady-state concentration can be obtained any time after the second day of dosing (5 half-lives = 5 · 9 h = 45 h). Quinidine serum concentrations should also be measured if the patient experiences a return of arrhythmia, or if the patient develops potential signs or symptoms of quinidine toxicity.

Literature-Based Recommended Dosing

• Because of the large amount of variability in quinidine pharmacokinetics, even when concurrent disease states and conditions are identified, many clinicians believe that the use of standard quinidine doses for various situations is warranted. The original computations of these doses were based on the pharmacokinetic dosing method described in the previous section, and the doses subsequently modified based on clinical experience.
• In general, the quinidine steady-state serum concentration expected from the lower end of the dosage range is 2–4 μg/ml, and it is 4–6 μg/ml for the upper end of the dosage range. Suggested oral quinidine maintenance doses are listed in Table 9-4.
• For pediatric use, the suggested dose of oral quinidine sulfate is 15–60 mg/kg/d, given every 6 hours. For intravenous use, the dose of quinidine gluconate injection is 2–10 mg/kg/dose, administered every 3–6 hours as needed. A 2-mg/kg test dose of oral quinidine sulfate or injectable quinidine gluconate (IM or IV) is recommended to determine if an idiosyncratic adverse effect will occur (maximum dose 200 mg).[34]
• When more than one disease state or condition is present in a patient, choosing the lowest daily dose will result in the safest, most conservative dosage recommendation.

TABLE 9-4 Literature-Based Recommended Oral Quinidine Initial Dosage Ranges for Various Disease States and Conditions

Disease state/ condition	Quinidine sulfate, immediate-release tablets	Quinidine sulfate, extended-release tablets	Quinidine gluconate extended-release tablets	Quinidine polygalacturonate tablets
Adult, normal liver function	200–300 mg every 6–8 h	600 mg every 8–12 h	324–648 mg every 8–12 h	275–413 mg every 6–8 h
Adult, liver cirrhosis or heart failure	100–200 mg every 6–8 h	300 mg every 8–12 h	324 mg every 8–12 h	138–275 mg every 6–8 h

- To illustrate the similarities and differences between this method of dosage calculation and the pharmacokinetic dosing method, the same examples used in the previous section will be used.

▶ *Example 1* LK is a 50-year-old, 75-kg (height 5′10″) male with ventricular tachycardia who requires therapy with oral quinidine gluconate. He has normal liver and cardiac function. Suggest an initial oral quinidine dosage regimen designed to achieve a steady-state quinidine concentration of 3 μg/ml.

1. *Choose quinidine dose based on disease states and conditions present in the patient.* A quinidine gluconate maintenance dose of 628 mg every 12 hours (1256 mg/d) is suggested for a patient without heart failure or liver disease who requires a quinidine steady-state serum concentration near the lower end of the therapeutic range.

    A steady-state quinidine serum concentration can be measured after steady-state is attained in 3–5 half- lives. Since the patient is expected to have a drug half-life of 7 hours, the quinidine steady-state concentration can be obtained any time after the second day of dosing (5 half-lives = 5 · 7 h = 35 h). Quinidine serum concentrations should also be measured if the patient experiences a return of arrhythmia, or if the patient develops potential signs or symptoms of quinidine toxicity.

▶ *Example 2* OI is a 60-year-old, 85-kg (height 6′1″) male with atrial fibrillation who requires therapy with oral quinidine sulfate. He has liver cirrhosis (Child-Pugh score = 11). Suggest an initial immediate-release quinidine sulfate dosage regimen designed to achieve a steady-state quinidine concentration of 2 μg/ml.

1. *Choose quinidine dose based on disease states and conditions present in the patient.* A quinidine sulfate maintenance dose of 100 mg every 6 hours (400 mg/d) is suggested for a patient with liver disease who requires a quinidine steady-state serum concentration near the lower end of the therapeutic range.

    A steady-state quinidine serum concentration can be measured after steady state is attained in 3–5 half- lives. Since the patient is expected to have a drug half-life of 9 hours, the quinidine steady-state concentration can be obtained any time after the second day of dosing (5 half-lives = 5 · 9 h = 45 h). Quinidine serum concentrations should also be measured if the patient experiences a return of arrhythmia, or if the patient develops potential signs or symptoms of quinidine toxicity.

USE OF QUINIDINE SERUM CONCENTRATIONS TO ALTER DOSES

- Because of the large amount of pharmacokinetic variability among patients, it is likely that doses computed using patient population characteristics will not always produce quinidine serum concentrations that are expected or desirable. Because of pharmacokinetic variability, the narrow therapeutic index of quinidine, and the desire to avoid adverse quinidine side effects, measurement of quinidine serum concentrations can be a useful adjunct for patients to ensure that therapeutic, nontoxic levels are present.
- Other important patient parameters (electrocardiogram, clinical signs and symptoms of the arrhythmia, potential quinidine side effects, etc.) should be followed to confirm that the patient is responding to treatment and not developing adverse drug reactions.

- When quinidine serum concentrations are measured in patients and a dosage change is necessary, clinicians should seek to use the simplest, most straightforward method available to determine a dose that will provide safe and effective treatment.

  - In most cases, a simple dosage ratio can be used to change quinidine doses, assuming the drug follows *linear pharmacokinetics.*
  - Sometimes it is useful to compute quinidine pharmacokinetic constants for a patient and base dosage adjustments on these parameters. In this case it may be possible to calculate and use *pharmacokinetic parameters* to alter the quinidine dose. Since steady-state concentrations are used, this technique will give the same dosage as the linear pharmacokinetics method. But since clearance is calculated, the value for the patient can be compared to the population average and previous measurements made in the patient.
  - In some situations it may be necessary to compute quinidine pharmacokinetic parameters for the patient as soon as possible, before steady-state conditions occur, and utilize these parameters to calculate the best drug dose. Computerized methods that incorporate expected population pharmacokinetic characteristics (*Bayesian pharmacokinetic computer programs*) can be used in difficult cases when serum concentrations are obtained at suboptimal times or the patient was not at steady state when serum concentrations were measured.

    - An additional benefit is that a complete pharmacokinetic workup (determination of clearance, volume of distribution, and half-life) can be done with one or more measured concentrations that do not have to be at steady state.

Linear Pharmacokinetics Method

- Because quinidine follows linear, dose-proportional pharmacokinetics in most patients, steady-state serum concentrations change in proportion to dose according to the following equation:

$$D_{new}/Css_{new} = D_{old}/Css_{old} \quad \text{or} \quad D_{new} = (Css_{new}/Css_{old})D_{old}$$

  where D is the dose, Css is the steady-state concentration, old indicates the dose that produced the steady-state concentration the patient is currently receiving, and new denotes the dose necessary to produce the desired steady-state concentration.
- The advantages of this method are that it is quick and simple. The main disadvantage is that steady-state concentrations are required.
- Because nonlinear pharmacokinetics for quinidine have been observed in some patients, suggested dosage increases greater than 75% using this method should be scrutinized by the prescribing clinician, and the risk versus benefit for the patient assessed before initiating large dosage increases (>75% over current dose).

▶ ***Example 1***   OI is a 60-year-old, 85-kg (height 6′1″) male with atrial fibrillation who requires therapy with oral quinidine sulfate extended-release tablets. He has liver cirrhosis (Child-Pugh score = 11). The patient's current steady-state quinidine concentration is 7.4 µg/ml at a dose of 600 mg every 12 hours. Compute a quinidine dose that will provide a steady-state concentration of 3 µg/ml.

  1. *Compute new dose to achieve desired serum concentration.* The patient can be expected to achieve steady-state conditions after 2 days ($5t_{1/2}$ = 5 · 9 h = 45 h) of therapy.

Using linear pharmacokinetics, the new dose to attain the desired concentration should be proportional to the old dose that produced the measured concentration (*Note:* Total daily dose = 600 mg/dose · 2 doses/day = 1200 mg/d):

$$D_{new} = (Css_{new}/Css_{old})D_{old} = (3\ \mu g/ml/7.4\ \mu g/ml)\ 1200\ mg/d$$
$$= 486\ mg/d, \text{rounded to } 600\ mg/d$$

The new suggested dose is 300 mg every 12 hours of quinidine sulfate extended-release tablets. If the patient experiences adverse drug effects, the new dosage regimen can be delayed for 1–2 estimated half-lives ($t_{1/2}$ = 9 h).

A steady-state quinidine serum concentration can be measured after steady state is attained in 3–5 half-lives. Since the patient is expected to have a drug half-life of 9 hours, the quinidine steady-state concentration can be obtained any time after the second day of dosing (5 half-lives = 5 · 9 h = 45 h). Quinidine serum concentrations should also be measured if the patient experiences a return of arrhythmia, or if the patient develops potential signs or symptoms of quinidine toxicity.

▶ *Example 2* MN is a 64-year-old, 78-kg (height 5′9″) male with ventricular tachycardia who requires therapy with oral quinidine sulfate immediate-release tablets. He has moderate heart failure (New York Heart Association CHF class III). The patient's current steady-state quinidine concentration is 2.2 μg/ml at a dose of 100 mg every 6 hours. Compute a quinidine dose that will provide a steady-state concentration of 4 μg/ml.

1. *Compute new dose to achieve desired serum concentration.* The patient can be expected to achieve steady-state conditions after 2 days ($5t_{1/2}$ = 5 · 7 h = 35 h) of therapy.

    Using linear pharmacokinetics, the new dose to attain the desired concentration should be proportional to the old dose that produced the measured concentration (*Note:* Total daily dose = 100 mg/dose · 4 doses/day = 400 mg/d):

$$D_{new} = (Css_{new}/Css_{old})D_{old} = (4\ \mu g/ml/2.2\ \mu g/ml)\ 400\ mg/d$$
$$= 727\ mg/d, \text{rounded to } 800\ mg/d \text{ or } 200\ mg \text{ every } 6\ h$$

The new suggested dose is 200 mg every 6 hours of quinidine sulfate immediate-release tablets, to begin immediately.

A steady-state quinidine serum concentration can be measured after steady state is attained in 3–5 half-lives. Since the patient is expected to have a drug half-life of 7 hours, the quinidine steady-state concentration can be obtained any time after the second day of dosing (5 half-lives = 5 · 7 h = 35 h). Quinidine serum concentrations should also be measured if the patient experiences a return of arrhythmia, or if the patient develops potential signs or symptoms of quinidine toxicity.

Pharmacokinetic Parameter Method

- The pharmacokinetic parameter method of adjusting drug doses allows the computation of an individual's own, unique pharmacokinetic constants and uses those to calculate a dose that achieves desired quinidine concentrations.

- If the patient is receiving oral quinidine therapy, quinidine clearance (Cl) can be calculated using the following formula:

$$Cl = \frac{F \cdot S(D / \tau)}{Css}$$

where F is the bioavailability fraction for the oral dosage form (F = 0.7 for most oral quinidine products), S is the fraction of the quinidine salt form that is active quinidine (S = 0.83 for quinidine sulfate, S = 0.62 for quinidine gluconate, S = 0.60 for quinidine polygalacturonate), D is the dose of quinidine salt in mg, Css is the steady-state quinidine concentration, and τ is the dosage interval in hours.

- Because this method also assumes linear pharmacokinetics, quinidine doses computed using the pharmacokinetic parameter method and the linear pharmacokinetic method should be identical.

▶ *Example 1*   OI is a 60-year-old, 85-kg (height 6′1″) male with atrial fibrillation who requires therapy with oral quinidine sulfate extended-release tablets. He has liver cirrhosis (Child-Pugh score = 11). The patient's current steady-state quinidine concentration is 7.4 µg/ml at a dose of 600 mg every 12 hours. Compute a quinidine dose that will provide a steady-state concentration of 3 µg/ml.

1. *Compute pharmacokinetic parameters.* The patient can be expected to achieve steady-state conditions after the second day ($5t_{1/2} = 5 \cdot 9$ h = 45 h) of therapy.

    Quinidine clearance can be computed using a steady-state quinidine concentration:

$$Cl = \frac{F \cdot S(D / \tau)}{Css} = \frac{0.7 \cdot 0.83(600 \, mg / 12h)}{7.4 \, mg / L} = 3.93 L / l$$

    (*Note:* µg/ml = mg/L, and this concentration unit was substituted for Css in the calculations so that unit conversion was not required.)

2. *Compute quinidine dose.* Quinidine clearance is used to compute the new dose:

$$D = \frac{Css \cdot Cl \cdot \tau}{F \cdot S} = \frac{3mg / L \cdot 3.93L / h \cdot 12h}{0.7 \cdot 0.83}$$

$$= 244 \, mg, \text{ rounded to } 300 \, mg \text{ every } 12h$$

The new quinidine dose should be instituted immediately.

   A steady-state quinidine serum concentration can be measured after steady state is attained in 3–5 half-lives. Since the patient is expected to have a drug half-life of 9 hours, the quinidine steady-state concentration can be obtained any time after the second day of dosing (5 half-lives = $5 \cdot 9$ h = 45 h). Quinidine serum concentrations should also be measured if the patient experiences a return of arrhythmia, or if the patient develops potential signs or symptoms of quinidine toxicity.

▶ *Example 2*   MN is a 64-year-old, 78-kg (height 5′9″) male with ventricular tachycardia who requires therapy with oral quinidine sulfate immediate-release tablets. He has moderate heart failure (NYHA CHF class III). The patient's current steady-state quinidine concentration is 2.2 µg/ml at a dose of 100 mg every 6 hours. Compute a quinidine dose that will provide a steady-state concentration of 4 µg/ml.

1. *Compute pharmacokinetic parameters.* The patient can be expected to achieve steady-state conditions after the second day ($5t_{1/2} = 5 \cdot 7$ h = 35 h) of therapy.

    Quinidine clearance can be computed using a steady-state quinidine concentration:

$$Cl = \frac{F \cdot S(D / \tau)}{Css} = \frac{0.7 \cdot 0.83(100mg / 6h)}{2.2mg / L} = 4.40L / l$$

(*Note:* µg/ml = mg/L and this concentration unit was substituted for Css in the calculations so that unnecessary unit conversion was not required.)

2. *Compute quinidine dose.* Quinidine clearance is used to compute the new dose:

$$D = \frac{Css \cdot Cl \cdot \tau}{F \cdot S} = \frac{4mg / L \cdot 4.40L / h \cdot 6h}{0.7 \cdot 0.83}$$
$$= 182 \text{ mg, rounded to 200 mg every 6h}$$

The new quinidine dose should be instituted immediately.

A steady-state quinidine serum concentration can be measured after steady state is attained in 3–5 half- lives. Since the patient is expected to have a drug half-life of 7 hours, the quinidine steady-state concentration can be obtained any time after the second day of dosing (5 half-lives = $5 \cdot 7$ h = 35 h). Quinidine serum concentrations should also be measured if the patient experiences a return of arrhythmia, or if the patient develops potential signs or symptoms of quinidine toxicity.

Bayesian Pharmacokinetic Computer Programs

• Computer programs are available that can assist in the computation of pharmacokinetic parameters for patients. The most reliable computer programs use a nonlinear regression algorithm that incorporates components of Bayes' theorem.

  • An advantage of this approach is that consistent dosage recommendations are made when several different practitioners are involved in therapeutic drug monitoring programs. However, since simpler dosing methods work just as well for patients with stable pharmacokinetic parameters and steady-state drug concentrations, many clinicians reserve the use of computer programs for more difficult situations. Those situations include serum concentrations that are not at steady state, serum concentrations not obtained at the specific times needed to employ simpler methods, and unstable pharmacokinetic parameters.
  • When only a limited number of quinidine concentrations are available, Bayesian pharmacokinetic computer programs can be used to compute a complete patient pharmacokinetic profile that includes clearance, volume of distribution, and half-life.

• Many Bayesian pharmacokinetic computer programs are available, and most should provide answers similar to the program used in the following examples. The program used to solve problems in this book is DrugCalc, written by Dr. Dennis Mungall and available at his Internet web site (www.clinpharmacologist.bigstep.com/consumersurvey.html).[41]

▶ *Example 1* OY is a 57-year-old, 79-kg (height 5′8″) male with ventricular tachycardia who requires therapy with oral quinidine gluconate. He has normal liver (bilirubin = 0.7 mg/dl, albumin = 4.0 gm/dl) and cardiac function. He started taking quinidine gluconate 648 mg every 12 hours at 0800 H. His quinidine serum concentration is 2.1 µg/ml at 0730 H on the second day of therapy, before the morning dose is given. Compute a quinidine gluconate dose that will provide a steady-state concentration of 4 µg/ml.

1. *Enter patient demographic, drug dosing, and serum concentration/time data into a Bayesian pharmacokinetic computer program.* In this case it is unlikely that the patient is at steady state, so the linear pharmacokinetics method cannot be used. The DrugCalc program requires quinidine salt doses be input in terms of quinidine base. A dose of 648 mg of quinidine gluconate is equivalent to 400 mg of quinidine base (400 mg quinidine base = 648 mg quinidine gluconate · 0.62).

2. *Compute pharmacokinetic parameters for the patient using the computer program.* The pharmacokinetic parameters computed by the program are a volume of distribution of 181 L, a half-life of 15.2 h, and a clearance of 8.21 L/h.

3. *Compute dose required to achieve desired quinidine serum concentrations.* The oral one-compartment-model equation used by the program to compute doses indicates that 972 mg of quinidine gluconate every 12 hours will produce a steady-state trough concentration of 4.7 µg/ml. (*Note:* DrugCalc uses salt form A and sustained-action options for quinidine gluconate.) This dose should be started immediately.

▶ *Example 2* SL is a 71-year-old, 82-kg (height 5′10″) male with atrial fibrillation who requires therapy with oral quinidine. He has liver cirrhosis (Child-Pugh score = 12, bilirubin = 3.2 mg/dl, albumin = 2.5 gm/dl) and normal cardiac function. He began taking quinidine sulfate extended-release tablets 600 mg every 12 hours at 0700 H. At 0700 H on the second day of therapy, before the morning dose is administered, the quinidine serum concentration is 4.5 µg/ml. Compute a quinidine sulfate dose that will provide a steady-state concentration of 4 µg/ml.

1. *Enter patient demographic, drug dosing, and serum concentration/time data into a Bayesian pharmacokinetic computer program.* In this case it is unlikely that the patient is at steady state, so the linear pharmacokinetics method cannot be used. The DrugCalc program requires quinidine salt doses be input in terms of quinidine base. A dose of 600 mg of quinidine sulfate is equivalent to 500 mg of quinidine base (500 mg quinidine base = 600 mg quinidine sulfate · 0.83).

2. *Compute pharmacokinetic parameters for the patient using the computer program.* The pharmacokinetic parameters computed by the program are a volume of distribution of 161 L, a half-life of 21.4 h, and a clearance of 5.24 L/h.

3. *Compute dose required to achieve desired quinidine serum concentrations.* The oral one-compartment-model equation used by the program to compute doses indicates that 300 mg of quinidine sulfate extended-release tablets every 12 hours will produce a steady-state trough concentration of 4.1 µg/ml. (*Note:* DrugCalc uses salt form B and sustained-action options for quinidine sulfate extended-release tablets.) This dose should be started immediately.

DOSING STRATEGIES

- Initial dose and dosage adjustment techniques using serum concentrations can be used in any combination as long as the limitations of each method are observed.
- Some dosing schemes link together logically when considered according to their basic approaches or philosophies. Dosage strategies that follow similar pathways are given in Table 9-5.

CONVERSION OF QUINIDINE DOSES FROM ONE SALT FORM TO ANOTHER

- Occasionally there is a need to convert a patient stabilized on quinidine therapy from one salt form to an equivalent amount of quinidine base using another salt form.
- In general, oral quinidine dosage forms, including most sustained-release tablets, have a bioavailability of 0.7. Assuming that equal quinidine serum concentrations are desired, this makes conversion between the two salt forms simple, since equivalent doses of drug are prescribed:

$$D_{new} = (D_{old} \cdot S_{old})/S_{new}$$

where D_{new} is the equivalent quinidine base dose for the new quinidine salt dosage form in mg/d, D_{old} is the dose of oral quinidine salt old dosage form in mg/d, and S_{old} and S_{new} are the fractions of the old and new quinidine salt dosage forms that are active quinidine.

▶ **Example 1**   JH is currently receiving oral extended-release quinidine sulfate 600 mg every 12 hours. She is responding well to therapy, has experienced no adverse drug effects, and has a steady-state quinidine concentration of 4.7 μg/ml. Suggest an equivalent dose of extended-release quinidine gluconate to be given to this patient every 8 hours.

1. *Calculate equivalent oral dose of quinidine.* The patient is currently receiving 600 mg every 12 hours, or 1200 mg/d (600 mg/dose · 2 doses/d = 1200 mg/d) of quinidine sulfate. The equivalent quinidine gluconate dose is

$$D_{new} = (D_{old} \cdot S_{old})/S_{new} = (1200 \text{ mg/d} \cdot 0.83)/0.62 = 1606 \text{ mg/d}$$

The dose should be rounded up to 1620 mg/d of quinidine gluconate, or 648 mg at 0700 H, 324 mg at 1500 H, and 648 mg at 2300 H.

TABLE 9-5 Dosing Strategies

Dosing approach/ philosophy	Initial dosing	Use of serum concentrations to alter doses
Pharmacokinetic parameters/ equations	Pharmacokinetic dosing method	Pharmacokinetic parameter method
Literature-based/ concept	Literature-based recommended dosing	Linear pharmacokinetic method
Computerized	Bayesian computer program	Bayesian computer programs

▶ *Example 2* LK is currently receiving oral extended-release quinidine gluconate 648 mg every 12 hours. He is responding well to therapy, has experienced no adverse drug effects, and has a steady-state quinidine concentration of 3.3 μg/ml. Suggest an equivalent dose of immediate-release oral quinidine sulfate for this patient.

1. *Calculate equivalent oral dose of quinidine.* The patient is currently receiving 648 mg every 12 hours or 1296 mg/d (648 mg/dose · 2 doses/d = 1296 mg/d) of quinidine gluconate. The equivalent quinidine sulfate dose is

$$D_{new} = (D_{old} \cdot S_{old})/S_{new} = (1296 \text{ mg/d} \cdot 0.62)/0.83 = 968 \text{ mg/d}$$

The dose should be rounded to 800 mg/d of quinidine sulfate, or 200 mg every 6 hours.

REFERENCES

1. Roden DM. Antiarrhythmic drugs. In: Hardman JG, Limbird LE, Gilman AG, eds. The pharmacological basis of therapeutics. 10th ed. New York: McGraw-Hill, 2001:933–70.
2. Bauman JL, Schoen MD. Arrhythmias. In: DiPiro JT, Talbert RL, Yee GC, Matzke GR, Wells BG, Posey LM, eds. Pharmacotherapy. 5th ed. New York: McGraw-Hill, 2002:273–304.
3. Ueda CT, Williamson BJ, Dzindzio BS. Absolute quinidine bioavailability. Clin Pharmacol Ther 1976;20(3):260–5.
4. Ueda CT, Hirschfeld DS, Scheinman MM, Rowland M, Williamson BJ, Dzindzio BS. Disposition kinetics of quinidine. Clin Pharmacol Ther 1976;19(1):30–6.
5. Woo E, Greenblatt DJ. A reevaluation of intravenous quinidine. Am Heart J 1978;96(6):829–32.
6. Greenblatt DJ, Pfeifer HJ, Ochs HR, et al. Pharmacokinetics of quinidine in humans after intravenous, intramuscular and oral administration. J Pharmacol Exp Ther 1977;202(2):365–78.
7. Ueda CT, Dzindzio BS. Quinidine kinetics in congestive heart failure. Clin Pharmacol Ther 1978;23(2):158–64.
8. Ueda CT, Dzindzio BS. Bioavailability of quinidine in congestive heart failure. Br J Clin Pharmacol 1981;11(6):571–7.
9. Covinsky JO, Russo J Jr, Kelly KL, Cashman J, Amick EN, Mason WD. Relative bioavailability of quinidine gluconate and quinidine sulfate in healthy volunteers. J Clin Pharmacol 1979;19(5–6):261–9.
10. Gibson DL, Smith GH, Koup JR, Stewart DK. Relative bioavailability of a standard and a sustained-release quinidine tablet. Clin Pharm 1982;1(4):366–8.
11. McGilveray IJ, Midha KK, Rowe M, Beaudoin N, Charette C. Bioavailability of 11 quinidine formulations and pharmacokinetic variation in humans. J Pharm Sci 1981;70(5):524–9.
12. Ochs HR, Greenblatt DJ, Woo E, Franke K, Pfeifer HJ, Smith TW. Single and multiple dose pharmacokinetics of oral quinidine sulfate and gluconate. Am J Cardiol 1978;41(4):770–7.
13. Woo E, Greenblatt DJ, Ochs HR. Short- and long-acting oral quinidine preparations: clinical implications of pharmacokinetic differences. Angiology 1978;29(3):243–50.
14. Drayer DE, Lowenthal DT, Restivo KM, Schwartz A, Cook CE, Reidenberg MM. Steady-state serum levels of quinidine and active metabolites in cardiac patients with varying degrees of renal function. Clin Pharmacol Ther 1978;24(1):31–9.
15. Drayer DE, Hughes M, Lorenzo B, Reidenberg MM. Prevalence of high (3S)-3-hydroxyquinidine/quinidine ratios in serum, and clearance of quinidine in cardiac patients with age. Clin Pharmacol Ther 1980;27(1):72–5.

16. Holford NH, Coates PE, Guentert TW, Riegelman S, Sheiner LB. The effect of quinidine and its metabolites on the electrocardiogram and systolic time intervals: concentration—effect relationships. Br J Clin Pharmacol 1981;11(2):187–95.

17. Rakhit A, Holford NH, Guentert TW, Maloney K, Riegelman S. Pharmacokinetics of quinidine and three of its metabolites in man. J Pharmacokinet Biopharm 1984;12(1):1–21.

18. Ueda CT, Dzindzio BS. Pharmacokinetics of dihydroquinidine in congestive heart failure patients after intravenous quinidine administration. Eur J Clin Pharmacol 1979;16(2):101–5.

19. Ueda CT, Williamson BJ, Dzindzio BS. Disposition kinetics of dihydroquinidine following quinidine administration. Res Commun Chem Pathol Pharmacol 1976; 14(2):215–25.

20. Narang PK, Crouthamel WG. Dihydroquinidine contamination of quinidine raw materials and dosage forms: rapid estimation by high-performance liquid chromatography. J Pharm Sci 1979;68(7):917–9.

21. Russo J Jr, Russo ME, Smith RA, Pershing LK. Assessment of quinidine gluconate for nonlinear kinetics following chronic dosing. J Clin Pharmacol 1982;22(5-6): 264–70.

22. Chen BH, Taylor EH, Ackerman BH, Olsen K, Pappas AA. Effect of pH on free quinidine [letter]. Drug Intell Clin Pharm 1988;22(10):826.

23. Mihaly GW, Cheng MS, Klein MB. Difference in the binding of quinine and quinidine to plasma proteins. Br J Clin Pharmacol 1987;24:769–74.

24. Woo E, Greenblatt DJ. Pharmacokinetic and clinical implications of quinidine protein binding. J Pharm Sci 1979;68(4):466–70.

25. Carliner NH, Crouthamel WG, Fisher ML, et al. Quinidine therapy in hospitalized patients with ventricular arrhythmias. Am Heart J 1979;98(6):708–15.

26. Conrad KA, Molk BL, Chidsey CA. Pharmacokinetic studies of quinidine in patients with arrhythmias. Circulation 1977;55(1):1–7.

27. Guentert TW, Holford NH, Coates PE, Upton RA, Riegelman S. Quinidine pharmacokinetics in man: choice of a disposition model and absolute bioavailability studies. J Pharmacokinet Biopharm 1979;7(4):315–30.

28. Kessler KM, Humphries WC Jr, Black M, Spann JF. Quinidine pharmacokinetics in patients with cirrhosis or receiving propranolol. Am Heart J 1978;96(5):627–35.

29. Powell JR, Okada R, Conrad KA, Guentert TW, Riegelman S. Altered quinidine disposition in a patient with chronic active hepatitis. Postgrad Med J 1982;58(676): 82–4.

30. Pugh RN, Murray-Lyon IM, Dawson JL, Pietroni MC, Williams R. Transection of the oesophagus for bleeding oesophageal varices. Br J Surg 1973;60(8):646–9.

31. Crouthamel WG. The effect of congestive heart failure on quinidine pharmacokinetics. Am Heart J 1975;90(3):335–9.

32. Kessler KM, Lowenthal DT, Warner H, Gibson T, Briggs W, Reidenberg MM. Quinidine elimination in patients with congestive heart failure or poor renal function. N Engl J Med 1974;290(13):706–9.

33. Ochs HR, Greenblatt DJ, Woo E, Smith TW. Reduced quinidine clearance in elderly persons. Am J Cardiol 1978;42(3):481–5.

34. Gunn VL, Nechyba C, eds. The Harriet Lane handbook: a manual for pediatric house officers. 16th ed. Philadelphia: Mosby, 2002.

35. Hall K, Meatherall B, Krahn J, Penner B, Rabson JL. Clearance of quinidine during peritoneal dialysis. Am Heart J 1982;104(3):646–7.

36. Chin TW, Pancorbo S, Comty C. Quinidine pharmacokinetics in continuous ambulatory peritoneal dialysis. Clin Exp Dial Apheresis 1981;5(4):391–7.

37. Hansten PD, Horn JR. Drug interactions analysis and management. Vancouver, WA: Applied Therapeutics, 1998.

38. Muralidharan G, Cooper JK, Hawes EM, Korchinski ED, Midha KK. Quinidine inhibits the 7-hydroxylation of chlorpromazine in extensive metabolisers of debrisoquine. Eur J Clin Pharmacol 1996;50(1-2):121–8.

39. von Moltke LL, Greenblatt DJ, Cotreau-Bibbo MM, Duan SX, Harmatz JS, Shader RI. Inhibition of desipramine hydroxylation in vitro by serotonin-reuptake-inhibitor antidepressants, and by quinidine and ketoconazole: a model system to predict drug interactions in vivo. J Pharmacol Exp Ther 1994;268(3):1278–83.

40. von Moltke LL, Greenblatt DJ, Duan SX, Daily JP, Harmatz JS, Shader RI. Inhibition of desipramine hydroxylation (Cytochrome P450-2D6) in vitro by quinidine and by viral protease inhibitors: relation to drug interactions in vivo. J Pharm Sci 1998;87(10):1184–9.

41. Wandell M, Mungall D. Computer assisted drug interpretation and drug regimen optimization. Am Assoc Clin Chem 1984;6:1–11.

42. Johnson JA, Parker RB, Patterson JH. Heart failure. In: DiPiro JT, Talbert RL, Yee GC, Matzke GR, Wells BG, Posey LM, eds. Pharmacotherapy—a pathophysiologic approach. 5th ed. New York: McGraw-Hill, 2002:185–218.

4 | ANTICONVULSANTS

10 | Phenytoin

Phenytoin is a hydantoin compound related to the barbiturates that is used for the treatment of seizures. It is an effective anticonvulsant for the chronic treatment of tonic-clonic (grand mal) or partial seizures and the acute treatment of generalized status epilepticus (Table 10-1).[1] Phenytoin is also a type 1B antiarrhythmic that is particularly useful in the treatment of digitalis-induced arrhythmias. It is also used in the treatment of trigeminal neuralgia.

- The antiseizure activity of phenytoin is related to its ability to inhibit the repetitive firing of action potentials caused by prolonged depolarization of neurons.[2,3] Additionally, phenytoin stops the spread of abnormal discharges from epileptic foci, thereby decreasing the spread of seizure activity throughout the brain.

THERAPEUTIC AND TOXIC CONCENTRATIONS

- The usual therapeutic range for total (unbound + bound) phenytoin serum concentrations when the drug is used in the treatment of seizures is 10–20 µg/ml. Since phenytoin is highly bound (~90%) to albumin, it is prone to plasma protein-binding displacement due to a large variety of factors.

  - The suggested therapeutic range for unbound phenytoin concentrations is based on the usual unbound fraction (10%) of phenytoin in individuals with normal plasma protein binding. Thus, the generally accepted therapeutic range for unbound phenytoin concentrations is 1–2 µg/ml.

- In the upper part of the therapeutic range (>15 µg/ml), some patients will experience minor central nervous system depression side effects such as drowsiness or fatigue.[2,3]

  - At total phenytoin concentrations above 20 µg/ml, nystagmus may occur and can be especially prominent upon lateral gaze.
  - When total concentrations exceed 30 µg/ml, ataxia, slurred speech, and/or incoordination can be observed.
  - If total phenytoin concentrations are above 40 µg/ml, mental status changes, including decreased mentation, severe confusion or lethargy, and coma are possible.
  - Drug-induced seizure activity has been observed at concentrations over 50–60 µg/ml.

- Because phenytoin follows nonlinear or saturable metabolism pharmacokinetics, it is possible to attain excessive drug concentrations with modest dosage increases.

CLINICAL USEFULNESS OF UNBOUND PHENYTOIN CONCENTRATIONS

- Total phenytoin serum concentrations are the mainstream way to gauge therapy with the anticonvulsant. In most patients without known or identifiable plasma protein-binding abnormalities, the unbound fraction of phenytoin will be normal (~10%) and unbound drug concentration measurement is unnecessary.

TABLE 10-1 International Classification of Epileptic Seizures[1]

Major class	Subset of class	Drug treatment for selected seizure type

Partial seizures (beginning locally)	1. Simple partial seizures (without impaired consciousness)
	   a. With motor symptoms
	   b. With somatosensory or special sensory symptoms
	   c. With autonomic symptoms
	   d. With psychological symptoms
		Carbamazepine
		Phenytoin
		Valproic acid
		Phenobarbital
		Primidone

	2. Complex partial seizures (with impaired consciousness)
	   a. Simple partial onset followed by impaired consciousness
	   b. Impaired consciousness at onset
		Carbamazepine
		Phenytoin
		Valproic acid
		Phenobarbital
		Primidone

	3. Partial seizures evolving into secondary generalized seizures	Carbamazepine Phenytoin Valproic acid Phenobarbital Primidone
Generalized seizures (convulsive or nonconvulsive)	1. Absence seizures (typical or atypical; also known as petite mal seizures)	Valproic acid Ethosuximide
	2. Tonic-clonic seizures (also known as grand mal seizures)	Carbamazepine Phenytoin Valproic acid Phenobarbital Primidone

- The relationship between total concentration (C), unbound or "free" concentration (C_f), and unbound or "free" fraction (f_B) is $C_f = f_B C$.

- Unbound phenytoin serum concentration monitoring should be restricted to those patients with known reasons to have altered drug plasma protein binding. Exceptions to this approach are patients with an augmented or excessive pharmacological response compared to their total phenytoin concentration.

  - If a patient has a satisfactory anticonvulsant response to a low total phenytoin concentration, one possible reason might be abnormal plasma protein binding ($f_B \geq 20\%$) for some unidentified reason.

- Unbound phenytoin serum concentrations should be measured in patients with factors known to alter phenytoin plasma protein binding. These factors fall into three broad categories: (1) lack of binding protein when there are insufficient plasma concentrations of albumin; (2) displacement of phenytoin from albumin-binding sites by endogenous compounds; and (3) displacement of phenytoin from albumin-binding sites by exogenous compounds (Table 10-2).[4–22]

  - Hypoalbuminemia can be found in patients with liver disease or the nephrotic syndrome, pregnant women, cystic fibrosis patients, burn patients, trauma patients, malnourished individuals, and the elderly.

TABLE 10-2 Disease States and Conditions That Alter Phenytoin Plasma Protein Binding

Insufficient albumin concentration (hypoalbuminemia)	Displacement by endogenous compounds	Displacement by exogenous compounds
Liver disease	Hyperbilirubinemia	Drug interactions
Nephrotic syndrome	Jaundice	Warfarin
Pregnancy	Liver disease	Valproic acid
Cystic fibrosis	Renal dysfunction	Aspirin (>2 g/d)
Burns		NSAIDs with high
Trauma		albumin binding
Malnourishment		
Elderly		

- Albumin concentrations below 3 g/dl are associated with high phenytoin unbound fractions in the plasma. Patients with albumin concentrations between 2.5 and 3 g/dl typically have phenytoin unbound fractions of 15–20%, while patients with albumin concentrations between 2.0 and 2.5 g/dl often have unbound phenytoin fractions > 20%.

- Displacement of phenytoin from plasma protein-binding sites by endogenous substances can occur in patients with hepatic or renal dysfunction.

  - Total bilirubin concentrations in excess of 2 mg/dl are associated with abnormal phenytoin plasma protein binding.
  - End-stage renal disease patients (creatinine clearance <10–15 ml/min) with uremia accumulate unidentified compound(s) in their blood that displace phenytoin from plasma protein-binding sites. Abnormal phenytoin binding persists in these patients even when dialysis procedures are instituted.

- Phenytoin plasma protein-binding displacement can also occur due to exogenously administered compounds such as drugs. Other drugs that are highly bound to albumin and cause plasma protein-binding displacement drug interactions with phenytoin include warfarin, valproic acid, aspirin (>2 g/d), and some highly bound nonsteroidal anti-inflammatory agents.

- Once the free fraction (f_B) has been determined for a patient with altered phenytoin plasma protein binding ($f_B = C_f/C$, where C is the total concentration and C_f is the unbound concentration), it is often not necessary to obtain additional unbound drug concentrations. If the situations that caused altered plasma protein binding are stable (albumin or bilirubin concentration, hepatic or renal function, other drug doses, etc.), total phenytoin concentrations can be converted to concurrent unbound values and used for therapeutic drug monitoring purposes.

  - If the disease state status or drug therapy changes, a new unbound phenytoin fraction will be present and needs to be remeasured using an unbound/total phenytoin concentration pair.

- When unbound phenytoin concentrations are unavailable, several methods have been suggested to estimate the value or a surrogate measure of the value. The most common surrogate is an estimation of the equivalent total phenytoin concentration that would provide the same unbound phenytoin

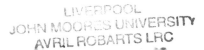

concentration if the patient had a normal unbound fraction value of 10%. These calculations "normalize" the total phenytoin concentration so that it can be compared to the usual phenytoin therapeutic range of 10–20 μg/ml and used for dosage-adjustment purposes.

- These equations provide only estimates of their respective concentrations, and actual unbound phenytoin concentrations should be measured whenever possible in patients with suspected abnormal phenytoin plasma protein binding.
- The equation for hypoalbuminemia is

$$C_{Normal\ Binding} = C/(X \cdot Alb + 0.1)$$

where $C_{Normal\ Binding}$ is the normalized total phenytoin concentration in μg/ml, C is the actual measured phenytoin concentration in μg/ml, X is a constant equal to 0.2 if protein-binding measurements were conducted at 37°C or 0.25 if conducted at 25°C, and Alb is the albumin concentration in g/dl.[23,24] [*Note:* In most experimental laboratories, protein binding is determined at normal body temperature (37°C); in most clinical laboratories, protein binding is determined at room temperature (25°C).]

  - If the patient has end-stage renal disease (creatinine clearance <10–15 ml/min), the same equation is used with a different constant value (X = 0.1).[23]
  - Because these methods assume that the normal unbound fraction of phenytoin is 10%, the estimated unbound phenytoin concentration (C_{fEST}) is computed using the following formula:

$$(C_{fEST}) = 0.1\ C_{Normal\ Binding}$$

- A different approach is taken with the equations used for patients receiving concurrent valproic acid administration. In this case, the unbound phenytoin concentration (C_{fEST}) is estimated using simultaneously measured total phenytoin (PHT in μg/ml) and valproic acid (VPA in μg/ml) concentrations:[25,26]

$$C_{fEST} = (0.095 + 0.001 \cdot VPA)PHT$$

This value is compared to the usual therapeutic range for unbound phenytoin concentrations (1–2 μg/ml) and used for dosage-adjustment purposes.

▶ *Example 1*   JM is an epileptic patient being treated with phenytoin. He has hypoalbuminemia (albumin = 2.2 g/dl) and normal renal function (creatinine clearance = 90 ml/min). His total phenytoin concentration is 7.5 μg/ml. Assuming that any unbound concentrations performed by the clinical laboratory will be conducted at 25°C, compute an estimated normalized phenytoin concentration for this patient.

1. *Choose an appropriate equation to estimate normalized total phenytoin concentration at the appropriate temperature.*

$$C_{Normal\ Binding} = C/(0.25 \cdot Alb + 0.1) = (7.5\ \mu g/ml)/(0.25 \cdot 2.2\ g/dl + 0.1)$$
$$= 11.5\ \mu g/ml$$

$$(C_{fEST}) = 0.1 C_{Normal\ Binding} = 0.1 \cdot 11.5\ \mu g/ml = 1.2\ \mu g/ml$$

This patient's estimated normalized total phenytoin concentration is expected to provide an unbound concentration equivalent to a total phenytoin concentration of 11.5 μg/ml for a patient with normal drug protein binding (C_{fEST} = 1.2 µg/ml). Because the estimated total value is within the therapeutic range 10–20 µg/ml, it is likely that the patient has an unbound phenytoin concentration within the therapeutic range. If possible, this should be confirmed by obtaining an actual, measured unbound phenytoin concentration.

▶ *Example 2* LM is an epileptic patient being treated with phenytoin. He has hypoalbuminemia (albumin = 2.2 g/dl) and poor renal function (creatinine clearance = 10 ml/min). His total phenytoin concentration is 7.5 µg/ml. Compute an estimated normalized phenytoin concentration for this patient.

1. *Choose an appropriate equation to estimate normalized total phenytoin concentration.*

$$C_{Normal\ Binding} = C/(0.1 \cdot Alb + 0.1) = (7.5\ µg/ml)/(0.1 \cdot 2.2\ g/dl + 0.1)$$
$$= 23.4\ µg/ml$$
$$(C_{fEST}) = 0.1\ C_{Normal\ Binding} = 0.1 \cdot 23.4\ µg/ml = 2.3\ µg/ml$$

This patient's estimated normalized total phenytoin concentration is expected to provide an unbound concentration equivalent to a total phenytoin concentration of 23.4 µg/ml for a patient with normal drug protein binding (C_{fEST} = 2.3 µg/ml). Because the estimated total value is above the therapeutic range 10–20 µg/ml, it is likely that the patient has an unbound phenytoin concentration above the therapeutic range. If possible, this should be confirmed by obtaining an actual, measured unbound phenytoin concentration.

▶ *Example 3* PM is an epileptic patient being treated with phenytoin and valproic acid. He has a normal albumin concentration (albumin = 4.2 g/dl) and normal renal function (creatinine clearance = 90 ml/min). His steady-state total phenytoin and valproic acid concentrations are 7.5 µg/ml and 100 µg/ml, respectively. Compute an estimated unbound phenytoin concentration for this patient.

1. *Choose an appropriate equation to estimate unbound phenytoin concentration.*

$$C_{fEST} = (0.095 + 0.001 \cdot VPA)PHT$$
$$= (0.095 + 0.001 \cdot 100\ µg/ml)(7.5\ µg/ml) = 1.5\ µg/ml$$

This patient's estimated unbound phenytoin concentration is expected to be within the therapeutic range for unbound concentrations. If possible, this should be confirmed by obtaining an actual, measured unbound phenytoin concentration.

CLINICAL MONITORING PARAMETERS

• The goal of therapy with anticonvulsants is to reduce seizure frequency and maximize quality of life with a minimum of adverse drug effects.[3] While it is desirable to entirely abolish seizure episodes, it may not be possible to accomplish this in many patients.
• Patients should be monitored for concentration-related side effects (drowsiness, fatigue, nystagmus, ataxia, slurred speech, incoordination, mental status changes, decreased mentation, confusion, lethargy, coma) as well as adverse reactions associated with long-term use (behavioral changes,

cerebellar syndrome, connective tissue changes, coarse facies, skin thickening, folate deficiency, gingival hyperplasia, lymphadenopathy, hirsutism, osteomalacia). Idiosyncratic side effects include skin rash, Stevens-Johnson syndrome, bone marrow suppression, systemic lupus-like reactions, and hepatitis.

- Phenytoin serum concentrations should be measured in most patients and are valuable tools to optimize therapy and to avoid adverse drug effects. Because phenytoin follows nonlinear or saturable pharmacokinetics, it is fairly easy to attain toxic concentrations with modest changes in drug dose.

BASIC CLINICAL PHARMACOKINETIC PARAMETERS

- Phenytoin is primarily eliminated by hepatic metabolism (>95%). Hepatic metabolism is mainly via the CYP2C9 enzyme system, with a smaller amount metabolized by CYP2C19. About 5% of a phenytoin dose is recovered in the urine as unchanged drug.
- Phenytoin follows Michaelis-Menten or saturable pharmacokinetics.[27,28] This is the type of nonlinear pharmacokinetics that occurs when the number of drug molecules overwhelms or saturates the enzyme's ability to metabolize the drug. When this occurs, steady-state drug serum concentrations increase in a disproportionate manner after a dosage increase (Figure 10-1).

  - The rate of drug removal is described by the classic Michaelis-Menten relationship that is used for all enzyme systems:

  $$\text{Rate of metabolism} = (V_{max} \cdot C)/(K_m + C)$$

  where V_{max} is the maximum rate of metabolism in mg/d, C is the phenytoin concentration in μg/ml, and K_m is the substrate concentration in μg/ml and the rate of metabolism = $V_{max}/2$.

  - The clinical implication of Michaelis-Menten pharmacokinetics is that the clearance of phenytoin is not a constant as it is with linear pharmacokinetics,

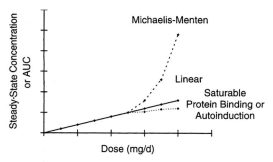

FIG. 10-1   If a drug follows linear pharmacokinetics, Css or area under the curve (AUC) increases proportionally with dose, resulting in a straight line on the plot. Nonlinear pharmacokinetics occurs when the Css or AUC/dose plot results in something other than a straight line. If a drug follows Michaelis-Menten pharmacokinetics (e.g., phenytoin, aspirin), as steady-state drug concentrations approach K_m, serum concentrations increase more than expected due to dose increases. If a drug follows nonlinear protein binding (e.g., valproic acid, disopyramide), total steady-state drug concentrations increase less than expected as dose increases.

but is concentration- or dose-dependent. As the dose or concentration of phenytoin increases, the clearance rate (Cl) decreases as the enzyme approaches saturable conditions:

$$Cl = V_{max}/(K_m + C)$$

This is the reason concentrations increase disproportionately after a phenytoin dosage increase.

- There is so much interpatient variability in Michaelis-Menten pharmacokinetic parameters for phenytoin (typically, V_{max} = 100–1000 mg/d and K_m = 1–15 μg/ml) that dosing the drug is extremely difficult.

- Phenytoin volume of distribution (V = 0.7 L/kg) is unaffected by saturable metabolism and is still determined by the physiological volume of blood (V_B) and tissues (V_T) as well as the unbound concentration of drug in the blood (f_B) and tissues (f_T):

$$V = V_B + (f_B/f_T)V_T$$

- Half-life ($t_{1/2}$) is still related to clearance and volume of distribution using the same equation as for linear pharmacokinetics:

$$t_{1/2} = (0.693 \cdot V)/Cl$$

However, since clearance is dose- or concentration-dependent, half-life also changes with phenytoin dosage or concentration changes.

- As doses or concentrations increase for a drug that follows Michaelis-Menten pharmacokinetics, clearance decreases and half-life becomes longer for the drug.
- The clinical implication of this finding is that the time to steady state (3–5 half-lives) is longer for phenytoin as the dose or concentration is increased. On average, the time to steady-state serum concentrations is approximately 5 days at a dosage of 300 mg/d and 15 days at a dosage of 400 mg/d.[27]

- Under steady-state conditions the rate of drug administration equals the rate of drug removal.[29] Therefore, the Michaelis-Menten equation can be used to compute the maintenance dose (MD in mg/d) required to achieve a target steady-state phenytoin serum concentration (Css in μg/ml or mg/L):

$$MD = \frac{V_{max} \cdot Css}{K_m + Css}$$

or, solved for Css,

$$Css = \frac{K_m \cdot MD}{V_{max} - MD}$$

- When K_m >> Css, phenytoin follows linear pharmacokinetics. First-order pharmacokinetics is another name for linear pharmacokinetics.
- When Css >> K_m, the rate of phenytoin metabolism becomes a constant equal to V_{max}. This situation is known as zero-order pharmacokinetics.

- For parenteral use, phenytoin is available in two different dosage forms.

- Phenytoin sodium contains 92% phenytoin by weight. To facilitate dissolution, ethanol and propylene glycol are added to the vehicle, and the pH of the solution is a adjusted to between 10 and 12. When phenytoin sodium is given intravenously, injection rates should not exceed 50 mg/min to avoid hypotension. Even at lower infusion rates, profound hypotension can result in patients with unstable blood pressure or shock.

- Phenytoin sodium injection can be given by slow intravenous push of undiluted drug, or added to normal saline at a concentration of 10 mg/ml or less and infused at <50 mg/min. When the drug is added to normal saline, it should be given as soon as possible after being mixed to avoid precipitation, and a 0.22-μm inline filter should be used to remove any drug crystals before they reach the patient.

- To avoid many of the problems associated with phenytoin sodium injection, a water-soluble phosphate ester prodrug of phenytoin, fosphenytoin, has been developed. Conversion of fosphenytoin to phenytoin is rapid, with a fosphenytoin half-life of approximately 15 minutes. To avoid confusion, fosphenytoin is prescribed in terms of phenytoin sodium equivalents (PEs). Thus, 100 mg PE of fosphenytoin is equivalent to 100 mg of phenytoin sodium.

  - Hypotension during intravenous administration fosphenytoin is much less of a problem than with phenytoin sodium.
  - The maximal intravenous infusion rate is 150 mg PE/min. Transient pruritus and paresthesia are associated with this route of administration.
  - Intramuscular absorption is rapid, with a peak concentration occurring about 30 minutes after injection, and bioavailability via this route of administration is 100%.
  - Fosphenytoin is much more expensive that phenytoin sodium injection, and this has limited its widespread use. Most clinicians reserve fosphenytoin use for patients who require intramuscular phenytoin, or patients with unstable or low blood pressure who require intravenous phenytoin therapy.

- For oral use, capsules contain phenytoin sodium (92% phenytoin, by weight), while tablets and suspensions contain phenytoin.

  - Phenytoin sodium capsules are labeled as either extended phenytoin sodium capsules or prompt phenytoin capsules.

    - Extended phenytoin capsules release phenytoin slowly from the gastrointestinal tract into the systemic circulation. The extended-release characteristics of this dosage form are due to the slow dissolution of the drug in gastric juices and not the result of extended-release dosage-form technology. Extended phenytoin sodium capsules are available in 30-, 100-, 200-, and 300-mg strengths.
    - Prompt phenytoin sodium capsules are absorbed fairly quickly from the gastrointestinal tract because they contain microcrystalline phenytoin sodium, which dissolves more quickly in gastric juices. As a result of their sustained-release properties, phenytoin doses given as extended phenytoin sodium capsules can be given every once or twice daily, but prompt phenytoin sodium capsules must be given multiple times daily.

  - Phenytoin tablets (50 mg, chewable) and suspension (125 mg/5 ml and 30 mg/5 ml) for oral use are available as the acid form of the drug. Both the tablet and suspension dosage forms are absorbed more rapidly than extended phenytoin sodium capsules, and once-daily dosing with these may not be possible in some patients.

- Because phenytoin follows nonlinear pharmacokinetics, an 8% difference in dose between dosage forms containing phenytoin (suspension and tablets, 100 mg = 100 mg phenytoin) and phenytoin sodium (capsules and injection, 100 mg = 92 mg phenytoin) can result in major changes in phenytoin serum concentrations.

  - Usually, phenytoin doses are not fine-tuned to the point of accounting directly for the difference in phenytoin content. Rather, clinicians are aware that when phenytoin dosage forms are changed, phenytoin content may change, and they anticipate that the drug concentration may increase or decrease because of this. Therefore, most clinicians recheck phenytoin serum concentrations after a dosage-form change is instituted.

- The oral bioavailability of phenytoin is very good for capsule, tablet, and suspension dosage forms and approximates 100%.[30–33] At larger amounts, there is some dose dependency on absorption characteristics.[34]

  - Single oral doses of 800 mg or more produce longer times for maximal concentrations to occur (T_{max}) and decreased bioavailability. Since larger oral doses also produce a higher incidence of gastrointestinal side effects (primarily nausea and vomiting due to local irritation), it is prudent to break maintenance doses larger than 800 mg/d into multiple doses.
  - If oral phenytoin loading doses are given, a common total dose is 1000 mg given as 400 mg, 300 mg, and 300 mg, separated by 2–6-hour time intervals.

- Enteral feedings given by nasogastric tube interfere with phenytoin absorption.[35–38] The solution to this problem is to stop the feedings, when possible, for 1–2 hours before and after phenytoin administration, and increase the oral phenytoin dose. It is not unusual for phenytoin oral dosage requirements to double or triple while the patient receives concurrent nasogastric feedings.

  - Intravenous phenytoin, or intravenous or intramuscular fosphenytoin doses, can also be substituted while nasogastric feedings are being administered.

- Although it is poorly documented, phenytoin oral malabsorption may also occur in patients with severe diarrhea, malabsorption syndromes, or gastric resection.
- The typical recommended loading dose for phenytoin is 15–20 mg/kg, resulting in 1000 mg for most adult patients.
- Usual initial maintenance doses are 5–10 mg/kg/d for children (6 months–16 years old) and 4–6 mg/kg/d for adults.

  - For adults, the most often prescribed dose is 300–400 mg/d of phenytoin. Because of an increased incidence of adverse effects in older patients (>65 years old), many clinicians prescribe a maximum of 200 mg/d as an initial dose for these individuals.[39,40]

EFFECT OF ALTERED PLASMA PROTEIN BINDING ON PHENYTOIN PHARMACOKINETICS

- For phenytoin, a drug with a low hepatic extraction ratio, plasma protein-binding displacement drug interactions cause major pharmacokinetic alterations but are not clinically significant because the pharmacological effect of the drug does not change (Figure 10-2A).

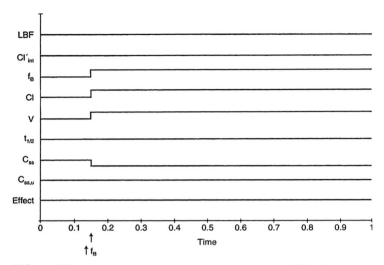

FIG. 10-2A   Schematic representation of physiological (LBF = liver blood flow, Cl'_{int} = intrinsic or unbound clearance, f_B = unbound fraction of drug in blood/plasma), pharmacokinetic (Cl = clearance; V = volume of distribution; $t_{1/2}$ = half-life; Css = total steady-state drug concentration; Css_u = unbound steady-state drug concentration), and pharmacodynamic (Effect = pharmacodynamic effect) changes that occur with decreased protein binding of phenytoin (arrow denotes $\uparrow f_B$).

- Because the clearance of the drug is dependent on the fraction of unbound drug in the blood and intrinsic clearance for an agent with a low hepatic extraction ratio, a decrease in plasma protein binding and an increase in unbound fraction will increase clearance ($\uparrow Cl = \uparrow f_B Cl'_{int}$) and volume of distribution [$\uparrow V = V_B + (\uparrow f_B/f_T)V_T$].
- Since half-life depends on clearance and volume of distribution, it is likely that because both increase, half-life will not change substantially [$t_{1/2} = (0.693 \cdot \uparrow V)/\uparrow Cl$]. However, it is possible that if either clearance or volume of distribution changes disproportionately, half-life will change.
- The total steady-state concentration will decline because of the increase in clearance ($\downarrow Css = k_0/\uparrow Cl$, where k_0 is the infusion rate of the drug). However, the unbound steady-state concentration will remain unaltered because the free fraction of drug in the blood is higher than it was before the increase in unbound fraction occurred ($Css_u = \uparrow f_B \downarrow Css$).
- The pharmacological effect of the drug does not change, because the free concentration of drug in the blood is unchanged.

- Clinicians need to be on the outlook for situations like this, because the total drug concentration (bound + unbound) can be misleading and can cause an unwarranted increase in drug dosage. Unbound drug concentrations should be used to convince clinicians that a drug dosage increase is not needed, even though total concentrations decline as a result of this interaction.

EFFECTS OF DISEASE STATES AND CONDITIONS ON PHARMACOKINETICS AND DOSING

- Measurement of V_{max} and K_m for phenytoin is very difficult to accomplish for research or clinical purposes. Therefore, the effects of disease states and conditions on these parameters is largely unknown. By necessity, this discussion will be in qualitative terms for phenytoin.
- Adults without the disease states and conditions discussed later in this section, with normal liver and renal function as well as normal plasma protein binding (~90%), have an average phenytoin V_{max} of 7 mg/kg/d (range 1.5–14 mg/kg/d) and a K_m of 4 µg/ml (range 1–15 µg/ml).[28]

Infants/Children

- Michaelis-Menten parameters for younger children ($\frac{1}{2}$–6 years) are $V_{max} = 12$ mg/kg/d and $K_m = 6$ µg/ml, while for older children (7–16 years), $V_{max} = 9$ mg/kg/d and $K_m = 6$ µg/ml.[41–46]

Liver Dysfunction

- Patients with liver cirrhosis or acute hepatitis have reduced phenytoin clearance because of destruction of liver parenchyma. This loss of functional hepatic cells reduces the amount of CYP2C9 and CYP2C19 available to metabolize the drug and decreases V_{max}. The volume of distribution is larger because of reduced plasma protein binding. Protein binding is reduced and unbound fraction is increased due to hypoalbuminemia and/or hyperbilirubinemia (especially albumin ≤3 g/dl and/or total bilirubin ≥2 mg/dl).

  - The effects that liver disease have on phenytoin pharmacokinetics are highly variable and difficult to predict accurately. It is possible for a patient with liver disease to have relatively normal or grossly abnormal phenytoin clearance and volume of distribution.

  - An index of liver dysfunction can be gained by applying the Child-Pugh clinical classification system (Table 10-3).[47] Child-Pugh scores are discussed more fully in Chapter 3 (Drug Dosing in Special Populations: Renal and Hepatic Disease, Dialysis, Heart Failure, Obesity, and Drug Interactions).

    - The Child-Pugh score consists of five laboratory tests or clinical symptoms: serum albumin, total bilirubin, prothrombin time, ascites, and hepatic encephalopathy. Each of these areas is given a score of 1 (normal) to 3 (severely abnormal; Table 10-3), and the scores for the five areas are summed.

TABLE 10-3 Child-Pugh Scores for Patients with Liver Disease[47]

Test/symptom	Score 1 point	Score 2 points	Score 3 points
Total bilirubin (mg/dl)	<2.0	2.0–3.0	>3.0
Serum albumin (g/dl)	>3.5	2.8–3.5	<2.8
Prothrombin time (seconds prolonged over control)	<4	4–6	>6
Ascites	Absent	Slight	Moderate
Hepatic Encephalopathy	None	Moderate	Severe

- The Child-Pugh score for a patient with normal liver function is 5, while the score for a patient with grossly abnormal serum albumin, total bilirubin, and prothrombin time values in addition to severe ascites and hepatic encephalopathy is 15. A Child-Pugh score greater than 8 is grounds for a decrease of 25–50% in the initial daily drug dose for phenytoin.
- As in any patient, with or without liver dysfunction, initial doses are meant as starting points for dosage titration based on patient response and avoidance of adverse effects. Phenytoin serum concentrations and the presence of adverse drug effects should be monitored frequently in patients with liver cirrhosis.

Trauma/Burns

- Trauma and burn patients have an increased ability to metabolize phenytoin beginning 3–7 days after their initial injury.[48,49] At this time, these patients become hypermetabolic, and the V_{max} for phenytoin increases. If caloric needs are not met during this phase of recovery for trauma patients, many become hypoalbuminemic and phenytoin plasma protein binding decreases, resulting in an increase unbound fraction.
- Phenytoin dosage requirements are increased while trauma and burn patients are in their hypermetabolic phase, and unbound concentration monitoring is indicated when patients have low albumin concentrations (especially for albumin levels ≤3 g/dl).

Pregnancy

- Pregnant women taking phenytoin have increased dosage requirements, particularly during the third trimester (>26 weeks).[4,5,50–54] There are several reasons for this change, including malabsorption of drug resulting in decreased bioavailability, increased metabolism of phenytoin, and decreased protein binding due to low albumin concentrations.
- Aggressive drug serum concentration monitoring, including the measurement of unbound phenytoin concentrations if the patient is hypoalbuminemic, is necessary to avoid seizures and subsequent harm to the unborn fetus. An additional concern when administering phenytoin to pregnant patients is the development of fetal hydantoin syndrome by the baby.

Elderly

- Individuals over the age of 65 have a decreased capacity to metabolize phenytoin, possibly due to age-related losses of liver parenchyma resulting in decreased amounts of CYP2C9 and CYP2C19.[39,40] Older patients also may have hypoalbuminemia with resulting decreases in plasma protein binding and increases in unbound fraction.[21,22]
- Many elderly patients also seem to have an increased propensity for central nervous system side effects due to phenytoin, and because of these pharmacokinetic and pharmacodynamic changes, clinicians tend to prescribe lower initial phenytoin doses for older patients (~200 mg/d).

Renal Dysfunction

- End-stage renal disease patients with creatinine clearances <10–15 ml/min have an unidentified substance in their blood that displaces phenytoin from

its plasma protein-binding sites.[14–18,20] This unknown compound is not removed by dialysis.[19]
- These patients also tend to have hypoalbuminemia, which increases the unbound fraction of phenytoin even further. Unbound phenytoin serum concentration monitoring is very helpful in determining dosage requirements for renal failure patients.

Hypoalbuminemia

- Other patients are also prone to hypoalbuminemia, including patients with the nephrotic syndrome, cystic fibrosis patients, and malnourished individuals. Unbound phenytoin concentration monitoring should be considered in these patients, especially when albumin concentrations are ≤3 g/dl.

Dialysis

- Hemodialysis does not remove enough phenytoin that supplemental post-dialysis doses are necessary.[55] The typical sieving coefficient during hemoperfusion for phenytoin is 0.45, so in some cases supplemental phenytoin doses may be needed.[56,57] Because of pharmacokinetic variability, phenytoin concentrations in patients receiving hemoperfusion should be checked.

Hyperbilirubinemia

- High bilirubin concentrations can also be found in patients with biliary tract obstruction or hemolysis. Unbound phenytoin concentration monitoring should be considered in these patients, especially when total bilirubin concentrations are ≥2 mg/dl.

DRUG INTERACTIONS

- Because phenytoin is so highly metabolized in the liver by CYP2C9 and CYP2C19, it is prone to drug interactions that inhibit hepatic microsomal enzymes.[58] Cimetidine, valproic acid, amiodarone, chloramphenicol, isoniazid, disulfiram, and omeprazole have been reported to inhibit phenytoin metabolism and increase phenytoin serum concentrations.
- Phenytoin is also a broad-based hepatic enzyme inducer that affects most cytochrome P450 systems. Drugs with narrow therapeutic ranges that can have their metabolism increased by concurrent phenytoin administration include carbamazepine, phenobarbital, cyclosporin, tacrolimus, and warfarin. When phenytoin therapy is added to the medication regimen for a patient, a comprehensive review for drug interactions should be conducted.
- Valproic acid, aspirin (>2 g/d), some highly protein-bound nonsteroidal antiinflammatory drugs, and warfarin can displace phenytoin from plasma protein-binding sites, necessitating monitoring of unbound phenytoin concentrations.

  - The drug interaction between valproic acid and phenytoin deserves special mention because of its complexity and because these two agents are regularly used together for the treatment of seizures.[6–9] The drug interaction involves the plasma protein-binding displacement and intrinsic clearance inhibition of phenytoin by valproic acid. What makes this interaction so difficult to detect and understand is that these two changes do not occur

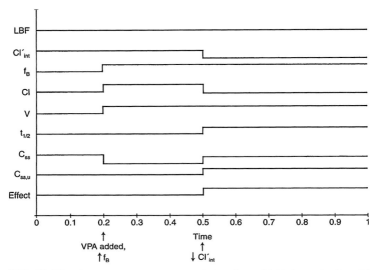

FIG. 10-2B Schematic representation of the effect of initiating valproic acid (VPA) treatment in an individual stabilized on phenytoin therapy (see Figure 10-2A legend for symbols). Initially, valproic acid decreases phenytoin plasma protein binding via competitive displacement for binding sites on albumin (arrow denotes ↑f_B). As valproic acid concentrations increase, the hepatic enzyme inhibition component of the drug interaction comes into play (arrow denotes ↓Cl'_{int}). The net result is total phenytoin concentrations that are largely unchanged from baseline, but unbound phenytoin concentrations and pharmacological effect increase.

simultaneously, so the impression left by the drug interaction depends on when in time it is observed in a patient (Figure 10-2B).

INITIAL DOSAGE DETERMINATION METHODS

- Several methods to initiate phenytoin therapy are available:

  - The *pharmacokinetic dosing method* is the most flexible of the techniques. It allows individualized target serum concentrations to be chosen for a patient, and each pharmacokinetic parameter can be customized to reflect specific disease states and conditions present in the patient.

    - Unfortunately, specific values for Michaelis-Menten pharmacokinetic variables are not known for many disease states and conditions because they are difficult to measure. Even when values are available, there is 10–15-fold variation for each parameter. Also, the pharmacokinetic dosing method is computationally intensive.

  - *Literature-based recommended dosing* is a very commonly used method to prescribe initial doses of phenytoin. Doses are based on those that commonly produce steady-state concentrations in the lower part of the therapeutic range, although there is a wide variation in the actual concentrations for specific patients.

Pharmacokinetic Dosing Method

- The goal of initial dosing with phenytoin is to compute the best dose possible for the patient given the set of disease states and conditions that influence phenytoin pharmacokinetics. The optimal way to accomplish this goal is to use average parameters measured in other patients with similar disease state and condition profiles as estimates of pharmacokinetic constants for the patient currently being treated with the drug.

  - Unfortunately, because of the difficulty in computing Michaelis-Menten parameters, accurate estimates of V_{max} and K_m are not available for many important patient populations.
  - Even if average population Michaelis-Menten constants are available, the 10–15-fold variation in these parameters means that initial doses derived from these parameters will not be successful in achieving desired goals in all patients.
  - Phenytoin serum concentration monitoring, including unbound concentration measurement if altered plasma protein binding is suspected, is an important component of therapy for this drug.
  - If the patient has significant hepatic dysfunction (Child-Pugh score ≥ 8), maintenance doses computed using this method should be decreased by 25–50%, depending on how aggressive therapy is required to be for the individual.

Michaelis-Menten Parameter Estimates

- Normal adults with normal liver and renal function as well as normal plasma protein binding have an average phenytoin V_{max} of 7 mg/kg/d and a K_m of 4 µg/ml. Michaelis-Menten parameters for younger children ($\frac{1}{2}$–6 years) are $V_{max} = 12$ mg/kg/d and $K_m = 6$ µg/ml, while for older children (7–16 years), $V_{max} = 9$ mg/kg/d and $K_m = 6$ µg/ml.

Volume of Distribution Estimates

- The volume of distribution for patients with normal phenytoin plasma protein binding is estimated at 0.7 L/kg for adults. For obese individuals, 30% or more above their ideal body weight, the volume of distribution can be estimated using the following equation:

$$V = 0.7 \text{ L/kg } [\text{IBW} + 1.33(\text{TBW} - \text{IBW})]$$

where IBW is ideal body weight in kg [$\text{IBW}_{females}$ (in kg) = 45 + 2.3(Ht − 60) or IBW_{males} (in kg) = 50 + 2.3(Ht − 60)], Ht is height in inches, and TBW is total body weight in kg.[59]

  - This parameter is used to estimate the loading dose (LD in mg) for phenytoin, if one is indicated:

$$LD = Css \cdot V$$

where Css is the desired total phenytoin concentration in mg/L (*Note:* mg/L = µg/ml, and this conversion was made directly to avoid unit conversion) and V is volume of distribution in L.

Selection of Appropriate Pharmacokinetic Model and Equations

- When phenytoin is given by short-term intravenous infusion or orally, the drug follows a one-compartment pharmacokinetic model. When oral therapy is required, most clinicians utilize an extended phenytoin capsule dosage form that has good bioavailability ($F = 1$), supplies a continuous release of phenytoin into the gastrointestinal tract, and provides a smooth phenytoin serum concentration/time curve that emulates an intravenous infusion after once- or twice-daily dosing.

  - The Michaelis-Menten pharmacokinetic equation that computes the average phenytoin steady-state serum concentration (Css in µg/ml = mg/L) is widely used and allows maintenance dosage calculation:

$$MD = \frac{V_{max} \cdot Css}{S(K_m + Css)}$$

  or, solved for Css;

$$Css = \frac{K_m \cdot (S \cdot MD)}{V_{max} - (S \cdot MD)}$$

  where V_{max} is the maximum rate of metabolism in mg/d, S is the fraction of the phenytoin salt form that is active phenytoin (0.92 for phenytoin sodium injection and capsules; 0.92 for fosphenytoin because doses are prescribed as a phenytoin sodium equivalent or PE, 1.0 for phenytoin acid suspensions and tablets), MD is the maintenance dose of the phenytoin salt contained in the dosage form in mg/d, Css is the phenytoin concentration in mg/L (which equals µg/ml), and K_m is the substrate concentration in mg/L (which equals µg/ml) where the rate of metabolism = $V_{max}/2$.

- The equation used to calculate loading doses (LD in mg) is based on a simple one-compartment model:

$$LD = (Css \cdot V)/S$$

  where Css is the desired phenytoin steady-state concentration in µg/ml which is equivalent to mg/L, V is the phenytoin volume of distribution, and S is the fraction of the phenytoin salt form that is active (0.92 for phenytoin sodium injection and capsules; 0.92 for fosphenytoin because doses are prescribed as a phenytoin sodium equivalent or PE, 1.0 for phenytoin acid suspensions and tablets).

- Intravenous phenytoin sodium doses should be short-term infusions given no faster than 50 mg/min, and intravenous fosphenytoin doses should be short-term infusions given no faster than 150 mg/min PE.

Steady-State Concentration Selection

- The generally accepted therapeutic ranges for total and unbound phenytoin concentrations are 10–20 and 1–2 µg/ml, respectively, for the treatment of seizures.

  - Unbound concentrations represent the portion of phenytoin that is in equilibrium with the central nervous system and should most accurately reflect drug concentration at the site of action. Thus, for patients with altered phenytoin plasma protein binding, it is more important to have the unbound concentration within its therapeutic range than the total concentration.

- To establish that the unbound fraction (f_B) is altered for a patient, phenytoin total and unbound concentrations should be measured simultaneously from the same blood sample: $f_B = C_f/C$, where C is the total phenytoin concentration in µg/ml and C_f is the unbound, or "free," phenytoin concentration in µg/ml.
- As long as the disease states or conditions that caused altered phenytoin plasma protein binding are stable, a previously measured unbound fraction can be used to convert newly measured total phenytoin concentrations to their unbound equivalent ($C_f = f_B C$).

▶ **Example 1** TD is a 50-year-old, 75-kg (height 5'10") male with simple partial seizures who requires therapy with oral phenytoin. He has normal liver and renal function. Suggest an initial phenytoin dosage regimen designed to achieve a steady-state phenytoin concentration of 12 µg/ml.

1. *Estimate Michaelis-Menten constants according to disease states and conditions present in the patient.* The V_{max} for a nonobese adult patient with normal liver and renal function is 7 mg/kg/d. For a 75-kg patient, $V_{max} = 525$ mg/d:

$$V_{max} = 7 \text{ mg/kg/d} \cdot 75 \text{ kg} = 525 \text{ mg/d}$$

For this individual, $K_m = 4$ mg/L.

2. *Compute dosage regimen.* Oral extended phenytoin sodium capsules will be prescribed to this patient (F = 1, S = 0.92). The initial dosage interval (τ) will be set to 24 hours. (*Note:* µg/ml = mg/L, and this concentration unit was substituted for Css in the calculations so that unit conversion was not required.) The dosage equation for phenytoin is

$$MD = \frac{V_{max} \cdot Css}{S(K_m + Css)} = \frac{525 \text{ mg/d} \cdot 12 \text{ mg/L}}{0.92(4 \text{ mg/L} + 12 \text{ mg/L})}$$

$$= 428 \text{ mg/d, rounded to 400 mg/d}$$

A steady-state trough total phenytoin serum concentration should be measured after steady-state is attained in 7–14 days. Phenytoin serum concentrations should also be measured if the patient experiences an exacerbation of epilepsy, or if the patient develops potential signs or symptoms of phenytoin toxicity.

▶ **Example 2** UO is a 10-year-old, 40-kg male with simple partial seizures who requires therapy with oral phenytoin. He has normal liver and renal function. Suggest an initial phenytoin dosage regimen designed to achieve a steady-state phenytoin concentration of 12 µg/ml.

1. *Estimate Michaelis-Menten constants according to disease states and conditions present in the patient.* The V_{max} for a 7–16-year-old adolescent patient with normal liver and renal function is 9 mg/kg/d. For a 40-kg patient, $V_{max} = 360$ mg/d:

$$V_{max} = 9 \text{ mg/kg/d} \cdot 40 \text{ kg} = 360 \text{ mg/d}$$

For this individual, $K_m = 6$ mg/L.

2. *Compute dosage regimen.* Oral phenytoin suspension will be prescribed to this patient (F = 1, S = 1). The initial dosage interval (τ) will be set to 12 hours. (*Note:* µg/ml = mg/L, and this concentration unit was

substituted for Css in the calculations so that unit conversion was not required.) The dosage equation for phenytoin is

$$MD = \frac{V_{max} \cdot Css}{S(K_m + Css)} = \frac{360 \text{ mg/d} \cdot 12 \text{ mg/L}}{1.0(6 \text{ mg/L} + 12 \text{ mg/L})}$$
$$= 240 \text{ mg/d, rounded to } 250 \text{ mg/d}$$

Phenytoin suspension, 125 mg every 12 hours, should be prescribed for the patient. A steady-state trough total phenytoin serum concentration should be measured after steady state is attained in 7–14 days. Phenytoin serum concentrations should also be measured if the patient experiences an exacerbation of epilepsy, or if the patient develops potential signs or symptoms of phenytoin toxicity.

• To illustrate the differences and similarities between oral and intravenous phenytoin dosage regimen design, the same cases will be used to compute intravenous phenytoin or fosphenytoin loading and maintenance doses.

▶ *Example 3*   TD is a 50-year-old, 75-kg (height 5′10″) male with simple partial seizures who requires therapy with intravenous phenytoin sodium. He has normal liver and renal function. Suggest an initial phenytoin dosage regimen designed to achieve a steady-state phenytoin concentration of 12 μg/ml.

1. *Estimate Michaelis-Menten and volume of distribution constants according to disease states and conditions present in the patient.* The V_{max} for a nonobese adult patient with normal liver and renal function is 7 mg/kg/d. For a 75-kg patient, V_{max} = 525 mg/d:

$$V_{max} = 7 \text{ mg/kg/d} \cdot 75 \text{ kg} = 525 \text{ mg/d}$$

For this individual, K_m = 4 mg/L. The volume of distribution for this patient is 53 L:

$$V = 0.7 \text{ L/kg} \cdot 75 \text{ kg} = 53 \text{ L}$$

2. *Compute dosage regimen.* Intravenous phenytoin sodium will be prescribed to this patient (F = 1, S = 0.92). If a loading dose is needed, it is computed using the following equation:

$$LD = (V \cdot Css)/S = (53 \text{ L} \cdot 12 \text{ mg/L})/0.92$$
$$= 691 \text{ mg, rounded to } 700 \text{ mg at a maximal rate of } 50 \text{ mg/min}$$

(*Note:* μg/ml = mg/L, and this concentration unit was substituted for Css in the calculations so that unit conversion was not required.)

For the maintenance dose, the initial dosage interval (τ) will be set to 12 hours. The dosage equation for phenytoin is

$$MD = \frac{V_{max} \cdot Css}{S(K_m + Css)} = \frac{525 \text{ mg/d} \cdot 12 \text{ mg/L}}{0.92(4 \text{ mg/L} + 12 \text{ mg/L})}$$
$$= 428 \text{ mg/d, rounded to } 400 \text{ mg/d}$$

The patient should be prescribed 200 mg of phenytoin sodium injection every 12 hours using an infusion rate no faster than 50 mg/min.

A steady-state trough total phenytoin serum concentration should be measured after steady state is attained in 7–14 days. Phenytoin serum concentrations should also be measured if the patient experiences an exacerbation of epilepsy, or if the patient develops potential signs or symptoms of phenytoin toxicity.

▶ **Example 4**   UO is a 10-year-old, 40-kg male with simple partial seizures who requires therapy with intravenous fosphenytoin. He has normal liver and renal function. Suggest an initial fosphenytoin dosage regimen designed to achieve a steady-state phenytoin concentration of 12 μg/ml.

1. *Estimate Michaelis-Menten and volume of distribution constants according to disease states and conditions present in the patient.* The V_{max} for a 7–16-year-old adolescent patient with normal liver and renal function is 9 mg/kg/d. For a 40-kg patient, V_{max} = 360 mg/d:

$$V_{max} = 9 \text{ mg/kg/d} \cdot 40 \text{ kg} = 360 \text{ mg/d}$$

For this individual, K_m = 6 mg/L. The volume of distribution for this patient is 28 L:

$$V = 0.7 \text{ L/kg} \cdot 40 \text{ kg} = 28 \text{ L}$$

2. *Compute dosage regimen.* Intravenous fosphenytoin will be prescribed, in phenytoin sodium equivalents or PE, to this patient (F = 1, S = 0.92). If a loading dose is needed, it is computed using the following equation:

$$LD = (V \cdot Css)/S = (28 \text{ L} \cdot 12 \text{ mg/L})/0.92$$
$$= 365 \text{ mg, rounded to 350 mg at a maximal rate of 150 mg/min PE}$$

(*Note:* μg/ml = mg/L, and this concentration unit was substituted for Css in the calculations so that unit conversion was not required.) The dosage equation for phenytoin is

$$MD = \frac{V_{max} \cdot Css}{S(K_m + Css)} = \frac{360 \text{ mg/d} \cdot 12 \text{ mg/L}}{0.92(6 \text{ mg/L} + 12 \text{ mg/L})}$$
$$= 261 \text{ mg/d, rounded to 250 mg/d}$$

Intravenous fosphenytoin, 125 mg PE every 12 hours, given no faster than 150 mg/min PE, should be prescribed for the patient. A steady-state trough total phenytoin serum concentration should be measured after steady state is attained in 7–14 days. Phenytoin serum concentrations should also be measured if the patient experiences an exacerbation of epilepsy, or if the patient develops potential signs or symptoms of phenytoin toxicity.

Literature-Based Recommended Dosing

• Because of the large amount of variability in phenytoin pharmacokinetics, even when concurrent disease states and conditions are identified, many clinicians believe that the use of standard phenytoin doses for various situations is warranted. The original computations of these doses were based on the pharmacokinetic dosing methods described in the previous section, and the doses subsequently modified based on clinical experience. In general, the expected phenytoin steady-state serum concentrations used to compute these doses was 10–15 μg/ml.
• Suggested phenytoin maintenance doses are 4–6 mg/kg/d for adults and 5–10 mg/kg/d for children ($\frac{1}{2}$–16 years old). Phenytoin loading doses are 15–20 mg/kg.

- For obese individuals (>30% over ideal body weight), adjusted body weight (ABW) should be used to compute loading doses:

$$ABW \text{ (in kg)} = IBW + 1.33(TBW - IBW)$$

where IBW is ideal body weight in kg [$IBW_{females}$ (in kg) = 45 + 2.3(Ht − 60) or IBW_{males} (in kg) = 50 + 2.3(Ht − 60)], Ht is height in inches, and TBW is total body weight in kg.[59] Although clearance probably is increased in obese individuals, precise information regarding the best weight factor is lacking for maintenance dose computation, so most clinicians use ideal body weight to calculate this dose.

- If the patient has significant hepatic dysfunction (Child-Pugh score ≥ 8), maintenance doses prescribed using this method should be decreased by 25–50%, depending on how aggressive therapy is required to be for the individual.

- To illustrate the similarities and differences between this method of dosage calculation and the pharmacokinetic dosing method, the same examples used in the previous section will be used.

▶ *Example 1*   TD is a 50-year-old, 75-kg (height 5′10″) male with simple partial seizures who requires therapy with oral phenytoin. He has normal liver and renal function. Suggest an initial phenytoin dosage regimen designed to achieve a steady-state phenytoin concentration of 12 µg/ml.

1. *Estimate phenytoin dose according to disease states and conditions present in the patient.* The suggested initial dosage rate for extended phenytoin sodium capsules in an adult patient is 4–6 mg/kg/d. Using a rate of 5 mg/kg/d, the initial dose is 400 mg/d:

    5 mg/kg/d · 75 kg = 375 mg/d, rounded to 400 mg/d

    Using a dosage interval of 24 hours, the prescribed dose should be 400 mg of extended phenytoin sodium capsules daily.

    A steady-state trough total phenytoin serum concentration should be measured after steady state is attained in 7–14 days. Phenytoin serum concentrations should also be measured if the patient experiences an exacerbation of epilepsy, or if the patient develops potential signs or symptoms of phenytoin toxicity.

▶ *Example 2*   UO is a 10-year-old, 40-kg male with simple partial seizures who requires therapy with oral phenytoin. He has normal liver and renal function. Suggest an initial phenytoin dosage regimen designed to achieve a steady-state phenytoin concentration of 12 µg/ml.

1. *Estimate phenytoin dose according to disease states and conditions present in the patient.* The suggested initial dosage rate for phenytoin suspension in an adolescent patient is 5–10 mg/kg/d. Using a rate of 6 mg/kg/d, the initial dose is 250 mg/d:

    6 mg/kg/d · 40 kg = 240 mg/d, rounded to 250 mg/d

    Using a dosage interval of 12 hours, the prescribed dose should be 125 mg of phenytoin suspension every 12 hours.

    A steady-state trough total phenytoin serum concentration should be measured after steady state is attained in 7–14 days. Phenytoin serum concentrations should also be measured if the patient experiences an exacerbation of epilepsy, or if the patient develops potential signs or symptoms of phenytoin toxicity.

- To illustrate the differences and similarities between oral and intravenous phenytoin dosage regimen design, the same cases will be used to compute intravenous phenytoin or fosphenytoin loading and maintenance doses.

▶ **Example 3**   TD is a 50-year-old, 75-kg (height 5′10″) male with simple partial seizures who requires therapy with intravenous phenytoin sodium. He has normal liver and renal function. Suggest an initial phenytoin dosage regimen designed to achieve a steady-state phenytoin concentration of 12 μg/ml.

1. *Estimate phenytoin dose according to disease states and conditions present in the patient.* The suggested initial dosage rate for phenytoin sodium injection in an adult patient is 4–6 mg/kg/d. Using a rate of 5 mg/kg/d, the initial dose is 400 mg/d:

$$5 \text{ mg/kg/d} \cdot 75 \text{ kg} = 375 \text{ mg/d, rounded to } 400 \text{ mg/d}$$

Using a dosage interval of 12 hours, the prescribed dose should be 200 mg of phenytoin sodium injection every 12 hours. If loading dose administration is necessary, the suggested amount is 15–20 mg/kg. Using 15 mg/kg, the suggested loading dose is 1250 mg of phenytoin sodium injection given no more quickly than 50 mg/min:

$$15 \text{ mg/kg} \cdot 75 \text{ kg} = 1125 \text{ mg, rounded to } 1250 \text{ mg}$$

A steady-state trough total phenytoin serum concentration should be measured after steady state is attained in 7–14 days. Phenytoin serum concentrations should also be measured if the patient experiences an exacerbation of epilepsy, or if the patient develops potential signs or symptoms of phenytoin toxicity.

▶ **Example 4**   UO is a 10-year-old, 40-kg male with simple partial seizures who requires therapy with intravenous fosphenytoin. He has normal liver and renal function. Suggest an initial phenytoin dosage regimen designed to achieve a steady-state phenytoin concentration of 12 μg/ml.

1. *Estimate phenytoin dose according to disease states and conditions present in the patient.* The suggested initial dosage rate for fosphenytoin injection in an adolescent patient is 5–10 mg/kg/d PE. Using a rate of 6 mg/kg/d, the initial dose is 250 mg/d PE:

$$6 \text{ mg/kg/d} \cdot 40 \text{ kg} = 240 \text{ mg/d, rounded to } 250 \text{ mg/d}$$

Using a dosage interval of 12 hours, the prescribed dose should be 125 mg of fosphenytoin injection every 12 hours. If loading dose administration is necessary, the suggested amount is 15–20 mg/kg PE. Using 15 mg/kg, the suggested loading dose is 600 mg PE of fosphenytoin injection given no more quickly than 150 mg/min PE:

$$15 \text{ mg/kg} \cdot 40 \text{ kg} = 600 \text{ mg}$$

A steady-state trough total phenytoin serum concentration should be measured after steady state is attained in 7–14 days. Phenytoin serum concentrations should also be measured if the patient experiences an exacerbation of epilepsy, or if the patient develops potential signs or symptoms of phenytoin toxicity.

USE OF PHENYTOIN SERUM CONCENTRATIONS TO ALTER DOSES

- Because of the large amount of pharmacokinetic variability among patients, it is likely that doses computed using patient population characteristics will not always produce phenytoin serum concentrations that are expected or desirable. Because of pharmacokinetic variability, the Michaelis-Menten pharmacokinetics followed by the drug, the narrow therapeutic index of phenytoin, and the desire to avoid adverse side effects of phenytoin, measurement of phenytoin serum concentrations is conducted for almost all patients to ensure that therapeutic, nontoxic levels are present.
- In addition to phenytoin serum concentrations, important patient parameters (seizure frequency, potential phenytoin side effects, etc.) should be followed to confirm that the patient is responding to treatment and not developing adverse drug reactions.
- When phenytoin serum concentrations are measured in patients and a dosage change is necessary, clinicians should seek to use the simplest, most straightforward method available to determine a dose that will provide safe and effective treatment.

  - A variety of methods are used to estimate new maintenance doses when one steady-state phenytoin serum concentration is available.

    - Based on typical Michaelis-Menten parameters, it is possible to adjust phenytoin doses with a one or more steady-state concentrations using the *empiric dosing method*. This technique is widely used by experienced clinicians to adjust doses.
    - The *Graves-Cloyd method* allows adjustment of phenytoin doses using one steady-state concentration. Because it uses a power function, it is computationally intensive.
    - The *Vozeh-Sheiner method* utilizes a specialized graph and Bayesian pharmacokinetic concepts to individualize phenytoin doses using a single steady-state concentration. Therefore, graph paper with population orbits must be available, and plotting the data is time-consuming.

  - Sometimes it is useful to compute phenytoin pharmacokinetic constants for a patient and base dosage adjustments on these. If two or more steady-state phenytoin serum concentrations are available from two or more different daily dosage rates, it may be possible to calculate and use *pharmacokinetic parameters* to alter the phenytoin dose.

    - Two graphical methods allow the computation of V_{max} and K_m for patients receiving phenytoin, but they are cumbersome and time-consuming.

      - The *Mullen method* uses the same specialized graph as the Vozeh-Sheiner method, but computes the patient's own Michaelis-Menten parameters instead of Bayesian pharmacokinetic estimates.
      - The *Ludden method* uses standard graph paper to plot the concentration/time data, and V_{max} and K_m are computed from the intercept and slope of the resulting line.

  - Computerized methods that incorporate expected population pharmacokinetic characteristics (*Bayesian pharmacokinetic computer programs*) can be used in difficult cases, when serum concentrations are obtained at suboptimal times or the patient was not at steady state when serum concentrations were measured. An additional benefit of this method is that a complete pharmacokinetic workup (V_{max}, K_m, V) can be done with one or more measured concentrations.

• So that results from the different methods can be compared, the same cases are used to compute adjusted doses for phenytoin.

Single Total Phenytoin Steady-State Serum Concentration Methods

Empiric Dosing Method

• Based on knowledge of population Michaelis-Menten pharmacokinetic parameters, it is possible to suggest empiric dosage increases for phenytoin when one steady-state serum concentration is available (Table 10-4).[60] The lower part of the suggested dosage range for each category tends to produce more conservative increases in steady-state concentration, while the upper part of the suggested dosage range tends to produce more aggressive increases.

• These dosage changes are suggested for outpatients, in whom avoiding adverse drug reactions is paramount. For hospitalized patients or patients who require aggressive treatment, larger empiric dosage adjustments may be needed. When dosage increases >100 mg/d are recommended, phenytoin concentrations and patient response should be carefully monitored.

• Whenever possible, clinicians should avoid prescribing more than one solid dosage form strength (i.e., 30- and 100-mg extended phenytoin capsules, etc.) for a patient. An effective way to increase the phenytoin dose for an individual who requires an increase of 50 mg/d when using the 100-mg extended phenytoin sodium capsule dosage form is to increase the dose by 100 mg every other day.

• For example, if a dosage increase of 50 mg/d is desired for an individual receiving 300 mg/d of extended phenytoin sodium capsule, a dosage increase of 300 mg/d alternating with 400 mg/d is possible if the patient is able to comply with a more complex dosage schedule. Alternate daily dosages are possible because of the extended-release characteristics of extended phenytoin capsules and the long half-life of phenytoin.

▶ **Example 1**   TD is a 50-year-old, 75-kg (height 5'10") male with simple partial seizures who requires therapy with oral phenytoin. He has normal liver and renal function. The patient has been prescribed 400 mg/d of extended phenytoin sodium capsules for 1 month, and his steady-state phenytoin total concentration is 6.2 μg/ml. The patient is assessed to be compliant with his dosage

TABLE 10-4 Empiric Phenytoin Dosage Increases Based on a Single Total Steady-State Concentration[60]

Measured phenytoin total serum concentration (μg/ml)	Suggested dosage increase[a]
<7	100 mg/d or more
7–12	50–100 mg/d
>12	30–50 mg/d

[a]Higher dosage used if more aggressive therapy desired, lower dosage used if less aggressive therapy desired.
Source: Modified from Mauro et al.

regimen. Suggest a new phenytoin dosage regimen designed to achieve a steady-state phenytoin concentration within the therapeutic range.

1. *Use Table 10-4 to suggest a new phenytoin dose.* The table suggests a dosage increase of ≥100 mg/d for this patient. The dose should be increased to 500 mg/d.

   A steady-state trough total phenytoin serum concentration should be measured after steady state is attained in 7–14 days. Phenytoin serum concentrations should also be measured if the patient experiences an exacerbation of epilepsy, or if the patient develops potential signs or symptoms of phenytoin toxicity.

▶ ***Example 2*** GF is a 35-year-old, 55-kg female (height 5′4″) with tonic-clonic seizures who requires therapy with oral phenytoin. She has normal liver and renal function. The patient has been prescribed 300 mg/d of extended phenytoin sodium capsules for 1 month, and her steady-state phenytoin total concentration is 10.7 μg/ml. The patient is assessed to be compliant with her dosage regimen. Suggest a new phenytoin dosage regimen designed to achieve a steady-state phenytoin concentration within the middle of the therapeutic range.

1. *Use Table 10-4 to suggest a new phenytoin dose.* The table suggests a dosage increase of 50–100 mg/d for this patient. The dose should be increased to 300 mg/d alternating with 400 mg/d.

   A steady-state trough total phenytoin serum concentration should be measured after steady state is attained in 7–14 days. Phenytoin serum concentrations should also be measured if the patient experiences an exacerbation of epilepsy, or if the patient develops potential signs or symptoms of phenytoin toxicity.

Pseudo-Linear Pharmacokinetics Method

- A simple, easy way to approximate new total serum concentrations after a reasonable phenytoin dosage adjustment has been made is to temporarily assume linear pharmacokinetics, then add 15–33% for a dosage increase or subtract 15–33% for a dosage decrease to account for Michaelis-Menten pharmacokinetics:

$$Css_{new} = (D_{new}/D_{old})Css_{old}$$

where Css_{new} is the expected steady-state concentration from the new phenytoin dose in μg/ml, Css_{old} is the measured steady-state concentration from the old phenytoin dose in μg/ml, D_{new} is the new phenytoin dose to be prescribed in mg/d, and D_{old} is the currently prescribed phenytoin dose in mg/d.[61]

  - *Note:* This method is only intended to provide a rough approximation of the resulting phenytoin steady-state concentration after an appropriate dosage adjustment, such as that suggested by the Mauro dosage chart, has been made. The pseudo-linear pharmacokinetics method should never be used to compute a new dose based on measured and desired phenytoin concentrations.

▶ ***Example 3*** TD is a 50-year-old, 75-kg (height 5′10″) male with simple partial seizures who requires therapy with oral phenytoin. He has normal liver and renal function. The patient has been prescribed 400 mg/d of extended phenytoin sodium capsules for 1 month, and his steady-state phenytoin total concentration is 6.2 μg/ml. The patient is assessed to be compliant with his dosage regimen. Suggest a new phenytoin dosage regimen designed to achieve a steady-state phenytoin concentration within the therapeutic range.

1. *Use pseudo-linear pharmacokinetics to predict the new concentration for the dosage increase, then adjust by 15–33% to account for Michaelis-Menten pharmacokinetics.* Since the patient is receiving extended phenytoin sodium capsules, an appropriate dosage change according to the Mauro dosage chart would be 100 mg/d, so an increase to 500 mg/d is suggested. Using pseudo-linear pharmacokinetics, the resulting total steady-state phenytoin serum concentration is:

$$Css_{new} = (D_{new}/D_{old})Css_{old} = [(500 \text{ mg/d})/(400 \text{ mg/d})](6.2 \text{ μg/ml})$$
$$= 7.8 \text{ μg/ml}$$

Because of Michaelis-Menten pharmacokinetics, the serum concentration is expected to increase by 15%, or 1.15 times, to 33%, or 1.33 times, more than that predicted by linear pharmacokinetics:

$$Css = 7.8 \text{ μg/ml} \cdot 1.15 = 9.0 \text{ μg/ml} \qquad \text{or}$$
$$Css = 7.8 \text{ μg/ml} \cdot 1.33 = 10.4 \text{ μg/ml}$$

Thus, a dosage increase of 100 mg/d can be expected to yield a total phenytoin steady-state serum concentration between 9 and 10 μg/ml.

A steady-state trough total phenytoin serum concentration should be measured after steady state is attained in 7–14 days. Phenytoin serum concentrations should also be measured if the patient experiences an exacerbation of epilepsy, or if the patient develops potential signs or symptoms of phenytoin toxicity.

▶ *Example 4*   GF is a 35-year-old, 55-kg female (height 5′4″) with tonic-clonic seizures who requires therapy with oral phenytoin. She has normal liver and renal function. The patient has been prescribed 300 mg/d of extended phenytoin sodium capsules for 1 month, and her steady-state phenytoin total concentration is 10.7 μg/ml. The patient is assessed to be compliant with her dosage regimen. Suggest a new phenytoin dosage regimen designed to achieve a steady-state phenytoin concentration within the middle of the therapeutic range.

1. *Use pseudo-linear pharmacokinetics to predict the new concentration for the dosage increase, then adjust by 15–33% to account for Michaelis-Menten pharmacokinetics.* Since the patient is receiving extended phenytoin sodium capsules, an appropriate dosage change according to the Mauro dosage chart would be 100 mg/d, so an increase to 400 mg/d is suggested. Using pseudo-linear pharmacokinetics, the resulting total steady-state phenytoin serum concentration is:

$$Css_{new} = (D_{new}/D_{old})Css_{old} = [(400 \text{ mg/d})/(300 \text{ mg/d})](10.7 \text{ μg/ml})$$
$$= 14.3 \text{ μg/ml}$$

Because of Michaelis-Menten pharmacokinetics, the serum concentration can be expected to increase by 15%, or 1.15 times, to 33%, or 1.33 times, more than that predicted by linear pharmacokinetics:

$$Css = 14.3 \text{ μg/ml} \cdot 1.15 = 16.4 \text{ μg/ml} \qquad \text{or}$$
$$Css = 14.3 \text{ μg/ml} \cdot 1.33 = 19.0 \text{ μg/ml}$$

Thus, a dosage increase of 100 mg/d can be expected to yield a total phenytoin steady-state serum concentration between 16 and 19 µg/ml.

A steady-state trough total phenytoin serum concentration should be measured after steady state is attained in 7–14 days. Phenytoin serum concentrations should also be measured if the patient experiences an exacerbation of epilepsy, or if the patient develops potential signs or symptoms of phenytoin toxicity.

Graves-Cloyd Method

• The Graves-Cloyd dosage adjustment method uses a steady-state phenytoin serum concentration to compute the patient's own phenytoin clearance rate $(D_{old}/Css_{old}$, where D_{old} is the administered phenytoin dose in mg/d and Css_{old} is the resulting measured total phenytoin steady-state concentration in µg/ml) at the dosage being given, then uses the measured concentration and desired concentration (Css_{new} in µg/ml) to estimate a new dose (D_{new} in mg/d) for the patient:[62]

$$D_{new} = (D_{old}/Css_{old}) \cdot Css_{new}^{0.199} \cdot Css_{old}^{0.804}$$

▶ **Example 5**   TD is a 50-year-old, 75-kg (height 5'10") male with simple partial seizures who requires therapy with oral phenytoin. He has normal liver and renal function. The patient has been prescribed 400 mg/d of extended phenytoin sodium capsules for 1 month, and his steady-state phenytoin total concentration is 6.2 µg/ml. The patient is assessed to be compliant with his dosage regimen. Suggest a new phenytoin dosage regimen designed to achieve a steady-state phenytoin concentration within the therapeutic range.

1. *Use the Graves-Cloyd method to estimate a new phenytoin dose for the desired steady-state concentration.* Phenytoin sodium 400 mg equals 368 mg of phenytoin (400 mg · 0.92 = 368 mg). A new total phenytoin steady-state serum concentration equal to 10 µg/ml is chosen for the patient:

$$D_{new} = (D_{old}/Css_{old}) \cdot Css_{new}^{0.199} \cdot Css_{old}^{0.804}$$
$$= [(368 \text{ mg/d})/(6.2 \text{ mg/L})] \cdot (10 \text{ mg/L})^{0.199} \cdot (6.2 \text{ mg/L})^{0.804}$$
$$= 407 \text{ mg/d}$$

This dose is equivalent to 442 mg/d of phenytoin sodium (407 mg/0.92 = 442 mg) rounded to 450 mg/d, or 400 mg/d on even days alternating with 500 mg/d on odd days.

A steady-state trough total phenytoin serum concentration should be measured after steady state is attained in 7–14 days. Phenytoin serum concentrations should also be measured if the patient experiences an exacerbation of epilepsy, or if the patient develops potential signs or symptoms of phenytoin toxicity.

▶ **Example 6**   GF is a 35-year-old, 55-kg female (height 5'4") with tonic-clonic seizures who requires therapy with oral phenytoin. She has normal liver and renal function. The patient has been prescribed 300 mg/d of extended phenytoin sodium capsules for 1 month, and her steady-state phenytoin total concentration is 10.7 µg/ml. The patient is assessed to be compliant with her dosage regimen. Suggest a new phenytoin dosage regimen designed to achieve a steady-state phenytoin concentration of 18 µg/ml.

1. *Use the Graves-Cloyd method to estimate a new phenytoin dose for the desired steady-state concentration.* Phenytoin sodium 300 mg equals 276 mg of phenytoin (300 mg · 0.92 = 276 mg). A new total phenytoin steady-state serum concentration equal to 18 µg/ml is chosen for the patient:

$$D_{new} = (D_{old}/Css_{old}) \cdot Css_{new}^{0.199} \cdot Css_{old}^{0.804}$$

$$= [(276 \text{ mg/d})/(10.7 \text{ mg/L})] \cdot (18 \text{ mg/L})^{0.199} \cdot (10.7 \text{ mg/L})^{0.804}$$

$$= 308 \text{ mg/d}$$

This dose is equivalent to 335 mg/d of phenytoin sodium (308 mg/0.92 = 335 mg) rounded to 350 mg/d, or 300 mg/d on odd days alternating with 400 mg/d on even days.

A steady-state trough total phenytoin serum concentration should be measured after steady state is attained in 7–14 days. Phenytoin serum concentrations should also be measured if the patient experiences an exacerbation of epilepsy, or if the patient develops potential signs or symptoms of phenytoin toxicity.

Vozeh-Sheiner or Orbit Graph Method

- A graphical method that employs population Michaelis-Menten information and using Bayes' theorem can also be used to adjust phenytoin doses using a single steady-state total concentration.[63] This method employs a series of orbs encompassing 50%, 75%, 90%, etc., of the population parameter combinations for V_{max} and K_m on the plot suggested by Mullen for use with multiple steady-state/dosage pairs (Figure 10-3). The use of the population's parameter orbs allows the plot to be used with one phenytoin steady-state concentration/dose pair.
- The graph is divided into two sectors. On the left side of the *x* axis, a steady-state total phenytoin concentration is plotted. On the *y* axis, the phenytoin dosage rate (in mg/kg/d of phenytoin; S = 0.92 for phenytoin sodium and fosphenytoin PE dosage forms) is plotted.

  - A straight line is drawn between these two points, extended into the right sector, and through the orbs contained in the right sector. If the line intersects more than one orb, the innermost orb is selected, and the midpoint of the line within that orb is found and marked.
  - The midpoint within the orb and the desired steady-state phenytoin total concentration (on the left portion of the *x* axis) are connected by a straight line. The intersection of this line with the *y* axis is the new phenytoin dose required to achieve the new phenytoin concentration. If needed, the phenytoin dose is converted to phenytoin sodium or fosphenytoin amounts.
  - If a line parallel to the *y* axis is drawn down to the *x* axis from the midpoint of the line within the orb, an estimate of K_m (in µg/ml) is obtained. Similarly, if a line parallel to the *x* axis is drawn to the left to the *y* axis from the midpoint of the line within the orb, an estimate of V_{max} (in mg/kg/d) is obtained.

► *Example 7*   TD is a 50-year-old, 75-kg (height 5′10″) male with simple partial seizures who requires therapy with oral phenytoin. He has normal liver and renal function. The patient has been prescribed 400 mg/d of extended phenytoin sodium capsules for 1 month, and his steady-state phenytoin total

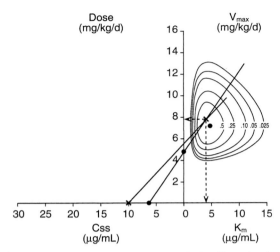

FIG. 10-3 Vozeh-Sheiner or orbit graph employing Bayesian feedback to estimate Michaelis-Menten parameters and phenytoin dose using one steady-state dose/concentration pair (Example 7 data shown). The orbs represent 50%, 75%, 90%, etc., of the population parameter combinations for V_{max} and K_m. The drug dose is converted into a phenytoin amount (in mg/kg/d) and plotted on the y axis (circle, 4.9 mg/kg/d). The concurrent steady-state phenytoin serum concentration is plotted on the left portion of the x axis (circle, 6.2 μg/ml), and the two points are joined with a straight line across the orbs. If the line intersects more than one orb, the innermost orb is selected, and the midpoint of the line within that orb is found and marked (x mark within orbs). The new desired steady-state concentration is identified on the left portion of the x axis (x mark on x axis, 10 μg/ml), and the two x marks are connected by a straight line. The required phenytoin dose is identified at the intersection of the drawn line and the y axis (5.5 mg/kg/d). If necessary, the dose can be converted to phenytoin sodium or fosphenytoin amounts. Estimates of V_{max} (7.9 mg/kg/d) and K_m (4 μg/ml) are obtained by extrapolating parallel lines to the y and x axes, respectively.

concentration is 6.2 μg/ml. The patient is assessed to be compliant with his dosage regimen. Suggest a new phenytoin dosage regimen designed to achieve a steady-state phenytoin concentration within the therapeutic range.

1. *Use the Vozeh-Sheiner method to estimate a new phenytoin dose for the desired steady-state concentration.* A new total phenytoin steady-state serum concentration equal to 10 μg/ml is chosen for the patient. Using the orbit graph, the serum concentration/dose information is plotted (*Note:* phenytoin dose = 0.92 · phenytoin sodium dose = 0.92 · 400 mg/d = 368 mg/d; (368 mg/d)/(75 kg) = 4.9 mg/kg/d; Figure 10-3). According to the graph, a dose of 5.5 mg/kg/d of phenytoin is required to achieve a steady-state concentration of 10 μg/ml. This equals an extended phenytoin sodium capsule dose of 450 mg/d, administered by alternating 400 mg/d on even days and 500 mg/d on odd days: (5.5 mg/kg/d · 75 kg)/0.92 = 448 mg/d, rounded to 450 mg/d.

A steady-state trough total phenytoin serum concentration should be measured after steady state is attained in 7–14 days. Phenytoin serum concentrations should also be measured if the patient experiences an exacerbation of epilepsy, or if the patient develops potential signs or symptoms of phenytoin toxicity.

▶ *Example 8* GF is a 35-year-old, 55-kg female (height 5′4″) with tonic-clonic seizures who requires therapy with oral phenytoin. She has normal liver and renal function. The patient has been prescribed 300 mg/d of extended phenytoin sodium capsules for 1 month, and her steady-state phenytoin total concentration equals 10.7 μg/ml. The patient is assessed to be compliant with her dosage regimen. Suggest a new phenytoin dosage regimen designed to achieve a steady-state phenytoin concentration of 18 μg/ml.

1. *Use the Vozeh-Sheiner method to estimate a new phenytoin dose for the desired steady-state concentration.* A new total phenytoin steady-state serum concentration equal to 18 μg/ml is chosen for the patient. Using the orbit graph, the serum concentration/dose information is plotted (*Note:* phenytoin dose = 0.92 · phenytoin sodium dose = 0.92 · 300 mg/d = 276 mg/d; (276 mg/d)/(55 kg) = 5.0 mg/kg/d; Figure 10-4). According to the graph, a dose of 5.7 mg/kg/d of phenytoin is required to achieve a steady-state concentration of 18 μg/ml. This equals an extended phenytoin sodium capsule dose of 350 mg/d, administered by alternating 300 mg/d on even days and 400 mg/d on odd days: (5.7 mg/kg/d · 55 kg)/0.92 = 341 mg/d, rounded to 350 mg/d.

A steady-state trough total phenytoin serum concentration should be measured after steady state is attained in 7–14 days. Phenytoin serum

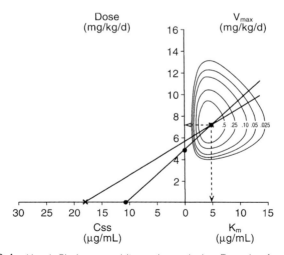

FIG. 10-4 Vozeh-Sheiner or orbit graph employing Bayesian feedback to estimate Michaelis-Menten parameters and phenytoin dose using one steady-state dose/concentration pair. The graph shows the solution for Example 8.

concentrations should also be measured if the patient experiences an exacerbation of epilepsy, or if the patient develops potential signs or symptoms of phenytoin toxicity.

Methods for Two or More Phenytoin Steady-State Serum Concentrations at Two or More Dosage Levels

• In order to utilize each of the dosage schemes in this section, at least two phenytoin steady-state serum concentrations at different dosage rates are needed. This requirement can be difficult to achieve.

Empiric Dosing Method

• Based on knowledge of population Michaelis-Menten pharmacokinetic parameters, it is possible to suggest empiric dosage increases for phenytoin when two or more steady-state serum concentrations at two or more dosage levels are available.[61] For instance, if a patient has steady-state phenytoin concentrations of 11.2 μg/ml on 300 mg/d of phenytoin sodium and 25.3 μg/ml on 400 mg/d of phenytoin sodium, it is obvious that a dose of 350 mg/d of phenytoin sodium will probably produce a steady-state phenytoin serum concentration in the mid to upper part of the therapeutic range.

• Similarly, if a patient has steady-state phenytoin concentrations of 11.2 μg/ml on 300 mg/d of phenytoin sodium and 15.0 μg/ml on 400 mg/d of phenytoin sodium, it is apparent that a dose of 450 mg/d of phenytoin sodium will probably produce a steady-state phenytoin serum concentration in the upper part of the therapeutic range. In this situation, Table 10-4 can be useful to suggest dosage increases.

▶ **Example 1**   TD is a 50-year-old, 75-kg (height 5′10″) male with simple partial seizures who requires therapy with oral phenytoin. He has normal liver and renal function. The patient was prescribed 400 mg/d of extended phenytoin sodium capsules for 1 month, and his steady-state phenytoin total concentration was 6.2 μg/ml. The dosage was increased to 500 mg/d of extended phenytoin sodium capsules for another month, after which the patient's steady-state phenytoin total concentration was 22.0 μg/ml and he had some lateral-gaze nystagmus. The patient is assessed to be compliant with his dosage regimen. Suggest a new phenytoin dosage regimen designed to achieve a steady-state phenytoin concentration within the mid to upper part of the therapeutic range.

1. *Empirically suggest a new phenytoin dose.* The next logical dose to prescribe is phenytoin sodium 450 mg/d to be taken by the patient as 400 mg/d on even days and 500 mg/d on odd days.

   A steady-state trough total phenytoin serum concentration should be measured after steady state is attained in 7–14 days. Phenytoin serum concentrations should also be measured if the patient experiences an exacerbation of epilepsy, or if the patient develops potential signs or symptoms of phenytoin toxicity.

▶ **Example 2**   GF is a 35-year-old, 55-kg female (height 5′4″) with tonic-clonic seizures who requires therapy with oral phenytoin. She has normal liver and renal function. The patient was prescribed 300 mg/d of extended phenytoin sodium capsules for 1 month, and her steady-state phenytoin total concentration was 10.7 μg/ml. At that time, the dose was increased to

350 mg/d of extended phenytoin sodium capsules for an additional month, and the resulting steady-state concentration was 15.8 µg/ml. The patient is assessed to be compliant with her dosage regimen. Suggest a new phenytoin dosage regimen increase designed to achieve a steady-state phenytoin concentration within the upper part of the therapeutic range.

1. *Empirically suggest a new phenytoin dose.* The next logical dose to pre-scribe is phenytoin sodium 400 mg/d (Table 10-4).

    A steady-state trough total phenytoin serum concentration should be measured after steady state is attained in 7–14 days. Phenytoin serum concentrations should also be measured if the patient experiences an exacerbation of epilepsy, or if the patient develops potential signs or symptoms of phenytoin toxicity.

Mullen Method

- The Mullen method dosage approach uses the same dose/concentration plot as that described for the Vozeh-Sheiner or orbit graph method, but the population orbs denoting the Bayesian distribution of V_{max} and K_m are omitted.[64,65]
- The graph is divided into two sectors. On the left side of the x axis, a steady-state total phenytoin concentration is plotted. On the y axis, the phenytoin dosage rate (in mg/kg/d of phenytoin; S = 0.92 for phenytoin sodium and fosphenytoin PE dosage forms) is plotted. A straight line is drawn between these two points and extended into the right sector.
- This process is repeated for all steady-state dose/concentrations pairs that are available. The intersection of these lines in the right sector provides the Michaelis-Menten constant values for the patient.

  - If a line parallel to the y axis is drawn down to the x axis from the intersection point, K_m (in µg/ml) is obtained. Similarly, if a line parallel to the x axis is drawn to the left to the y axis from the intersection point, an estimate of V_{max} (in mg/kg/d) is obtained.

- To compute the new phenytoin dose, the intersection point and the desired steady-state phenytoin total concentration (on the left portion of the x axis) are connected by a straight line. The intersection of this line with the y axis is the new phenytoin dose required to achieve the new phenytoin concentration. If needed, the phenytoin dose is converted to phenytoin sodium or fosphenytoin amounts.

▶ *Example 3* TD is a 50-year-old, 75-kg (height 5′10″) male with simple partial seizures who requires therapy with oral phenytoin. He has normal liver and renal function. The patient was prescribed 400 mg/d of extended phenytoin sodium capsules for 1 month, and his steady-state phenytoin total concentration was 6.2 µg/ml. The dosage was increased to 500 mg/d of extended phenytoin sodium capsules for another month, after which the patient's steady-state phenytoin total concentration was 22.0 µg/ml and he had some lateral-gaze nystagmus. The patient is assessed to be compliant with his dosage regimen. Suggest a new phenytoin dosage regimen designed to achieve a steady-state phenytoin concentration within the therapeutic range.

1. *Use the Mullen method to estimate a new phenytoin dose for the desired steady-state concentration.* The serum concentration/dose information is plotted on the graph. (*Note:* Phenytoin dose = 0.92 · phenytoin

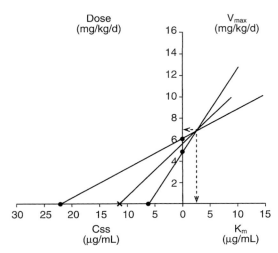

FIG. 10-5 Mullen graph used to compute Michaelis-Menten parameters and phenytoin dose using two or more steady-state dose/concentration pairs (Example 3 data shown). The first dose and concentration are plotted as circles on the y (4.9 mg/kg/d) and x axes (6.2 μg/ml), respectively, and joined by a straight line. This process is repeated for the second dose/concentration pair (6.1 mg/kg/d, 22 μg/ml) plus any others that are available. The intersection of the lines in the right sector of the graph is used to compute a new dose by drawing a straight line between the intersection and the new desired steady-state concentration on the left portion of the x axis (x on x axis, 11.5 μg/ml). The required dose is the intersection of this new line with the y axis (5.5 mg/kg/d). Estimates of V_{max} (6.8 mg/kg/d) and K_m (2.2 μg/ml) are obtained by extrapolating parallel lines to the y and x axes, respectively.

sodium dose = 0.92 · 400 mg/d = 368 mg/d, (368 mg/d)/(75 kg) = 4.9 mg/kg/d; phenytoin dose = 0.92 · phenytoin sodium dose = 0.92 · 500 mg/d = 460 mg/d, (460 mg/d)/(75 kg) = 6.1 mg/kg/d; Figure 10-5). According to the graph, a dose of 5.5 mg/kg/d of phenytoin is required to achieve a steady-state concentration of 11.5 μg/ml. This equals an extended phenytoin sodium capsule dose of 450 mg/d, administered by alternating 400 mg/d on even days and 500 mg/d on odd days: (5.5 mg/kg/d · 75 kg)/0.92 = 448 mg/d, rounded to 450 mg/d. V_{max} = 6.8 mg/kg/d and K_m = 2.2 μg/ml for this patient.

A steady-state trough total phenytoin serum concentration should be measured after steady state is attained in 7–14 days. Phenytoin serum concentrations should also be measured if the patient experiences an exacerbation of epilepsy, or if the patient develops potential signs or symptoms of phenytoin toxicity.

► **Example 4** GF is a 35-year-old, 55-kg female (height 5′4″) with tonic-clonic seizures who requires therapy with oral phenytoin. She has normal liver and renal function. The patient was prescribed 300 mg/d of extended phenytoin sodium capsules for 1 month, and her steady-state phenytoin total

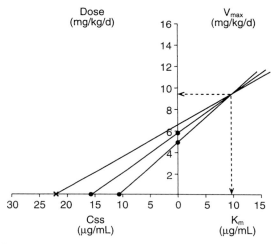

FIG. 10-6   Mullen graph used to estimate Michaelis-Menten parameters and phenytoin dose using two or more steady-state dose/concentration pairs. The graph shows the solution for Example 4.

concentration was 10.7 µg/ml. At that time, the dose was increased to 350 mg/d of extended phenytoin sodium capsules for an additional month, and the resulting steady-state concentration was 15.8 µg/ml. The patient is assessed to be compliant with her dosage regimen. Suggest a new phenytoin dosage regimen increase designed to achieve a steady-state phenytoin concentration within the upper part of the therapeutic range.

1. *Use the Mullen method to estimate a new phenytoin dose for the desired steady-state concentration.* The serum concentration/dose information is plotted on the graph. (*Note:* Phenytoin dose = 0.92 · phenytoin sodium dose = 0.92 · 300 mg/d = 276 mg/d, (276 mg/d)/(55 kg) = 5 mg/kg/d; phenytoin dose = 0.92 · Phenytoin sodium dose = 0.92 · 350 mg/d = 322 mg/d, (322 mg/d)/(55 kg) = 5.9 mg/kg/d; Figure 10-6). According to the graph, a dose of 6.7 mg/kg/d of phenytoin is required to achieve a steady-state concentration of 22 µg/ml. This equals an extended phenytoin sodium capsule dose of 400 mg/d: (6.7 mg/kg/d · 55 kg)/0.92 = 401 mg/d, rounded to 400 mg/d. V_{max} = 9.4 mg/kg/d and K_m = 9.5 µg/ml for this patient.

    A steady-state trough total phenytoin serum concentration should be measured after steady state is attained in 7–14 days. Phenytoin serum concentrations should also be measured if the patient experiences an exacerbation of epilepsy, or if the patient develops potential signs or symptoms of phenytoin toxicity.

Ludden Method

• The Ludden method involves the arrangement of the Michaelis-Menten equation so that two or more maintenance doses (MD, in mg/d of phenytoin) and steady-state concentrations (Css in mg/L = μg/ml) can be used to obtain graphical solutions for V_{max} and K_m.[29]

$$MD = -K_m(MD/Css) + V_{max}$$

When the maintenance dose is plotted on the y axis and MD/Css is plotted on the x axis of Cartesian graph paper, a straight line with a y intercept of V_{max} and a slope equal to $-K_m$ is found. If three or more dose/concentration pairs are available, it is best to actually plot the data so the best straight line can be drawn through the points.

- If only two dose/concentration pairs are available, a direct mathematical solution can be found. The slope for a simple linear equation is the quotient of the change in the y-axis values (Δy) and the change in the x-axis values (Δx): slope = $\Delta y / \Delta x$. Applying this to the above rearrangement of the Michaels-Menten equation,

$$-K_m = (MD_1 - MD_2)/[(MD_1/Css_1) - (MD_2/Css_2)]$$

where the subscript 1 indicates the higher dose and the subscript 2 indicates the lower dose. Once this has been accomplished, V_{max} can be solved for in the rearranged Michaelis-Menten equation: $V_{max} = MD + K_m(MD/Css)$. The Michaelis-Menten equation can be used to compute steady-state concentrations for a given dose or vice versa.

▶ **Example 5**   TD is a 50-year-old, 75-kg (height 5'10") male with simple partial seizures who requires therapy with oral phenytoin. He has normal liver and renal function. The patient was prescribed 400 mg/d of extended phenytoin sodium capsules for 1 month, and his steady-state phenytoin total concentration was 6.2 μg/ml. The dosage was increased to 500 mg/d of extended phenytoin sodium capsules for another month after which the patient's, steady-state phenytoin total concentration was 22.0 μg/ml and he had some lateral-gaze nystagmus. The patient is assessed to be compliant with his dosage regimen. Suggest a new phenytoin dosage regimen designed to achieve a steady-state phenytoin concentration within the therapeutic range.

1. *Use the Ludden method to estimate V_{max} and K_m.* The serum concentration/dose information is plotted on the graph. (*Note:* Phenytoin dose = 0.92 · phenytoin sodium dose = 0.92 · 400 mg/d = 368 mg/d, (368 mg/d)/ (75 kg) = 4.9 mg/kg/d; phenytoin dose = 0.92 · phenytoin sodium dose = 0.92 · 500 mg/d = 460 mg/d, (460 mg/d)/(75 kg) = 6.1 mg/kg/d; Figure 10-7). According to the graph, V_{max} = 510 mg/d and K_m = 2.4 mg/L.
   Because only two dose/steady-state concentrations pairs are available, a direct mathematical solution can also be found:

$$-K_m = (MD_1 - MD_2)/[(MD_1/Css_1) - (MD_2/Css_2)]$$
$$= (460 \text{ mg/d} - 368 \text{ mg/d})/\{[(460 \text{ mg/d})/(22 \text{ mg/L})]$$
$$-[(368 \text{ mg/d})/(6.2 \text{ mg/L})]\} = -2.4 \text{ mg/L}$$

$$K_m = 2.4 \text{ mg/L}$$

$$V_{max} = MD + K_m(MD/Css)$$
$$= 368 \text{ mg/d} + \{2.4[(368 \text{ mg/d})/(6.2 \text{ mg/L})]\} = 510 \text{ mg/d}$$

2. *Use the Michaelis-Menten equation to compute a new phenytoin dose for the desired steady-state concentration.* According to the Michaelis-Menten

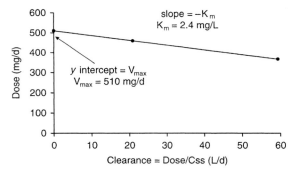

FIG. 10-7 Ludden graph used to compute Michaelis-Menten parameters and phenytoin dose using two or more steady-state dose/concentration pairs (Example 5 data shown). Dose is plotted on the *y* axis and clearance (Dose/Css) is plotted on the *x* axis for each data pair. The best straight line is drawn through the points. Slope equals $-K_m$, and V_{max} is the *y* intercept. These values are then used to compute the required maintenance dose (MD) for any desired steady-state serum concentration: MD = $(V_{max} \cdot Css)/[S(K_m + Css)]$.

equation, a dose equal to 450 mg of phenytoin sodium is required to achieve a steady-state concentration of 10.4 µg/ml:

$$Css = \frac{K_m \cdot (S \cdot MD)}{V_{max} - (S \cdot MD)} = \frac{2.4 \text{ mg/L} \cdot (0.92 \cdot 450 \text{ mg/d})}{510 \text{ mg/d} - (0.92 \cdot 450 \text{ mg/d})} = 10.4 \text{ mg/L}$$

This dose would administered by alternating 400 mg/d on even days and 500 mg/d on odd days.

A steady state trough total phenytoin serum concentration should be measured after steady state is attained in 7–14 days. Phenytoin serum concentrations should also be measured if the patient experiences an exacerbation of epilepsy, or if the patient develops potential signs or symptoms of phenytoin toxicity.

▶ **Example 6** GF is a 35-year-old, 55-kg female (height 5′4″) with tonic-clonic seizures who requires therapy with oral phenytoin. She has normal liver and renal function. The patient was prescribed 300 mg/d of extended phenytoin sodium capsules for 1 month, and her steady-state phenytoin total concentration was 10.7 µg/ml. At that time, the dose was increased to 350 mg/d of extended phenytoin sodium capsules for an additional month, and the resulting steady-state concentration was 15.8 µg/ml. The patient is assessed to be compliant with her dosage regimen. Suggest a new phenytoin dosage regimen increase designed to achieve a steady-state phenytoin concentration within the upper part of the therapeutic range.

1. *Use the Ludden method to estimate V_{max} and K_m.* The serum concentration/dose information is plotted on the graph. (*Note:* Phenytoin dose = 0.92 · phenytoin sodium dose = 0.92 · 300 mg/d = 276 mg/d, phenytoin dose = 0.92 · phenytoin sodium dose = 0.92 · 350 mg/d = 322 mg/d; Figure 10-8). According to the graph, V_{max} = 495 mg/d and K_m = 8.5 mg/L.

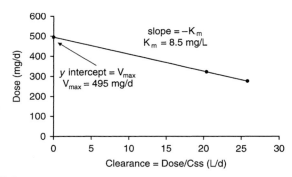

FIG. 10-8   Ludden graph used to compute Michaelis-Menten parameters and phenytoin dose using two or more steady-state dose/concentration pairs. The graph shows the solution for Example 6.

Because only two dose/steady-state concentrations pairs are available, a direct mathematical solution can also be found:

$$-K_m = (MD_1 - MD_2)/[(MD_1/Css_1) - (MD_2/Css_2)]$$
$$= (322 \text{ mg/d} - 276 \text{ mg/d})/\{[(322 \text{ mg/d})/(15.8 \text{ mg/L})]$$
$$-[(276 \text{ mg/d})/(10.7 \text{ mg/L})]\} = -8.5 \text{ mg/L}$$

$$K_m = 8.5 \text{ mg/L}$$

$$V_{max} = MD + K_m(MD/Css)$$
$$= 322 \text{ mg/d} + \{8.5 \text{ mg/L}[(322 \text{ mg/d})/(15.8 \text{ mg/L})]\} = 495 \text{ mg/d}$$

2. *Use the Michaelis-Menten equation to compute a new phenytoin dose for the desired steady-state concentration.* According to the Michaelis-Menten equation, a dose equal to 400 mg of phenytoin sodium is required to achieve a steady-state concentration of 24.6 μg/ml:

$$Css = \frac{K_m \cdot (S \cdot MD)}{V_{max} - (S \cdot MD)} = \frac{8.5 \text{ mg/L} \cdot (0.92 \cdot 400 \text{ mg/d})}{495 \text{ mg/d} - (0.92 \cdot 400 \text{ mg/d})} = 24.6 \text{ mg/L}$$

A steady-state trough total phenytoin serum concentration should be measured after steady state is attained in 7–14 days. Phenytoin serum concentrations should also be measured if the patient experiences an exacerbation of epilepsy, or if the patient develops potential signs or symptoms of phenytoin toxicity.

BAYESIAN PHARMACOKINETIC COMPUTER PROGRAMS

• Computer programs are available that can assist in the computation of pharmacokinetic parameters for patients. The most reliable computer programs use a nonlinear regression algorithm that incorporates components of Bayes' theorem.

  • An advantage of this approach is that consistent dosage recommendations are made when several different practitioners are involved in therapeutic drug monitoring programs. However, since simpler dosing methods work just as well for patients with stable pharmacokinetic parameters and steady-state drug concentrations, many clinicians reserve the use of computer programs for more difficult situations. Those situations include serum concentrations that are not at steady state, serum concentrations not obtained at the specific times needed to employ simpler methods, and unstable pharmacokinetic parameters.

- When only a limited number of phenytoin concentrations are available, Bayesian pharmacokinetic computer programs can be used to compute a complete patient pharmacokinetic profile that includes V_{max}, K_m, and volume of distribution. This is a distinct advantage compared to other methods used to adjust phenytoin dose based on one or more steady-state serum concentrations.

- Many Bayesian pharmacokinetic computer programs are available, and most should provide answers similar to the program used in the following examples. The program used to solve problems in this book is DrugCalc, written by Dr. Dennis Mungall and available at his Internet web site (www.clinpharmacologist.bigstep.com/consumersurvey.html).[66]

▶ **Example 1** TD is a 50-year-old, 75-kg (height 5′10″) male with simple partial seizures who requires therapy with oral phenytoin. He has normal liver and renal function (total bilirubin = 0.5 mg/dl, albumin = 4.0 g/dl, serum creatinine = 0.9 mg/dl). The patient has been prescribed 400 mg/d of extended phenytoin sodium capsules for 1 month, and his steady-state phenytoin total concentration is 6.2 µg/ml. The patient is assessed to be compliant with his dosage regimen. Suggest a new phenytoin dosage regimen designed to achieve a steady-state phenytoin concentration within the therapeutic range.

1. *Enter patient demographic, drug dosing, and serum concentration/time data into a Bayesian pharmacokinetic computer program.* DrugCalc requires doses to be entered in terms of phenytoin. A 400-mg dose of phenytoin sodium is equal to 368 mg of phenytoin (400 mg phenytoin sodium · 0.92 = 368 mg phenytoin). Extended phenytoin sodium capsules are input as a slow-release dosage form.

2. *Compute pharmacokinetic parameters for the patient using the computer program.* The pharmacokinetic parameters computed by the program are a volume of distribution of 53 L, a V_{max} of 506 mg/d, and a K_m of 4.3 mg/L.

3. *Compute the dose required to achieve desired phenytoin serum concentrations.* The one-compartment-model Michaelis-Menten equations used by the program to compute doses indicates that a dose of 414 mg/d of phenytoin will produce a total steady-state concentration of 12.1 µg/ml. This is equivalent to 450 mg/d of phenytoin sodium (414 mg/d phenytoin/ 0.92 = 450 mg/d phenytoin sodium). Extended phenytoin sodium capsules would be prescribed as 400 mg/d on even days alternating with 500 mg/d on odd days.

   A steady-state trough total phenytoin serum concentration should be measured after steady state is attained in 7–14 days. Phenytoin serum concentrations should also be measured if the patient experiences an exacerbation of epilepsy, or if the patient develops potential signs or symptoms of phenytoin toxicity.

▶ **Example 2** GF is a 35-year-old, 55-kg (height 5′4″) tall female with tonic-clonic seizures who requires therapy with oral phenytoin. She has normal liver and renal function (total bilirubin = 0.6 mg/dl, albumin = 4.6 g/dl, serum creatinine = 0.6 mg/dl). The patient has been prescribed 300 mg/d of extended phenytoin sodium capsules for 1 month, and her steady-state phenytoin total concentration is 10.7 µg/ml. The patient is assessed to be compliant with her dosage regimen. Suggest a new phenytoin dosage regimen designed to achieve a steady-state phenytoin concentration of 18 µg/ml.

1. *Enter patient demographic, drug dosing, and serum concentration/time data into a Bayesian pharmacokinetic computer program.* DrugCalc requires doses to be entered in terms of phenytoin. A 300-mg dose of phenytoin sodium is equal to 276 mg of phenytoin (300 mg phenytoin sodium · 0.92 = 276 mg phenytoin). Extended phenytoin sodium capsules are input as a slow-release dosage form.

2. *Compute pharmacokinetic parameters for the patient using the computer program.* The pharmacokinetic parameters computed by the program are a volume of distribution of 34 L, a V_{max} of 354 mg/d, and a K_m of 5.8 mg/L.

3. *Compute the dose required to achieve desired phenytoin serum concentrations.* The one-compartment-model Michaelis-Menten equations used by the program to compute doses indicates that a dose of 304 mg/d of phenytoin will produce a total steady-state concentration of 19.6 µg/ml. This is equivalent to 330 mg/d of phenytoin sodium (304 mg/d phenytoin/ 0.92 = 330 mg/d phenytoin sodium). Extended phenytoin sodium capsules would be prescribed as 330 mg/d (three 100-mg capsules + one 30-mg capsule).

A steady-state trough total phenytoin serum concentration should be measured after steady state is attained in 7–14 days. Phenytoin serum concentrations should also be measured if the patient experiences an exacerbation of epilepsy, or if the patient develops potential signs or symptoms of phenytoin toxicity.

▶ *Example 3*   TY is a 27-year-old, 60-kg (height 5′6″) female with complex partial seizures who requires therapy with oral phenytoin. She has normal liver and renal function (total bilirubin = 0.8 mg/dl, albumin = 5.1 g/dl, serum creatinine = 0.4 mg/dl). The patient was prescribed 300 mg/d of extended phenytoin sodium capsules for 1 month, and her steady-state phenytoin total concentration was 8.7 µg/ml. At that time, the patient's dose was increased to 400 mg/d of extended phenytoin sodium capsules for an additional month, and her resulting steady-state concentration was 13.2 µg/ml. The patient is assessed to be compliant with her dosage regimen. Suggest a new phenytoin dosage regimen designed to achieve a steady-state phenytoin concentration within the upper part of the therapeutic range.

1. *Enter patient demographic, drug dosing, and serum concentration/time data into a Bayesian pharmacokinetic computer program.* DrugCalc requires doses to be entered in terms of phenytoin. A 300-mg dose of phenytoin sodium is equal to 276 mg of phenytoin (300 mg phenytoin sodium · 0.92 = 276 mg phenytoin), while a 400-mg dose of phenytoin sodium equals 368 mg of phenytoin (400 mg phenytoin sodium · 0.92 = 368 mg phenytoin). Extended phenytoin sodium capsules are input as a slow-release dosage form.

2. *Compute pharmacokinetic parameters for the patient using the computer program.* The pharmacokinetic parameters computed by the program are a volume of distribution of 43 L, a V_{max} of 586 mg/d, and a K_m of 13.2 mg/L.

3. *Compute the dose required to achieve the desired phenytoin serum concentrations.* The one-compartment-model Michaelis-Menten equations

TABLE 10-5 Dosing Strategies

Dosing approach/ philosophy	Initial dosing	Use of serum concentrations to alter doses
Pharmacokinetic parameters/ equations	Pharmacokinetic dosing method	Vozeh-Sheiner method (1 concentration/ dose pair) or Mullen method (≥2 concentration/ dose pairs) or Ludden method (≥2 concentration/ dose pairs)
Literature-based/ concept	Literature-based recommended dosing	Empiric dosing method
Mathematical	___a	Graves-Cloyd method (1 concentration/ dose pair)
Computerized	Bayesian computer program	Bayesian computer program

aAny initial dosing method appropriate for the patient.

used by the program to compute doses indicates that a dose of 396 mg/d of phenytoin will produce a total steady-state concentration of 20.4 μg/ml. This is equivalent to 430 mg/d of phenytoin sodium (396 mg/d phenytoin/ 0.92 = 430 mg/d phenytoin sodium). Extended phenytoin sodium capsules would be prescribed as 430 mg/d (four 100-mg capsules + one 30-mg capsule).

A steady-state trough total phenytoin serum concentration should be measured af measured after steady state is attained in 7–14 days. Phenytoin serum concentrations should also be measured if the patient experiences an exacerbation of epilepsy, or if the patient develops potential signs or symptoms of phenytoin toxicity.

DOSING STRATEGIES

- Initial dose and dosage adjustment techniques using serum concentrations can be used in any combination as long as the limitations of each method are observed.
- Some dosing schemes link together logically when considered according to their basic approaches or philosophies. Dosage strategies that follow similar pathways are given in Table 10-5.

USE OF PHENYTOIN BOOSTER DOSES TO IMMEDIATELY INCREASE SERUM CONCENTRATIONS

- If a patient has a subtherapeutic phenytoin serum concentration in an acute situation, it may be desirable to increase the phenytoin concentration as quickly as possible. A rational way to increase the serum concentrations rapidly is to administer a booster dose of phenytoin, a process also known as "reloading" the patient with phenytoin, computed using pharmacokinetic techniques.

- A modified loading-dose equation is used to accomplish computation of the booster dose (BD) which takes into account the current phenytoin concentration present in the patient:

$$BD = [(C_{desired} - C_{actual})V]/S$$

where $C_{desired}$ is the desired phenytoin concentration, C_{actual} is the actual current phenytoin concentration for the patient, S is the fraction of the phenytoin salt form that is active phenytoin (0.92 for phenytoin sodium injection and capsules; 0.92 for fosphenytoin because doses are prescribed as a phenytoin sodium equivalent or PE, 1.0 for phenytoin acid suspensions and tablets), and V is the volume of distribution for phenytoin.

- If the volume of distribution for phenytoin is known for the patient, it can be used in the calculation. However, this value is not usually known and is assumed to equal the population average of 0.7 L/kg.

  - For obese individuals, 30% or more above their ideal body weight, the volume of distribution can be estimated using the following equation:

  $$V = 0.7 \text{ L/kg}[IBW + 1.33(TBW - IBW)]$$

  where IBW is ideal body weight in kg [$IBW_{females}$ (in kg) = 45 + 2.3(Ht − 60) or IBW_{males} (in kg) = 50 + 2.3(Ht − 60)], Ht is height in inches, and TBW is total body weight in kg.

- Concurrent with the administration of the booster dose, the maintenance dose of phenytoin is usually increased. Clinicians need to recognize that the administration of a booster dose does not alter the time required to achieve steady-state conditions when a new phenytoin dosage rate is prescribed. It still requires a sufficient time period to attain steady state when the dosage rate is changed. However, usually the difference between the post–booster dose phenytoin concentration and the ultimate steady-state concentration is reduced by giving the extra dose of drug.

▶ *Example 1*   BN is a 22-year-old, 85-kg (height 6′2″) male with complex partial seizures who is receiving therapy with intravenous phenytoin sodium. He has normal liver and renal function. After receiving an initial loading dose of phenytoin sodium (1000 mg) and a maintenance dose of 300 mg/d of phenytoin sodium for 5 days, his phenytoin concentration was measured at 5.6 μg/ml immediately after seizure activity was observed. Compute a booster dose of phenytoin to achieve a phenytoin concentration of 15 μg/ml.

1. *Estimate volume of distribution according to disease states and conditions present in the patient.* In the case of phenytoin, the population average volume of distribution is 0.7 L/kg, and this value will be used to estimate the parameter for the patient. The patient is not obese, so his actual body weight will be used in the computation:

$$V = 0.7 \text{ L/kg} \cdot 85 \text{ kg} = 60 \text{ L}$$

2. *Compute booster dose.* The booster dose is computed using the following equation:

$$BD = [(C_{desired} - C_{actual})V]/S = [(15 \text{ mg/L} - 5.6 \text{ mg/L})60 \text{ L}]/0.92 = 613 \text{ mg}$$

This value is rounded to 600 mg of phenytoin sodium infused no faster than 50 mg/min. (*Note:* μg/ml = mg/L, and this concentration unit was substituted for Css in the calculations so that unit conversion was not required.) If the maintenance dose is increased, it will take additional time for a new steady-state condition to be achieved. Phenytoin serum concentrations should be measured at this time.

REFERENCES

1. Brodie MJ, Dichter MA. Antiepileptic drugs. N Engl J Med 1996;334(3):168–75.
2. McNamara JO. Drugs effective in the therapy of the epilepsies. In: Hardman JG, Limbird LE, Gilman AG, eds. The pharmacological basis of therapeutics. 10th ed. New York: McGraw-Hill, 2001:521–48.
3. Gidal BE, Garnett WR, Graves NM. Epilepsy. In: DiPiro JT, Talbert RL, Yee GC, Matzke GR, Wells BG, Posey LM, eds. Pharmacotherapy. 5th ed. New York: McGraw-Hill, 2002:1031–60.
4. Chen SS, Perucca E, Lee JN, Richens A. Serum protein binding and free concentration of phenytoin and phenobarbitone in pregnancy. Br J Clin Pharmacol 1982;13(4):547–52.
5. Knott C, Williams CP, Reynolds F. Phenytoin kinetics during pregnancy and the puerperium. Br J Obstet Gynaecol 1986;93(10):1030–7.
6. Perucca E, Hebdige S, Frigo GM, Gatti G, Lecchini S, Crema A. Interaction between phenytoin and valproic acid: plasma protein binding and metabolic effects. Clin Pharmacol Ther 1980;28(6):779–89.
7. Pisani FD, Di Perri RG. Intravenous valproate: effects on plasma and saliva phenytoin levels. Neurology 1981;31(4):467–70.
8. Riva R, Albani F, Contin M, et al. Time-dependent interaction between phenytoin and valproic acid. Neurology 1985;35(4):510–5.
9. Frigo GM, Lecchini S, Gatti G, Perucca E, Crema A. Modification of phenytoin clearance by valproic acid in normal subjects. Br J Clin Pharmacol 1979;8(6): 553–6.
10. Paxton JW. Effects of aspirin on salivary and serum phenytoin kinetics in healthy subjects. Clin Pharmacol Ther 1980;27(2):170–8.
11. Leonard RF, Knott PJ, Rankin GO, Robinson DS, Melnick DE. Phenytoin-salicylate interaction. Clin Pharmacol Ther 1981;29(1):56–60.
12. Fraser DG, Ludden TM, Evens RP, Sutherland EWd. Displacement of phenytoin from plasma binding sites by salicylate. Clin Pharmacol Ther 1980;27(2):165–9.
13. Olanow CW, Finn AL, Prussak C. The effects of salicylate on the pharmacokinetics of phenytoin. Neurology 1981;31(3):341–2.
14. Mabuchi H, Nakahashi H. A major inhibitor of phenytoin binding to serum protein in uremia. Nephron 1988;48(4):310–4.
15. Dasgupta A, Malik S. Fast atom bombardment mass spectrometric determination of the molecular weight range of uremic compounds that displace phenytoin from protein binding: absence of midmolecular uremic toxins. Am J Nephrol 1994;14(3): 162–8.
16. Odar-Cederlof I, Borga O. Kinetics of diphenylhydantoin in uraemic patients: consequences of decreased plasma protein binding. Eur J Clin Pharmacol 1974;7:31–7.
17. Odar-Cederlof I, Borga O. Impaired plasma protein binding of phenytoin in uremia and displacement effect of salicylic acid. Clin Pharmacol Ther 1976;20(1):36–47.
18. Odar-Cederlof I. Plasma protein binding of phenytoin and warfarin in patients undergoing renal transplantation. Clin Pharmacokin 1977;2:147–53.
19. Dodson WE, Loney LC. Hemodialysis reduces the unbound phenytoin in plasma. J Pediatr 1982;101(3):465–8.
20. Kinniburgh DW, Boyd ND. Isolation of peptides from uremic plasma that inhibit phenytoin binding to normal plasma proteins. Clin Pharmacol Ther 1981;30(2): 276–80.
21. Peterson GM, McLean S, Aldous S, Von Witt RJ, Millingen KS. Plasma protein binding of phenytoin in 100 epileptic patients. Br J Clin Pharmacol 1982;14(2):298–300.

22. Patterson M, Heazelwood R, Smithurst B, Eadie MJ. Plasma protein binding of phenytoin in the aged: in vivo studies. Br J Clin Pharmacol 1982;13(3):423–5.
23. Winter ME, Tozer TN. Phenytoin. In: Evans WE, Schentag JJ, Jusko WJ, eds. Applied pharmacokinetics. 3rd ed. Vancouver, WA: Applied Therapeutics 1992;25:1–44.
24. Anderson GD, Pak C, Doane KW, et al. Revised Winter-Tozer equation for normalized phenytoin concentrations in trauma and elderly patients with hypoalbuminemia. Ann Pharmacother 1997;31(3):279–84.
25. Haidukewych D, Rodin EA, Zielinski JJ. Derivation and evaluation of an equation for prediction of free phenytoin concentration in patients co-medicated with valproic acid. Ther Drug Monit 1989;11(2):134–9.
26. Kerrick JM, Wolff DL, Graves NM. Predicting unbound phenytoin concentrations in patients receiving valproic acid: a comparison of two prediction methods. Ann Pharmacother 1995;29(5):470–4.
27. Allen JP, Ludden TM, Burrow SR, Clementi WA, Stavchansky SA. Phenytoin cumulation kinetics. Clin Pharmacol Ther 1979;26(4):445–8.
28. Grasela TH, Sheiner LB, Rambeck B, et al. Steady-state pharmacokinetics of phenytoin from routinely collected patient data. Clin Pharmacokin 1983;8:355–64.
29. Ludden TM, Allen JP, Valutsky WA, et al. Individualization of phenytoin dosage regimens. Clin Pharmacol Ther 1977;21(3):287–93.
30. Jusko WJ, Koup JR, Alvan G. Nonlinear assessment of phenytoin bioavailability. J Pharmacokinet Biopharm 1976;4(4):327–36.
31. Gugler R, Manion CV, Azarnoff DL. Phenytoin: pharmacokinetics and bioavailability. Clin Pharmacol Ther 1976;19(2):135–42.
32. Smith TC, Kinkel A. Absorption and metabolism of phenytoin from tablets and capsules. Clin Pharmacol Ther 1976;20(6):738–42.
33. Chakrabarti S, Belpaire F, Moerman E. Effect of formulation on dissolution and bioavailability of phenytoin tablets. Pharmazie 1980;35(10):627–9.
34. Jung D, Powell JR, Walson P, Perrier D. Effect of dose on phenytoin absorption. Clin Pharmacol Ther 1980;28(4):479–85.
35. Fleisher D, Sheth N, Kou JH. Phenytoin interaction with enteral feedings administered through nasogastric tubes. J Parenter Enteral Nutr 1990;14(5):513–6.
36. Cacek AT, DeVito JM, Koonce JR. In vitro evaluation of nasogastric administration methods for phenytoin. Am J Hosp Pharm 1986;43(3):689–92.
37. Bauer LA. Interference of oral phenytoin absorption by continuous nasogastric feedings. Neurology 1982;32(5):570–2.
38. Ozuna J, Friel P. Effect of enteral tube feeding on serum phenytoin levels. J Neurosurg Nurs 1984;16(6):289–91.
39. Bach B, Molholm Hansen J, Kampmann JP, Rasmussen SN, Skovsted L. Disposition of antipyrine and phenytoin correlated with age and liver volume in man. Clin Pharmacokinet 1981;6:389–96.
40. Bauer LA, Blouin RA. Age and phenytoin kinetics in adult epileptics. Clin Pharmacol Ther 1982;31(3):301–4.
41. Blain PG, Mucklow JC, Bacon CJ, Rawlins MD. Pharmacokinetics of phenytoin in children. Br J Clin Pharmacol 1981;12(5):659–61.
42. Chiba K, Ishizaki T, Miura H, Minagawa K. Apparent Michaelis-Menten kinetic parameters of phenytoin in pediatric patients. Pediatr Pharmacol 1980;1(2):171–80.
43. Chiba K, Ishizaki T, Miura H, Minagawa K. Michaelis-Menten pharmacokinetics of diphenylhydantoin and application in the pediatric age patient. J Pediatr 1980;96(3 pt 1):479–84.
44. Dodson WE. Nonlinear kinetics of phenytoin in children. Neurology 1982;32(1):42–8.
45. Leff RD, Fischer LJ, Roberts RJ. Phenytoin metabolism in infants following intravenous and oral administration. Dev Pharmacol Ther 1986;9(4):217–23.
46. Bauer LA, Blouin RA. Phenytoin Michaelis-Menten pharmacokinetics in Caucasian paediatric patients. Clin Pharmacokinet 1983;8(6):545–9.

47. Pugh RN, Murray-Lyon IM, Dawson JL, Pietroni MC, Williams R. Transection of the oesophagus for bleeding oesophageal varices. Br J Surg 1973;60(8):646–9.
48. Bauer LA, Edwards WA, Dellinger EP, Raisys VA, Brennan C. Importance of unbound phenytoin serum levels in head trauma patients. J Trauma 1983;23(12): 1058–60.
49. Boucher BA, Rodman JH, Jaresko GS, Rasmussen SN, Watridge CB, Fabian TC. Phenytoin pharmacokinetics in critically ill trauma patients. Clin Pharmacol Ther 1988;44(6):675–83.
50. Chiba K, Ishizaki T, Tabuchi T, Wagatsuma T, Nakazawa Y. Antipyrine disposition in relation to lowered anticonvulsant plasma level during pregnancy. Obstet Gynecol 1982;60(5):620–6.
51. Dickinson RG, Hooper WD, Wood B, Lander CM, Eadie MJ. The effect of pregnancy in humans on the pharmacokinetics of stable isotope labelled phenytoin. Br J Clin Pharmacol 1989;28(1):17–27.
52. Lander CM, Smith MT, Chalk JB, et al. Bioavailability and pharmacokinetics of phenytoin during pregnancy. Eur J Clin Pharmacol 1984;27(1):105–10.
53. Kochenour NK, Emery MG, Sawchuk RJ. Phenytoin metabolism in pregnancy. Obstet Gynecol 1980;56(5):577–82.
54. Landon MJ, Kirkley M. Metabolism of diphenylhydantoin (phenytoin) during pregnancy. Br J Obstet Gynaecol 1979;86(2):125–32.
55. Aronoff GR, Berns JS, Brier ME, Golper TA, Morrison G, Singer I, Swan SK, Bennett WM. Drug prescribing in renal failure—dosing guidelines for adults. 4th ed. Philadelphia: American College of Physicians, 1999.
56. Golper TA. Update on drug sieving coefficients and dosing adjustments during continuous renal replacement therapies. Contrib Nephrol 2001(132):349–53.
57. Golper TA, Marx MA. Drug dosing adjustments during continuous renal replacement therapies. Kidney Int Suppl 1998;66:S165–8.
58. Hansten PD, Horn JR. Drug interactions analysis and management. Vancouver, WA: Applied Therapeutics, 1999.
59. Abernethy DR, Greenblatt DJ. Phenytoin disposition in obesity. Determination of loading dose. Arch Neurol 1985;42(5):468–71.
60. Mauro LS, Mauro VF, Bachmann KA, Higgins JT. Accuracy of two equations in determining normalized phenytoin concentrations. Drug Intel Clin Pharm 1989;23(1):64–8.
61. Bauer LA. Clinical pharmacokinetics and pharmacodynamics. In: DiPiro JT, Talbert RL, Yee GC, Matzke GR, Wells BG, Posey LM, eds. Pharmacotherapy. 6th ed. New York: McGraw-Hill, 2006:51–73.
62. Graves N, Cloyd J, Leppik I. Phenytoin dosage predictions using population clearances. Ann Pharmacother 1982;16:473–8.
63. Vozeh S, Muir KT, Sheiner LB, Follath F. Predicting individual phenytoin dosage. J Pharmacokinet Biopharm 1981;9(2):131–46.
64. Mullen PW. Optimal phenytoin therapy: a new technique for individualizing dosage. Clin Pharmacol Ther 1978;23(2):228–32.
65. Mullen PW, Foster RW. Comparative evaluation of six techniques for determining the Michaelis-Menten parameters relating phenytoin dose and steady-state serum concentrations. J Pharm Pharmacol 1979;31(2):100–4.
66. Wandell M, Mungall D. Computer assisted drug interpretation and drug regimen optimization. Am Assoc Clin Chem 1984;6:1–11.

11 | Carbamazepine

Carbamazepine is an iminostilbene derivative related to the tricyclic antidepressants that is used in the treatment of tonic-clonic (grand mal), partial or secondarily generalized seizures (Table 11-1).[1,2] Carbamazepine is also a useful agent to treat trigeminal neuralgia and bipolar affective disorders.[2]

- The antiseizure activity of carbamazepine is related to its ability to decrease transmission in the nucleus ventralis anterior section of the thalamus, an area of the brain thought to be involved in the generalization and propagation of epileptic discharges.[1,2]

THERAPEUTIC AND TOXIC CONCENTRATIONS

- The accepted therapeutic range for carbamazepine is 4–12 mg/ml when the drug is used for the treatment of seizures.
- Carbamazepine plasma protein binding is quite variable among individuals because it is bound to both albumin and α_1-acid glycoprotein (AAG). In patients with normal concentrations of these proteins, plasma protein binding is 75–80%, resulting in a free fraction of drug of 20–25%.[3–5]

  - AAG is classified as an acute-phase reactant protein that is present in lower amounts in all individuals but is secreted in large amounts in response to certain stresses and disease states such as trauma, heart failure, and myocardial infarction. In patients with these disease states, carbamazepine binding to AAG can be even larger, resulting in an unbound fraction as low as 10–15%.

- Little prospective work has been done to establish the therapeutic range for unbound carbamazepine serum concentrations or the clinical situations in which unbound carbamazepine serum concentration measurements are useful. As an initial guide, 25% of the total carbamazepine therapeutic range has been used to establish a preliminary desirable range for unbound carbamazepine serum concentrations of 1–3 µg/ml.

  - Although carbamazepine is highly plasma protein-bound, it is harder to displace this agent to the extent that a clinically important change in protein binding takes place. Generally speaking, a doubling of unbound fraction in the plasma is required to produce such an alteration.
  - It is very difficult to change the protein binding of carbamazepine from 80% to 60% to achieve the same doubling of unbound fraction in the plasma (20% to 40%). As a result, the use of unbound carbamazepine serum concentrations is currently limited to those patients who have total concentrations within the therapeutic range but who experience adverse effects usually seen at higher concentrations, or those patients who have total concentrations below the therapeutic range but who have a therapeutic response usually observed at higher concentrations.

- Carbamazepine-10,11-epoxide is an active metabolite of carbamazepine that contributes to both the therapeutic and toxic effects of the drug, and can be measured in serum samples at a limited number of epilepsy centers.[6–12]

TABLE 11-1 International Classification of Epileptic Seizures [39]

Major class	Subset of class	Drug treatment for selected seizure type
Partial seizures (beginning locally)	1. Simple partial seizures (without impaired consciousness) a. With motor symptoms b. With somatosensory or special sensory symptoms c. With autonomic symptoms d. With psychological symptoms	Carbamazepine Phenytoin Valproic acid Phenobarbital Primidone
	2. Complex partial seizures (with impaired consciousness) a. Simple partial onset followed by impaired consciousness b. Impaired consciousness at onset	Carbamazepine Phenytoin Valproic acid Phenobarbital Primidone
	3. Partial seizures evolving into secondary generalized seizures	Carbamazepine Phenytoin Valproic acid Phenobarbital Primidone
Generalized seizures (convulsive or nonconvulsive)	1. Absence seizures (typical or atypical; also known as petite mal seizures)	Valproic acid Ethosuximide
	2. Tonic-clonic seizures (also known as grand mal seizures)	Carbamazepine Phenytoin Valproic acid Phenobarbital Primidone

- Epoxide concentrations tend to be higher in patients taking enzyme inducers and lower in patients taking enzyme inhibitors. The ratio of epoxide to parent drug (expressed as a percentage) in chronically treated patients averages about 12% for carbamazepine monotherapy, 14% when carbamazepine is taken with phenobarbital, 18% when carbamazepine is taken with phenytoin, and about 25% when carbamazepine is taken with both phenytoin and phenobarbital.
- The therapeutic range of carbamazepine-10,11-epoxide is not known, although a suggested range of 0.4–4 μg/ml is used by several research centers.
- In the upper part of the therapeutic range (>8 mg/ml), some patients begin to experience the concentration-related adverse effects of carbamazepine treatment: nausea, vomiting, lethargy, dizziness, drowsiness, headache, blurred vision, diplopia, unsteadiness, ataxia, incoordination.
- Because carbamazepine induces its own hepatic metabolism, these adverse effects can also be seen early during dosage titration periods, soon after

dosage increases are made. To improve patient acceptance, it is important to initiate and titrate carbamazepine doses at a slow rate to minimize side effects.

CLINICAL MONITORING PARAMETERS

- The goal of therapy with anticonvulsants is to reduce seizure frequency and maximize quality of life with a minimum of adverse drug effects. While it is desirable to abolish seizure episodes entirely, it may not be possible to accomplish this in many patients.
- Patients should be monitored for concentration-related side effects (nausea, vomiting, lethargy, dizziness, drowsiness, headache, blurred vision, diplopia, unsteadiness, ataxia, incoordination).
- Because carbamazepine has antidiuretic effects associated with reduced levels of antidiuretic hormone, some patients may develop hyponatremia during chronic therapy with carbamazepine, and serum sodium concentrations may need to be measured periodically.
- Hematological adverse effects can be divided into two types.

  - The first is a leukopenia that occurs in many patients and requires no therapeutic intervention. The typical clinical picture is an individual with a normal white blood cell count who develops a transient decrease in this index. In a few patients, a decreased, stable white blood cell count of 3000 cells/mm^2 or less may persist but does not appear to cause any deleterious effects.
  - The second hematological effect is severe and usually requires discontinuation of the drug. Thrombocytopenia, leukopenia (trend downward in white blood cell count with <2500 cells/mm^2 or absolute neutrophil count <1000 cells/mm^2), or anemia are in this category. Rarely, aplastic anemia and agranulocytosis have been reported during carbamazepine treatment.

- Drug-induced hepatitis due to carbamazepine therapy has also been reported.
- The severe hematological and hepatic adverse effects tend to occur early in treatment. Therefore, many clinicians do a complete blood cell count and liver function tests monthly for the first 3–6 months after a patient begins carbamazepine treatment, and repeats these tests every 3–6 months for the first year.
- Other idiosyncratic side effects include skin rash, Stevens-Johnson syndrome, and systemic lupus-like reactions.
- Carbamazepine serum concentrations should be measured in most patients. Because epilepsy is an episodic disease state, patients do not experience seizures on a continuous basis. Thus, during dosage titration it is difficult to tell if the patient is responding to drug therapy or simply is not experiencing any abnormal central nervous system discharges at that time.
- Carbamazepine serum concentrations are also valuable tools for avoiding adverse drug effects. Patients are more likely to accept drug therapy if adverse reactions are held to the absolute minimum. Because carbamazepine induces its own hepatic metabolism, it is fairly easy to attain toxic concentrations with modest increases in drug dose before maximal enzyme induction has occurred.

BASIC CLINICAL PHARMACOKINETIC PARAMETERS

- Carbamazepine is eliminated primarily by hepatic metabolism (>99%), mainly via the CYP3A4 enzyme system.[13,14]

- Altogether, 33 metabolites have been identified, with carbamazepine-10,11-epoxide being the major species. The epoxide metabolite is active and probably contributes to both the therapeutic and toxic side effects observed during therapy.
- Carbamazepine is a potent inducer of hepatic drug-metabolizing enzymes, and induces its own metabolism, a process known as autoinduction (Figure 11-1).[15–19] As a result, patients cannot initially be placed on the dose of carbamazepine that will ultimately result in a safe and effective outcome.

- At first, patients are started on $\frac{1}{4}$–$\frac{1}{3}$ of the desired maintenance dose. This exposes hepatic drug-metabolizing enzymes to carbamazepine and begins the induction process. The dose is increased by a similar amount every 2–3 weeks until the total desired daily dose is ultimately given.
- This gradual exposure to carbamazepine allows liver enzyme induction and carbamazepine clearance increases to occur over a 6–12-week time period.
- Therapeutic effect and steady-state carbamazepine serum concentrations can be assessed 2–3 weeks after the final dosage increase.
- Autoinduction continues to occur in patients who are stabilized on a carbamazepine dose but who require a dosage increase. It appears that a 2–3-week time period is also needed under chronic dosing conditions for maximal autoinduction to occur after a dosage increase. The effects of autoinduction are reversible even when doses are discontinued for as few as 6 days.[20]

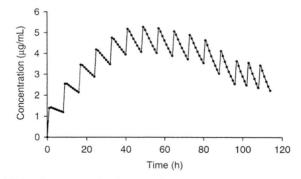

FIG. 11-1 Carbamazepine induces its own metabolism via the hepatic microsomal enzyme system CYP3A4 system. This process is known as autoinduction. When dosing is initiated, serum concentrations increase according to the baseline clearance and half-life. After a few doses of carbamazepine, enough autoinduction has occurred that clearance increases, half-life decreases, and drug accumulation slows down. With additional exposure of liver tissue to carbamazepine, clearance continues to increase and half-life continues to shorten. As a result of these pharmacokinetic changes, carbamazepine concentrations decline and ultimately stabilize in accord with the new clearance and half-life values. Maximal autoinduction usually occurs 2–3 weeks after dosing commences. Because of the autoinduction phenomenon, the ultimate desired maintenance dose cannot be started with the first dose. Additional autoinduction occurs with subsequent increases in dose.

- An injectable form of carbamazepine is not available.
- For oral use, the drug is available as immediate-release tablets (chewable 100 mg, regular 200 mg), sustained-release tablets (100-, 200-, and 400-mg tablets; 300-mg capsule) and suspension (100 mg/5 ml).

  - The rapid-release dosage forms are erratically absorbed from the gastrointestinal tract, resulting in peak concentrations between 2 and 24 hours after a single dose of tablets (average 6 hours). In multiple-dose studies after maximal autoinduction has taken place, peak concentrations occur about 3 hours after tablet administration.
  - Peak concentrations after multiple doses of the sustained-release dosage forms are observed 3–12 hours after administration.

- Rectal administration of an extemporaneously compounded carbamazepine retention enema results in similar serum concentrations as that produced by a comparable immediate-release tablet.[21,22]
- The absolute oral bioavailability of carbamazepine is not known, because no intravenous form of the drug is available for comparison. Based on the best estimates available, carbamazepine bioavailability is good and averages about 85–90%.

  - The relative bioavailability of other dosage forms (chewable tablet, suspension, sustained-release tablets and capsule) compared to the immediate-release tablet approaches 100%.
  - If a patient is receiving a stable dose of carbamazepine on one dosage form, the same total daily dose of another dosage form can typically be substituted without adjustment.
  - Some bioequivalence problems have been reported with generic carbamazepine products.[23–26] Until further data are available, therapeutic serum carbamazepine concentrations should be confirmed in patients after a switch has been made to tablets of a different manufacture.

- Usual initial maintenance doses are 10–20 mg/kg/d for children under 6 years of age, 200 mg/d for children 6–12 years old, and 400 mg/d for adults. Twice-daily dosing is used initially, until autoinduction takes place.
- Dosage increases to allow for autoinduction are made every 2–3 weeks, depending on response and adverse effects.
- Most adults require 800–1200 mg/d of carbamazepine, while older children require 400–800 mg/d.
- Although some minor side effects occur, single loading doses of 8 mg/kg have been given to adults as suspension or immediate-release tablets in order to achieve therapeutic concentrations within 2–4 hours after administration.[27]

EFFECTS OF DISEASE STATES AND CONDITIONS ON PHARMACOKINETICS AND DOSING

- After single doses of carbamazepine, the oral clearance (Cl/F) is 11–26 ml/h/kg, and half-life is 35 hours for adults.[28–30]
- During multiple dosing after maximal autoinduction has taken place, oral clearance is 50–100 mg/h/kg, and half-life is 5–27 hours.
- In children 6–12 years old, oral clearance and half-life are 50–200 ml/h/kg and 3–15 hours, respectively, during chronic dosing.

- Clearance rates can be higher and half-lives shorter in patients receiving other hepatic drug-metabolizing enzyme inducers (phenytoin, phenobarbital, rifampin).[31–33]
- Carbamazepine volume of distribution using immediate-release tablets (V/F) is 1–2 L/kg.

Liver Dysfunction

- Patients with liver cirrhosis or acute hepatitis have reduced carbamazepine clearance because of destruction of liver parenchyma. This loss of functional hepatic cells reduces the amount of CYP3A4 available to metabolize the drug and decreases clearance.
- The volume of distribution may be larger because of reduced plasma protein binding. Protein binding may be reduced and unbound fraction maybe increased due to hypoalbuminemia and/or hyperbilirubinemia (especially albumin ≤3 g/dl and/or total bilirubin ≥2 mg/dl).
- The effects of liver disease on carbamazepine pharmacokinetics are highly variable and difficult to predict accurately. It is possible for a patient with liver disease to have relatively normal or grossly abnormal carbamazepine clearance and volume of distribution. A liver disease patient who has relatively normal albumin and bilirubin concentrations can have a normal volume of distribution for carbamazepine.
- An index of liver dysfunction can be gained by applying the Child-Pugh clinical classification system to the patient (Table 11-2).[34] Child-Pugh scores are discussed more fully in Chapter 3 (Drug Dosing in Special Populations: Renal and Hepatic Disease, Dialysis, Heart Failure, Obesity, and Drug Interactions).

  - The Child-Pugh score consists of five laboratory tests or clinical symptoms: serum albumin, total bilirubin, prothrombin time, ascites, and hepatic encephalopathy. Each of these areas is given a score of 1 (normal) to 3 (severely abnormal; Table 11-2), and the scores for the five areas are summed.
  - The Child-Pugh score for a patient with normal liver function is 5, while the score for a patient with grossly abnormal serum albumin, total bilirubin, and prothrombin time values in addition to severe ascites and hepatic encephalopathy is 15.
  - A Child-Pugh score greater than 8 is grounds for a decrease of 25–50% in the initial daily drug dose for carbamazepine.

- As in any patient, with or without liver dysfunction, initial doses are meant as starting points for dosage titration based on patient response and avoidance of

TABLE 11-2 Child-Pugh Scores for Patients with Liver Disease [34]

Test/symptom	Score 1 point	Score 2 points	Score 3 points
Total bilirubin (mg/dl)	<2.0	2.0–3.0	>3.0
Serum albumin (g/dl)	>3.5	2.8–3.5	<2.8
Prothrombin time (seconds prolonged over control)	<4	4–6	>6
Ascites	Absent	Slight	Moderate
Hepatic Encephalopathy	None	Moderate	Severe

adverse effects. Carbamazepine serum concentrations and the presence of adverse drug effects should be monitored frequently in patients with liver cirrhosis.

Other Disease States and Conditions

- Elderly patients have lower carbamazepine oral clearance rates than younger adults, so lower initial doses (100 mg/d) may be used in older individuals.
- During the third trimester of pregnancy, oral clearance of carbamazepine may decrease and require dosage adjustment.
- Doses of carbamazepine do not require adjustment for patients with renal failure, and the drug is not removed by dialysis.[35,36]
- Breast milk concentrations of carbamazepine are about 60% of concurrent serum concentrations.

DRUG INTERACTIONS

- Carbamazepine is a potent inducer of hepatic drug-metabolizing enzyme systems.[37] The CYP1A2, CYP2C9, and CYP3A4 enzyme systems are all induced by carbamazepine, and drug substrates for other enzyme systems also have known drug interactions with carbamazepine.

  - Other antiepileptic drugs for which clearance rates are increased and steady-state concentrations decreased by carbamazepine-related enzyme induction include felbamate, lamotrigine, phenytoin, primidone, tiagabine, topiramate, and valproic acid.
  - Carbamazepine therapy also increases the clearance and decreases steady-state concentrations of many other drugs, including oral contraceptives, calcium channel blockers, tricyclic antidepressants, cyclosporin, tacrolimus, theophylline, and warfarin.
  - As a general rule, when carbamazepine is added to a patient's drug regimen, loss of therapeutic effect due to one of the other drugs must be considered as a possible drug interaction with carbamazepine.

- Carbamazepine is a substrate for CYP3A4, and other drugs can affect carbamazepine clearance and steady-state serum concentrations.[37]

  - Phenytoin and phenobarbital can increase carbamazepine clearance and decrease carbamazepine steady-state serum concentrations.
  - Cimetidine, macrolide antibiotics, azole antifungals, fluoxetine, fluvoxamine, nefazodone, cyclosporin, diltiazem, verapamil, indinavir, and ritonavir are examples of drugs that decrease carbamazepine clearance and increase carbamazepine steady-state concentrations.
  - Administration of single doses of carbamazepine with grapefruit juice increases both area under the serum concentration/time curve (AUC) and maximal serum concentration (C_{max}) of carbamazepine by about 40%.

INITIAL DOSAGE DETERMINATION METHODS

- Because of the large amount of variability in carbamazepine pharmacokinetics, even when concurrent disease states and conditions are identified, most clinicians believe that the use of standard carbamazepine doses for various situations is warranted.
- The original computations of these doses were based on pharmacokinetic dosing methods, and the doses were subsequently modified based on clinical experience. In general, the expected carbamazepine steady-state serum concentrations used to compute these doses are 6–8 μg/ml.

- Usual initial maintenance doses are 10–20 mg/kg/d for children under 6 years of age, 200 mg/d for children 6–12 years old, and 400 mg/d for adults. Twice-daily dosing is used initially, until autoinduction takes place. Dosage increases to allow for autoinduction are made every 2–3 weeks, depending on response and adverse effects.
- Most adults require 800–1200 mg/d of carbamazepine, while older children require 400–800 mg/d.
- If the patient has significant hepatic dysfunction (Child-Pugh score ≥8), maintenance doses prescribed using this method should be decreased by 25–50%, depending on how aggressive therapy is required to be for the individual.

▶ *Example 1* KL is a 51-year-old, 75-kg (height 5′10″) male with simple partial seizures who requires therapy with oral carbamazepine. He has normal liver function. Suggest an initial carbamazepine dosage regimen designed to achieve a steady-state carbamazepine concentration of 6–8 mg/ml.

1. *Estimate carbamazepine dose according to disease states and conditions present in the patient.* The suggested initial dosage rate for immediate-release carbamazepine tablets in an adult patient is 200 mg twice daily (400 mg/d). This dose would be titrated upward in 200-mg increments every 2–3 weeks while monitoring for adverse and therapeutic effects. The goal of therapy includes maximal suppression of seizures, avoidance of side effects, and a target drug range of 800–1200 mg/d.

    A steady-state trough total carbamazepine serum concentration should be measured after steady state is achieved in 2–3 weeks at the highest dosage rate attained. Carbamazepine serum concentrations should also be measured if the patient experiences an exacerbation of epilepsy, or if the patient develops potential signs or symptoms of carbamazepine toxicity.

▶ *Example 2* UO is a 10-year-old, 40-kg male with simple partial seizures who requires therapy with oral carbamazepine. He has normal liver function. Suggest an initial carbamazepine dosage regimen designed to achieve a steady-state carbamazepine concentration of 6–8 µg/ml.

1. *Estimate carbamazepine dose according to disease states and conditions present in the patient.* The suggested initial dosage rate for immediate-release carbamazepine tablets for a child in this age range is 100 mg twice daily (200 mg/d). This dose would be titrated upward in 100-mg increments every 2–3 weeks while monitoring for adverse and therapeutic effects. The goal of therapy includes maximal suppression of seizures, avoidance of side effects, and a target drug range of 400–800 mg/d.

    A steady-state trough total carbamazepine serum concentration should be measured after steady state is achieved in 2–3 weeks at the highest dosage rate attained. Carbamazepine serum concentrations should also be measured if the patient experiences an exacerbation of epilepsy, or if the patient develops potential signs or symptoms of carbamazepine toxicity.

USE OF CARBAMAZEPINE SERUM CONCENTRATIONS TO ALTER DOSES

- Because of the large amount of pharmacokinetic variability among patients, it is likely that doses computed using patient population characteristics will not always produce carbamazepine serum concentrations that are expected or desirable.

- Because of pharmacokinetic variability, the autoinduction pharmacokinetics followed by the drug, the narrow therapeutic index of carbamazepine, and the desire to avoid adverse side effects of carbamazepine, measurement of carbamazepine serum concentrations is conducted for almost all patients to ensure that therapeutic, nontoxic levels are present.
- In addition to carbamazepine serum concentrations, important patient parameters (seizure frequency, potential carbamazepine side effects, etc.) should be followed to confirm that the patient is responding to treatment and not developing adverse drug reactions.
- When carbamazepine serum concentrations are measured in patients and a dosage change is necessary, clinicians should seek to use the simplest, most straightforward method available to determine a dose that will provide safe and effective treatment.

Pseudo-Linear Pharmacokinetics Method

- A simple, easy way to approximate new total serum concentrations after a dosage adjustment with carbamazepine is to temporarily assume linear pharmacokinetics, then subtract 10–20% for a dosage increase or add 10–20% for a dosage decrease to account for autoinduction pharmacokinetics:

$$Css_{new} = (D_{new} / D_{old})Css_{old}$$

where Css_{new} is the expected steady-state concentration from the new carbamazepine dose in $\mu g/ml$, Css_{old} is the measured steady-state concentration from the old carbamazepine dose in $\mu g/ml$, D_{new} is the new carbamazepine dose to be prescribed in mg/d, and D_{old} is the currently prescribed carbamazepine dose in mg/d.

- *Note:* This method is only intended to provide a rough approximation of the resulting carbamazepine steady-state concentration after an appropriate dosage adjustment, such as 100–200 mg/d, has been made. The pseudo-linear pharmacokinetics method should never be used to compute a new dose based on measured and desired carbamazepine concentrations.

▶ ***Example 1*** KL is a 51-year-old, 75-kg (height 5′10″) male with simple partial seizures who requires therapy with oral carbamazepine. He has normal liver function. After dosage titration, the patient was prescribed 200 mg in the morning, 200 mg in the afternoon, and 400 mg at bedtime (800 mg/d) of carbamazepine tablets for 1 month, after which his steady-state carbamazepine total concentration was 3.8 µg/ml. The patient is assessed to be compliant with his dosage regimen. Suggest a carbamazepine dosage regimen designed to achieve a steady-state carbamazepine concentration within the therapeutic range.

1. *Use pseudo-linear pharmacokinetics to predict the new concentration for a dosage increase, then adjust by* 10–20% *to account for autoinduction pharmacokinetics.* Since the patient is receiving carbamazepine tablets, a convenient dosage change would be 200 mg/d, and an increase to 1000 mg/d (400 mg in the morning and at bedtime, 200 mg in the afternoon) is suggested. Using pseudo-linear pharmacokinetics, the resulting total steady-state carbamazepine serum concentration is

$$Css_{new} = (D_{new}/D_{old})Css_{old} = [(1000 \text{ mg/d})/(800 \text{ mg/d})](3.8 \text{ µg/ml})$$
$$= 4.8 \text{ µg/ml}$$

Because of autoinduction pharmacokinetics, the serum concentration can be expected to increase 10% less, or 0.90 times, to 20%, or 0.80 times, less than that predicted by linear pharmacokinetics:

$$Css = 4.8 \text{ μg/ml} \cdot 0.90 = 4.3 \text{ μg/ml and}$$

$$Css = 4.8 \text{ μg/ml} \cdot 0.80 = 3.8 \text{ μg/ml}$$

Thus, a dosage increase of 200 mg/d can be expected to yield a total carbamazepine steady-state serum concentration between 3.8 and 4.3 μg/ml.

A steady-state trough total carbamazepine serum concentration should be measured after steady state is attained in 2–3 weeks. Carbamazepine serum concentrations should also be measured if the patient experiences an exacerbation of epilepsy, or if the patient develops potential signs or symptoms of carbamazepine toxicity.

▶ *Example 2*   UO is a 10-year-old, 40-kg male with simple partial seizures who requires therapy with oral carbamazepine. He has normal liver function. After dosage titration, the patient was prescribed 200 mg three times daily (600 mg/d) of carbamazepine tablets for 1 month, after which his steady-state carbamazepine total concentration was 5.1 μg/ml. The patient is assessed to be compliant with his dosage regimen. Suggest a carbamazepine dosage regimen designed to achieve a steady-state carbamazepine concentration in the middle of the therapeutic range.

1. *Use pseudo-linear pharmacokinetics to predict the new concentration for a dosage increase, then adjust by* 10–20% *to account for autoinduction pharmacokinetics.* Since the patient is receiving carbamazepine tablets, a convenient dosage change would be 200 mg/d, and an increase to 800 mg/d (300 mg in the morning and at bedtime, 200 mg in the afternoon) is suggested. Using pseudo-linear pharmacokinetics, the resulting total steady-state carbamazepine serum concentration is

$$Css_{new} = (D_{new}/D_{old})Css_{old} = [(800 \text{ mg/d})/(600 \text{ mg/d})](5.1 \text{ μg/ml})$$
$$= 6.8 \text{ μg/ml}$$

Because of autoinduction pharmacokinetics, the serum concentration can be expected to increase 10% less, or 0.90 times, to 20%, or 0.80 times, less than that predicted by linear pharmacokinetics:

$$Css = 6.8 \text{ μg/ml} \cdot 0.90 = 6.1 \text{ μg/ml and}$$

$$Css = 6.8 \text{ μg/ml} \cdot 0.80 = 5.4 \text{ μg/ml}$$

Thus, a dosage increase of 200 mg/d can be expected to yield a total carbamazepine steady-state serum concentration between 5.4 and 6.1 μg/ml.

A steady-state trough total carbamazepine serum concentration should be measured after steady state is attained in 2–3 weeks. Carbamazepine serum concentrations should also be measured if the patient experiences an exacerbation of epilepsy, or if the patient develops potential signs or symptoms of carbamazepine toxicity.

BAYESIAN PHARMACOKINETIC COMPUTER PROGRAMS

• Computer programs are available that can assist in the computation of pharmacokinetic parameters for patients.[38] The most reliable computer programs use a nonlinear regression algorithm that incorporates components of Bayes' theorem.

- Unfortunately, these computer programs have not been able to give acceptable solutions unless four or more carbamazepine concentrations are available. This is due to the complexity of the autoinduction pharmacokinetics that carbamazepine follows under chronic dosing conditions. Because of the large number of concentrations needed, this dosage adjustment approach cannot be recommended at this time.

REFERENCES

1. Gidal BE, Graves NM, Garnett WR. Epilepsy. In: DiPiro JT, Talbert RL, Yee GC, Matzke GR, Wells BG, Posey LM, eds. Pharmacotherapy. 5th ed. New York: McGraw-Hill, 2002:1031–60.
2. McNamara JO. Drugs effective in the therapy of the epilepsies. In: Hardman JG, Limbird LE, Gilman AG, eds. The pharmacological basis of therapeutics. 10th ed. New York: McGraw-Hill, 2001:521–48.
3. Hooper WD, Dubetz DK, Bochner F, et al. Plasma protein binding of carbamazepine. Clin Pharmacol Ther 1975;17(4):433–40.
4. Lawless LM, DeMonaco HJ, Muido LR. Protein binding of carbamazepine in epileptic patients. Neurology 1982;32(4):415–8.
5. Paxton JW, Donald RA. Concentrations and kinetics of carbamazepine in whole saliva, parotid saliva, serum ultrafiltrate, and serum. Clin Pharmacol Ther 1980;28(5):695–702.
6. Rane A, Hojer B, Wilson JT. Kinetics of carbamazepine and its 10,11-epoxide metabolite in children. Clin Pharmacol Ther 1976;19(3):276–83.
7. McKauge L, Tyrer JH, Eadie MJ. Factors influencing simultaneous concentrations of carbamazepine and its epoxide in plasma. Ther Drug Monit 1981;3(1):63–70.
8. Brodie MJ, Forrest G, Rapeport WG. Carbamazepine 10,11 epoxide concentrations in epileptics on carbamazepine alone and in combination with other anticonvulsants. Br J Clin Pharmacol 1983;16(6):747–9.
9. Eichelbaum M, Bertilsson L, Lund L, Palmer L, Sjoqvist F. Plasma levels of carbamazepine and carbamazepine-10,11-epoxide during treatment of epilepsy. Eur J Clin Pharmacol 1976;09(5-6):417–21.
10. MacKichan JJ, Duffner PK, Cohen ME. Salivary concentrations and plasma protein binding of carbamazepine and carbamazepine 10,11-epoxide in epileptic patients. Br J Clin Pharmacol 1981;12(1):31–7.
11. Hundt HK, Aucamp AK, Muller FO, Potgieter MA. Carbamazepine and its major metabolites in plasma: a summary of eight years of therapeutic drug monitoring. Ther Drug Monit 1983;5(4):427–35.
12. Elyas AA, Patsalos PN, Agbato OA, Brett EM, Lascelles PT. Factors influencing simultaneous concentrations of total and free carbamazepine and carbamazepine-10,11-epoxide in serum of children with epilepsy. Ther Drug Monit 1986;8(3):288–92.
13. Bertilsson L, Tybring G, Widen J, Chang M, Tomson T. Carbamazepine treatment induces the CYP3A4 catalysed sulphoxidation of omeprazole, but has no or less effect on hydroxylation via CYP2C19. Br J Clin Pharmacol 1997;44(2):186–9.
14. Kerr BM, Thummel KE, Wurden CJ, et al. Human liver carbamazepine metabolism. Role of CYP3A4 and CYP2C8 in 10,11-epoxide formation. Biochem Pharmacol 1994;47(11):1969.
15. Perucca E, Bittencourt P, Richens A. Effect of dose increments on serum carbamazepine concentration in epileptic patients. Clin Pharmacokinet 1980;5(6):576–82.
16. McNamara PJ, Colburn WA, Gibaldi M. Time course of carbamazepine self-induction. J Pharmacokinet Biopharm 1979;7(1):63–8.
17. Eichelbaum M, Kothe KW, Hoffmann F, von Unruh GE. Use of stable labelled carbamazepine to study its kinetics during chronic carbamazepine treatment. Eur J Clin Pharmacol 1982;23(3):241–4.
18. Pitlick WH, Levy RH, Tropin AS, Green JR. Pharmacokinetic model to describe self-induced decreases in steady-state concentrations of carbamazepine. J Pharm Sci 1976;65(3):462.

19. Bertilsson L, Hojer B, Tybring G, Osterloh J, Rane A. Autoinduction of carbamazepine metabolism in children examined by a stable isotope technique. Clin Pharmacol Ther 1980;27(1):83–8.
20. Schaffler L, Bourgeois BF, Luders HO. Rapid reversibility of autoinduction of carbamazepine metabolism after temporary discontinuation. Epilepsia 1994;35(1):195–8.
21. Neuvonen PJ, Tokola O. Bioavailability of rectally administered carbamazepine mixture. Br J Clin Pharmacol 1987;24(6):839–41.
22. Graves NM, Kriel RL, Jones-Saete C, Cloyd JC. Relative bioavailability of rectally administered carbamazepine suspension in humans. Epilepsia 1985;26(5):429–33.
23. Hartley R, Aleksandrowicz J, Ng PC, McLain B, Bowmer CJ, Forsythe WI. Breakthrough seizures with generic carbamazepine: a consequence of poorer bioavailability? Br J Clin Pract 1990;44(7):270–3.
24. Meyer MC, Straughn AB, Mhatre RM, Shah VP, Williams RL, Lesko LJ. The relative bioavailability and in vivo-in vitro correlations for four marketed carbamazepine tablets. Pharm Res 1998;15(11):1787–91.
25. Olling M, Mensinga TT, Barends DM, Groen C, Lake OA, Meulenbelt J. Bioavailability of carbamazepine from four different products and the occurrence of side effects. Biopharm Drug Dispos 1999;20(1):19–28.
26. Yacobi A, Zlotnick S, Colaizzi JL, et al. A multiple-dose safety and bioequivalence study of a narrow therapeutic index drug: a case for carbamazepine. Clin Pharmacol Ther 1999;65(4):389–94.
27. Cohen H, Howland MA, Luciano DJ, et al. Feasibility and pharmacokinetics of carbamazepine oral loading doses. Am J Health Syst Pharm 1998;55(11):1134–40.
28. Cotter LM, Eadie MJ, Hooper WD, Lander CM, Smith GA, Tyrer JH. The pharmacokinetics of carbamazepine. Eur J Clin Pharmacol 1977;12(6):451–6.
29. Levy RH, Pitlick WH, Troupin AS, Green JR, Neal JM. Pharmacokinetics of carbamazepine in normal man. Clin Pharmacol Ther 1975;17(6):657–68.
30. Rawlins MD, Collste P, Bertilsson L, Palmer L. Distribution and elimination kinetics of carbamazepine in man. Eur J Clin Pharmacol 1975;8(2):91–6.
31. Monaco F, Riccio A, Benna P, et al. Further observations on carbamazepine plasma levels in epileptic patients. Relationships with therapeutic and side effects. Neurology 1976;26(10):936–73.
32. Battino D, Bossi L, Croci D, et al. Carbamazepine plasma levels in children and adults: influence of age, dose, and associated therapy. Ther Drug Monit 1980;2(4):315–22.
33. Eichelbaum M, Kothe KW, Hoffman F, von Unruh GE. Kinetics and metabolism of carbamazepine during combined antiepileptic drug therapy. Clin Pharmacol Ther 1979;26(3):366–71.
34. Pugh RN, Murray-Lyon IM, Dawson JL, Pietroni MC, Williams R. Transection of the oesophagus for bleeding oesophageal varices. Br J Surg 1973;60(8):646–9.
35. Lee CS, Wang LH, Marbury TC, Bruni J, Perchalski RJ. Hemodialysis clearance and total body elimination of carbamazepine during chronic hemodialysis. Clin Toxicol 1980;17(3):429–38.
36. Kandrotas RJ, Oles KS, Gal P, Love JM. Carbamazepine clearance in hemodialysis and hemoperfusion. Drug Intel Clin Pharm 1989;23(2):137–40.
37. Hansten PD, Horn JR. Drug interactions analysis and management. Vancouver, WA: Applied Therapeutics, 1999.
38. Wandell M, Mungall D. Computer assisted drug interpretation and drug regimen optimization. Am Assoc Clin Chem 1984;6:1–11.
39. Brodie MJ, Dichter MA. Antiepileptic drugs. N Engl J Med 1996;334(3):168–75.

12 | Valproic Acid

Valproic acid is an agent that is chemically related to free fatty acids and is used in the treatment of generalized, partial, and absence (petit mal) seizures.[1] As such, it has the widest spectrum of activity compared to the other currently available antiepileptic drugs (Table 12-1).

- Valproic acid is available in intravenous and oral dosage forms, and can be used for the acute treatment and chronic prophylaxis of seizures. Valproic acid is also a useful agent for the treatment of bipolar affective disorders.
- Although the precise mechanism of action of valproic acid is unknown, its antiepileptic effect is thought to be due to its ability to increase concentrations of the neuroinhibitor γ-aminobutyric acid (GABA), to potentate the postsynaptic response to GABA, or to exert a direct effect on cellular membranes.[2]

THERAPEUTIC AND TOXIC CONCENTRATIONS

- The generally accepted therapeutic range for total valproic acid steady-state concentrations is 50–100 μg/ml, although some clinicians suggest drug concentrations as high as 175 μg/ml with appropriate monitoring of serum concentrations and possible adverse effects.
- Valproic acid is highly protein-bound to albumin, with typical values of 90–95%.[3,4]

  - Plasma protein binding of valproic acid is saturable within the therapeutic range, which results in less protein binding and higher unbound fraction of drug at higher concentrations. The concentration-dependent protein binding of valproic acid causes the drug to follow nonlinear pharmacokinetics (Figure 12-1).
  - This type of nonlinear pharmacokinetics is fundamentally different from that observed during phenytoin administration. Phenytoin hepatic metabolism becomes saturated, which causes Michaelis-Menten pharmacokinetics to take place. As a result, when phenytoin doses are increased total and unbound steady-state concentrations increase more than a proportional amount (e.g., when the dose is doubled, serum concentrations may increase 3–5-fold or more).
  - In the case of valproic acid, when the dose is increased, total drug steady-state concentration increases less than expected, but unbound steady-state drug concentration increases in a proportional fashion (e.g., when the dose is doubled, total serum concentration increases 1.6–1.9 times but unbound steady-state serum concentration doubles; Figure 12-2). The pharmacokinetic rational for these changes is explained fully under Basic Clinical Pharmacokinetic Parameters, later in this chapter.

- Insufficient prospective work has been done to establish the therapeutic range for unbound valproic acid steady-state serum concentrations.

  - As an initial guide, 5% of the lower end and 10% of the upper end of the total concentration therapeutic range is used to construct the preliminary unbound steady-state concentration therapeutic range for valproic acid of 2.5–10 μg/ml.

304

TABLE 12-1 International Classification of Epileptic Seizures [1]

Major class	Subset of class	Drug treatment for selected seizure type
Partial seizures (beginning locally)	1. Simple partial seizures (without impaired consciousness) *a.* With motor symptoms *b.* With somatosensory or special sensory symptoms *c.* With autonomic symptoms *d.* With psychological symptoms	Carbamazepine Phenytoin Valproic acid Phenobarbital Primidone
	2. Complex partial seizures (with impaired consciousness) *a.* Simple partial onset followed by impaired consciousness *b.* Impaired consciousness at onset	Carbamazepine Phenytoin Valproic acid Phenobarbital Primidone
	3. Partial seizures evolving into secondary generalized seizures	Carbamazepine Phenytoin Valproic acid Phenobarbital Primidone
Generalized seizures (convulsive or nonconvulsive)	1. Absence seizures (typical or atypical; also known as petite mal seizures)	Valproic acid Ethosuximide
	2. Tonic-clonic seizures (also known as grand mal seizures)	Phenytoin Carbamazepine Valproic acid Phenobarbital Primidone

- The percent used for each case is the average unbound fraction of drug at the appropriate concentration.
- More information is available that identifies the clinical situations in which unbound valproic acid serum concentration measurement is useful. As is the case with phenytoin, measurement of unbound valproic acid serum concentrations should be considered in patients with factors known to alter valproic acid plasma protein binding.[4–8]
- These factors fall into three broad categories: (1) lack of binding protein when there are insufficient plasma concentrations of albumin, (2) displacement of valproic acid from albumin-binding sites by endogenous compounds, and (3) displacement of valproic acid from albumin-binding sites by exogenous compounds (Table 12-2).
- Low albumin concentrations, known as hypoalbuminemia, can be found in patients with liver disease or the nephrotic syndrome, pregnant women, cystic fibrosis patients, burn patients, trauma patients, malnourished individuals, and the elderly.

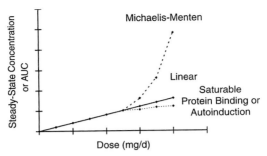

FIG. 12-1 If a drug follows linear pharmacokinetics, Css or area under the curve (AUC) increases proportionally with dose, resulting in a straight line on the plot. Nonlinear pharmacokinetics occurs when the plot of Css or AUC versus dose results in something other than a straight line. If a drug follows Michaelis-Menten pharmacokinetics (e.g., phenytoin, aspirin), as steady-state drug concentrations approach K_m, serum concentrations increase more than expected due to dose increases. If a drug follows nonlinear protein binding (e.g., valproic acid, disopyramide), total steady-state drug concentrations increase less than expected as dose increases.

- Albumin concentrations below 3 g/dl are associated with high valproic acid unbound fractions in the plasma.
- Albumin is manufactured by the liver, so patients with hepatic disease may have difficulty synthesizing the protein.
- Patients with nephrotic syndrome waste albumin by eliminating it in the urine.
- Malnourished patients can be so nutritionally deprived that albumin production is impeded.

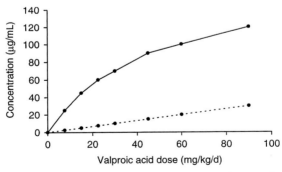

FIG. 12-2 Although total valproic acid concentrations increase in a nonlinear fashion with dosage increases (solid line), unbound, or "free" valproic acid concentrations increase in a linear fashion with dosage increases (dashed line). Valproic acid is a low-extraction-ratio drug, and its unbound serum concentrations are a function of intrinsic clearance (Cl'_{int}) only: $Css_u = (D/\tau)/Cl'_{int}$, where D is valproic acid dose in mg, τ is the dosage interval in hours, and Css_u is the unbound steady-state valproic acid concentration.

TABLE 12-2 Disease States and Conditions That Alter Valproic Acid Plasma Protein Binding

Insufficient albumin concentration (hypoalbuminemia)	Displacement by endogenous compounds	Displacement by exogenous compounds
Liver disease	Hyperbilirubinemia	Drug interactions
Nephrotic syndrome	Jaundice	Warfarin
Pregnancy	Liver disease	Phenytoin
Cystic fibrosis	Renal dysfunction	Aspirin (>2 g/d)
Burns		NSAIDs with high
Trauma		albumin binding
Malnourishment		
Elderly		

- Malnourishment is the reason for hypoalbuminemia in some elderly patients, although there is a general downtrend in albumin concentrations in older patients. However, the unbound fraction of valproic acid is higher in elderly patients even if albumin concentrations are within the normal range.
- While they are recovering from their injuries, burn and trauma patients can become hypermetabolic and albumin concentrations can decrease if enough calories are not supplied during this phase of their disease state.
- Albumin concentrations may decline during pregnancy as maternal reserves are shifted to the developing fetus; such findings are especially prevalent during the third trimester.

- Displacement of valproic acid from plasma protein-binding sites by endogenous substances can occur in patients with hepatic or renal dysfunction. The mechanism is competition for albumin plasma protein-binding sites between the exogenous substances and valproic acid.

- Bilirubin (a by-product of heme metabolism) is broken down by the liver, so patients with hepatic disease can have excessive bilirubin concentrations. Total bilirubin concentrations in excess of 2 mg/dl are associated with abnormal valproic acid plasma-protein binding.
- End-stage renal disease patients (creatinine clearance <10–15 ml/min) with uremia (blood urea nitrogen concentrations >80–100 mg/dl) accumulate unidentified compound(s) in their blood that displace valproic acid from plasma protein-binding sites. Abnormal valproic acid binding persists in these patients even when dialysis procedures are instituted.

- Valproic acid plasma protein-binding displacement can also occur due to exogenously administered compounds such as drugs. In this case, the mechanism is competition for albumin-binding sites between valproic acid and other agents.

- Other drugs that are highly bound to albumin and cause plasma protein-binding displacement drug interactions with valproic acid include warfarin, phenytoin, aspirin (>2 g/d), and some highly bound nonsteroidal anti-inflammatory agents.

- At the upper end of the therapeutic range (>75 μg/ml), some patients will begin to experience the concentration-dependent adverse effects of valproic acid therapy: ataxia, sedation, lethargy, and tiredness.

  - In many individuals, these side effects dissipate with continued dosing, and slow dosage titration may assist in minimizing these adverse reactions in newly treated patients.
  - Other concentration-related side effects of valproic acid therapy include tremor at concentrations >100 μg/ml, and stupor or coma at concentrations >175 μg/ml.
  - Valproic acid-associated thrombocytopenia can usually be limited by a decrease in drug dose.

CLINICAL MONITORING PARAMETERS

- The goal of therapy with anticonvulsants is to reduce seizure frequency and maximize quality of life with a minimum of adverse drug effects. While it is desirable to abolish seizure episodes entirely, it may not be possible to accomplish this in many patients.
- Patients should be monitored for concentration-related side effects (ataxia, sedation, lethargy, tiredness, tremor, stupor, coma, thrombocytopenia) as well as gastrointestinal upset associated with local irritation of gastric mucosa (nausea, vomiting, anorexia).[9]
- Elevated liver function tests, increased serum ammonia, alopecia, and weight gain, have been reported during chronic valproic acid treatment.
- Serious, but rare, idiosyncratic side effects include hepatotoxicity, pancreatitis, pitting edema, systemic lupus-like reactions, and leukopenia with bone marrow changes.
- Valproic acid serum concentrations should be measured in most patients.

  - Because epilepsy is an episodic disease state, patients do not experience seizures on a continuous basis. Thus, during dosage titration it is difficult to tell if the patient is responding to drug therapy or simply is not experiencing any abnormal central nervous system discharges at that time.
  - Valproic acid serum concentrations are also valuable tools for avoiding adverse drug effects. Patients are more likely to accept drug therapy if adverse reactions are held to the absolute minimum.

BASIC CLINICAL PHARMACOKINETIC PARAMETERS

- Valproic acid is eliminated primarily by hepatic metabolism (>95%). Hepatic metabolism is via glucuronidation, beta-oxidation, and alpha-hydroxylation. About 1–5% of a valproic acid dose is recovered in the urine as unchanged drug.

  - More than 10 metabolites have been identified for valproic acid, and the 4-en-valproic acid metabolite may be associated with the drug's propensity to cause hepatotoxicity.

- Valproic acid follows nonlinear pharmacokinetics due to saturable, or concentration-dependent, plasma protein binding. This is the type of nonlinear pharmacokinetics that occurs when the number of drug molecules overwhelms or saturates albumin's ability to bind the drug in the plasma.

  - Total steady-state drug serum concentrations increase in a disproportionate manner after a dosage increase, but unbound steady-state drug serum concentrations increase in a proportional fashion (Figure 12-2).

- Valproic acid is eliminated almost completely by hepatic metabolism, and it has a low hepatic extraction ratio. The hepatic clearance rate is described by the classic relationship that is used to describe hepatic clearance:

$$Cl_H = [LBF \cdot (f_B Cl'_{int})]/(LBF + f_B Cl'_{int})$$

where LBF is liver blood flow, f_B is the unbound fraction of drug in the blood, and Cl'_{int} is the intrinsic ability of the enzyme system to metabolize the drug.

- Since valproic acid has a low hepatic extraction ratio, this expression for hepatic clearance simplifies to $Cl_H = f_B Cl'_{int}$.

- The clinical implication of concentration-dependent plasma protein-binding pharmacokinetics is that the clearance of valproic acid is not a constant as it is with linear pharmacokinetics, but is concentration- or dose-dependent.

- As the dose or concentration of valproic acid increases, the clearance rate (Cl) increases because more unbound drug is available to hepatic enzymes for metabolism: $\uparrow Cl_H = \uparrow f_B Cl'_{int}$. This is why total steady-state concentrations increase disproportionately after a valproic acid dosage increase: $\uparrow Css = [F(\Uparrow D/\tau)]/\uparrow Cl_H$, where F is valproic acid bioavailability, D is valproic acid dose, τ is the dosage interval, and Cl_H is hepatic clearance.
- When valproic acid dose is increased, the unbound fraction increases and causes an increase in hepatic clearance. Because dose and hepatic clearance increase simultaneously, total valproic acid concentrations increase, but by an amount that is smaller than expected.
- There is so much interpatient variability in concentration-dependent plasma protein-binding parameters for valproic acid that predicting changes in unbound fraction and hepatic clearance is extremely difficult.
- Since unbound steady-state concentrations are influenced only by intrinsic clearance, unbound concentrations increase in a proportional amount to dose:

$$Css_u = [F(D/\tau)]/Cl'_{int}$$

- Valproic acid volume of distribution ($V = 0.15$–0.2 L/kg) is also affected by concentration-dependent plasma protein binding and is determined by the physiological volume of blood (V_B) and tissues (V_T) as well as the unbound fraction of drug in the blood (f_B) and tissues (f_T):

$$V = V_B + (f_B/f_T)V_T$$

- As valproic acid concentrations increase, unbound fraction of drug in the blood increases, which causes an increase in the volume of distribution for the drug:

$$\uparrow V = V_B + (\uparrow f_B/f_T)V_T$$

- Half-life ($t_{1/2}$) is related to clearance and volume of distribution using the same equation as for linear pharmacokinetics:

$$t_{1/2} = (0.693 \cdot V)/Cl$$

However, since clearance and volume of distribution are functions of dose- or concentration-dependent plasma protein binding for valproic acid, half-life also changes with drug dosage or concentration changes.

- As doses or concentrations increase for a drug that follows concentration-dependent plasma protein-binding pharmacokinetics, clearance and volume of distribution simultaneously increase, and half-life changes are variable depending on the relative changes in clearance and volume of distribution: $\leftrightarrow t_{1/2} = (0.693 \cdot \uparrow V)/\uparrow Cl$.
- The clinical implication of this finding is that the time to steady state (3–5 half-lives) is variable as the dose or concentration is increased for valproic acid. On average, valproic acid half-life is 12–18 hours in adult patients with total concentrations within the therapeutic range.

- Valproic acid is available as three different entities, and all of them are prescribed as valproic acid equivalents: valproic acid, sodium valproate (the sodium salt of valproic acid), and divalproex sodium (a stable coordination compound consisting of a 1:1 ratio of valproic acid and sodium valproate).

  - For parenteral use, valproic acid is available as a 100-mg/ml solution. When it is given intravenously, it should be diluted in at least 50 ml of intravenous solution, and given over 1 hour (injection rates should not exceed 20 mg/min).
  - For oral use, a syrup (50 mg/ml), soft capsule (250 mg), enteric-coated capsules (125, 250, and 500 mg), and sprinkle capsules (125 mg, used to sprinkle into foods) are available.

    - The enteric-coated capsules are not sustained-release products, but only delay the absorption of drug after ingestion. As a result, there are fewer gastrointestinal side effects with the enteric-coated product.
    - The oral bioavailability of valproic acid is very good for all dosage forms and approximates 100%. Therefore, the same total daily dose of valproic acid can be used regardless of whether intravenous or oral valproic acid is administered to a patient.

- The typical maintenance dose for valproic acid is 15 mg/kg/d, resulting in 1000 mg/d or 500 mg twice daily for most adult patients. However, because age and coadministration of other antiepileptic drugs that are enzyme inducers (e.g., carbamazepine, phenytoin, phenobarbital) affect valproic acid pharmacokinetics, many clinicians recommend the administration of 7.5 mg/kg/d for adults or 10 mg/kg/d for children under 12 years of age receiving monotherapy and 15 mg/kg/d for adults or 20 mg/kg/d for children under 12 years old receiving other drugs that are enzyme inducers.[10]

EFFECTS OF DISEASE STATES AND CONDITIONS ON PHARMACOKINETICS AND DOSING

- For valproic acid, oral clearance (Cl/F) is 7–12 ml/h/kg and half-life is 12–18 hours for adults.[11] In children 6–12 years old, oral clearance and half-life are 10–20 ml/h/kg and 6–8 hours, respectively.[12]
- Clearance rates may be higher and half-lives shorter in patients receiving other hepatic drug metabolizing enzyme inducers (phenytoin, phenobarbital, carbamazepine).

  - For adults receiving other antiepileptic drugs that are enzyme inducers, valproic acid clearance for adults is 15–18 ml/h/kg and half-lives range from 4 to 12 hours.
  - If children receive therapy with other antiepileptic drugs that are enzyme inducers, clearance is 20–30 ml/h/kg and half-life is 4–6 h.[13,14]

- Valproic acid volume of distribution (V/F) is 0.15–0.2 L/kg.[11,15]
- Valproic acid serum concentrations exhibit some diurnal variation in patients, so the time that steady-state serum concentrations should be noted when comparing multiple values.[4,16]

Liver Dysfunction

- Patients with liver cirrhosis or acute hepatitis have reduced valproic acid clearance because of destruction of liver parenchyma.[17] This loss of functional hepatic cells reduces the amount of enzymes available to metabolize the drug and decreases clearance.
- Valproic acid clearance in patients with liver disease is 3–4 ml/h/kg.
- The volume of distribution may be larger because of reduced plasma protein binding (free fraction ≈29%).
- Protein binding may be reduced and unbound fraction may be increased due to hypoalbuminemia and/or hyperbilirubinemia (especially albumin ≤3 g/dl and/or total bilirubin ≥2 mg/dl).
- Average half-life for valproic acid in patients with liver disease is 25 hours.
- The effects of liver disease on valproic acid pharmacokinetics are highly variable and difficult to predict accurately. It is possible for a patient with liver disease to have relatively normal or grossly abnormal valproic acid clearance and volume of distribution.
- An index of liver dysfunction can be gained by applying the Child-Pugh clinical classification system to the patient (Table 12-3).[18] Child-Pugh scores are discussed more fully in Chapter 3 (Drug Dosing in Special Populations: Renal and Hepatic Disease, Dialysis, Heart Failure, Obesity, and Drug Interactions).

  - The Child-Pugh score consists of five laboratory tests or clinical symptoms: serum albumin, total bilirubin, prothrombin time, ascites, and hepatic encephalopathy. Each of these areas is given a score of 1 (normal) to 3 (severely abnormal; Table 12-3), and the scores for the five areas are summed.
  - The Child-Pugh score for a patient with normal liver function is 5, while the score for a patient with grossly abnormal serum albumin, total bilirubin, and prothrombin time values in addition to severe ascites and hepatic encephalopathy is 15.
  - A Child-Pugh score greater than 8 is grounds for a decrease of 25–50% in the initial daily drug dose of valproic acid.

TABLE 12-3 Child-Pugh Scores for Patients with Liver Disease[18]

Test/symptom	Score 1 point	Score 2 points	Score 3 points
Total bilirubin (mg/dl)	<2.0	2.0–3.0	>3.0
Serum albumin (g/dl)	>3.5	2.8–3.5	<2.8
Prothrombin time (seconds prolonged over control)	<4	4–6	>6
Ascites	Absent	Slight	Moderate
Hepatic Encephalopathy	None	Moderate	Severe

- As in any patient, with or without liver dysfunction, initial doses are meant as starting points for dosage titration based on patient response and avoidance of adverse effects. Valproic acid serum concentrations and the presence of adverse drug effects should be monitored frequently in patients with liver cirrhosis.

Other Disease States and Conditions

- Elderly patients have lower valproic acid oral clearance rates and higher unbound fractions than younger adults, so lower initial doses may be used in older individuals.[4]
- During the third trimester of pregnancy, oral clearance of valproic acid may decrease and require dosage adjustment.[19] Breast milk concentrations of valproic acid are about 10% of concurrent serum concentrations.
- Doses of valproic acid do not require adjustment for patients with renal failure, and the drug is not removed by dialysis.[20]

DRUG INTERACTIONS

- Valproic acid is a potent inhibitor of hepatic drug-metabolizing enzyme systems and glucuronidation.[21–23]

  - Other antiepileptic drugs for which clearance rates are decreased and steady-state concentrations increased by valproic acid-related enzyme inhibition include clonazepam, carbamazepine, phenytoin, primidone, lamotrigine, and ethosuximide.
  - Valproic acid therapy also decreases the clearance and increases steady-state concentrations of other drugs, including zidovudine, amitriptyline and nortriptyline.
  - When valproic acid is added to a patient's drug regimen, an adverse effect due to one of the other drugs must be considered as a possible drug interaction with valproic acid.

- Other drugs can affect valproic acid clearance and steady-state serum concentrations.[21]

  - Phenytoin, lamotrigine, rifampin, and carbamazepine can increase valproic acid clearance and decrease valproic acid steady-state serum concentrations.
  - Cimetidine, chlorpromazine, and felbamate are examples of drugs that decrease valproic acid clearance and increase valproic acid steady-state concentrations.

- Because valproic acid is highly protein-bound, plasma protein-binding drug interactions can occur with other drugs that are highly bound to albumin.[21] Aspirin, warfarin, and phenytoin all have plasma protein-binding drug interactions with valproic acid, and these drugs have higher unbound fractions when given concurrently with valproic acid.

  - The drug interaction between valproic acid and phenytoin deserves special examination because of its complexity and because these two agents are regularly used together for the treatment of seizures.[24–27] The drug interaction involves the plasma protein-binding displacement and intrinsic clearance inhibition of phenytoin by valproic acid. What makes this

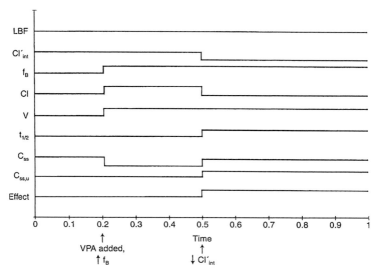

FIG. 12-3   Schematic representation of the effect on physiological (LBF = liver blood flow, Cl'_{int} = intrinsic or unbound clearance, f_B = unbound fraction of drug in blood/plasma), pharmacokinetic (Cl = clearance; V = volume of distribution; $t_{1/2}$ = half-life; Css = total steady-state drug concentration; Css_u = unbound steady-state drug concentration), and pharmacodynamic (Effect = pharmacodynamic effect) parameters that occur when initiating valproic acid (VPA) treatment in an individual stabilized on phenytoin therapy. Initially, valproic acid decreases phenytoin plasma protein binding via competitive displacement for binding sites on albumin (arrow denotes $\uparrow f_B$). As valproic acid concentrations increase, the hepatic enzyme inhibition component of the drug interaction comes into play (arrow denotes $\downarrow Cl'_{int}$). The net result is that total phenytoin concentrations are largely unchanged from baseline, but unbound phenytoin concentrations and pharmacological effect increase.

interaction so difficult to detect and understand is that these two changes do not occur simultaneously, so the impression left by the drug interaction depends on when in time it is observed in a patient (Figure 12-3).

INITIAL DOSAGE DETERMINATION METHODS

• Several methods to initiate valproic acid therapy are available:

   • The *pharmacokinetic dosing method* is the most flexible of the techniques. It allows individualized target serum concentrations to be chosen for a patient, and each pharmacokinetic parameter can be customized to reflect specific disease states and conditions present in the patient.
   • *Literature-based recommended dosing* is a very commonly used method of prescribing initial doses of valproic acid. Doses are based on those that commonly produce steady-state concentrations near the lower end of the therapeutic range, although there is a wide variation in the actual concentrations for a specific patient.

Pharmacokinetic Dosing Method

- The goal of initial dosing of valproic acid is to compute the best dose possible for the patient given the set of disease states and conditions that influence valproic acid pharmacokinetics and the epileptic disorder being treated. In order to do this, pharmacokinetic parameters for the patient are estimated using average parameters measured in other patients with similar disease state and condition profiles.

Clearance Estimate

- Valproic acid is metabolized predominately by the liver. Unfortunately, there is no good way to estimate the elimination characteristics of liver-metabolized drugs using an endogenous marker of liver function in the same manner that serum creatinine and estimated creatinine clearance are used to estimate the elimination of agents that are eliminated renally.

  - Therefore, a patient is categorized according to the disease states and conditions that are known to change valproic acid clearance, and clearance previously measured in studies is used as an estimate of the current patient's clearance.
  - To produce the most conservative valproic acid doses in patients with multiple concurrent disease states or conditions that affect valproic acid pharmacokinetics, the disease state or condition with the smallest clearance should be used to compute doses. This approach will avoid accidental overdosage as much as is currently possible.

Volume of Distribution Estimate

- Valproic acid volume of distribution is assumed to be 0.15 L/kg for adults and 0.2 L/kg for children under 12 years of age. Patients with cirrhosis or renal failure may have larger volumes of distribution due to decreased plasma protein binding.

Half-Life and Elimination Rate Constant Estimate

- Once the correct clearance and volume of distribution estimates have been identified for the patient, they can be converted into valproic acid half-life ($t_{1/2}$) and elimination rate constant (k) estimates using the following equations:

$$t_{1/2} = (0.693 \cdot V)/Cl$$
$$k = 0.693/t_{1/2} = Cl/V$$

Selection of Appropriate Pharmacokinetic Model and Equations

- When given by intravenous injection or orally, valproic acid follows a one-compartment pharmacokinetic model.

  - When oral therapy is required, valproic acid has good bioavailability (F = 1), and dosing every 8–12 hours provides a relatively smooth serum concentration/time curve that emulates an intravenous infusion.
  - A very simple pharmacokinetic equation that computes the average valproic acid steady-state serum concentration (Css in μg/ml = mg/L) is

widely used and allows maintenance dosage calculation:

$$\text{Css} = [F(D/\tau)]/\text{Cl} \qquad \text{or} \qquad D = (\text{Css} \cdot \text{Cl} \cdot \tau)/F$$

where F is the bioavailability fraction for the oral dosage form (F = 1 for oral valproic acid products), D is the dose of valproic acid in mg, and τ is the dosage interval in hours. Cl is valproic acid clearance in L/h.

- When intravenous therapy is required, the same pharmacokinetic equation is widely used:

$$\text{Css} = (D/\tau)/\text{Cl} \qquad \text{or} \qquad D = \text{Css} \cdot \text{Cl} \cdot \tau$$

where D is the dose of valproic acid in mg, and τ is the dosage interval in hours. Cl is valproic acid clearance in L/h.

  - The equation used to calculate an intravenous loading dose (LD in mg) is based on a simple one-compartment model:

$$\text{LD} = \text{Css} \cdot V$$

where Css is the desired valproic acid steady-state concentration in μg/ml, which is equivalent to mg/L, and V is the valproic acid volume of distribution Intravenous valproic acid doses should be infusions over at least 60 minutes ($\leq$20 mg/min).

▶ **Example 1**   KL is a 51-year-old, 75-kg (height 5'10") male with tonic-clonic seizures who requires therapy with oral valproic acid. He has normal liver function and takes no medications that induce hepatic enzymes. Suggest an initial valproic acid dosage regimen designed to achieve a steady-state valproic acid concentration of 50 μg/ml.

1. *Estimate clearance and volume of distribution according to disease states and conditions present in the patient.* The clearance rate for an adult patient who is not taking other drugs that induce hepatic drug metabolism is 7–12 ml/h/kg. Using a value of 10 ml/h/kg, the estimated clearance is

$$\text{Cl} = 75 \text{ kg} \cdot 10 \text{ ml/h/kg} = 750 \text{ ml/h or } 0.75 \text{ L/h}$$

Using 0.15 L/kg, the estimated volume of distribution is

$$75 \text{ kg} \cdot 0.15 \text{ L/kg} = 11 \text{ L}$$

2. *Estimate half-life and elimination rate constant.* Once the correct clearance and volume of distribution estimates have been identified for the patient, they can be converted into the valproic acid half-life ($t_{1/2}$) and elimination rate constant (k) estimates using the following equations:

$$t_{1/2} = (0.693 \cdot V)/\text{Cl} = (0.693 \cdot 11 \text{ L})/0.75 \text{ L/h} = 10 \text{ h}$$
$$k = 0.693/t_{1/2} = 0.693/10 \text{ h} = 0.069 \text{ h}^{-1}$$

3. *Compute dosage regimen.* Oral enteric-coated divalproex sodium tablets will be prescribed to this patient (F = 1). (*Note:* μg/ml = mg/L, and this concentration unit was substituted for Css in the calculations so that unit conversion was not required.) The dosage equation for oral valproic acid is

$$D = (\text{Css} \cdot \text{Cl} \cdot \tau)/F = (50 \text{ mg/L} \cdot 0.75 \text{ L/h} \cdot 12 \text{ h})/1$$
$$= 450 \text{ mg, rounded to } 500 \text{ every } 12 \text{ h}$$

A steady-state trough valproic acid serum concentration should be measured after steady state is attained in 3–5 half-lives. Since the drug is expected to have a half-life of 10 hours, a valproic acid steady-state concentration can be obtained any time after the second day of dosing (5 half-lives = 5 · 10 h = 50 h). Valproic acid serum concentrations should also be measured if the patient experiences an exacerbation of epilepsy, or if the patient develops potential signs or symptoms of valproic acid toxicity.

▶ **Example 2** UO is a 10-year-old, 40-kg male with absence seizures who requires therapy with oral valproic acid. He has normal liver function and currently takes carbamazepine. Suggest an initial valproic acid dosage regimen designed to achieve a steady-state valproic acid concentration of 50 µg/ml.

1. *Estimate clearance and volume of distribution according to disease states and conditions present in the patient.* The clearance rate for a child who takes other drugs that induce hepatic drug metabolism is 20–30 ml/h/kg. Using a value of 25 ml/h/kg, the estimated clearance is

$$Cl = 40 \text{ kg} \cdot 25 \text{ ml/h/kg} = 1000 \text{ ml/h or 1 L/h}$$

Using 0.2 L/kg, the estimated volume of distribution is

$$40 \text{ kg} \cdot 0.2 \text{ L/kg} = 8 \text{ L}$$

2. *Estimate half-life and elimination rate constant.* Once the correct clearance and volume of distribution estimates have been identified for the patient, they can be converted into the valproic acid half-life ($t_{1/2}$) and elimination rate constant (k) estimates using the following equations:

$$t_{1/2} = (0.693 \cdot V)/Cl = (0.693 \cdot 8 \text{ L})/1 \text{ L/h} = 6 \text{ h}$$
$$k = 0.693/t_{1/2} = 0.693/6 \text{ h} = 0.116 \text{ h}^{-1}$$

3. *Compute dosage regimen.* Oral valproic acid syrup will be prescribed to this patient (F = 1). (*Note:* µg/ml = mg/L, and this concentration unit was substituted for Css in the calculations so that unit conversion was not required.) The dosage equation for oral valproic acid is

$$D = (Css \cdot Cl \cdot \tau)/F = (50 \text{ mg/L} \cdot 1 \text{ L/h} \cdot 8 \text{ h})/1$$
$$= 400 \text{ mg, or 400 mg every 8 h}$$

A steady-state trough valproic acid serum concentration should be measured after steady state is attained in 3–5 half-lives. Since the drug is expected to have a half-life of 6 hours, a valproic acid steady-state concentration can be obtained any time after the first day of dosing (5 half-lives = 5 · 6 h = 30 h). Valproic acid serum concentrations should also be measured if the patient experiences an exacerbation of epilepsy, or if the patient develops potential signs or symptoms of valproic acid toxicity.

▶ **Example 3** HU is a 25-year-old, 85-kg (height 6′2″) male with tonic-clonic seizures who requires therapy with intravenous valproic acid. He has normal liver function and takes no medications that induce hepatic enzymes. Suggest an initial valproic acid dosage regimen designed to achieve a steady-state valproic acid concentration of 75 µg/ml.

1. *Estimate clearance and volume of distribution according to disease states and conditions present in the patient.* The clearance rate for an adult patient who is not taking other drugs that induce hepatic drug metabolism is 7–12 ml/h/kg. Using a value of 10 ml/h/kg, the estimated clearance is

$$Cl = 85 \text{ kg} \cdot 10 \text{ ml/h/kg} = 850 \text{ ml/h or 0.85 L/h}$$

Using 0.15 L/kg, the estimated volume of distribution is

$$85 \text{ kg} \cdot 0.15 \text{ L/kg} = 13 \text{ L}$$

2. *Estimate half-life and elimination rate constant.* Once the correct clearance and volume of distribution estimates have been identified for the patient, they can be converted into the valproic acid half-life ($t_{1/2}$) and elimination rate constant (k) estimates using the following equations:

$$t_{1/2} = (0.693 \cdot V)/Cl = (0.693 \cdot 13 \text{ L})/0.85 \text{ L/h} = 11 \text{ h}$$
$$k = 0.693/t_{1/2} = 0.693/11 \text{ h} = 0.063 \text{ h}^{-1}$$

3. *Compute dosage regimen.* Valproic acid injection will be prescribed to this patient (F = 1). (*Note:* µg/ml = mg/L, and this concentration unit was substituted for Css in the calculations so that unit conversion was not required.) The maintenance dosage equation for valproic acid is

$$D = (Css \cdot Cl \cdot \tau)/F = (75 \text{ mg/L} \cdot 0.85 \text{ L/h} \cdot 8 \text{ h})/1$$
$$= 510 \text{ mg, rounded to 500 every 8 h}$$

The loading-dose (LD) equation for valproic acid is

$$LD = Css \cdot V = 75 \text{ mg/L} \cdot 13 \text{ L} = 975 \text{ mg, rounded to 1000 mg}$$

Intravenous doses should be given over 1 h ($\leq$20 mg/min).

A steady-state trough valproic acid serum concentration should be measured after steady state is attained in 3–5 half-lives. Since the drug is expected to have a half-life of 11 hours, a valproic acid steady-state concentration can be obtained any time after the second day of dosing (5 half-lives = 5 · 11 h = 55 h). Valproic acid serum concentrations should also be measured if the patient experiences an exacerbation of epilepsy, or if the patient develops potential signs or symptoms of valproic acid toxicity.

Literature-Based Recommended Dosing

- Because of the large amount of variability in valproic acid pharmacokinetics, even when concurrent disease states and conditions are identified, most clinicians believe that the use of standard valproic acid doses for various situations is warranted. The original computations of these doses were based on the pharmacokinetic dosing methods, and the doses were subsequently modified based on clinical experience. In general, the expected valproic acid steady-state serum concentrations used to compute these doses was 50 µg/ml.
- Usual initial maintenance doses for pediatric patients are 10 mg/kg/d if the child is not taking a hepatic enzyme inducer (phenytoin, phenobarbital, carbamazepine, rifampin), or 20 mg/kg/d if the child is taking a hepatic enzyme inducer.
- For adults, initial maintenance doses are 7.5 mg/kg/d if the patient is not taking hepatic enzyme inducers, or 15 mg/kg/d if a hepatic enzyme inducer is concurrently being administered.
- Two or three divided daily doses are used initially for these total doses. To avoid gastrointestinal side effects, doses over 1500 mg given at one time should be avoided.
- Dosage increases of 5–10 mg/kg/d are made every 1–2 weeks, depending on response and adverse effects. Most adults require 1500–3000 mg/d of valproic acid, and most children require 30–60 mg/kg/d.
- If the patient has significant hepatic dysfunction (Child-Pugh score $\geq$8), maintenance doses prescribed using this method should be decreased by

25–50%, depending on how aggressive therapy is required to be for the individual.

- To illustrate the similarities and differences between this method of dosage calculation and the pharmacokinetic dosing method, the same examples used in the previous section will be used.

▶ *Example 4*   KL is a 51-year-old, 75-kg (height 5′10″) male with tonic-clonic seizures who requires therapy with oral valproic acid. He has normal liver function and takes no medications that induce hepatic enzymes. Suggest an initial valproic acid dosage regimen for this patient.

1. *Estimate valproic acid dose according to disease states and conditions present in the patient.* Oral enteric-coated divalproex sodium tablets will be prescribed to this patient. The suggested initial maintenance dosage rate for valproic acid in an adult patient who is not taking enzyme inducers is

$$75 \text{ kg} \cdot 7.5 \text{ mg/kg/d} = 563 \text{ mg/d or } 250 \text{ mg every } 12 \text{ h}$$

This dose would be titrated upward in 5–10-mg/kg/d increments every 1–2 weeks while monitoring for adverse and therapeutic effects. The goals of therapy include maximal suppression of seizures and avoidance of side effects.

A steady-state trough total valproic acid serum concentration should be measured after steady state is attained in 1–2 weeks. Valproic acid serum concentrations should also be measured if the patient experiences an exacerbation of epilepsy, or if the patient develops potential signs or symptoms of valproic acid toxicity.

▶ *Example 5*   UO is a 10-year-old, 40-kg male with absence seizures who requires therapy with oral valproic acid. He has normal liver function and currently takes carbamazepine. Suggest an initial valproic acid dosage regimen for this patient.

1. *Estimate valproic acid dose according to disease states and conditions present in the patient.* Oral valproic acid syrup will be prescribed to this patient. The suggested initial maintenance dosage rate for valproic acid for a child who is taking enzyme inducers is

$$40 \text{ kg} \cdot 20 \text{ mg/kg/d} = 800 \text{ mg/d, rounded to } 750 \text{ mg/d or}$$
$$250 \text{ mg every } 8 \text{ h}$$

This dose would be titrated upward in 5–10-mg/kg/d increments every 1–2 weeks while monitoring for adverse and therapeutic effects. The goals of therapy include maximal suppression of seizures and avoidance of side effects.

A steady-state trough total valproic acid serum concentration should be measured after steady state is attained in 1–2 weeks. Valproic acid serum concentrations should also be measured if the patient experiences an exacerbation of epilepsy, or if the patient develops potential signs or symptoms of valproic acid toxicity.

▶ *Example 6*   HU is a 25-year-old, 85-kg (height 6′2″) male with tonic-clonic seizures who requires therapy with intravenous valproic acid. He has normal liver function and takes no medications that induce hepatic enzymes. Suggest an initial valproic acid dosage regimen for this patient.

1. *Estimate valproic acid dose according to disease states and conditions present in the patient.* Intravenous valproic acid injection will

be prescribed to this patient. The suggested initial maintenance dosage rate for an adult patient who is not taking enzyme inducers is

$$85 \text{ kg} \cdot 7.5 \text{ mg/kg/d} = 638 \text{ mg/d, rounded to } 750 \text{ mg/d or}$$
$$250 \text{ mg every 8 h}$$

This dose would be titrated upward in 5–10-mg/kg/d increments every 1–2 weeks while monitoring for adverse and therapeutic effects. If needed, a loading dose of 7.5 mg/kg could be given as the first dose:

$$85 \text{ kg} \cdot 7.5 \text{ mg/kg/d} = 638 \text{ mg, rounded to } 750 \text{ mg}$$

Intravenous doses should be administered over 1 hour (≤ 20 mg/min). The goals of therapy include maximal suppression of seizures and avoidance of side effects.

A steady-state trough total valproic acid serum concentration should be measured after steady state is attained in 1–2 weeks. Valproic acid serum concentrations should also be measured if the patient experiences an exacerbation of epilepsy, or if the patient develops potential signs or symptoms of valproic acid toxicity.

USE OF VALPROIC ACID SERUM CONCENTRATIONS TO ALTER DOSES

- Because of the large amount of pharmacokinetic variability among patients, it is likely that doses computed using patient population characteristics will not always produce valproic acid serum concentrations that are expected or desirable. Because of pharmacokinetic variability, the nonlinear pharmacokinetics followed by the drug due to concentration-dependent plasma protein binding, the narrow therapeutic index of valproic acid, and the desire to avoid adverse side effects of valproic acid, valproic acid serum concentrations are measured for most patients, to ensure that therapeutic, nontoxic levels are present.
- In addition to valproic acid serum concentrations, important patient parameters (seizure frequency, potential valproic acid side effects, etc.) should be followed to confirm that the patient is responding to treatment and not developing adverse drug reactions.
- When valproic acid serum concentrations are measured in patients and a dosage change is necessary, clinicians should seek to use the simplest, most straightforward method available to determine a dose that will provide safe and effective treatment.

  - In most cases, a simple dosage ratio can be used to change valproic acid doses by temporarily assuming that valproic acid follows linear pharmacokinetics (*pseudo-linear pharmacokinetics method*). An empiric adjustment is made in the estimated steady-state concentrations to adjust for nonlinear, concentration-dependent plasma protein binding.
  - In some situations it may be necessary or desirable to compute the valproic acid *pharmacokinetic parameters* for the patient and utilize these to calculate the best drug dose.
  - Computerized methods that incorporate expected population pharmacokinetic characteristics (*Bayesian pharmacokinetic computer programs*) can be used in difficult cases in which serum concentrations are obtained at suboptimal times, or the patient was not at steady state when serum concentrations were measured.

Pseudo-Linear Pharmacokinetics Method

- A simple, easy way to approximate new total serum concentrations after a dosage adjustment with valproic acid is to temporarily assume linear pharmacokinetics, then subtract 10–20% for a dosage increase or add 10–20% for a dosage decrease to account for nonlinear, concentration-dependent plasma protein-binding pharmacokinetics:

$$D_{new} = (Css_{new}/Css_{old})D_{old}$$

where Css_{new} is the expected steady-state concentration from the new valproic acid dose in $\mu g/ml$, Css_{old} is the measured steady-state concentration from the old valproic acid dose in $\mu g/ml$, D_{new} is the new valproic acid dose to be prescribed in mg/d, and D_{old} is the currently prescribed valproic acid dose in mg/d.
- As expected, unbound steady-state concentrations increase or decrease in a linear fashion with dose.

  - *Note:* This method is only intended to provide a rough approximation of the resulting valproic acid total steady-state concentration after an appropriate dosage adjustment has been made.

▶ *Example 7* KL is a 51-year-old, 75-kg (height 5′10″) male with tonic-clonic seizures who requires therapy with oral valproic acid. After dosage titration, the patient was prescribed 500 mg every 12 hours of enteric-coated divalproex sodium tablets (1000 mg/d) for 1 month, after which his steady-state valproic acid total concentration was 38 $\mu g/ml$. The patient is assessed to be compliant with his dosage regimen. Suggest a valproic acid dosage regimen designed to achieve a steady-state valproic acid concentration of 80 $\mu g/ml$.

1. *Use pseudo-linear pharmacokinetics to predict the new concentration for a dosage increase, then adjust by 10–20% to account for nonlinear, concentration-dependent plasma protein-binding pharmacokinetics.* Using pseudo-linear pharmacokinetics, the resulting new dose is

$$D_{new} = (Css_{new}/Css_{old})D_{old} = [(80 \ \mu g/ml)/(38 \ \mu g/ml)](1000 \ mg/d)$$
$$= 2105 \ mg/d, \text{ rounded to } 2000 \ mg/d \text{ or } 1000 \ mg \text{ every } 12 \ h$$

Because of nonlinear, concentration-dependent protein-binding pharmacokinetics, the total steady-state serum concentration is expected to be 10% less, or 0.90 times, to 20% less, or 0.80 times, that predicted by linear pharmacokinetics:

$$Css = 80 \ \mu g/ml \cdot 0.90 = 72 \ \mu g/ml \qquad \text{or}$$
$$Css = 80 \ \mu g/ml \cdot 0.80 = 64 \ \mu g/ml$$

Thus, a dosage rate of 2000 mg/d is expected to yield a total valproic acid steady-state serum concentration between 64 and 72 $\mu g/ml$.

A steady-state trough total valproic acid serum concentration should be measured after steady state is attained in 1–2 weeks. Valproic acid serum concentrations should also be measured if the patient experiences an exacerbation of epilepsy, or if the patient develops potential signs or symptoms of valproic acid toxicity.

► **Example 8**   UO is a 10-year-old, 40-kg male with absence seizures who requires therapy with oral valproic acid. He has normal liver function. After dosage titration, the patient was prescribed 400 mg three times daily (1200 mg/d) of valproic acid syrup for 1 month, after which his steady-state valproic acid total concentration was 130 µg/ml. The patient is assessed to be compliant with his dosage regimen. Suggest a valproic acid dosage regimen designed to achieve a steady-state valproic acid concentration of 75 µg/ml.

1. *Use pseudo-linear pharmacokinetics to predict the new concentration for a dosage decrease, then adjust by 10–20% to account for nonlinear, concentration-dependent plasma protein-binding pharmacokinetics.* Using pseudo-linear pharmacokinetics, the resulting new dose is

$$D_{new} = (Css_{new}/Css_{old})D_{old} = [(75 \text{ µg/ml})/(130 \text{ µg/ml})](1200 \text{ mg/d})$$
$$= 692 \text{ mg/d, rounded to } 750 \text{ mg/d or } 250 \text{ mg every } 8 \text{ h}$$

Because of nonlinear, concentration-dependent protein binding pharmacokinetics, the total steady-state serum concentration is expected to be 10% greater, or 1.10 times, to 20% greater, or 1.2 times, that predicted by linear pharmacokinetics:

$$Css = 75 \text{ µg/ml} \cdot 1.10 = 83 \text{ µg/ml} \quad \text{or}$$
$$Css = 75 \text{ µg/ml} \cdot 1.20 = 90 \text{ µg/ml}$$

Thus, a dosage rate of 750 mg/d is expected to yield a total valproic acid steady-state serum concentration between 83 and 90 µg/ml.

A steady-state trough total valproic acid serum concentration should be measured after steady state is attained in 1–2 weeks. Valproic acid serum concentrations should also be measured if the patient experiences an exacerbation of epilepsy, or if the patient develops potential signs or symptoms of valproic acid toxicity.

Pharmacokinetic Parameter Method

- The pharmacokinetic parameter method of adjusting drug doses was among the first techniques available to change doses using serum concentrations. It allows the computation of an individual's own, unique pharmacokinetic constants and uses those to calculate a dose that achieves desired valproic acid concentrations.
- The pharmacokinetic parameter method requires that steady state has been achieved and uses only a steady-state valproic acid concentration (Css).

  - During intravenous dosing, the following equation is used to compute valproic acid clearance (Cl):

  $$Cl = (D/\tau)/Css$$

  where D is the dose of valproic acid in mg, Css is the steady-state valproic acid concentration in mg/L, and τ is the dosage interval in hours.
  - If the patient is receiving oral valproic acid therapy, valproic acid clearance (Cl) can be calculated using the following formula:

  $$Cl = [F(D/\tau)]/Css$$

  where F is the bioavailability fraction for the oral dosage form (F = 1 for oral valproic acid products), D is the dose of valproic acid in mg, Css is the steady-state valproic acid concentration in mg/L, and τ is the dosage interval in hours.

- Occasionally, valproic acid serum concentrations are obtained before and after an intravenous dose.

  - Assuming a one-compartment model, the volume of distribution (V) is calculated using the following equation:

$$V = D/(C_{postdose} - C_{predose})$$

    where D is the dose of valproic acid in mg, $C_{postdose}$ is the post–loading dose concentration in mg/L, and $C_{predose}$ is the concentration before the loading dose was administered in mg/L. ($C_{predose}$ should be obtained within 30 minutes of dosage administration; $C_{postdose}$ should be obtained 30–60 minutes after the end of infusion, to avoid the distribution phase.)
  - If the predose concentration was also a steady-state concentration, valproic acid clearance can also be computed. If both clearance (Cl) and volume of distribution (V) have been measured using these techniques, the half-life $[t_{1/2} = (0.693 \cdot V)/Cl]$ and elimination rate constant $(k = 0.693/t_{1/2} = Cl/V)$ can be computed.
  - The clearance, volume of distribution, elimination rate constant, and half-life measured using these techniques are the patient's own, unique valproic acid pharmacokinetic constants and can be used in one-compartment-model equations to compute the required dose to achieve any desired serum concentration.

- Because this method also assumes linear pharmacokinetics, valproic acid doses computed using the pharmacokinetic parameter method and the pseudo-linear pharmacokinetic method should be identical.
- As with the previous method, to account for nonlinear, concentration-dependent plasma protein-binding pharmacokinetics, 10–20% for a dosage increase can be subtracted or 10–20% for a dosage decrease can be added to the expected steady-state serum concentration.
- To illustrate the similarities and differences between this method of dosage calculation and the pharmacokinetic parameter method, the same examples used in the previous section will be used.

▶ **Example 9**   KL is a 51-year-old, 75-kg (height 5'10") male with tonic-clonic seizures who requires therapy with oral valproic acid. After dosage titration, the patient was prescribed 500 mg every 12 hours of enteric-coated divalproex sodium tablets (1000 mg/d) for 1 month, after which his steady-state valproic acid total concentration was 38 μg/ml. The patient is assessed to be compliant with his dosage regimen. Suggest a valproic acid dosage regimen designed to achieve a steady-state valproic acid concentration of 80 μg/ml.

1. *Compute pharmacokinetic parameters.* The patient can be expected to achieve steady-state conditions after 2–3 days of therapy. Valproic acid clearance can be computed using a steady-state valproic acid concentration:

$$Cl = [F(D/\tau)]/Css = [1(500 \text{ mg}/12 \text{ h})]/(38 \text{ mg/L}) = 1.1 \text{ L/h}$$

   (*Note:* μg/ml = mg/L, and this concentration unit was substituted for Css in the calculations so that unit conversion was not required.)
2. *Compute valproic acid dose.* Valproic acid clearance is used to compute the new dose:

$$D = (Css \cdot Cl \cdot \tau)/F = (80 \text{ mg/L} \cdot 1.1 \text{ L/h} \cdot 12 \text{ h})/1$$
$$= 1056 \text{ mg, rounded to } 1000 \text{ mg every } 12 \text{ h}$$

Because of valproic acid's nonlinear, concentration-dependent protein-binding pharmacokinetics, the total steady-state serum concentration can be expected to be 10% less, or 0.90 times, to 20% less, or 0.80 times, that predicted by linear pharmacokinetics:

$$Css = 80 \ \mu g/ml \cdot 0.90 = 72 \ \mu g/ml \qquad \text{or}$$
$$Css = 80 \ \mu g/ml \cdot 0.80 = 64 \ \mu g/ml$$

Thus, a dosage rate of 2000 mg/d can be expected to yield a total valproic acid steady-state serum concentration between 64 and 72 μg/ml.

A steady-state trough total valproic acid serum concentration should be measured after steady state is attained in 1–2 weeks. Valproic acid serum concentrations should also be measured if the patient experiences an exacerbation of epilepsy, or if the patient develops potential signs or symptoms of valproic acid toxicity.

▶ *Example 10*   UO is a 10-year-old, 40-kg male with absence seizures who requires therapy with oral valproic acid. He has normal liver function. After dosage titration, the patient was prescribed 400 mg three times daily (1200 mg/d) of valproic acid syrup for 1 month, after which his steady-state valproic acid total concentration was 130 μg/ml. The patient is assessed to be compliant with his dosage regimen. Suggest a valproic acid dosage regimen designed to achieve a steady-state valproic acid concentration of 75 μg/ml.

1. *Compute pharmacokinetic parameters.* The patient can be expected to achieve steady-state conditions after 2–3 days of therapy. Valproic acid clearance can be computed using a steady-state valproic acid concentration:

$$Cl = [F(D/\tau)]/Css = [1(400 \ mg/8 \ h)]/(130 \ mg/L) = 0.38 \ L/h$$

(*Note:* μg/ml = mg/L, and this concentration unit was substituted for Css in the calculations so that unit conversion was not required.)

2. *Compute valproic acid dose.* Valproic acid clearance is used to compute the new dose:

$$D = (Css \cdot Cl \cdot \tau)/F = (75 \ mg/L \cdot 0.38 \ L/h \cdot 8 \ h)/1$$
$$= 228 \ mg, \text{ rounded to 250 mg every 8 h}$$

Because of valproic acid's nonlinear, concentration-dependent protein-binding pharmacokinetics, the total steady-state serum concentration can be expected to be 10% more, or 1.10 times, to 20%, or 1.20 times, more than that predicted by linear pharmacokinetics:

$$Css = 75 \ \mu g/ml \cdot 1.10 = 83 \ \mu g/ml \qquad \text{or}$$
$$Css = 75 \ \mu g/ml \cdot 1.2 = 90 \ \mu g/ml$$

Thus, a dosage rate of 750 mg/d can be expected to yield a total valproic acid steady-state serum concentration between 83 and 90 μg/ml.

A steady-state trough total valproic acid serum concentration should be measured after steady state is attained in 1–2 weeks. Valproic acid serum concentrations should also be measured if the patient experiences an exacerbation of epilepsy, or if the patient develops potential signs or symptoms of valproic acid toxicity.

▶ *Example 11*   PP is a 59-year-old, 65-kg (height 5′8″) male with tonic-clonic seizures who is receiving valproic acid injection 500 mg every 8 hours. His current steady-state valproic acid concentration (obtained 30 minutes before "booster" dose administration) is 40 µg/ml. Compute a valproic acid maintenance dose that will provide a steady-state concentration of 75 µg/ml. Additionally, in an attempt to boost valproic acid concentrations as soon as possible, an additional, single valproic acid "booster" dose of 500 mg over 60 minutes was given before the maintenance dosage rate was increased. The valproic acid total serum concentration 30 minutes after the additional dose was 105 µg/ml.

1. *Compute pharmacokinetic parameters.* The patient can be expected to achieve steady-state conditions after 2–3 days of therapy. Valproic acid clearance can be computed using a steady-state valproic acid concentration:

$$Cl = [F(D/\tau)]/Css = [1(500 \text{ mg/8 h})]/(40 \text{ mg/L}) = 1.6 \text{ L/h}$$

(*Note:* µg/ml = mg/L, and this concentration unit was substituted for Css in the calculations so that unit conversion was not required.)

Valproic acid volume of distribution can be computed using the pre–bolus dose (Css = 40 µg/ml) and post–bolus dose concentrations:

$$V = D/(C_{postdose} - C_{predose}) = 500 \text{ mg}/(105 \text{ mg/L} - 40 \text{ mg/L}) = 8 \text{ L}$$

(*Note:* µg/ml = mg/L, and this concentration unit was substituted for Css in the calculations so that unit conversion was not required.)

Valproic acid half-life $(t_{1/2})$ and elimination rate constant (k) can also be computed:

$$t_{1/2} = (0.693 \cdot V)/Cl = (0.693 \cdot 8 \text{ L})/(1.6 \text{ L/h}) = 3.5 \text{ h}$$
$$k = Cl/V = (1.6 \text{ L/h})/(8 \text{ L}) = 0.20 \text{ h}^{-1}$$

2. *Compute valproic acid dose.* Valproic acid clearance is used to compute the new valproic acid maintenance dose:

$$D = (Css \cdot Cl \cdot \tau) = (75 \text{ mg/L} \cdot 1.6 \text{ L/h} \cdot 8 \text{ h})$$
$$= 960 \text{ mg, rounded to } 1000 \text{ mg every 8 h}$$

Because of valproic acid's nonlinear, concentration-dependent protein binding pharmacokinetics, the total steady-state serum concentration can be expected to be 10% less, or 0.90 times, to 20% less, or 0.80 times, that predicted by linear pharmacokinetics:

$$Css = 75 \text{ µg/ml} \cdot 0.90 = 68 \text{ µg/ml} \qquad \text{or}$$
$$Css = 75 \text{ µg/ml} \cdot 0.80 = 60 \text{ µg/ml}$$

Thus, a dosage rate of 3000 mg/d can be expected to yield a total valproic acid steady-state serum concentration between 60 and 68 µg/ml.

The new valproic acid maintenance dose should be instituted one dosage interval after the additional "booster" dose was given.

A valproic acid serum concentration should be measured after steady state is attained in 3–5 half-lives. Since the drug has a half-life of 3.5 hours, a valproic acid steady-state concentration can be obtained after 1 day of continuous dosing (5 half-lives = 5 · 3.5 h = 17.5 h). Valproic acid serum concentrations should also be measured if the patient experiences an exacerbation of epilepsy, or if the patient develops potential signs or symptoms of valproic acid toxicity.

BAYESIAN PHARMACOKINETIC COMPUTER PROGRAMS

- Computer programs are available that can assist in the computation of pharmacokinetic parameters for patients. The most reliable computer programs use a nonlinear regression algorithm that incorporates components of Bayes' theorem.[28]

  - An advantage of this approach is that consistent dosage recommendations can be made when several different practitioners are involved in therapeutic drug monitoring programs. However, since simpler dosing methods work just as well for patients with stable pharmacokinetic parameters and steady-state drug concentrations, many clinicians reserve the use of computer programs for more difficult situations. Those situations include serum concentrations that are not at steady state, serum concentrations not obtained at the specific times needed to employ simpler methods, and unstable pharmacokinetic parameters.
  - When only a limited number of valproic acid concentrations are available, Bayesian pharmacokinetic computer programs can be used to compute a complete patient pharmacokinetic profile that includes clearance, half-life, and volume of distribution. This is a distinct advantage compared to the other methods used to adjust valproic acid dose based on one or more steady-state serum concentrations.

- Many Bayesian pharmacokinetic computer programs are available, and most should provide answers similar to the program used in the following examples. The program used to solve problems in this book is DrugCalc, written by Dr. Dennis Mungall and available at his Internet web site (www.clinpharmacologist.bigstep.com/consumersurvey.html).[28]

▶ **Example 12**   LK is a 50-year-old, 75-kg (height 5′10″) male with complex partial seizures who is receiving 500 mg of oral enteric-coated valproic acid tablets every 8 hours. He has normal liver (bilirubin = 0.7 mg/dl, albumin = 4.0 g/dl) function, and also takes 1200 mg/d of carbamazepine. The patient's current steady-state valproic acid concentration is 31 μg/ml. Compute a valproic acid dose that will provide a steady-state concentration of 70 μg/ml.

1. *Enter patient demographic, drug dosing, and serum concentration/time data into a Bayesian pharmacokinetic computer program.*
2. *Compute pharmacokinetic parameters for the patient using the computer program.* The pharmacokinetic parameters computed by the program are a volume of distribution of 8.6 L, a half-life of 5.2 hours, and a clearance of 1.13 L/h.
3. *Compute dose required to achieve desired valproic acid serum concentrations.* The one-compartment-model first-order absorption equations used by the program to compute doses indicates that a dose of 1000 mg every 8 hours will produce a steady-state valproic acid concentration of 68 μg/ml.

▶ **Example 13**   HJ is a 62-year-old, 87-kg (height 6′1″) male with tonic-clonic seizures who was given a new prescription of 500 mg of oral valproic acid capsules every 12 hours. He has liver cirrhosis (Child-Pugh score = 12, bilirubin = 3.2 mg/dl, albumin = 2.5 g/dl). The patient's trough valproic acid concentration before the seventh dose was 72 μg/ml, and he is experiencing some minor adverse effects (sedation, lethargy, tiredness). Compute a valproic acid dose that will provide a total steady-state concentration of 50 μg/ml.

1. *Enter patient demographic, drug dosing, and serum concentration/time data into a Bayesian pharmacokinetic computer program.* In this case it

is unlikely that the patient is at steady state, so the pseudo-linear pharmacokinetics method cannot be used.

2. *Compute pharmacokinetic parameters for the patient using the computer program.* The pharmacokinetic parameters computed by the program are a volume of distribution of 12.5 L, a half-life of 19 hours, and a clearance of 0.46 L/h.

3. *Compute dose required to achieve desired valproic acid serum concentrations.* The one-compartment first-order absorption equations used by the program to compute doses indicates that a dose of 750 mg every 24 hours will produce a steady-state concentration of 46 µg/ml.

▶ ***Example 14***   JB is a 50-year-old, 60-kg (5'7") male with tonic-clonic seizures who was started on 500 mg of valproic acid every 8 hours intravenously after being administered an intravenous loading dose of 750 mg of valproic acid at 0800 H over 60 minutes. The valproic acid concentration was 30 µg/ml before the third maintenance dose. What valproic acid dose is needed to achieve Css = 75 µg/ml?

1. *Enter patient demographic, drug dosing, and serum concentration/time data into a Bayesian pharmacokinetic computer program.* In this case it is unlikely that the patient is at steady state, so the linear pharmacokinetics method cannot be used. Valproic acid doses will be input as intravenous bolus doses.

2. *Compute pharmacokinetic parameters for the patient using the computer program.* The pharmacokinetic parameters computed by the program are a volume of distribution of 8.9 L, a half-life of 15 hours, and clearance of 0.42 L/h.

3. *Compute dose required to achieve desired valproic acid serum concentrations.* The one-compartment-model intravenous bolus equations used by the program to compute doses indicates that a dose of 300 mg of valproic acid every 8 hours will produce a steady-state concentration of 75 µg/ml.

DOSING STRATEGIES

- Initial dose and dosage adjustment techniques using serum concentrations can be used in any combination as long as the limitations of each method are observed.
- Some dosing schemes link together logically when considered according to their basic approaches or philosophies. Dosage strategies that follow similar pathways are given in Table 12-4.

TABLE 12-4 Dosing Strategies

Dosing approach/ philosophy	Initial dosing	Use of serum concentrations to alter doses
Pharmacokinetic parameters/ equations	Pharmacokinetic dosing method	Pharmacokinetic parameter method
Literature-based/ concept	Literature-based recommended dosing	Empiric dosing changes with Pseudo-linear pharmacokinetic method
Computerized	Bayesian computer programs	Bayesian computer programs

REFERENCES

1. Brodie MJ, Dichter MA. Antiepileptic drugs. N Engl J Med 1996;334(3):168–75.
2. McNamara JO. Drugs effective in the therapy of the epilepsies. In: Hardman JG, Limbird LE, Gilman AG, eds. The pharmacological basis of therapeutics. 10th ed. New York: McGraw-Hill, 2001:521–48.
3. Kodama Y, Koike Y, Kimoto H, et al. Binding parameters of valproic acid to serum protein in healthy adults at steady state. Ther Drug Monit 1992;14(1):55–60.
4. Bauer LA, Davis R, Wilensky A, Raisys V, Levy RH. Valproic acid clearance: unbound fraction and diurnal variation in young and elderly adults. Clin Pharmacol Ther 1985;37(6):697–700.
5. Urien S, Albengres E, Tillement JP. Serum protein binding of valproic acid in healthy subjects and in patients with liver disease. Int J Clin Pharmacol Ther Toxicol 1981;19(7):319–25.
6. Brewster D, Muir NC. Valproate plasma protein binding in the uremic condition. Clin Pharmacol Ther 1980;27(1):76–82.
7. Bruni J, Wang LH, Marbury TC, Lee CS, Wilder BJ. Protein binding of valproic acid in uremic patients. Neurology 1980;30(5):557–9.
8. Gugler R, Mueller G. Plasma protein binding of valproic acid in healthy subjects and in patients with renal disease. Br J Clin Pharmacol 1978;5(5):441–6.
9. Gidal BE, Graves NM, Garnett WR. Epilepsy. In: DiPiro JT, Talbert RL, Yee GC, Matzke GR, Wells BG, Posey LM, eds. Pharmacotherapy. 5th ed. New York: McGraw-Hill, 2002:1031–60.
10. Garnett WR. Antiepileptics. In: Schumacher GE, ed. Therapeutic drug monitoring. 1st ed. Stamford, CT: Appleton & Lange, 1995:345–95.
11. Zaccara G, Messori A, Moroni F. Clinical pharmacokinetics of valproic acid—1988. Clin Pharmacokinet 1988;15(6):367–89.
12. Hall K, Otten N, Johnston B, Irvine-Meek J, Leroux M, Seshia S. A multivariable analysis of factors governing the steady-state pharmacokinetics of valproic acid in 52 young epileptics. J Clin Pharmacol 1985;25(4):261–8.
13. Cloyd JC, Kriel RL, Fischer JH. Valproic acid pharmacokinetics in children. II. Discontinuation of concomitant antiepileptic drug therapy. Neurology 1985;35(11):1623–7.
14. Chiba K, Suganuma T, Ishizaki T, et al. Comparison of steady-state pharmacokinetics of valproic acid in children between monotherapy and multiple antiepileptic drug treatment. J Pediatr 1985;106(4):653–8.
15. Gugler R, von Unruh GE. Clinical pharmacokinetics of valproic acid. Clin Pharmacokinet 1980;5(1):67–83.
16. Bauer LA, Davis R, Wilensky A, Raisys V, Levy RH. Diurnal variation in valproic acid clearance. Clin Pharmacol Ther 1984;35(4):505–9.
17. Klotz U, Rapp T, Muller WA. Disposition of valproic acid in patients with liver disease. Eur J Clin Pharmacol 1978;13(1):55–60.
18. Pugh RN, Murray-Lyon IM, Dawson JL, Pietroni MC, Williams R. Transection of the oesophagus for bleeding oesophageal varices. Br J Surg 1973;60(8):646–9.
19. Omtzigt JG, Nau H, Los FJ, Pijpers L, Lindhout D. The disposition of valproate and its metabolites in the late first trimester and early second trimester of pregnancy in maternal serum, urine, and amniotic fluid: effect of dose, co-medication, and the presence of spina bifida. Eur J Clin Pharmacol 1992;43(4):381–8.
20. Kandrotas RJ, Love JM, Gal P, Oles KS. The effect of hemodialysis and hemoperfusion on serum valproic acid concentration. Neurology 1990;40(9):1456–8.
21. Hansten PD, Horn JR. Drug interactions analysis and management. Vancouver, WA: Applied Therapeutics, 1999.
22. Bauer LA, Harris C, Wilensky AJ, Raisys VA, Levy RH. Ethosuximide kinetics: possible interaction with valproic acid. Clin Pharmacol Ther 1982;31(6):741–5.
23. Trapnell CB, Klecker RW, Jamis-Dow C, Collins JM. Glucuronidation of 3′-azido-3′-deoxythymidine (zidovudine) by human liver microsomes: relevance to clinical pharmacokinetic interactions with atovaquone, fluconazole, methadone, and valproic acid. Antimicrob Agents Chemother 1998;42(7):1592–6.

24. Pisani FD, Di Perri RG. Intravenous valproate: effects on plasma and saliva phenytoin levels. Neurology 1981;31(4):467–70.

25. Perucca E, Hebdige S, Frigo GM, Gatti G, Lecchini S, Crema A. Interaction between phenytoin and valproic acid: plasma protein binding and metabolic effects. Clin Pharmacol Ther 1980;28(6):779–89.

26. Riva R, Albani F, Contin M, et al. Time-dependent interaction between phenytoin and valproic acid. Neurology 1985;35(4):510–5.

27. Frigo GM, Lecchini S, Gatti G, Perucca E, Crema A. Modification of phenytoin clearance by valproic acid in normal subjects. Br J Clin Pharmacol 1979;8(6):553–6.

28. Wandell M, Mungall D. Computer assisted drug interpretation and drug regimen optimization. Am Assoc Clin Chem 1984;6:1–11.

13 | **Phenobarbital/Primidone**

Phenobarbital is a barbiturate and primidone is a deoxybarbiturate that are effective in the treatment of generalized tonic-clonic and partial seizures (Table 13-1).[1] Phenobarbital is available as a separate agent, but it is also an active metabolite produced via hepatic metabolism during primidone treatment. Therefore, and because they share a similar antiseizure spectrum, these two drugs are considered together in this chapter.

- The probable mechanism of action of phenobarbital is elevation of seizure threshold by interacting with γ-aminobutyric acid$_A$ (GABA$_A$) postsynaptic receptors, which potentates synaptic inhibition.[2,3]
- Although the exact mechanism of action for the antiepileptic effect of primidone is not known, a portion of its antiseizure activity is due to its active metabolites, phenobarbital and phenylethylmalonamide (PEMA).[2,3]

THERAPEUTIC AND TOXIC CONCENTRATIONS

- The therapeutic ranges of phenobarbital and primidone are defined by most laboratories as 15–40 µg/ml and 5–12 µg/ml, respectively. When primidone is given, sufficient doses are usually administered to produce therapeutic concentrations of both phenobarbital and primidone.

  - Concentrations of the other possible active metabolite of primidone, PEMA, are not routinely measured.
  - Although animal experiments indicate that primidone has inherent antiseizure activity, some clinicians believe that phenobarbital is the predominant species responsible for the therapeutic effect of primidone in humans.[4] Because phenobarbital and PEMA are produced via hepatic metabolism of primidone, it is very difficult to study the antiepileptic activity of primidone alone in patients.

- The most common concentration-related adverse effects of phenobarbital involve the central nervous system: ataxia, headache, unsteadiness, sedation, confusion, and lethargy.[2,5] Other concentration-related side effects are nausea and, in children, irritability and hyperactivity.

  - At phenobarbital concentrations >60 µg/ml, stupor and coma have been reported.
  - During long-term treatment with phenobarbital, changes in behavior, porphyria, decreased cognitive function, and osteomalacia can occur.

- Concentration-related side effects of primidone include nausea, vomiting, diplopia, dizziness, sedation, unsteadiness, and ataxia.[2,5] Generally, slow dosage titration, administration of smaller doses, and more frequent dosing of the drug produce relief from these side effects.

  - Long-term treatment with primidone is associated with behavioral changes, decreased cognitive function, and disorders of the connective tissue.
  - Some of the adverse effects noted during treatment with primidone may be due to phenobarbital.

329

TABLE 13-1 International Classification of Epileptic Seizures[1]

Major class	Subset of class	Drug treatment for selected seizure type

Partial seizures (beginning locally)	1. Simple partial seizures (without impaired consciousness)
	  a. With motor symptoms
	  b. With somatosensory or special sensory symptoms
	  c. With autonomic symptoms
	  d. With psychological symptoms
		Carbamazepine
		Phenytoin
		Valproic acid
		Phenobarbital
		Primidone

	2. Complex partial seizures (with impaired consciousness)
	  a. Simple partial onset followed by impaired consciousness
	  b. Impaired consciousness at onset
		Carbamazepine
		Phenytoin
		Valproic acid
		Phenobarbital
		Primidone

	3. Partial seizures evolving into secondary generalized seizures	Carbamazepine Phenytoin Valproic acid Phenobarbital Primidone
Generalized seizures (convulsive or nonconvulsive)	1. Absence seizures (typical or atypical; also known as petite mal seizures)	Ethosuximide Valproic acid
	2. Tonic-clonic seizures (also known as grand mal seizures)	Phenytoin Carbamazepine Valproic acid Phenobarbital Primidone

- Idiosyncratic side effects that are independent of concentration for both drugs include skin rashes and blood dyscrasias.

CLINICAL MONITORING PARAMETERS

- The goal of therapy with anticonvulsants is to reduce seizure frequency and maximize quality of life with a minimum of adverse drug effects. While it is desirable to abolish seizure episodes entirely, it may not be possible to accomplish this in many patients.
- Patients should be monitored for concentration-related side effects (diplopia, ataxia, dizziness, headache, unsteadiness, sedation, confusion, lethargy) as well as gastrointestinal upset (nausea, vomiting) when receiving these drugs. Serious, but rare, idiosyncratic side effects include connective tissue disorders, blood dyscrasias, and skin rashes.
- Phenobarbital serum concentrations, or primidone plus phenobarbital serum concentrations for patients receiving primidone therapy, should be measured in most patients. Because epilepsy is an episodic disease state, patients do not experience seizures on a continuous basis. Thus, during dosage titration it is difficult to tell if the patient is responding to drug therapy or simply is not experiencing any abnormal central nervous system discharges at that time.

- Serum concentrations are also valuable tools for avoiding adverse drug effects. Patients are more likely to accept drug therapy if adverse reactions are held to the absolute minimum.

BASIC CLINICAL PHARMACOKINETIC PARAMETERS

- Phenobarbital is eliminated primarily (65–70%) by hepatic metabolism to inactive metabolites.[6] About 30–35% of a phenobarbital dose is recovered as unchanged drug in the urine. Renal excretion of unchanged phenobarbital is pH-dependent, with alkaline urine increasing renal clearance.

  - Phenobarbital is about 50% bound to plasma proteins.
  - The absolute bioavailability of oral phenobarbital in humans approaches 100%.[7]
  - Phenobarbital is available in tablet (15, 16, 30, 60, 100 mg), capsule (16 mg), elixir (15 mg/5 ml, 20 mg/5 ml), and injectable (30, 60, 65, and 130 mg/ml for intravenous or intramuscular use) forms.
  - The typical maintenance dose of phenobarbital is 2.5–5 mg/kg/d for neonates, 3–4.5 mg/kg/d for pediatric patients (<10 years old), and 1.5–2 mg/kg/d for older patients.[2,5] For the acute treatment of status epilepticus, intravenous phenobarbital doses of 15–20 mg/kg are used.

- Primidone is eliminated by hepatic metabolism (40–60%) and renal excretion of unchanged drug (40–60%).[8]

  - In adults, approximately 15–20% of a primidone dose is converted by the liver into phenobarbital.
  - Phenylethylmalonamide is another active metabolite of primidone.[8,9] When starting treatment with primidone, PEMA concentrations are detectable after the first dose, but phenobarbital concentrations may not be measurable for 5–7 days (Figure 13-1).

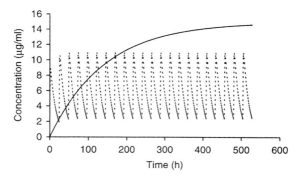

FIG. 13-1   Primidone and phenobarbital concentrations after administration of primidone. Primidone concentrations fluctuate over the dosage interval with a half-life of 8–15 hours, but phenobarbital concentrations accumulate slowly with an average half-life of 100 hours in adults as primidone is converted to phenobarbital. As a result, primidone concentrations reach steady-state conditions long before phenobarbital concentrations reach steady state. In order to measure steady-state serum concentrations of both drugs, one must wait at least 3–4 weeks after a primidone dosage change.

- Primidone does not bind significantly to plasma proteins in humans. Because an intravenous form of the drug is not available commercially, the absolute bioavailability of primidone in humans is not known.
- Primidone is available as tablets (50 and 250 mg) and an oral suspension (250 mg/5 ml). Usual maintenance doses of primidone are 12–20 mg/kg/d for neonates, 12–23 mg/kg/d for pediatric patients (<15 years old), and 10–25 mg/kg/d for older patients.

EFFECTS OF DISEASE STATES AND CONDITIONS ON PHARMACOKINETICS AND DOSING

Phenobarbital

- The clearance rate (Cl) of phenobarbital for older children (≥12 years old) and adults is 4 ml/h/kg, and for children it is 8 ml/h/kg.[5,7,10]

  - Phenobarbital volume of distribution (V) is 0.7 L/kg, and its half-life averages 120 hours in neonates (0–4 weeks old), 60 hours in children (≥2 months old), and 100 hours in adults.

Liver Dysfunction

- Although only limited studies in patients with hepatic disease are available, a 50% increase in half-life is seen in adults with liver cirrhosis or acute viral hepatitis.[11] Patients with liver cirrhosis or acute hepatitis may have reduced phenobarbital clearance because of destruction of liver parenchyma. This loss of functional hepatic cells reduces the amount of enzymes available to metabolize the drug and decreases clearance.

  - An index of liver dysfunction can be gained by applying the Child-Pugh clinical classification system to the patient (Table 13-2).[12] Child-Pugh scores are discussed more fully in Chapter 3 (Drug Dosing in Special Populations: Renal and Hepatic Disease, Dialysis, Heart Failure, Obesity, and Drug Interactions).
  - The Child-Pugh score consists of five laboratory tests or clinical symptoms: serum albumin, total bilirubin, prothrombin time, ascites, and hepatic encephalopathy. Each of these areas is given a score of 1 (normal) to 3 (severely abnormal; Table 13-2), and the scores for the five areas are summed.
  - The Child-Pugh score for a patient with normal liver function is 5, while the score for a patient with grossly abnormal serum albumin, total bilirubin, and prothrombin time values in addition to severe ascites and hepatic encephalopathy is 15.

TABLE 13-2 Child-Pugh Scores for Patients with Liver Disease[12]

Test/symptom	Score 1 point	Score 2 points	Score 3 points
Total bilirubin (mg/dl)	<2.0	2.0–3.0	>3.0
Serum albumin (g/dl)	>3.5	2.8–3.5	<2.8
Prothrombin time (seconds prolonged over control)	<4	4–6	>6
Ascites	Absent	Slight	Moderate
Hepatic Encephalopathy	None	Moderate	Severe

- A Child-Pugh score greater than 8 is grounds for a decrease of 25–50% in the initial daily drug dose for phenobarbital.
- As in any patient, with or without liver dysfunction, initial doses are meant as starting points for dosage titration based on patient response and avoidance of adverse effects. Phenobarbital serum concentrations and the presence of adverse drug effects should be monitored frequently in patients with liver cirrhosis.

Renal Dysfunction

- Because phenobarbital is also eliminated by the kidneys, patients with renal dysfunction (creatinine clearance <30 ml/min) who are receiving phenobarbital should be closely monitored.

Dialysis and Hemoperfusion

- Phenobarbital is significantly removed (~30% of total body amount) by hemodialysis, and supplemental doses may need to be given after a dialysis session. Phenobarbital is significantly removed by hemoperfusion, with a sieving coefficient of 0.8.[13,14] Supplemental dosing during hemoperfusion should be guided by serum concentration monitoring.

Lactation

- Phenobarbital enters breast milk, so nursing infants should be monitored for possible adverse drug reactions.[15]

Primidone

- The clearance rate (Cl/F) of primidone for older patients (≥12 years old) taking primidone alone is 35 ml/h/kg.[16] However, the primidone clearance rate increases to 50 ml/h/kg for older patients if they are receiving concurrent therapy with phenytoin or carbamazepine.[16] For children, primidone clearance averages 125 ml/h/kg.[17]
- Primidone volume of distribution (V/F) is 0.7 L/kg, and its half-life averages 8 hours in adults taking concurrent phenytoin or carbamazepine or children (<12 years old), and 15 hours in adults taking primidone alone.[5,16,17]

Liver/Renal Dysfunction

- Although no studies in patients with hepatic or renal disease are available, because almost equal amounts of primidone are eliminated by the liver and kidneys, patients with renal or hepatic dysfunction who are receiving primidone should be closely monitored. A Child-Pugh score greater than 8 or creatinine clearance <30 ml/min are grounds for a decrease of 25–50% in the initial daily drug dose for primidone.
- As in any patient, with or without liver or renal dysfunction, initial doses are meant as starting points for dosage titration based on patient response and avoidance of adverse effects. Primidone and phenobarbital serum concentrations as well as the presence of adverse drug effects should be monitored frequently in patients with liver or kidney disease who are taking primidone.

Dialysis

- Primidone is significantly removed (~30% of total body amount) by hemodialysis, and supplemental doses may need to be given after a dialysis session.

DRUG INTERACTIONS

- Phenobarbital is a potent inducer of hepatic drug metabolism for the CYP1A2, CYP2C9, and CYP3A4 enzyme systems.[18] Because phenobarbital is also a metabolite produced during primidone therapy, primidone has similar drug interaction potential.

    - Because phenobarbital is such a broad-based hepatic enzyme inducer, patients should be monitored closely for drug interactions whenever either of these agents is added to their therapeutic regimen.
    - A brief list of the compounds whose metabolism and clearance are increased by concurrent phenobarbital treatment includes carbamazepine, lamotrigine, valproic acid, cyclosporin, nifedipine, diltiazem, verapamil, oral contraceptives, tricyclic antidepressants, quinidine, theophylline, and warfarin.
    - Other anticonvulsants that decrease the metabolism and clearance of phenobarbital are felbamate and valproic acid.
    - Phenytoin may also exhibit a co-interaction with phenobarbital, in which the two agents change the metabolism and clearance of each other. The net result of this drug interaction is quite variable and can result in an increase, decrease, or no change in the steady-state concentrations of both drugs.

- Primidone metabolism and clearance are increased by carbamazepine and phenytoin treatment, while valproic acid therapy decreases primidone metabolism and clearance.

INITIAL DOSAGE DETERMINATION METHODS

- Several methods to initiate phenobarbital or primidone therapy are available.

    - The *pharmacokinetic dosing method* is the most flexible of the techniques. It allows individualized target serum concentrations to be chosen for a patient, and each pharmacokinetic parameter can be customized to reflect specific disease states and conditions present in the patient.
    - *Literature-based recommended dosing* is a very commonly used method to prescribe initial doses of phenobarbital or primidone. Doses are based on those that commonly produce steady-state concentrations near the lower end of the therapeutic range, although there is a wide variation in the actual concentrations for a specific patient.

Pharmacokinetic Dosing Method

- The goal of initial dosing with phenobarbital or primidone is to compute the best dose possible for the patient given the set of disease states and conditions that influence pharmacokinetics of the drugs and the epileptic disorder being treated. In order to do this, pharmacokinetic parameters for the patient are estimated using average parameters measured in other patients with similar disease state and condition profiles.

Clearance Estimate

- Phenobarbital is metabolized predominantly by the liver, while primidone is about 50% hepatically eliminated. Unfortunately, there is no good way to estimate the elimination characteristics of liver-metabolized drugs using an endogenous marker of liver function in the same manner that serum creatinine and estimated creatinine clearance are used to estimate the elimination of agents that are eliminated renally.

- As a result, a patient is categorized according to the disease states and conditions that are known to change drug clearance, and the clearance previously measured in these studies is used as an estimate of the current patient's clearance.
- To produce the most conservative phenobarbital or primidone doses in patients with multiple concurrent disease states or conditions that affect their respective pharmacokinetics, the disease state or condition with the smallest clearance should be used to compute doses. This approach will avoid accidental overdosage as much as is currently possible.

Volume of Distribution Estimate

- The volume of distribution of both drugs is assumed to be 0.7 L/kg for adults and children.

Half-Life and Elimination Rate Constant Estimate

- Once the correct clearance and volume of distribution estimates have been identified for the patient, they can be converted into the half-life ($t_{1/2}$) and elimination rate constant (k) estimates using the following equations:

$$t_{1/2} = (0.693 \cdot V)/Cl$$
$$k = 0.693/t_{1/2} = Cl/V$$

Selection of Appropriate Pharmacokinetic Model and Equations

- Primidone and phenobarbital follow a one-compartment pharmacokinetic model. When oral therapy of either drug or intramuscular treatment with phenobarbital is required, both anticonvulsants have good bioavailability (assume F = 1), and once-daily dosing of phenobarbital or multiple daily dosing of primidone provides a relatively smooth serum concentration/time curve that emulates an intravenous infusion.

  - A very simple pharmacokinetic equation that computes the average phenobarbital or primidone steady-state serum concentration (Css in μg/ml = mg/L) is widely used and allows maintenance dosage calculation:

  $$Css = [F(D/\tau)]/Cl \qquad or \qquad D = (Css \cdot Cl \cdot \tau)/F$$

  where F is the bioavailability fraction for the oral dosage form (F = 1 for both drugs), D is the dose of the anticonvulsant in mg, Cl is anticonvulsant clearance in L/h, and τ is the dosage interval in hours.
  - When intravenous therapy with phenobarbital is required, a similar pharmacokinetic equation is widely used:

  $$Css = (D/\tau)/Cl \qquad or \qquad D = Css \cdot Cl \cdot \tau$$

  where D is the dose of phenobarbital in mg, and τ is the dosage interval in hours. Cl is phenobarbital clearance in L/h.

- The equation used to calculate an intravenous loading dose for phenobarbital (LD in mg) is based on a simple one-compartment model:

$$LD = Css \cdot V$$

where Css is the desired phenobarbital steady-state concentration in μg/ml, which is equivalent to mg/L, and V is the phenobarbital volume of distribution. Intravenous phenobarbital doses should be administered no faster than 100 mg/minute.

▶ *Example 1*   GO is a 50-year-old, 75-kg (height 5′10″) male with tonic-clonic seizures who requires therapy with oral phenobarbital. He has normal liver and renal function. Suggest an initial phenobarbital dosage regimen designed to achieve a steady-state concentration of 20 μg/ml.

1. *Estimate clearance and volume of distribution according to disease states and conditions present in the patient.* The clearance rate for an adult patient is 4 ml/h/kg. Using this value, the estimated clearance is

$$Cl = 75 \text{ kg} \cdot 4 \text{ ml/h/kg} = 300 \text{ ml/h or } 0.3 \text{ L/h}$$

The estimated volume of distribution is

$$75 \text{ kg} \cdot 0.7 \text{ L/kg} = 53 \text{ L}$$

2. *Estimate half-life and elimination rate constant.* Once the correct clearance and volume of distribution estimates have been identified for the patient, they can be converted into the phenobarbital half-life ($t_{1/2}$) and elimination rate constant (k) estimates using the following equations:

$$t_{1/2} = (0.693 \cdot V)/Cl = (0.693 \cdot 53 \text{ L})/(0.3 \text{ L/h}) = 122 \text{ h}$$
$$k = Cl/V = (0.3 \text{ L/h})/(53 \text{ L}) = 0.0057 \text{ h}^{-1}$$

3. *Compute dosage regimen.* Oral phenobarbital tablets will be prescribed for this patient (F = 1). (*Note:* μg/ml = mg/L, and this concentration unit was substituted for Css in the calculations so that unit conversion was not required.) The dosage equation for oral phenobarbital is

$$D = (Css \cdot Cl \cdot \tau)/F = [(20 \text{ mg/L} \cdot (0.3 \text{ L/h}) \cdot 24 \text{ h})]/1$$
$$= 144 \text{ mg, rounded to } 120 \text{ every } 24 \text{ h}$$

A steady-state trough phenobarbital serum concentration should be measured after steady state is attained in 3–5 half-lives. Since the drug is expected to have a half-life of 122 hours, a phenobarbital steady-state concentration can be obtained at any time after 4 weeks of dosing (5 half-lives = 5 · 122 h = 610 h or 25 d). Phenobarbital serum concentrations should also be measured if the patient experiences an exacerbation of epilepsy, or if the patient develops potential signs or symptoms of phenobarbital toxicity.

▶ *Example 2*   GO is a 50-year-old, 75-kg (height 5′10″) male with tonic-clonic seizures who requires therapy with intravenous phenobarbital. He has normal liver and renal function. Suggest an initial phenobarbital dosage regimen designed to achieve a steady-state concentration of 20 μg/ml.

1. *Estimate clearance and volume of distribution according to disease states and conditions present in the patient.* The clearance rate for an adult patient is 4 ml/h/kg. Using this value, the estimated clearance is

$$Cl = 75 \text{ kg} \cdot 4 \text{ ml/h/kg} = 300 \text{ ml/h or } 0.3 \text{ L/h}$$

The estimated volume of distribution is

$$75 \text{ kg} \cdot 0.7 \text{ L/kg} = 53 \text{ L}$$

2. *Estimate half-life and elimination rate constant.* Once the correct clearance and volume of distribution estimates have been identified for the patient, they can be converted into the phenobarbital half-life ($t_{1/2}$) and elimination rate constant (k) estimates using the following equations:

$$t_{1/2} = (0.693 \cdot V)/Cl = (0.693 \cdot 53 \text{ L})/(0.3 \text{ L/h}) = 122 \text{ h}$$
$$k = Cl/V = (0.3 \text{ L/h})/(53 \text{ L}) = 0.0057 \text{ h}^{-1}$$

3. *Compute dosage regimen.* Intravenous phenobarbital will be prescribed for this patient. (*Note:* µg/ml = mg/L, and this concentration unit was substituted for Css in the calculations so that unit conversion was not required.) The dosage equation for intravenous phenobarbital is

$$D = Css \cdot Cl \cdot \tau = 20 \text{ mg/L} \cdot 0.3 \text{ L/h} \cdot 24 \text{ h}$$
$$= 144 \text{ mg, rounded to 120 every 24 h}$$

If needed, an intravenous loading dose could also be computed for the patient:

$$LD = Css \cdot V = 20 \text{ mg/L} \cdot 53 \text{ L} = 1060 \text{ mg, rounded to 1000 mg}$$

Intravenous loading doses should be administered no faster than 100 mg/min.

A steady-state trough phenobarbital serum concentration should be measured after steady state is attained in 3–5 half-lives. Since the drug is expected to have a half-life of 122 hours, a phenobarbital steady-state concentration can be obtained at any time after 4 weeks of dosing (5 half-lives = 5 · 122 h = 610 h or 25 d). Phenobarbital serum concentrations should also be measured if the patient experiences an exacerbation of epilepsy, or if the patient develops potential signs or symptoms of phenobarbital toxicity.

▶ *Example 3*   BI is a 23-year-old, 65-kg (height 5′6″) male with complex partial seizures who requires therapy with oral primidone. He has normal liver and renal function and takes carbamazepine. Suggest an initial primidone dosage regimen designed to achieve a steady-state primidone concentration of 6 µg/ml.

1. *Estimate clearance and volume of distribution according to disease states and conditions present in the patient.* The clearance rate for an adult patient taking carbamazepine is 50 ml/h/kg. Using this value, the estimated clearance is

$$Cl = 65 \text{ kg} \cdot 50 \text{ ml/h/kg} = 3250 \text{ ml/h or 3.25 L/h}$$

The estimated volume of distribution is

$$65 \text{ kg} \cdot 0.7 \text{ L/kg} = 46 \text{ L}$$

2. *Estimate half-life and elimination rate constant.* Once the correct clearance and volume of distribution estimates have been identified for the patient, they can be converted into the primidone half-life ($t_{1/2}$) and

elimination rate constant (k) estimates using the following equations:

$$t_{1/2} = (0.693 \cdot V)/Cl = (0.693 \cdot 46 \text{ L})/(3.25 \text{ L/h}) = 10 \text{ h}$$

$$k = Cl/V = (3.25 \text{ L/h})/(46 \text{ L}) = 0.071 \text{ h}^{-1}$$

3. *Compute dosage regimen.* Oral primidone tablets will be prescribed to this patient (F = 1). (*Note:* μg/ml = mg/L, and this concentration unit was substituted for Css in the calculations so that unit conversion was not required.) The dosage equation for oral primidone is

$$D = (Css \cdot Cl \cdot \tau)/F = [(6 \text{ mg/L} \cdot 3.25 \text{ L/h} \cdot 12 \text{ h})]/1$$

$$= 234 \text{ mg, rounded to } 250 \text{ mg every } 12 \text{ h}$$

To avoid side effects, the starting dose should be 50% of this anticipated maintenance dose (125 mg every 12 hours) and the dose titrated to the full dose over 1–2 weeks.

Steady-state trough primidone and phenobarbital serum concentrations should be measured after steady state for both agents is attained in 3–5 half-lives. Since the patient is expected to have a phenobarbital half-life of 100 hours or more, steady-state concentrations can be obtained at any time after 3–4 weeks of dosing at the full primidone maintenance dose (5 phenobarbital half-lives = 5 · 100 h = 500 h or 21 d). Primidone and phenobarbital serum concentrations should also be measured if the patient experiences an exacerbation of epilepsy, or if the patient develops potential signs or symptoms of primidone toxicity.

Literature-Based Recommended Dosing

- Because of the large amount of variability in phenobarbital and primidone pharmacokinetics, even when concurrent disease states and conditions are identified, most clinicians believe that the use of standard drug doses for various situations is warranted. The original computations of these doses were based on pharmacokinetic dosing methods, and the doses were subsequently modified based on clinical experience. In general, the expected steady-state serum concentrations used to compute these doses was near the lower end of the therapeutic range for each drug (Table 13-3).
- Phenobarbital is usually administered once or twice daily, while primidone is given 2–4 times daily. To avoid side effects, primidone doses are started at 25–50% of the ultimate desired maintenance dose, with dosage increases made every 1–2 weeks depending on response and adverse effects.
- If the patient has significant hepatic dysfunction (Child-Pugh score ≥8) or renal disease (creatinine clearance <30 ml/min), maintenance doses prescribed using this method should be decreased by 25–50%, depending on how aggressive therapy is required to be for the individual.

TABLE 13-3 Literature-Based Initial Doses for Phenobarbital and Primidone

Patient profile	Phenobarbital dose (mg/kg/d)	Primidone dose (mg/kg/d)
Neonates	2.5–5	12–20
Children	3–4.5	12–23
Adult	1.5–2	10–25

Note: Intravenous loading doses for phenobarbital are 15–20 mg/kg for status epilepticus.

- To illustrate the similarities and differences between this method of dosage calculation and the pharmacokinetic dosing method, the same examples used in the previous section will be used.

▶ *Example 4*   GO is a 50-year-old, 75-kg (height 5′10″) male with tonic-clonic seizures who requires therapy with oral phenobarbital. He has normal liver and renal function. Suggest an initial phenobarbital dosage regimen designed to achieve a steady-state concentration of 20 µg/ml.

1. *Estimate phenobarbital dose according to disease states and conditions present in the patient.* Oral phenobarbital tablets will be prescribed for this patient. The suggested initial maintenance dosage rate for phenobarbital in an adult patient is 1.5–2 mg/kg/d. Using 1.5 mg/kg/d, the dose is

$$75 \text{ kg} \cdot 1.5 \text{ mg/kg/d} = 113 \text{ mg/d, rounded to } 120 \text{ mg/d}$$

   Trough phenobarbital serum concentrations should be measured after steady state is attained in 3–5 half-lives. Since the patient is expected to have a phenobarbital half-life of 100 hours or more, steady-state concentrations can be obtained at any time after 3–4 weeks of dosing (5 phenobarbital half-lives = 5 · 100 h = 500 h or 21 d). Phenobarbital serum concentrations should also be measured if the patient experiences an exacerbation of epilepsy, or if the patient develops potential signs or symptoms of phenobarbital toxicity.

▶ *Example 5*   GO is a 50-year-old, 75-kg (height 5′10″) male with tonic-clonic seizures who requires therapy with intravenous phenobarbital. He has normal liver and renal function. Suggest an initial phenobarbital dosage regimen designed to achieve a steady-state concentration of 20 µg/ml.

1. *Estimate phenobarbital dose according to disease states and conditions present in the patient.* Intravenous phenobarbital will be prescribed for this patient. The suggested initial maintenance dosage rate for phenobarbital in an adult patient is 1.5–2 mg/kg/d. Using 1.5 mg/kg/d, the maintenance dose is

$$75 \text{ kg} \cdot 1.5 \text{ mg/kg/d} = 113 \text{ mg/d, rounded to } 120 \text{ mg/d}$$

   If it is needed, the loading-dose range is 15–20 mg/kg. Using 15 mg/kg, the loading dose is

$$75 \text{ kg} \cdot 15 \text{ mg/kg} = 1125 \text{ mg, rounded to } 1000 \text{ mg}$$

   A steady-state trough phenobarbital serum concentration should be measured after steady state is attained in 3–4 weeks. Phenobarbital serum concentrations should also be measured if the patient experiences an exacerbation of epilepsy, or if the patient develops potential signs or symptoms of phenobarbital toxicity.

▶ *Example 6*   BI is a 23-year-old, 65-kg (height 5′6″) male with complex partial seizures who requires therapy with oral primidone. He has normal liver and renal function and takes carbamazepine. Suggest an initial primidone dosage regimen designed to achieve a steady-state primidone concentration of 6 µg/ml.

1. *Estimate primidone dose according to disease states and conditions present in the patient.* Oral primidone tablets will be prescribed for this patient. The suggested initial maintenance dosage rate for primidone in an adult patient is 10–25 mg/kg/d. Because the patient is taking carbamazepine,

which is known to induce primidone metabolism, a dose of 15 mg/kg/d will be used to compute the initial dose:

$$65 \text{ kg} \cdot 15 \text{ mg/kg/d} = 975 \text{ mg/d, rounded to } 1000 \text{ mg/d}$$

This dose will be given as 250 mg every 6 hours. To avoid side effects, the starting dose should be 50% of this anticipated maintenance dose (125 mg every 6 hours), and the dose should be titrated to the full dose over 1–2 weeks according to response and adverse effects.

Steady-state trough primidone and phenobarbital serum concentrations should be measured after steady state for both agents is attained in 3–5 half-lives. Since the patient is expected to have a phenobarbital half-life of 100 hours or more, steady-state concentrations can be obtained at any time after 3–4 weeks of dosing at the full primidone maintenance dose (5 phenobarbital half-lives = 5 · 100 h = 500 h or 21 d). Primidone and phenobarbital serum concentrations should also be measured if the patient experiences an exacerbation of epilepsy, or if the patient develops potential signs or symptoms of primidone toxicity.

USE OF PHENOBARBITAL AND PRIMIDONE SERUM CONCENTRATIONS TO ALTER DOSES

- Because of the large amount of pharmacokinetic variability among patients, it is likely that doses computed using patient population characteristics will not always produce phenobarbital or primidone serum concentrations that are expected or desirable. Because of pharmacokinetic variability, the narrow therapeutic index of phenobarbital and primidone, and the desire to avoid adverse side effects, serum concentrations of these anticonvulsants are measured for most patients, to ensure that therapeutic, nontoxic levels are present.
- In addition to phenobarbital or primidone serum concentrations, important patient parameters (seizure frequency, potential side effects, etc.) should be followed to confirm that the patient is responding to treatment and not developing adverse drug reactions.
- When phenobarbital or primidone serum concentrations are measured in patients and a dosage change is necessary, clinicians should seek to use the simplest, most straightforward method available to determine a dose that will provide safe and effective treatment.

  - In most cases a simple dosage ratio can be used to change doses, since phenobarbital and primidone follow *linear pharmacokinetics*. Sometimes it is not possible simply to change the dose because of the limited number of oral dosage strengths, and the dosage interval must also be changed.
  - In some situations it may be necessary or desirable to compute the phenobarbital or primidone *pharmacokinetic parameters* for the patient and utilize these to calculate the best drug dose.
  - Computerized methods that incorporate expected population pharmacokinetic characteristics (*Bayesian pharmacokinetic computer programs*) can be used in difficult cases, when renal function is changing, serum concentrations are obtained at suboptimal times, or the patient was not at steady state when serum concentrations were measured.

Linear Pharmacokinetics Method

- Because phenobarbital and primidone follow linear, dose-proportional pharmacokinetics, steady-state serum concentrations change in proportion to dose according to the following equation:

$$D_{new}/Css_{new} = D_{old}/Css_{old} \quad \text{or} \quad D_{new} = (Css_{new}/Css_{old})D_{old}$$

where D is the dose, Css is the steady-state concentration, old indicates the dose that produced the steady-state concentration the patient is currently receiving, and new denotes the dose necessary to produce the desired steady-state concentration.

- The advantages of this method are that it is quick and simple.
- The disadvantages are that steady-state concentrations are required, and primidone may undergo some induction of its hepatic clearance at higher doses as phenobarbital concentrations increase.
- This method works for phenobarbital regardless of the route of administration.
- When primidone is administered to a patient, phenobarbital is produced as an active metabolite, and the new phenobarbital concentration resulting from a primidone dosage changes in a linear fashion.

  - The phenobarbital concentration resulting from a primidone dosage change can be estimated using a rearrangement of the above equation:

$$Css_{new} = (D_{new}/D_{old})Css_{old}$$

  where D is the primidone dose, Css is the steady-state phenobarbital concentration, old indicates the primidone dose that produced the steady-state phenobarbital concentration the patient is currently receiving, and new denotes the primidone dose necessary to produce the desired steady-state phenobarbital concentration.

▶ *Example 7*   LK is a 13-year-old, 47-kg (height 5′1″) female with complex partial seizures who requires therapy with oral primidone. After dosage titration, the patient was prescribed 250 mg of primidone tablets every 8 hours (750 mg/d) for 1 month, after which her steady-state primidone and phenobarbital concentrations were 3 µg/ml and 15 µg/ml, respectively. The patient is assessed to be compliant with her dosage regimen. Suggest a primidone dosage regimen designed to achieve a steady-state primidone concentration of 6 µg/ml.

1. *Compute new dose to achieve desired serum concentration.* Using linear pharmacokinetics, the primidone dose necessary to cause the required change in steady-state concentration is

$$D_{new} = (Css_{new}/Css_{old})D_{old} = [(6 \text{ µg/ml})/(3 \text{ µg/ml})](750 \text{ mg/d})$$
$$= 1500 \text{ mg/d, or } 500 \text{ mg every 8 h}$$

The dosage regimen should be titrated to this value over a period of 1–2 weeks to avoid adverse effects. Using linear pharmacokinetics, the resulting steady-state phenobarbital serum concentration is

$$Css_{new} = (D_{new}/D_{old})Css_{old}$$
$$= [(1500 \text{ mg/d})/(750 \text{ mg/d})](15 \text{ µg/ml}) = 30 \text{ µg/ml}$$

Steady-state trough primidone and phenobarbital serum concentrations should be measured after steady state is attained in 3–4 weeks. Primidone and phenobarbital serum concentrations should also be measured if the patient experiences an exacerbation of epilepsy, or if the patient develops potential signs or symptoms of primidone toxicity.

▶ *Example 8*   HI is a 42-year-old, 75-kg (height 5′10″) male with tonic-clonic seizures who requires therapy with oral phenobarbital. After dosage titration, the patient was prescribed 120 mg daily of phenobarbital tablets for 1 month, after which his steady-state phenobarbital concentration was 20 μg/ml. The patient is assessed to be compliant with his dosage regimen. Suggest a phenobarbital dosage regimen designed to achieve a steady-state phenobarbital concentration of 30 μg/ml.

1. *Compute new dose to achieve desired serum concentration.* Using linear pharmacokinetics, the resulting steady-state phenobarbital serum concentration is

$$D_{new} = (Css_{new}/Css_{old})D_{old}$$
$$= [(30 \text{ μg/ml})/(20 \text{ μg/ml})](120 \text{ mg/d}) = 180 \text{ mg/d}$$

A steady-state trough phenobarbital serum concentration should be measured after steady state is attained in 3–4 weeks. Phenobarbital serum concentrations should also be measured if the patient experiences an exacerbation of epilepsy, or if the patient develops potential signs or symptoms of phenobarbital toxicity.

Pharmacokinetic Parameter Method

- The pharmacokinetic parameter method of adjusting drug doses was among the first techniques available to change doses using serum concentrations. It allows the computation of an individual's own, unique pharmacokinetic constants and uses those to calculate a dose that achieves desired phenobarbital or primidone concentrations.
- For patients who are receiving oral phenobarbital, the pharmacokinetic parameter method requires that steady state has been achieved and uses only a steady-state phenobarbital concentration (Css).

  - Phenobarbital clearance (Cl) can be calculated using the following formula:

  $$Cl = [F(D/\tau)]/Css$$

  where F is the bioavailability fraction for the oral dosage form (F = 1 for oral phenobarbital products), D is the dose of phenobarbital in mg, Css is the steady-state phenobarbital concentration in mg/L, and τ is the dosage interval in hours.
  - Phenobarbital clearance during intravenous therapy can be computed using an equivalent formula:

  $$Cl = (D/\tau)/Css$$

  where D is the dose of phenobarbital in mg, Css is the steady-state phenobarbital concentration in mg/L, and τ is the dosage interval in hours.
- If the patient is receiving oral primidone, primidone clearance (Cl) is computed using the same equation:

  $$Cl = [F(D/\tau)]/Css$$

  where F is the bioavailability fraction for the oral dosage form (F = 1 for oral primidone products), D is the dose of primidone in mg, Css is the steady-state primidone concentration in mg/L, and τ is the dosage interval in hours.

  - The phenobarbital concentration resulting from a primidone dosage change can be estimated using the following equation:

  $$Css_{new} = (D_{new}/D_{old})Css_{old}$$

  where D is the primidone dose, Css is the steady-state phenobarbital concentration, old indicates the primidone dose that produced the steady-state

phenobarbital concentration the patient is currently receiving, and new denotes the primidone dose necessary to produce the desired steady-state phenobarbital concentration.

• To illustrate the similarities and differences between this method of dosage calculation and the pharmacokinetic parameter method, the same examples used in the previous section will be used.

▶ *Example 9* LK is a 13-year-old, 47-kg (height 5′1″) female with complex partial seizures who requires therapy with oral primidone. After dosage titration, the patient was prescribed 250 mg of primidone tablets every 8 hours (750 mg/d) for 1 month, after which her steady-state primidone and phenobarbital concentrations were 3 µg/ml and 15 µg/ml, respectively. The patient is assessed to be compliant with her dosage regimen. Suggest a primidone dosage regimen designed to achieve a steady-state primidone concentration of 6 µg/ml.

1. *Compute pharmacokinetic parameters.* The patient can be expected to achieve steady-state conditions for both primidone and phenobarbital after 3–4 weeks of therapy. Primidone clearance can be computed using a steady-state primidone concentration:

$$Cl = [F(D/\tau)]/Css = [1(250 \text{ mg/8 h})]/(3 \text{ mg/L}) = 10 \text{ L/h}$$

(*Note:* µg/ml = mg/L, and this concentration unit was substituted for Css in the calculations so that unit conversion was not required.)

2. *Compute primidone dose and resulting phenobarbital concentration.* Primidone clearance is used to compute the new dose:

$$D = (Css \cdot Cl \cdot \tau)/F = (6 \text{ mg/L} \cdot 10 \text{ L/h} \cdot 8 \text{ h})/1$$
$$= 480 \text{ mg, rounded to 500 mg every 8 h}$$

Using linear pharmacokinetics, the resulting steady-state phenobarbital serum concentration is

$$Css_{new} = (D_{new}/D_{old})Css_{old}$$
$$= [(1500 \text{ mg/d})/(750 \text{ mg/d})](15 \text{ µg/ml}) = 30 \text{ µg/ml}$$

Steady-state trough primidone and phenobarbital serum concentrations should be measured after steady-state is attained in 3–4 weeks. Primidone and phenobarbital serum concentrations should also be measured if the patient experiences an exacerbation of epilepsy, or if the patient develops potential signs or symptoms of primidone toxicity.

▶ *Example 10* HI is a 42-year-old, 75-kg (height 5′10″) male with tonic-clonic seizures who requires therapy with oral phenobarbital. After dosage titration, the patient was prescribed 120 mg of phenobarbital tablets daily for 1 month, after which his steady-state phenobarbital concentration was 20 µg/ml. The patient is assessed to be compliant with his dosage regimen. Suggest a phenobarbital dosage regimen designed to achieve a steady-state phenobarbital concentration of 30 µg/ml.

1. *Compute pharmacokinetic parameters.* The patient can be expected to achieve steady-state conditions after 3–4 weeks of therapy. Phenobarbital

clearance can be computed using a steady-state phenobarbital concentration:

$$Cl = [F(D/\tau)]/Css = [1(120 \text{ mg}/24 \text{ h})]/(20 \text{ mg/L}) = 0.25 \text{ L/h}$$

(*Note:* μg/ml = mg/L, and this concentration unit was substituted for Css in the calculations so that unit conversion was not required.)

2. *Compute phenobarbital dose.* Phenobarbital clearance is used to compute the new dose:

$$D = (Css \cdot Cl \cdot \tau)/F = (30 \text{ mg/L} \cdot 0.25 \text{ L/h} \cdot 24 \text{ h})/1$$

$$= 180 \text{ mg every } 24 \text{ h}$$

A steady-state trough phenobarbital serum concentration should be measured after steady state is attained in 3–4 weeks. Phenobarbital serum concentrations should also be measured if the patient experiences an exacerbation of epilepsy, or if the patient develops potential signs or symptoms of phenobarbital toxicity.

BAYESIAN PHARMACOKINETIC COMPUTER PROGRAMS

- Computer programs are available that can assist in the computation of pharmacokinetic parameters for patients. The most reliable computer programs use a nonlinear regression algorithm that incorporates components of Bayes' theorem.

  - An advantage of this approach is that consistent dosage recommendations can be made when several different practitioners are involved in therapeutic drug monitoring programs. However, since simpler dosing methods work just as well for patients with stable pharmacokinetic parameters and steady-state drug concentrations, many clinicians reserve the use of computer programs for more difficult situations. Those situations include serum concentrations that are not at steady state, serum concentrations not obtained at the specific times needed to employ simpler methods, and unstable pharmacokinetic parameters.
  - When only a limited number of steady-state concentrations are available, Bayesian pharmacokinetic computer programs can be used to compute a complete patient pharmacokinetic profile that includes clearance, volume of distribution, and half-life.

- Many Bayesian pharmacokinetic computer programs are available, and most should provide answers similar to the program used in the following examples. The program used to solve problems in this book is DrugCalc, written by Dr. Dennis Mungall and available at his Internet web site (www.clinpharmacologist.bigstep.com/consumersurvey.html).[19] Currently, this program is available only for phenobarbital, not for primidone.

- ▶ ***Example 11*** HI is a 42-year-old, 75-kg (height 5′10″) male with tonic-clonic seizures who requires therapy with oral phenobarbital. After dosage titration, the patient was prescribed 120 mg of phenobarbital tablets daily for 1 month, after which his steady-state phenobarbital concentration was 20 μg/ml. The patient is assessed to be compliant with his dosage regimen. Suggest a phenobarbital dosage regimen designed to achieve a steady-state phenobarbital concentration of 30 μg/ml.

  1. *Enter patient demographic, drug dosing, and serum concentration/time data into a Bayesian pharmacokinetic computer program.*

2. *Compute pharmacokinetic parameters for the patient using the computer program.* The pharmacokinetic parameters computed by the program are a volume of distribution of 51 L, a half-life of 185 h, and a clearance of 0.19 L/h.
3. *Compute dose required to achieve desired phenobarbital serum concentrations.* The one-compartment-model first-order absorption equation used by the program to compute doses indicates that a dose of 180 mg every 24 hours will produce a steady-state phenobarbital concentration of 36 µg/ml.

▸ *Example 12* JB is an 8-year-old, 35-kg (height 4′2″) male with simple partial seizures who was started on 100 mg of phenobarbital syrup every 24 hours. The phenobarbital concentration before the tenth maintenance dose was 12 µg/ml. What phenobarbital dose is needed to achieve Css = 25 µg/ml?

1. *Enter patient demographic, drug dosing, and serum concentration/time data into a Bayesian pharmacokinetic computer program.* In this case it is unlikely that the patient is at steady state, so the linear pharmacokinetics method cannot be used.
2. *Compute pharmacokinetic parameters for the patient using the computer program.* The pharmacokinetic parameters computed by the program are a volume of distribution of 26 L, a half-life of 82 h, and clearance of 0.22 L/h.
3. *Compute dose required to achieve desired phenobarbital serum concentrations.* The one-compartment-model equations used by the program to compute doses indicates that a dose of phenobarbital 175 mg every 24 hours will produce a steady-state concentration of 26 µg/ml.

DOSING STRATEGIES

- Initial dose and dosage adjustment techniques using serum concentrations can be used in any combination as long as the limitations of each method are observed.
- Some dosing schemes link together logically when considered according to their basic approaches or philosophies. Dosage strategies that follow similar pathways are given in Table 13-4.

TABLE 13-4 Dosing Strategies

Dosing approach/ philosophy	Initial dosing	Use of serum concentrations to alter doses
Pharmacokinetic parameters/ equations	Pharmacokinetic dosing method	Pharmacokinetic parameter method
Literature-based/ concepts	Literature-based recommended dosing method	Linear pharmacokinetics method
Computerized	Bayesian computer program	Bayesian computer program

REFERENCES

1. Brodie MJ, Dichter MA. Antiepileptic drugs. N Engl J Med 1996;334(3):168–75.
2. Gidal BE, Graves NM, Garnett WR. Epilepsy. In: DiPiro JT, Talbert RL, Yee GC, Matzke GR, Wells BG, Posey LM, eds. Pharmacotherapy. 5th ed. New York: McGraw-Hill, 2002:1031–60.
3. McNamara JO. Drugs effective in the therapy of the epilepsies. In: Hardman JG, Limbird LE, Gilman AG, eds. The pharmacological basis of therapeutics. 10th ed. New York: McGraw-Hill, 2001:521–48.
4. Smith DB. Primidone: Clinical Use. In: Levy R, Mattson R, Meldrum B, eds. Antiepileptic Drugs. 3rd ed. New York: Raven, 1989:423–38.
5. Garnett WR. Antiepileptics. In: Schumacher GE, ed. Therapeutic drug monitoring. 1st ed. Stamford, CT: Appleton & Lange, 1995:345–95.
6. Browne TR, Evans JE, Szabo GK, Evans BA, Greenblatt DJ. Studies with stable isotopes II: phenobarbital pharmacokinetics during monotherapy. J Clin Pharmacol 1985;25(1):51–8.
7. Nelson E, Powell JR, Conrad K, et al. Phenobarbital pharmacokinetics and bioavailability in adults. J Clin Pharmacol 1982;22(2–3):141–8.
8. Streete JM, Berry DJ, Pettit LI, Newbery JE. Phenylethylmalonamide serum levels in patients treated with primidone and the effects of other antiepileptic drugs. Ther Drug Monit 1986;8(2):161–5.
9. Baumel IP, Gallagher BB, Mattson RH. Phenylethylmalonamide (PEMA). An important metabolite of primidone. Arch Neurol 1972;27(1):34–41.
10. Heimann G, Gladtke E. Pharmacokinetics of phenobarbital in childhood. Eur J Clin Pharmacol 1977;12(4):305–10.
11. Alvin J, McHorse T, Hoyumpa A, Bush MT, Schenker S. The effect of liver disease in man on the disposition of phenobarbital. J Pharmacol Exp Ther 1975;192(1):224–35.
12. Pugh RN, Murray-Lyon IM, Dawson JL, Pietroni MC, Williams R. Transection of the oesophagus for bleeding oesophageal varices. Br J Surg 1973;60(8):646–9.
13. Golper TA. Update on drug sieving coefficients and dosing adjustments during continuous renal replacement therapies. Contrib Nephrol 2001(132):349–53.
14. Golper TA, Marx MA. Drug dosing adjustments during continuous renal replacement therapies. Kidney Int Suppl 1998;66:S165–8.
15. Rust RS, Dodson WE. Phenobarbital: absorption, distribution, and excretion. In: Levy RH, Mattson R, Meldrum B, eds. Antiepileptic Drugs. 3rd ed. New York: Raven, 1989:293–304.
16. Cloyd JC, Miller KW, Leppik IE. Primidone kinetics: effects of concurrent drugs and duration of therapy. Clin Pharmacol Ther 1981;29(3):402–7.
17. Kauffman RE, Habersang R, Lansky L. Kinetics of primidone metabolism and excretion in children. Clin Pharmacol Ther 1977;22(2):200–5.
18. Hansten PD, Horn JR. Drug interactions analysis and management. Vancouver, WA: Applied Therapeutics, 1999.
19. Wandell M, Mungall D. Computer assisted drug interpretation and drug regimen optimization. Am Assoc Clin Chem 1984;6:1–11.

14 | **Ethosuximide**

Ethosuximide is a succinimide compound that is effective in the treatment of absence (petit mal) seizures (Table 14-1).[1] Although the exact mechanism of action is not known, the antiepileptic effect of ethosuximide is thought to be due to its ability to decrease low-threshold calcium currents in thalamic neurons.[2] The thalamus has a key role in the production of 3-Hz spike-wave rhythms that are a hallmark of absence seizures. Ethosuximide may also inhibit the sodium-potassium ATPase system and NADPH-linked aldehyde reductase.[3]

THERAPEUTIC AND TOXIC CONCENTRATIONS

- The therapeutic range for ethosuximide is defined by most laboratories as 40–100 μg/ml, although some clinicians suggest drug concentrations as high as 150 μg/ml with appropriate monitoring of serum concentrations and possible side effects.[4]
- The most common adverse effects of ethosuximide are gastric distress, nausea, vomiting, and anorexia, but these gastrointestinal problems appear to be due to local irritation of gastric mucosa. Generally, administration of smaller doses and more frequent dosing of the drug produce relief from these side effects.
- At the upper end of the therapeutic range (>70 μg/ml), some patients will begin to experience the concentration-dependent adverse effects of ethosuximide treatment: drowsiness, fatigue, lethargy, dizziness, ataxia, hiccups, euphoria, and headaches.
- Idiosyncratic side effects that are independent of concentration include rash, systemic lupus-like syndromes, and blood dyscrasias (leukopenia, pancytopenia).

CLINICAL MONITORING PARAMETERS

- The goal of therapy with anticonvulsants is to reduce seizure frequency and maximize quality of life with a minimum of adverse drug effects. While it is desirable to abolish seizure episodes entirely, it may not be possible to accomplish this in many patients.
- Patients should be monitored for concentration-related side effects (drowsiness, fatigue, lethargy, dizziness, ataxia, hiccups, euphoria, headaches) as well as gastrointestinal upset associated with local irritation of gastric mucosa (gastric distress, nausea, vomiting, anorexia).
- Serious, but rare, idiosyncratic side effects include systemic lupus-like syndromes, leukopenia, and pancytopenia.
- Ethosuximide serum concentrations should be measured in most patients. Because epilepsy is an episodic disease state, patients do not experience seizures on a continuous basis. Thus, during dosage titration it is difficult to tell if the patient is responding to drug therapy or simply is not experiencing any abnormal central nervous system discharges at that time.
- Ethosuximide serum concentrations are also valuable tools for avoiding adverse drug effects. Patients are more likely to accept drug therapy if adverse reactions are held to the absolute minimum.

TABLE 14-1 International Classification of Epileptic Seizures[1]

Major class	Subset of class	Drug treatment for selected seizure type

Partial seizures (beginning locally)	1. Simple partial seizures (without impaired consciousness)
	  a. With motor symptoms
	  b. With somatosensory or special sensory symptoms
	  c. With autonomic symptoms
	  d. With psychological symptoms
		Carbamazepine
		Phenytoin
		Valproic acid
		Phenobarbital
		Primidone

	2. Complex partial seizures (with impaired consciousness)
	  a. Simple partial onset followed by impaired consciousness
	  b. Impaired consciousness at onset
		Carbamazepine
		Phenytoin
		Valproic acid
		Phenobarbital
		Primidone

	3. Partial seizures evolving into secondary generalized seizures	Carbamazepine Phenytoin Valproic acid Phenobarbital Primidone
Generalized seizures (convulsive or nonconvulsive)	1. Absence seizures (typical or atypical; also known as petit mal seizures)	Ethosuximide Valproic acid
	2. Tonic-clonic seizures (also known as grand mal seizures)	Phenytoin Carbamazepine Valproic acid Phenobarbital Primidone

BASIC CLINICAL PHARMACOKINETIC PARAMETERS

- Ethosuximide is eliminated primarily by hepatic metabolism (70–80%) via hydroxylation and then conjugated to inactive metabolites.[5] About 20–30% of an ethosuximide dose is recovered as unchanged drug in the urine.[6] Ethosuximide is not significantly bound to plasma proteins.
- At concentrations exceeding 100 μg/ml, the drug may follow nonlinear pharmacokinetics, presumably due to Michaelis-Menten (concentration-dependent or saturable) metabolism.[7]
- Because an intravenous form of the drug is not available commercially, the absolute bioavailability in humans is not known. However, based on animal studies, ethosuximide oral bioavailability of capsules (250 mg) and syrup (250 mg/5 ml) is assumed to be 100%.[4]
- The typical maintenance dose for ethosuximide is 20 mg/kg/d for pediatric patients (<12 years old) and 15 mg/kg/d for older patients.[4]

EFFECTS OF DISEASE STATES AND CONDITIONS ON PHARMACOKINETICS AND DOSING

- Ethosuximide oral clearance rate (Cl/F) for older children (≥12 years old) and adults is 12 ml/h/kg, and for children it is 16 ml/h/kg.[4]
- Ethosuximide volume of distribution (V/F) is 0.7 L/kg, and its half-life averages 30 hours in children and 60 hours in adults.[4]

Hepatic Dysfunction

- Although studies in patients with hepatic disease are not available, 70–80% of the drug is eliminated by hepatic metabolism. As a result, patients with liver cirrhosis or acute hepatitis may have reduced ethosuximide clearance because of destruction of liver parenchyma. This loss of functional hepatic cells reduces the amount of enzymes available to metabolize the drug and decreases clearance.
- An index of liver dysfunction can be gained by applying the Child-Pugh clinical classification system to the patient (Table 14-2).[8] Child-Pugh scores are discussed more fully in Chapter 3 (Drug Dosing in Special Populations: Renal and Hepatic Disease, Dialysis, Heart Failure, Obesity, and Drug Interactions).

  - The Child-Pugh score consists of five laboratory tests or clinical symptoms: serum albumin, total bilirubin, prothrombin time, ascites, and hepatic encephalopathy. Each of these areas is given a score of 1 (normal) to 3 (severely abnormal; Table 14-2), and the scores for the five areas are summed.
  - The Child-Pugh score for a patient with normal liver function is 5, while the score for a patient with grossly abnormal serum albumin, total bilirubin, and prothrombin time values in addition to severe ascites and hepatic encephalopathy is 15. A Child-Pugh score greater than 8 is grounds for a decrease of 25–50% in the initial daily drug dose of ethosuximide.

- As in any patient, with or without liver dysfunction, initial doses are meant as starting points for dosage titration based on patient response and avoidance of adverse effects. Ethosuximide serum concentrations and the presence of adverse drug effects should be monitored frequently in patients with liver cirrhosis.

Renal Dysfunction

- A small amount (20–30%) of ethosuximide is usually eliminated unchanged by the kidneys, so patients with renal dysfunction (creatinine clearance <30 ml/min) who are receiving ethosuximide should be closely monitored.[6]

Dialysis

- Ethosuximide is significantly removed by hemodialysis, and supplemental doses may need to be given after a dialysis session.[9]

TABLE 14-2 Child-Pugh Scores for Patients with Liver Disease[8]

Test/symptom	Score 1 point	Score 2 points	Score 3 points
Total bilirubin (mg/dl)	<2.0	2.0–3.0	>3.0
Serum albumin (g/dl)	>3.5	2.8–3.5	<2.8
Prothrombin time (seconds prolonged over control)	<4	4–6	>6
Ascites	Absent	Slight	Moderate
Hepatic Encephalopathy	None	Moderate	Severe

Pregnancy/Lactation

• The drug crosses into the placenta and enters breast milk, achieving concentrations at both sites similar to concurrent maternal serum concentrations.[10–12]

DRUG INTERACTIONS

• Unlike other antiepileptic drugs, ethosuximide is not a hepatic enzyme inducer or inhibitor, and appears to cause no clinically important drug interactions.[13]
• Valproic acid can inhibit ethosuximide metabolism and increase steady-state concentrations, especially when ethosuximide serum concentrations are near the upper end of the therapeutic range.[7]

INITIAL DOSAGE DETERMINATION METHODS

• Several methods to initiate ethosuximide therapy are available.

  • The *pharmacokinetic dosing method* is the most flexible of the techniques. It allows individualized target serum concentrations to be chosen for a patient, and each pharmacokinetic parameter can be customized to reflect specific disease states and conditions present in the patient.
  • *Literature-based recommended dosing* is a very commonly used method to prescribe initial doses of ethosuximide. Doses are based on those that commonly produce steady-state concentrations near the lower end of the therapeutic range, although there is a wide variation in the actual concentrations for a specific patient.

Pharmacokinetic Dosing Method

• The goal of initial dosing of ethosuximide is to compute the best dose possible for the patient given the set of disease states and conditions that influence ethosuximide pharmacokinetics and the epileptic disorder being treated. In order to do this, pharmacokinetic parameters for the patient are estimated using average parameters measured in other patients with similar disease state and condition profiles.

Clearance Estimate

• Ethosuximide is metabolized predominately by the liver. Unfortunately, there is no good way to estimate the elimination characteristics of liver-metabolized drugs using an endogenous marker of liver function in the same manner that serum creatinine and estimated creatinine clearance are used to estimate the elimination of agents that are eliminated renally.

  • As a result, a patient is categorized according to the disease states and conditions that are known to change ethosuximide clearance, and clearances previously measured in studies are used as an estimate of the current patient's clearance.
  • To produce the most conservative ethosuximide doses in patients with multiple concurrent disease states or conditions that affect ethosuximide pharmacokinetics, the disease state or condition with the smallest clearance should be used to compute doses. This approach will avoid accidental overdosage as much as is currently possible.

Volume of Distribution Estimate

- Ethosuximide volume of distribution is assumed to be 0.7 L/kg for adults and children.

Half-life and Elimination Rate Constant Estimate

- Once the correct clearance and volume of distribution estimates have been identified for a patient, they can be converted into the ethosuximide half-life ($t_{1/2}$) and elimination rate constant (k) estimates using the following equations:

$$t_{1/2} = (0.693 \cdot V)/Cl$$

$$k = 0.693/t_{1/2} = Cl/V$$

Selection of Appropriate Pharmacokinetic Model and Equations

- Ethosuximide follows a one-compartment pharmacokinetic model. Ethosuximide has good bioavailability (F = 1), and once- or twice-daily dosing provides a relatively smooth serum concentration/time curve that emulates an intravenous infusion.

  - A very simple pharmacokinetic equation that computes the average ethosuximide steady-state serum concentration (Css in µg/ml = mg/L) is widely used and allows maintenance dosage calculation:

$$Css = [F(D/\tau)]/Cl \qquad or \qquad D = (Css \cdot Cl \cdot \tau)/F$$

  where F is the bioavailability fraction for the oral dosage form (F = 1 for oral ethosuximide products), D is the dose of ethosuximide in mg, Cl is ethosuximide clearance in L/h, and τ is the dosage interval in hours.

▶ *Example 1*   LK is a 13-year-old, 47-kg (height 5′1″) female with absence seizures who requires therapy with oral ethosuximide. She has normal liver and renal function. Suggest an initial ethosuximide dosage regimen designed to achieve a steady-state ethosuximide concentration equal to 50 µg/ml.

1. *Estimate clearance and volume of distribution according to disease states and conditions present in the patient.* The clearance rate for children 12 years and older, and among adults, is 12 ml/h/kg. Using this value, the estimated clearance is

$$Cl = 47 \text{ kg} \cdot 12 \text{ ml/h/kg} = 564 \text{ ml/h or } 0.564 \text{ L/h}$$

The estimated volume of distribution is

$$47 \text{ kg} \cdot 0.7 \text{ L/kg} = 33 \text{ L}$$

2. *Estimate half-life and elimination rate constant.* Once the correct clearance and volume of distribution estimates have been identified for the patient, they can be converted into the ethosuximide half-life ($t_{1/2}$) and elimination rate constant (k) estimates using the following equations:

$$t_{1/2} = (0.693 \cdot V)/Cl = (0.693 \cdot 33 \text{ L})/0.564 \text{ L/h} = 41 \text{ h}$$

$$k = Cl/V = (0.564 \text{ L/h})/33 \text{ L} = 0.017 \text{ h}^{-1}$$

3. *Compute dosage regimen.* Oral ethosuximide capsules will be prescribed for this patient (F = 1). (*Note:* µg/ml = mg/L, and this concentration unit

was substituted for Css in the calculations so that unit conversion was not required.) The dosage equation for oral ethosuximide is

$$D = (Css \cdot Cl \cdot \tau)/F = (50 \text{ mg/L} \cdot 0.564 \text{ L/h} \cdot 12 \text{ h})/1$$
$$= 338 \text{ mg, rounded to } 250 \text{ every } 12 \text{ h}$$

A steady-state trough ethosuximide serum concentration should be measured after steady state is attained in 3–5 half-lives. Since the drug is expected to have a half-life of 41 hours, an ethosuximide steady-state concentration can be obtained at any time after the ninth day of dosing (5 half-lives = $5 \cdot 41$ h = 205 h or 9 d). Ethosuximide serum concentrations should also be measured if the patient experiences an exacerbation of epilepsy, or if the patient develops potential signs or symptoms of ethosuximide toxicity.

► **Example 2** CT is a 10-year-old, 40-kg (height 4′2″) male with absence seizures who requires therapy with oral ethosuximide. He has normal liver and renal function. Suggest an initial ethosuximide dosage regimen designed to achieve a steady-state ethosuximide concentration of 50 µg/ml.

1. *Estimate clearance and volume of distribution according to disease states and conditions present in the patient.* The clearance rate for a child is 16 ml/h/kg. Using this value, the estimated clearance is

$$Cl = 40 \text{ kg} \cdot 16 \text{ ml/h/kg} = 640 \text{ ml/h or } 0.640 \text{ L/h}$$

Using 0.7 L/kg, the estimated volume of distribution is

$$40 \text{ kg} \cdot 0.7 \text{ L/kg} = 28 \text{ L}$$

2. *Estimate half-life and elimination rate constant.* Once the correct clearance and volume of distribution estimates have been identified for the patient, they can be converted into the ethosuximide half-life ($t_{1/2}$) and elimination rate constant (k) estimates using the following equations:

$$t_{1/2} = (0.693 \cdot V)/Cl = (0.693 \cdot 28 \text{ L})/0.640 \text{ L/h} = 30 \text{ h}$$

$$k = Cl/V = (0.640 \text{ L/h})/28 \text{ L} = 0.023 \text{ h}^{-1}$$

3. *Compute dosage regimen.* Oral ethosuximide syrup will be prescribed for this patient (F = 1). (*Note:* µg/ml = mg/L, and this concentration unit was substituted for Css in the calculations so that unit conversion was not required.) The dosage equation for oral ethosuximide is

$$D = (Css \cdot Cl \cdot \tau)/F = (50 \text{ mg/L} \cdot 0.640 \text{ L/h} \cdot 12 \text{ h})/1$$

$$= 384 \text{ mg, rounded to } 400 \text{ mg every } 12 \text{ h}$$

A steady-state trough ethosuximide serum concentration should be measured after steady state is attained in 3–5 half-lives. Since the drug is expected to have a half-life of 30 hours, an ethosuximide steady-state concentration can be obtained at any time after the sixth day of dosing (5 half-lives = $5 \cdot 30$ h = 150 h or 6 d). Ethosuximide serum concentrations should also be measured if the patient experiences an exacerbation of epilepsy, or if the patient develops potential signs or symptoms of ethosuximide toxicity.

Literature-Based Recommended Dosing

• Because of the large amount of variability in ethosuximide pharmacokinetics, even when concurrent disease states and conditions are identified, most clinicians believe that the use of standard ethosuximide doses for various situations is warranted. The original computations of these doses were based on pharmacokinetic dosing methods, and the doses were subsequently modified based on clinical experience. In general, the expected ethosuximide steady-state serum concentrations used to compute these doses was 40–50 µg/ml.

• The usual initial maintenance dose for pediatric patients (<12 years old) is 20 mg/kg/d. For older patients, the initial maintenance dose is 15 mg/kg/d. One or two divided daily doses are used initially for these total doses.

• To avoid gastrointestinal side effects, doses over 1500 mg given at one time should be avoided.

• Dosage increases of 3–7 mg/kg/d are made every 1–2 weeks, depending on response and adverse effects.

• While maximal doses are 40 mg/kg/d for children less than 12 years old and 30 mg/kg/d for older patients, ethosuximide serum concentrations and adverse effects should be used to judge optimal response to the drug.

• If the patient has significant hepatic dysfunction (Child-Pugh score ≥8), maintenance doses prescribed using this method should be decreased by 25–50%, depending on how aggressive therapy is required to be for the individual.

• To illustrate the similarities and differences between this method of dosage calculation and the pharmacokinetic dosing method, the same examples used in the previous section will be used.

▶ *Example 3*   LK is a 13-year-old, 47-kg (height 5′1″) female with absence seizures who requires therapy with oral ethosuximide. She has normal liver and renal function. Suggest an initial ethosuximide dosage regimen designed to achieve a steady-state ethosuximide concentration of 50 µg/ml.

1. *Estimate ethosuximide dose according to disease states and conditions present in the patient.* Oral ethosuximide capsules will be prescribed for this patient. The suggested initial maintenance dosage rate for ethosuximide in patients over 12 years is 15 mg/kg/d:

$$47 \text{ kg} \cdot 15 \text{ mg/kg/d} = 705 \text{ mg/d, rounded to } 750 \text{ mg/d}$$

This dose could be given as 250 mg in the morning and 500 mg in the evening. The dose should be titrated upward in 3–7-mg/kg/d increments every 1–2 weeks while monitoring for adverse and therapeutic effects. The goals of therapy include maximal suppression of seizures and avoidance of side effects.

A steady-state trough total ethosuximide serum concentration should be measured after steady state is attained in 1–2 weeks. Ethosuximide serum concentrations should also be measured if the patient experiences an exacerbation of epilepsy, or if the patient develops potential signs or symptoms of ethosuximide toxicity.

▶ *Example 4*   CT is a 10-year-old, 40-kg (height 4′2″) male with absence seizures who requires therapy with oral ethosuximide. He has normal liver and renal function. Suggest an initial ethosuximide dosage regimen designed to achieve a steady-state ethosuximide concentration of 50 µg/ml.

1. *Estimate ethosuximide dose according to disease states and conditions present in the patient.* Oral ethosuximide syrup will be prescribed for

this patient. The suggested initial maintenance dosage rate for ethosuximide for a child is 20 mg/kg/d:

$$40 \text{ kg} \cdot 20 \text{ mg/kg/d} = 800 \text{ mg/d or } 400 \text{ mg every } 12 \text{ h}$$

This dose should be titrated upward in 3–7-mg/kg/d increments every 1–2 weeks while monitoring for adverse and therapeutic effects. The goals of therapy include maximal suppression of seizures and avoidance of side effects.

A steady-state trough total ethosuximide serum concentration should be measured after steady state is attained in 1–2 weeks. Ethosuximide serum concentrations should also be measured if the patient experiences an exacerbation of epilepsy, or if the patient develops potential signs or symptoms of ethosuximide toxicity.

USE OF ETHOSUXIMIDE SERUM CONCENTRATIONS TO ALTER DOSES

- Because of the large amount of pharmacokinetic variability among patients, it is likely that doses computed using patient population characteristics will not always produce ethosuximide serum concentrations that are expected or desirable.

  - Because of pharmacokinetic variability, the possible nonlinear pharmacokinetics followed by the drug at high concentrations, the narrow therapeutic index of ethosuximide, and the desire to avoid adverse side effects of ethosuximide, ethosuximide serum concentrations are measured in most patients, to ensure that therapeutic, nontoxic levels are present.

- In addition to ethosuximide serum concentrations, important patient parameters (seizure frequency, potential ethosuximide side effects, etc.) should be followed to confirm that the patient is responding to treatment and not developing adverse drug reactions.
- When ethosuximide serum concentrations are measured in patients and a dosage change is necessary, clinicians should use the simplest, most straightforward method available to determine a dose that will provide safe and effective treatment.

  - In most cases a simple dosage ratio can be used to change doses, since ethosuximide follows *linear pharmacokinetics*. Sometimes it is not possible simply to change the dose because of the limited number of oral dosage strengths, and the dosage interval must also be changed.
  - In some situations it may be necessary or desirable to compute the ethosuximide *pharmacokinetic parameters* for the patient and utilize these to calculate the best drug dose.
  - Computerized methods that incorporate expected population pharmacokinetic characteristics (*Bayesian pharmacokinetic computer programs*) can be used in difficult cases, when serum concentrations are obtained at suboptimal times, or the patient was not at steady state when serum concentrations were measured.

Linear Pharmacokinetics Method

- Because ethosuximide follows linear, dose-proportional pharmacokinetics in most patients with concentrations within and below the therapeutic range, steady-state serum concentrations change in proportion to dose according to the following equation:

$$D_{new}/Css_{new} = D_{old}/Css_{old} \qquad or \qquad D_{new} = (Css_{new}/Css_{old})D_{old}$$

where D is the dose, Css is the steady-state concentration, old indicates the dose that produced the steady-state concentration the patient is currently receiving, and new denotes the dose necessary to produce the desired steady-state concentration.

- The advantages of this method are that it is quick and simple.
- The disadvantages are that steady-state concentrations are required, and the assumption of linear pharmacokinetics may not be valid in all patients.
- When steady-state serum concentrations increase more than expected after a dosage increase or decrease less than expected after a dosage decrease, non-linear ethosuximide pharmacokinetics is a possible explanation for the observation. Therefore, suggested dosage increases greater than 75% using this method should be scrutinized by the prescribing clinician, and the risk versus benefit for the patient assessed before initiating large dosage increases (>75% over current dose).

▶ *Example 5*   LK is a 13-year-old, 47-kg (height 5′1″) female with absence seizures who requires therapy with oral ethosuximide. After dosage titration, the patient was prescribed 500 mg of ethosuximide capsules every 12 hours (1000 mg/d) for 1 month, after which her steady-state ethosuximide total concentration was 38 µg/ml. The patient is assessed to be compliant with her dosage regimen. Suggest an ethosuximide dosage regimen designed to achieve a steady-state ethosuximide concentration of 80 µg/ml.

1. *Compute new dose to achieve desired serum concentration.* Using linear pharmacokinetics, the resulting total steady-state ethosuximide serum concentration is

$$D_{new} = (Css_{new}/Css_{old})D_{old}$$
$$= [(80 \ µg/ml)/(38 \ µg/ml)](1000 \ mg/d) = 2105 \ mg/d$$

This dose would be rounded to 2000 mg/d or 1000 mg every 12 hours.

A steady-state trough total ethosuximide serum concentration should be measured after steady state is attained in 1–2 weeks. Ethosuximide serum concentrations should also be measured if the patient experiences an exacerbation of epilepsy, or if the patient develops potential signs or symptoms of ethosuximide toxicity.

▶ *Example 6*   CT is a 10-year-old, 40-kg (height 4′2″) male with absence seizures who requires therapy with oral ethosuximide. After dosage titration, the patient was prescribed 500 mg of ethosuximide syrup twice daily (1000 mg/d) for 1 month, after which his steady-state ethosuximide total concentration was 130 µg/ml. The patient is assessed to be compliant with his dosage regimen. Suggest a ethosuximide dosage regimen designed to achieve a steady-state ethosuximide concentration of 75 µg/ml.

1. *Compute new dose to achieve desired serum concentration.* Using linear pharmacokinetics, the resulting total steady-state ethosuximide serum concentration is

$$D_{new} = (Css_{new}/Css_{old})D_{old}$$
$$= [(75 \ µg/ml)/(130 \ µg/ml)](1000 \ mg/d) = 577 \ mg/d$$

This dose would be rounded to 500 mg/d or 250 mg every 12 hours.

A steady-state trough total ethosuximide serum concentration should be measured after steady state is attained in 1–2 weeks. Ethosuximide serum concentrations should also be measured if the patient experiences an exacerbation of epilepsy, or if the patient develops potential signs or symptoms of ethosuximide toxicity.

Pharmacokinetic Parameter Method

- The pharmacokinetic parameter method of adjusting drug doses was among the first techniques available to change doses using serum concentrations. It allows the computation of an individual's own, unique pharmacokinetic constants and uses those to calculate a dose that achieves desired ethosuximide concentrations.
- The pharmacokinetic parameter method requires that steady state has been achieved and uses only a steady-state ethosuximide concentration (Css). Ethosuximide clearance (Cl) can be calculated using the following formula:

$$Cl = [F(D/\tau)]/Css$$

where F is the bioavailability fraction for the oral dosage form (F = 1 for oral ethosuximide products), D is the dose of ethosuximide in mg, Css is the steady-state ethosuximide concentration in mg/L, and τ is the dosage interval in hours.
- To illustrate the similarities and differences between this method of dosage calculation and the pharmacokinetic parameter method, the same examples used in the previous section will be used.

▶ **Example 7**   LK is a 13-year-old, 47-kg (height 5'1'') female with absence seizures who requires therapy with oral ethosuximide. After dosage titration, the patient was prescribed 500 mg of ethosuximide capsules every 12 hours (1000 mg/d) for 1 month, after which her steady-state ethosuximide total concentration was 38 µg/ml. The patient is assessed to be compliant with her dosage regimen. Suggest a ethosuximide dosage regimen designed to achieve a steady-state ethosuximide concentration of 80 µg/ml.

1. *Compute pharmacokinetic parameters.* The patient can be expected to achieve steady-state conditions after 1–2 weeks of therapy. Ethosuximide clearance can be computed using a steady-state ethosuximide concentration:

$$Cl = [F(D/\tau)]/Css = [1(500 \text{ mg}/12 \text{ h})]/(38 \text{ mg/L}) = 1.1 \text{ L/h}$$

(*Note:* µg/ml = mg/L, and this concentration unit was substituted for Css in the calculations so that unit conversion was not required.)

2. *Compute ethosuximide dose.* Ethosuximide clearance is used to compute the new dose:

$$D = (Css \cdot Cl \cdot \tau)/F = (80 \text{ mg/L} \cdot 1.1 \text{ L/h} \cdot 12 \text{ h})/1$$

$$= 1056 \text{ mg, rounded to } 1000 \text{ mg every } 12 \text{ h}$$

A steady-state trough total ethosuximide serum concentration should be measured after steady state is attained in 1–2 weeks. Ethosuximide serum concentrations should also be measured if the patient experiences an exacerbation of epilepsy, or if the patient develops potential signs or symptoms of ethosuximide toxicity.

▶ *Example 8*   CT is a 10-year-old, 40-kg (height 4′2″) male with absence seizures who requires therapy with oral ethosuximide. After dosage titration, the patient was prescribed 500 mg of ethosuximide syrup twice daily (1000 mg/d) for 1 month, after which his steady-state ethosuximide total concentration was 130 μg/ml. The patient is assessed to be compliant with his dosage regimen. Suggest a ethosuximide dosage regimen designed to achieve a steady-state ethosuximide concentration of 75 μg/ml.

1. *Compute pharmacokinetic parameters.* The patient can be expected to achieve steady-state conditions after 1–2 weeks of therapy. Ethosuximide clearance can be computed using a steady-state ethosuximide concentration:

$$Cl = [F(D/\tau)]/Css = [1(500 \text{ mg}/12 \text{ h})]/(130 \text{ mg/L}) = 0.32 \text{ L/h}$$

(*Note:* μg/ml = mg/L, and this concentration unit was substituted for Css in the calculations so that unit conversion was not required.)

2. *Compute ethosuximide dose.* Ethosuximide clearance is used to compute the new dose:

$$D = (Css \cdot Cl \cdot \tau)/F = (75 \text{ mg/L} \cdot 0.32 \text{ L/h} \cdot 12 \text{ h})/1$$
$$= 288 \text{ mg, rounded to } 250 \text{ mg every } 12 \text{ h}$$

     A steady-state trough total ethosuximide serum concentration should be measured after steady state is attained in 1–2 weeks. Ethosuximide serum concentrations should also be measured if the patient experiences an exacerbation of epilepsy, or if the patient develops potential signs or symptoms of ethosuximide toxicity.

BAYESIAN PHARMACOKINETIC COMPUTER PROGRAMS

- Computer programs are available that can assist in the computation of pharmacokinetic parameters for patients. The most reliable computer programs use a nonlinear regression algorithm that incorporates components of Bayes' theorem.[14]
- An advantage of this approach is that consistent dosage recommendations can be made when several different practitioners are involved in therapeutic drug monitoring programs. Since simpler dosing methods work just as well for patients with stable pharmacokinetic parameters and steady-state drug concentrations, many clinicians reserve the use of computer programs for more difficult situations. Those situations include serum concentrations that are not at steady state, serum concentrations not obtained at the specific times needed to employ simpler methods, and unstable pharmacokinetic parameters.
- Many Bayesian pharmacokinetic computer programs are available, and most should provide answers similar to the program used in the following examples. The program used to solve problems in this book is DrugCalc, written by Dr. Dennis Mungall and available at his Internet web site (www.clinpharmacologist.bigstep.com/consumersurvey.html).[14]

▶ *Example 9*   LK is a 13-year-old, 47-kg (height 5′1″) female with absence seizures who requires therapy with oral ethosuximide. The patient has normal liver and renal function (bilirubin = 0.5 mg/dl, albumin 4.6 mg/dl, serum creatinine = 0.5 mg/dl). After dosage titration, the patient was prescribed 500 mg of ethosuximide capsules every 12 hours (1000 mg/d) for 2 weeks, after which her steady-state ethosuximide total concentration was 38 μg/ml. The patient is assessed to be compliant with her dosage regimen.

Suggest a ethosuximide dosage regimen designed to achieve a steady-state ethosuximide concentration of 80 µg/ml.

1. *Enter patient demographic, drug dosing, and serum concentration/time data into a Bayesian pharmacokinetic computer program.*
2. *Compute pharmacokinetic parameters for the patient using the computer program.* The pharmacokinetic parameters computed by the program are a volume of distribution of 46 L, a half-life of 26 hours, and a clearance of 1.24 L/h.
3. *Compute dose required to achieve desired ethosuximide serum concentrations.* The one-compartment-model first-order absorption equation used by the program to compute doses indicates that a dose of 1000 mg every 12 hours will produce a steady-state ethosuximide concentration of 68 µg/ml.

▶ *Example 10* JB is an 8-year-old, 35-kg (height 4′2″) male with absence seizures who was started on 350 mg of ethosuximide syrup every 12 hours. His ethosuximide concentration was 25 µg/ml before the fifth maintenance dose. What ethosuximide dose is needed to achieve Css = 75 µg/ml?

1. *Enter patient demographic, drug dosing, and serum concentration/time data into a Bayesian pharmacokinetic computer program.* In this case it is unlikely that the patient is at steady state, so the linear pharmacokinetics method cannot be used.
2. *Compute pharmacokinetic parameters for the patient using the computer program.* The pharmacokinetic parameters computed by the program are a volume of distribution of 30 L, a half-life of 18 hours, and clearance of 1.12 L/h.
3. *Compute dose required to achieve desired ethosuximide serum concentrations.* The one-compartment-model oral equations used by the program to compute doses indicates that a dose of ethosuximide 1000 mg every 12 hours will produce a steady-state concentration of 69 µg/ml.

DOSING STRATEGIES

- Initial dose and dosage adjustment techniques using serum concentrations can be used in any combination as long as the limitations of each method are observed.
- Some dosing schemes link together logically when considered according to their basic approaches or philosophies. Dosage strategies that follow similar pathways are given in Table 14-3.

TABLE 14-3 Dosing Strategies

Dosing approach/ philosophy	Initial dosing	Use of serum concentrations to alter doses
Pharmacokinetic parameters/ equations	Pharmacokinetic dosing method	Pharmacokinetic parameter method
Literature-based/ concepts	Literature-based recommended dosing method	Linear pharmacokinetics method
Computerized	Bayesian computer program	Bayesian computer program

REFERENCES

1. Brodie MJ, Dichter MA. Antiepileptic drugs. N Engl J Med 1996;334(3):168–75.
2. McNamara JO. Drugs effective in the therapy of the epilepsies. In: Hardman JG, Limbird LE, Gilman AG, eds. The pharmacological basis of therapeutics. 10th ed. New York: McGraw-Hill, 2001:521–48.
3. Gidal BE, Graves NM, Garnett WR. Epilepsy. In: DiPiro JT, Talbert RL, Yee GC, Matzke GR, Wells BG, Posey LM, eds. Pharmacotherapy. 5th ed. New York: McGraw-Hill, 2002:1031–60.
4. Garnett WR. Antiepileptics. In: Schumacher GE, ed. Therapeutic drug monitoring. 1st ed. Stamford, CT: Appleton & Lange, 1995:345–95.
5. Chang T. Ethosuximide—biotransformation. In: Levy RH, Mattson R, Meldrum B, eds. Antiepileptic drugs. 3rd ed. New York: Raven, 1989:679–83.
6. Glazko AJ. Antiepileptic drugs: biotransformation, metabolism, and serum half-life. Epilepsia 1975;16(2):367–91.
7. Bauer LA, Harris C, Wilensky AJ, Raisys VA, Levy RH. Ethosuximide kinetics: possible interaction with valproic acid. Clin Pharmacol Ther 1982;31(6):741–5.
8. Pugh RN, Murray-Lyon IM, Dawson JL, Pietroni MC, Williams R. Transection of the oesophagus for bleeding oesophageal varices. Br J Surg 1973;60(8):646–9.
9. Marbury TC, Lee CS, Perchalski RJ, Wilder BJ. Hemodialysis clearance of ethosuximide in patients with chronic renal disease. Am J Hosp Pharm 1981;38(11):1757–60.
10. Chang T. Ethosuximide—absorption, distribution, and excretion. In: Levy RH, Mattson R, Meldrum B, eds. Antiepileptic drugs. 3rd ed. New York: Raven, 1989:679–83.
11. Rane A, Tunell R. Ethosuximide in human milk and in plasma of a mother and her nursed infant. Br J Clin Pharmacol 1981;12(6):855–8.
12. Koup JR, Rose JQ, Cohen ME. Ethosuximide pharmacokinetics in a pregnant patient and her newborn. Epilepsia 1978;19(6):535–9.
13. Hansten PD, Horn JR. Drug interactions analysis and management. Vancouver, WA: Applied Therapeutics, 1999.
14. Wandell M, Mungall D. Computer assisted drug interpretation and drug regimen optimization. Am Assoc Clin Chem 1984;6:1–11.

5 | IMMUNOSUPPRESSANTS

15 | Cyclosporine

Cyclosporine is a cyclic polypeptide with immunosuppressant properties that is used for the prevention of graft-versus-host disease in bone marrow transplant patients, for the prevention of graft rejection in solid-organ transplant patients, and for the treatment of psoriasis, rheumatoid arthritis, and a variety of other autoimmune diseases.[1-5]

- The immunomodulating properties of cyclosporine are due to its ability to block the production of intraleukin-2 and other cytokines secreted by T lymphocytes.[6] Cyclosporine binds to cyclophilin, an intracellular cytoplasmic protein found in T cells. The cyclosporine–cyclophilin complex interacts with calcineurin, inhibits the catalytic activity of calcineurin, and prevents the production of intermediaries involved with the expression of genes regulating the production of cytokines.

THERAPEUTIC AND TOXIC CONCENTRATIONS

- The therapeutic range of cyclosporine used by clinicians varies greatly according to the type of assay used to measure cyclosporine and whether blood or serum concentrations are determined by the clinical laboratory (Table 15-1).[1-5,7,8]

  - Because cyclosporine is bound to red blood cells, blood concentrations are higher than simultaneously measured serum or plasma concentrations.
  - High-pressure liquid chromatography (HPLC) assay techniques are specific for cyclosporine measurement in blood, serum, or plasma. However, older immunoassays conducted via fluorescence polarization (polyclonal TDx® assay, Abbott Diagnostics) or radioimmunoassay (polyclonal RIA, various manufacturers) are nonspecific and measure both cyclosporine and its metabolites. Newer monoclonal fluorescence polarization (monoclonal TDx® assay) and radioimmunoassays (various) are now available that are relatively specific for cyclosporine and produce results similar to the HPLC assay.

    - Cyclosporine concentrations measured simultaneously in a patient using the specific high-pressure liquid chromatography technique or one of the specific immunoassays will be lower than that determined using a nonspecific immunoassay.

- Since cyclosporine metabolites are excreted in bile, liver transplant patients who are immediately post–transplant surgery can have very high cyclosporine metabolite concentrations in the blood, serum, and plasma because bile production has not begun yet in the newly transplanted organ.

  - If nonspecific immunoassays are used to measure cyclosporine concentrations in liver transplant patients immediately after surgery, before the graft has begun to produce bile, the predominant species measured with this assay methodology may be cyclosporine metabolites and not cyclosporine.

- Desired cyclosporine concentrations differ among the various types of organ transplants, change with time during the posttransplantation phase, and are determined by protocols specific to the transplantation service and institution.[1-5,7,8]

TABLE 15-1 Cyclosporine Therapeutic Concentrations for Different Assay Techniques and Biological Fluids

Assay	Biological fluid	Therapeutic concentration (ng/ml)
High-pressure liquid chromatography (HPLC), monoclonal fluorescence polarization immunoassay (monoclonal TDx® assay, Abbott Diagnostics), or monoclonal radioimmunoassay (various manufacturers)	Blood	100–400
High-pressure liquid chromatography (HPLC), monoclonal fluorescence polarization immunoassay (monoclonal TDx® assay, Abbott Diagnostics), or monoclonal radioimmunoassay (various manufacturers)	Plasma	50–150
Polyclonal fluorescence polarization immunoassay (polyclonal TDx® assay, Abbott Diagnostics), or polyclonal radioimmunoassay (various manufacturers)	Blood	200–800
Polyclonal fluorescence polarization immunoassay (polyclonal TDx® assay, Abbott Diagnostics), or polyclonal radioimmunoassay (various manufacturers)	Plasma	100–400

- For patients receiving cyclosporine after a bone marrow transplant, the goal of therapy is to prevent graft-versus-host disease while avoiding adverse effects of immunosuppressant therapy.[4,7,8] Graft-versus-host disease is a result of donor T lymphocytes detecting antigens on host tissues and producing an immunological response against these antigens and host tissues.

  - To prevent acute graft-versus-host disease from occurring in allogenic bone marrow transplant patients with HCA-identical sibling donors, cyclosporine therapy is usually instituted on the day of marrow transplant (day 0), and doses are adjusted to provide therapeutic trough concentrations.

    - If prophylaxis of acute graft-versus-host disease is successful, cyclosporine doses can begin to be tapered on about posttransplant day 50, with the goal of drug discontinuation by about posttransplant day 180.

  - For allogeneic bone marrow transplant patients with HLA-mismatched or HLA-identical unrelated donors, the risk of acute graft-versus-host disease is higher, so cyclosporine therapy may be more prolonged for these patients.

  - After posttransplantation day 100, chronic graft-versus-host disease may occur and can also be treated with cyclosporine therapy.

- For patients receiving solid organ transplants such as kidney, liver, heart, lung, or heart–lung transplantation, the goal of cyclosporine therapy is to prevent acute or chronic rejection of the transplanted organ while minimizing drug side effects.[1-3,5,7,8]

  - Because cyclosporine can cause nephrotoxicity, many centers delay cyclosporine therapy in renal transplant patients for a few days or until the kidney begins functioning, to avoid untoward effects on the newly transplanted organ. Also, desired cyclosporine concentrations in renal transplant patients are generally lower than for other transplant patients, to avoid toxicity in the new renal graft (typically 100–200 ng/ml versus 150–300 ng/ml using whole blood with a specific, high-pressure liquid chromatograph assay).

- For other solid-organ transplant patients, cyclosporine therapy may be started several hours before surgery. During the immediate postoperative phase, intravenous cyclosporine may be given to these patients.

- For long-term management of immunosuppression in solid-organ tissue transplant patients, cyclosporine doses are gradually tapered to the lowest concentration and dose possible over a 6–12-month time period as long as rejection episodes do not occur.

- Hypertension, nephrotoxicity, hyperlipidemia, tremor, hirsutism, and gingival hyperplasia are all typical adverse effects of cyclosporine treatment.[1–5,7,8]

  - Hypertension is the most common side effect associated with cyclosporine therapy, and is treated with traditional antihypertensive drug therapy.
  - Nephrotoxicity is separated into acute and chronic varieties.

    - Acute nephrotoxicity is concentration- or dose-dependent and reverses with a dosage decrease. Renal damage in this situation is thought to be due to renal vasoconstriction which results in increased renal vascular resistance, decreased renal blood flow, and reduced glomerular filtration rate.
    - Chronic nephrotoxicity is accompanied by kidney tissue damage, including interstitial fibrosis, nonspecific tubular vacuolization, and structural changes in arteries, arterioles, and proximal tubular epithelium.
    - Increased serum creatinine and blood urea nitrogen (BUN) values, hyperkalemia, hyperuricemia, proteinuria, and increased renal sodium excretion occur with cyclosporine-induced nephrotoxicity.
    - The clinical features of cyclosporine nephrotoxicity and acute graft rejection in renal transplant patients are similar, so renal biopsies may be conducted to differentiate between these possibilities.[1] Because biopsy findings are similar between cyclosporine-induced nephrotoxicity and chronic rejection of kidney transplants, this technique is less helpful in this situation.

  - Hyperlipidemia is treated using dietary counseling and antilipid drug therapy.
  - Cyclosporine dosage decreases may be necessary to decrease tremor associated with drug therapy, while hirsutism is usually addressed using patient counseling.
  - Gingival hyperplasia can be minimized through the use of appropriate and regular dental hygiene and care.

CLINICAL MONITORING PARAMETERS

- Bone marrow transplant patients should be monitored for the signs and symptoms associated with graft-versus-host disease.[4] These include a generalized maculopapular skin rash, diarrhea, abdominal pain, ileus, hyperbilirubinemia, and increased liver function tests (serum transaminases and alkaline phosphatase). Patients with severe chronic graft-versus-host disease may have involvement of the skin, liver, eyes, mouth, esophagus, or other organs similar to what might be seen with systemic autoimmune diseases.

- Solid-organ transplant patients should be monitored for graft rejection consistent with the transplanted organ.

  - For renal transplant patients, increased serum creatinine, azotemia, hypertension, edema, weight gain secondary to fluid retention, graft tenderness, fever, and malaise may be due to an acute rejection episode.[1] Hypertension, proteinuria, a continuous decline in renal function (increases in serum creatinine and blood urea nitrogen levels), and uremia are indicative of chronic rejection in renal transplant patients.
  - For hepatic transplant patients, acute rejection signs and symptoms include fever, lethargy, graft tenderness, increased white blood cell count, change in bile color or amount, hyperbilirubinemia, and increased liver function tests.[5] Chronic rejection in a liver transplant patient may be accompanied only by increased liver function tests and jaundice.
  - For heart transplant patients, acute rejection is accompanied by low-grade fever, malaise, heart failure (presence of S_3 heart sound), or atrial arrhythmia.[2] Chronic rejection in heart transplant patients, also known as cardiac allograft vasculopathy, which is characterized by accelerated coronary artery atherosclerosis, may include the following symptoms: arrhythmias, decreased left ventricular function, heart failure, myocardial infarction, and sudden cardiac death.
  - For all solid-organ transplant patients, tissue biopsies may be taken from the transplanted tissue to confirm the diagnosis of organ rejection.[1-5]

- Typical adverse effects of cyclosporine treatment include hypertension, nephrotoxicity, hyperlipidemia, tremor, hirsutism, and gingival hyperplasia.[1-5,7,8] The management of these more common drug side effects are discussed in the previous section.

  - Other adverse drug reactions to cyclosporine that occur less frequently include gastrointestinal side effects (nausea, vomiting, diarrhea), headache, hepatotoxicity, hyperglycemia, acne, leukopenia, hyperkalemia, and hypomagnesemia.

- Because of the pivotal role that cyclosporine plays as an immunosuppressant in transplant patients, as well as the severity of its concentration- and dose-dependent side effects, cyclosporine concentrations should be measured in every patient receiving the drug.
- If a patient experiences signs or symptoms of graft-versus-host disease or organ rejection, a cyclosporine concentration should be checked to ensure that levels have not fallen below the therapeutic range.
- If a patient encounters a possible clinical problem that could be an adverse drug effect of cyclosporine therapy, a cyclosporine concentration should be measured to determine if levels are in the toxic range.
- During the immediate posttransplantation phase, cyclosporine concentrations are measured daily in most patients even though steady state may not yet have been achieved, in order to prevent acute rejection in solid-organ transplant patients or acute graft-versus-host disease in bone marrow transplant patients.
- After discharge from the hospital, cyclosporine concentrations continue to be obtained at most clinic visits.

- In patients receiving allogeneic bone marrow transplants from HLA-identical sibling donors, it is usually possible to decrease cyclosporine doses and concentrations about 2 months after the transplant and to stop cyclosporine therapy altogether after about 6 months posttransplant if no or only mild acute rejection episodes have taken place.
- In allogeneic bone marrow transplant patients with HLA-mismatched related or HLA-identical unrelated donors and all solid-organ transplant patients, chronic cyclosporine therapy is usually required. In these cases, cyclosporine doses and concentrations are decreased to the minimum required to prevent graft-versus-host reactions or rejection episodes, in order to decrease drug adverse effects.

- Although some newer data suggest that determination of cyclosporine area under the concentration/time curve using multiple concentrations[9,10] or 2-hour-postdose cyclosporine concentrations[11] may be useful in the future, most transplant centers continue to used predose trough cyclosporine concentration determinations to adjust drug doses.

BASIC CLINICAL PHARMACOKINETIC PARAMETERS

- Cyclosporine is eliminated almost completely by hepatic metabolism (>99%).[12] Hepatic metabolism is mainly via the CYP3A4 enzyme system, and the drug is a substrate for P-glycoprotein.
- There are more than 25 identified cyclosporine metabolites.[7,8] None of these metabolites appears to have significant immunosuppressive effects in humans. Most of the metabolites are eliminated in the bile.
- Less than 1% of a cyclosporine dose is recovered as unchanged drug in the urine.
- Within the therapeutic range, cyclosporine follows linear pharmacokinetics.[13]
- There is a large amount of intrasubject variability in cyclosporine concentrations obtained on a day-to-day basis, even when the patient should be at steady state. There are many reasons for this variability.

  - Cyclosporine has low water solubility, and its gastrointestinal absorption can be influenced by many variables.[7,8,14,15]

    - To improve the consistency of absorption rate and bioavailability for original dosage form (Sandimmune®, Novartis), a microemulsion version of the drug (Neoral®, Novartis) is marketed to help reduce absorption variability. While use of microemulsion cyclosporine does decrease steady-state concentration variability (10–30% for Neoral versus 16–38% for Sandimmune for trough concentrations), there are still substantial day-to-day changes in cyclosporine concentrations regardless of the dosage form used.[16]
    - The fat content of meals has an influence on the absorption of oral cyclosporine.[17] Foods containing large amounts of fat enhance the absorption of cyclosporine.
    - Oral cyclosporine solution is prepared with olive oil and alcohol to enhance the solubility of the drug. The solution is mixed in milk, chocolate milk, or orange juice, using a glass container, immediately before swallowing. When the entire dose has been given, the glass container should be rinsed with the diluting liquid and the contents immediately consumed.

- If microemulsion cyclosporine solution is administered, it should be mixed in a similar fashion using apple or orange juice.
- Grapefruit juice should not be used, since this vehicle inhibits CYP3A4 and/or P-glycoprotein in the gastrointestinal tract and markedly increases bioavailability.
- Variation in cyclosporine solution absorption is dependent on how accurately the administration technique for each dose is reproduced.

- After liver transplantation, bile production and flow may not begin immediately, or bile flow may be diverted from the gastrointestinal tract using a T-tube.[18,19] In the absence of bile salts, the absorption of cyclosporine can be greatly decreased. Bile appears to assist in the dissolution of cyclosporine, which increases the absorption of the drug.
- Diarrhea also impairs cyclosporine absorption,[20,21] and bone marrow transplantation patients may experience diarrhea as a part of graph-versus-host disease.[4]
- Other drug therapy can also increase or decrease the intestinal first-pass clearance of cyclosporine.[22]

- Cyclosporine is a drug with a low to moderate hepatic extraction ratio, and with an average liver extraction ratio of ~30%.[23] Thus its hepatic clearance is influenced by unbound fraction in the blood (f_B), intrinsic clearance (Cl'_{int}) and liver blood flow (LBF).

  - Cyclosporine binds primarily to erythrocytes and lipoproteins, yielding unbound fractions in the blood that are highly variable (1.4–12%).[24–29]

    - Erythrocyte concentrations vary in transplant patients, especially those who have received bone marrow or kidney transplants.
    - Lipoprotein concentrations also vary among patients, and hyperlipidemia is an adverse effect of cyclosporine.

  - Hepatic intrinsic clearance is different among individuals, and there is a large amount of variability in this value within individual liver transplant patients that changes according to the viability of the graft and time after transplantation surgery.
  - Other drug therapy can also increase or decrease the hepatic intrinsic clearance of cyclosporine.[22]
  - Liver blood flow exhibits a great deal of day-to-day intrasubject variability, which will also change the hepatic clearance of cyclosporine.
  - Changing the unbound fraction in the blood, hepatic intrinsic clearance, or liver blood flow will also change the hepatic first-pass metabolism of cyclosporine.

- Cyclosporine capsules and solution are available in regular (25-, 50-, and 100-mg capsules; 100-mg/ml solution) and microemulsion (25- and 100-mg capsules; 100-mg/ml solution) forms.

  - Although the oral absorption characteristics are more consistent and bioavailability is higher for microemulsion forms of cyclosporine, it is recommended that patients switched from cyclosporine to microemulsion cyclosporine have doses converted on a 1:1 basis. Subsequent microemulsion cyclosporine dosage adjustments are based on concentration monitoring.

- Cyclosporine injection for intravenous administration is available at a concentration of 50 mg/ml. Before administration, it should be diluted in 20–100 ml of normal saline or 5% dextrose, and the drug should be infused over 2–6 hours. Anaphylactic reactions have occurred with this dosage form, possibly due to the castor oil dilutant used to enhance dissolution of the drug.

- The initial dose of cyclosporine varies greatly among various transplant centers. Cyclosporine therapy is commonly started 4–12 hours before the transplantation procedure. According to a survey of transplant centers in the United States, the average initial oral doses (± standard deviation) for renal, liver, and heart transplant patients were 9 ± 3 mg/kg/d, 8 ± 4 mg/kg/d, and 7 ± 3 mg/kg/d.[16]

- For both rheumatoid arthritis and psoriasis, the recommended initial dose is 2.5 mg/kg/d, with a maximal recommended dose of 4 mg/kg/d.

EFFECTS OF DISEASE STATES AND CONDITIONS ON CYCLOSPORINE PHARMACOKINETICS AND DOSING

- Transplantation type does not appear to have a substantial effect on cyclosporine pharmacokinetics. The overall mean for all transplant groups is a clearance of 6 ml/min/kg, a volume of distribution of 5 L/kg, and a half-life of 10 hours for adults.[7,8,14,15]

- Average clearance is higher (10 ml/min/kg) and mean half-life is shorter (6 hours) in children (≤16 years old).[7,8,14,15]

- These results are based on a specific high-pressure liquid chromatography assay method conducted using whole blood samples.

- Because the drug is eliminated primarily by hepatic metabolism, clearance is lower (3 ml/min/kg) and half-life prolonged (20 hours) in patients with liver failure.[7,8,30] Immediately after liver transplantation, cyclosporine metabolism is depressed until the graft begins functioning in a stable manner.

  - Patients with transient liver dysfunction, regardless of transplantation type, will have decreased cyclosporine clearance and increased half-life values.

- Immediately after transplantation surgery, oral absorption of cyclosporine, especially in liver transplant patients with T-tubes, is highly variable.[18,19]

- Obesity does not influence cyclosporine pharmacokinetics, so doses for obese patients should be based on ideal body weight.[31–35]

- Renal failure does not change cyclosporine pharmacokinetics, and the drug is not significantly removed by hemodialysis or peritoneal dialysis.[36–38]

- The hemofiltration sieving coefficient for cyclosporine is 0.58, which indicates significant removal.[39,40] Replacement doses during hemoperfusion should be determined using cyclosporine concentrations.

DRUG INTERACTIONS

- Drug interactions with cyclosporine fall into two basic categories.

  - The first are agents known to cause nephrotoxicity when administered by themselves.[22] Drugs in this category of drug interactions include aminoglycoside antibiotics, vancomycin, cotrimoxazole (trimethoprim–sulfamethoxazole), amphotericin B, and anti-inflammatory drugs (azapropazon, diclofenac, naproxen, other nonsteroidal anti-inflammatory drugs). Other agents are melphalan, ketoconazole, cimetidine, ranitidine, and tacrolimus.

  - The second category of drug interactions involves inhibition or induction of cyclosporine metabolism. Cyclosporine is metabolized by CYP3A4 and is a substrate for P-glycoprotein, so the potential for many pharmacokinetic drug interactions exists with agents that inhibit these pathways or are also cleared by these mechanisms.[22]

- Because both of these drug elimination systems also exist in the gastrointestinal tract, inhibition drug interactions may also enhance cyclosporine oral bioavailability by diminishing the intestinal and hepatic first-pass effects.
- Drugs that inhibit cyclosporine clearance include the calcium channel blockers (verapamil, diltiazem, nicardipine), azole antifungals (fluconazole, itraconazole, ketoconazole), macrolide antibiotics (erythromycin, clarithromycin), antivirals (indinavir, nelfinavir, ritonavir, saquinavir), steroids (methylprednisolone, oral contraceptives, androgens), psychotropic agents (fluvoxamine, nefazodone), and as well as other agents (amiodarone, chloroquine, allopurinol, bromocriptine, metoclopramide, cimetidine, grapefruit juice).
- Inducing agents include other antibiotics (nafcillin, rifampin, rifabutin), anticonvulsants (phenytoin, carbamazepine, phenobarbital, primidone), barbiturates, aminoglutethimide, troglitazone, octreotide, and ticlopidine.

- Because of the large number of interacting agents, and the critical nature of the drugs involved in the treatment of transplant patients, complete avoidance of drug interactions with cyclosporine is not possible. Thus, most drug interactions with cyclosporine are managed using appropriate cyclosporine dosage modification, with cyclosporine concentration monitoring as a guide.

- Cyclosporine can also change the clearance of other drugs via competitive inhibition of CYP3A4 and/or P-glycoprotein.[22]

- Drugs that may exhibit decreased clearance and increased serum concentrations when given with cyclosporine include prednisolone, digoxin, calcium channel blockers (verapamil, diltiazem, bepridil, nifedipine and most other dihydropyridine analogs, sildenafil), ergot alkaloids, vinca alkaloids, simvastatin, and lovastatin.

INITIAL DOSAGE DETERMINATION METHODS

- Several methods to initiate cyclosporine therapy are available:

- The *pharmacokinetic dosing method* is the most flexible of the techniques. It allows individualized target serum concentrations to be chosen for a patient, and each pharmacokinetic parameter can be customized to reflect specific disease states and conditions present in the patient.
- *Literature-based recommended dosing* is a very commonly used method to prescribe initial doses of cyclosporine. Doses are based on those that commonly produce steady-state concentrations near the lower end of the therapeutic range, although there is a wide variation in the actual concentrations for a specific patient.

Pharmacokinetic Dosing Method

- The goal of initial dosing of cyclosporine is to compute the best dose possible for the patient in order to prevent graft rejection or graft-versus-host disease given the set of disease states and conditions that influence cyclosporine pharmacokinetics, while avoiding adverse drug reactions. In order to do this, pharmacokinetic parameters for the patient are estimated using average parameters measured in other patients with similar disease state and condition profiles.

Clearance Estimate

- Cyclosporine is almost completely metabolized by the liver. Unfortunately, there is no good way to estimate the elimination characteristics of liver-metabolized drugs using an endogenous marker of liver function in the same fashion that serum creatinine and estimated creatinine clearance are used to estimate the elimination of agents that are eliminated renally.

  - As a result, a patient is categorized according to the disease states and conditions that are known to change cyclosporine clearance, and clearances previously measured in studies are used as an estimate of the current patient's clearance rate.

Selection of Appropriate Pharmacokinetic Model and Equations

- When given by intravenous infusion or orally, cyclosporine follows a two-compartment model.[38]

  - When oral therapy is chosen, the drug is often absorbed erratically and with variable absorption rate, and some patients may exhibit a "double-peak" phenomenon, in which a maximum concentration is achieved 2–3 hours after dosage administration with a second maximum concentration 2–4 hours after that.[17,41]

    - Because of the complex absorption profile and the fact that the drug is usually administered twice daily, a very simple pharmacokinetic equation that calculates the average cyclosporine steady-state serum concentration (Css in ng/ml = µg/L) is widely used and allows maintenance dose computation:

$$Css = [F(D/\tau)]/Cl \qquad \text{or} \qquad D = (Css \cdot Cl \cdot \tau)/F$$

    where F is the bioavailability fraction for the oral dosage form (F averages 0.3 or 30% for most patient populations and oral dosage forms), D is the dose of cyclosporine in mg, Cl is cyclosporine clearance in L/h, and τ is the dosage interval in hours.

- If the drug is to be given intravenously as an intermittent infusion, the equivalent equation for that route of administration is

$$Css = (D/\tau)/Cl \qquad \text{or} \qquad D = Css \cdot Cl \cdot \tau$$

Steady-State Concentration Selection

- The generally accepted therapeutic ranges for cyclosporine in blood, serum, or plasma using various specific and nonspecific (parent drug + metabolite) assays are given in Table 15-1.

  - More important than these general guidelines are the specific requirements for each graft type as defined by the transplant center where the surgery was conducted. Clinicians should become familiar with the cyclosporine protocols used at the various institutions at which they practice.
  - Although it is unlikely that steady state has been achieved, cyclosporine concentrations are usually obtained on a daily basis, even when dosage changes were made the previous day, because of the critical nature of the therapeutic effect provided by the drug.

▶*Example 1*   HO is a 50-year-old, 75-kg (height 5′10″) male renal transplant patient 2 days posttransplant surgery. The patient's liver function tests are normal. Suggest an initial oral cyclosporine dose designed to achieve a steady-state cyclosporine trough blood concentration of 250 ng/ml.

1. *Estimate clearance according to disease states and conditions present in the patient.* The mean cyclosporine clearance for adult patients is 6 ml/min/kg. The cyclosporine blood clearance for this patient is expected to be

   $$Cl = 6 \text{ ml/min/kg} \cdot 75 \text{ kg} \cdot [(60 \text{ min/h})/(1000 \text{ ml/L})] = 27 \text{ L/h}$$

2. *Compute dosage regimen.* A 12-hour dosage interval will be used for this patient. (*Note:* ng/ml = µg/L, and this concentration is substituted for Css in the calculations so that unit conversion is not required. Also, a conversion constant of 1000 µg/mg is used to change the dose amount to mg.) The dosage equation for oral cyclosporine is

   $$D = (Css \cdot Cl \cdot \tau)/F = (250 \text{ µg/L} \cdot 27 \text{ L/h} \cdot 12 \text{ h})/(0.3 \cdot 1000 \text{ µg/mg})$$

   $$= 270 \text{ mg, rounded to } 300 \text{ mg every } 12 \text{ h}$$

Cyclosporine serum concentrations should be obtained on a daily basis, with steady state expected to occur in about 2 days (5 half-lives = 5 · 10 h = 50 h, or ~2 d.

▶*Example 2*   Same patient as in Example 1, except compute an initial dose using intravenous cyclosporine.

1. *Estimate clearance according to disease states and conditions present in the patient.* The mean cyclosporine clearance for adult patients is 6 ml/min/kg. The cyclosporine blood clearance for this patient is expected to be

   $$Cl = 6 \text{ ml/min/kg} \cdot 75 \text{ kg} \cdot [(60 \text{ min/h})/(1000 \text{ ml/L})] = 27 \text{ L/h}$$

2. *Compute dosage regimen.* A 12-hour dosage interval will be used for this patient. (*Note:* ng/ml = µg/L, and this concentration is substituted for Css in the calculations so that unit conversion was not required. Also, a conversion constant of 1000 µg/mg is used to change the dose amount to mg.) The dosage equation for intravenous cyclosporine is

   $$D = Css \cdot Cl \cdot \tau = (250 \text{ µg/L} \cdot 27 \text{ L/h} \cdot 12 \text{ h})/(1000 \text{ µg/mg})$$

   $$= 81 \text{ mg, rounded to } 75 \text{ mg every } 12 \text{ h}$$

Cyclosporine serum concentrations should be obtained on a daily basis, with steady state expected to occur in about 2 days (5 half-lives = 5 · 10 h = 50 h, or ~2 d).

Literature-Based Recommended Dosing

- Because of the large amount of variability in cyclosporine pharmacokinetics, even when concurrent disease states and conditions are identified, many clinicians believe that the use of standard cyclosporine doses for various situations is warranted.
- Most transplant centers use doses that are determined using a cyclosporine dosage protocol. The original computations of these doses were based on the pharmacokinetic dosing method described in the previous section, and the doses were subsequently modified based on clinical experience.

- The expected cyclosporine steady-state concentration used to compute these doses depends on the type of transplanted tissue and the posttransplantation time line.
- Initial oral doses of 8–18 mg/kg/d or intravenous doses of 3–6 mg/kg/d (one-third the oral dose, to account for ~30% oral bioavailability) are used, but vary greatly from institution to institution.[1–5,7,8,15]
- For obese individuals (>30% over ideal body weight), ideal body weight should be used to compute initial doses.[31–35]
- To illustrate how this technique is used, the same patient examples utilized in the previous section are repeated for this dosage approach for comparison purposes.

▶*Example 3*   HO is a 50-year-old, 75-kg (height 5′10″) male renal transplant patient 2 days posttransplant surgery. The patient's liver function tests are normal. Suggest an initial oral cyclosporine dose designed to achieve a steady-state cyclosporine trough blood concentration within the therapeutic range.

1. *Choose a cyclosporine dose based on disease states and conditions present in the patient and transplant type.* The cyclosporine oral dosage range for adult patients is 8–18 mg/kg/d. Because this is a renal transplant patient, a dose near the lower end of the range (8 mg/kg/d) will be used in order to avoid nephrotoxicity. The initial cyclosporine dose for this patient is 600 mg/d, given as 300 mg every 12 hours:

    Dose = 8 mg/kg/d · 75 kg = 600 mg/d or 300 mg every 12 h

    Cyclosporine serum concentrations should be obtained on a daily basis, with steady state expected to occur after 2 days (5 half-lives = 5 · 10 h = 50 h, or ~2 d) of treatment.

▶*Example 4*   Same patient as in Example 3, except compute an initial dose using intravenous cyclosporine.

1. *Choose a cyclosporine dose based on disease states and conditions present in the patient and transplant type.* The cyclosporine intravenous dosage range for adult patients is 3–6 mg/kg/d. Because this is a renal transplant patient, a dose near the lower end of the range (3 mg/kg/d) will be used in order to avoid nephrotoxicity. The initial cyclosporine dose for this patient is 200 mg/d, given as 100 mg every 12 hours:

    Dose = 3 mg/kg/d · 75 kg

    = 225 mg/d, rounded to 200 mg/d or 100 mg every 12 h

    Cyclosporine serum concentrations should be obtained on a daily basis, with steady state expected to occur after 2 days (5 half-lives = 5 · 10 h = 50 h, or ~2 d) of treatment.

USE OF CYCLOSPORINE CONCENTRATIONS TO ALTER DOSES

- Because of the large amount of pharmacokinetic variability among patients, it is likely that doses computed using patient population characteristics will not always produce cyclosporine concentrations that are expected or desirable.
- Because of pharmacokinetic variability, the narrow therapeutic index of cyclosporine, and the severity of adverse side effects of cyclosporine, measurement of cyclosporine concentrations is mandatory for patients, to ensure that therapeutic, nontoxic levels are present.

- In addition to cyclosporine concentrations, important patient parameters (transplanted organ function tests or biopsies, clinical signs and symptoms of graft rejection or graft-versus-host disease, potential cyclosporine side effects, etc.) should be followed to confirm that the patient is responding to treatment and not developing adverse drug reactions.
- When cyclosporine concentrations have been measured in patients and a dosage change is necessary, clinicians should use the simplest, most straightforward method available to determine a dose that will provide safe and effective treatment.

  - In most cases a simple dosage ratio can be used to change cyclosporine doses, assuming the drug follows *linear pharmacokinetics*.
  - Sometimes it is useful to compute cyclosporine pharmacokinetic constants for a patient and base dosage adjustments on these. In this case it may be possible to calculate and use *pharmacokinetic parameters* to alter the cyclosporine dose.
  - Computerized methods that incorporate expected population pharmacokinetic characteristics (*Bayesian pharmacokinetic computer programs*) can be used in difficult cases, when concentrations are obtained at suboptimal times or the patient was not at steady-state when concentrations were measured.

Linear Pharmacokinetics Method

- Because cyclosporine follows linear, dose-proportional pharmacokinetics,[13] steady-state concentrations change in proportion to dose according to the following equation:

$$D_{new}/Css_{new} = D_{old}/Css_{old} \quad \text{or} \quad D_{new} = (Css_{new}/Css_{old})D_{old}$$

where D is the dose, Css is the steady-state concentration, old indicates the dose that produced the steady-state concentration the patient is currently receiving, and new denotes the dose necessary to produce the desired steady-state concentration.

- The advantages of this method are that it is quick and simple. The main disadvantage is that steady-state concentrations are required.

▶*Example 5*   LK is a 50-year-old, 75-kg (height 5′10″) male renal transplant recipient who is receiving 400 mg of oral cyclosporine capsules every 12 hours. He has normal liver function. His current steady-state cyclosporine blood concentration is 375 ng/ml. Compute a cyclosporine dose that will provide a steady-state concentration of 200 ng/ml.

1. *Compute a new dose to achieve the desired concentration.* The patient can be expected to achieve steady-state conditions after the second day ($5t_{1/2} = 5 \cdot 10\ h = 50\ h$) of therapy. Using linear pharmacokinetics, the new dose to attain the desired concentration should be proportional to the old dose that produced the measured concentration (total daily dose = 400 mg/dose · 2 doses/d = 800 mg/d):

$$D_{new} = (Css_{new}/Css_{old})D_{old} = [(200\ ng/ml)/(375\ ng/ml)](800\ mg/d)$$
$$= 427\ mg/d,\ rounded\ to\ 400\ mg/d$$

The new suggested dose is 400 mg/d or 200 mg of cyclosporine capsules every 12 hours, to be started at the next scheduled dosing time.

A steady-state trough cyclosporine serum concentration should be measured after steady state is attained in 3–5 half-lives. Since the drug is expected to have a half-life of 10 hours, a cyclosporine steady-state concentration can be obtained at any time after the second day of dosing (5 half-lives = 5 · 10 h = 50 h). Cyclosporine concentrations should also be measured if the patient experiences signs or symptoms of graft rejection, or if the patient develops potential signs or symptoms of cyclosporine toxicity.

▶*Example 6*   FD is a 60-year-old, 85-kg (height 6′1″) male liver transplant patient who is receiving 75 mg of intravenous cyclosporine every 12 hours. His current steady-state cyclosporine concentration is 215 ng/ml. Compute a cyclosporine dose that will provide a steady-state concentration of 350 ng/ml.

1. *Compute a new dose to achieve the desired concentration.* The patient recently received a liver transplant and can be expected to have a longer cyclosporine half-life if the organ is not yet functioning at an optimal level ($t_{1/2}$ = 20 h). Therefore it may take up to 4 days of consistent cyclosporine therapy to achieve steady-state conditions ($5t_{1/2}$ = 5 · 20 h = 100 h or ~4 d).

   Using linear pharmacokinetics, the new dose to attain the desired concentration should be proportional to the old dose that produced the measured concentration (total daily dose = 75 mg/dose · 2 doses/d = 150 mg/d):

   $$D_{new} = (Css_{new}/Css_{old})D_{old} = [(350 \text{ ng/ml})/(215 \text{ ng/ml})](150 \text{ mg/d})$$
   $$= 244 \text{ mg/d, rounded to 250 mg/d or 125 mg every 12 h}$$

   A steady-state trough cyclosporine serum concentration should be measured after steady state is attained in 3–5 half-lives. Since the drug is expected to have a half-life of up to 20 hours, a cyclosporine steady-state concentration can be obtained at any time after the fourth day of dosing (5 half-lives = 5 · 20 h = 100 h or 4 d). Cyclosporine concentrations should also be measured if the patient experiences signs or symptoms of graft rejection, or if the patient develops potential signs or symptoms of cyclosporine toxicity.

2. If the patient in example 6 received cyclosporin as a continuous infusion at a rate of 6 mg/h, the equivalent dosage adjustment computation would be

   $$D_{new} = (Css_{new}/Css_{old})D_{old} = [(350 \text{ ng/ml})/(215 \text{ ng/ml})](6 \text{ mg/h})$$
   $$D_{new} = 9.8 \text{ mg/h, rounded to 10 mg/h}$$

Pharmacokinetic Parameter Method

- The pharmacokinetic parameter method of adjusting drug doses was among the first techniques available to change doses using drug concentrations. It allows the computation of an individual's own, unique pharmacokinetic constants and uses those to calculate a dose that achieves desired cyclosporine concentrations.
- The pharmacokinetic parameter method requires that steady state has been achieved and uses only a steady-state cyclosporine concentration.

  - Cyclosporine clearance can be measured using a single steady-state cyclosporine concentration and the following formula for orally administered drug:

    $$Cl = [F(D/\tau)]/Css$$

  where Cl is cyclosporine clearance in L/h, F is the bioavailability factor for cyclosporine (F = 0.3), τ is the dosage interval in hours, and Css is the cyclosporine steady-state concentration in ng/ml, which equals μg/L.

- If cyclosporine is administered intravenously, it is not necessary to take bioavailability into account:

$$Cl = (D/\tau)/Css$$

where Cl is cyclosporine clearance in L/h, τ is the dosage interval in hours, and Css is the cyclosporine steady-state concentration in ng/ml, which equals $\mu g/L$.

- Although this method does allow computation of cyclosporine clearance, it yields exactly the same cyclosporine dose as that supplied using linear pharmacokinetics. As a result, most clinicians prefer to calculate the new dose directly, using the simpler linear pharmacokinetics method.
- To demonstrate this point, the patient cases used to illustrate the linear pharmacokinetics method will be used as examples for the pharmacokinetic parameter method.

▶*Example 7* LK is a 50-year-old, 75-kg (height 5′10″) male renal transplant recipient who is receiving 400 mg of oral cyclosporine capsules every 12 hours. He has normal liver function. His current steady-state cyclosporine blood concentration is 375 ng/ml. Compute a cyclosporine dose that will provide a steady-state concentration of 200 ng/ml.

1. *Compute pharmacokinetic parameters.* The patient can be expected to achieve steady-state conditions after the second day ($5t_{1/2} = 5 \cdot 10$ h = 50 h or 2 d) of therapy. Cyclosporine clearance can be computed using a steady-state cyclosporine concentration:

$$Cl = [F(D/\tau)]/Css = [0.3 \cdot (400 \text{ mg}/12 \text{ h}) \cdot (1000 \text{ } \mu g/mg)]/(375 \text{ } \mu g/L)$$
$$= 26.7 \text{ L/h}$$

(*Note:* $\mu g/L$ = ng/ml, and this concentration unit was substituted for Css in the calculations so that unit conversion was not required.)

2. *Compute cyclosporine dose.* Cyclosporine clearance is used to compute the new dose:

$$D = (Css \cdot Cl \cdot \tau)/F = (200 \text{ } \mu g/L \cdot 26.7 \text{ L/h} \cdot 12 \text{ h})/(0.3 \cdot 1000 \text{ } \mu g/mg)$$
$$= 214 \text{ mg, rounded to } 200 \text{ mg every } 12 \text{ h}$$

A steady-state trough cyclosporine serum concentration should be measured after steady state is attained in 3–5 half-lives. Since the drug is expected to have a half-life of 10 hours, a cyclosporine steady-state concentration can be obtained at any time after the second day of dosing (5 half-lives = $5 \cdot 10$ h = 50 h). Cyclosporine concentrations should also be measured if the patient experiences signs or symptoms of graft rejection, or if the patient develops potential signs or symptoms of cyclosporine toxicity.

▶*Example 8* FD is a 60-year-old, 85-kg (height 6′1″) male liver transplant patient who is receiving 75 mg of intravenous cyclosporine every 12 hours. His current steady-state cyclosporine concentration is 215 ng/ml. Compute a cyclosporine dose that will provide a steady-state concentration of 350 ng/ml.

1. *Compute pharmacokinetic parameters.* The patient recently received a liver transplant and can be expected to have a longer cyclosporine half-life if the organ is not yet functioning at an optimal level ($t_{1/2} = 20$ h).

Therefore it may take up to 4 days of consistent cyclosporine therapy to achieve steady-state conditions ($5t_{1/2} = 5 \cdot 20$ h = 100 h or ~4 d).

Cyclosporine clearance can be computed using a steady-state cyclosporine concentration:

$$Cl = (D/\tau)/Css = [(75 \text{ mg}/12 \text{ h}) \cdot (1000 \text{ μg/mg})]/(215 \text{ μg/L})$$
$$= 29.1 \text{ L/h}$$

(*Note:* μg/L = ng/ml, and this concentration unit was substituted for Css in the calculations so that unit conversion was not required.)

2. *Compute cyclosporine dose.* Cyclosporine clearance is used to compute the new dose:

$$D = Css \cdot Cl \cdot \tau = [(350 \text{ μg/L} \cdot 29.1 \text{ L/h} \cdot 12 \text{ h})]/(1000 \text{ μg/mg})$$
$$= 122 \text{ mg, rounded to 125 mg every 12 h}$$

A steady-state trough cyclosporine serum concentration should be measured after steady state is attained in 3–5 half-lives. Since the drug is expected to have a half-life of up to 20 hours, a cyclosporine steady-state concentration can be obtained at any time after the fourth day of dosing (5 half-lives = $5 \cdot 20$ h = 100 h or 4 d). Cyclosporine concentrations should also be measured if the patient experiences signs or symptoms of graft rejection, or if the patient develops potential signs or symptoms of cyclosporine toxicity.

3. If the patient in example 8 received cyclosporin as a continuous infusion at a rate of 6 mg/h, the equivalent clearance and dosage adjustment computation would be:

$$Cl = K_o/Css = (6 \text{ mg/h} \cdot 1000 \text{ μg/mg})/(215 \text{ μg/L}) = 27.9 \text{ L/h}$$

$$K_o = Css \cdot Cl = (350 \text{ μg/L} \cdot 27.9 \text{ L/h})/(1000 \text{ μg/mg})$$
$$= 9.8 \text{ mg/h, rounded to 10 mg/h}$$

BAYESIAN PHARMACOKINETIC COMPUTER PROGRAMS

- Computer programs are available that can assist in the computation of pharmacokinetic parameters for patients.[42–44] The most reliable computer programs use a nonlinear regression algorithm that incorporates components of Bayes' theorem.

  - An advantage of this approach is that consistent dosage recommendations can be made when several different practitioners are involved in therapeutic drug monitoring programs. However, since simpler dosing methods work just as well for patients with stable pharmacokinetic parameters and steady-state drug concentrations, many clinicians reserve the use of computer programs for more difficult situations. Those situations include serum concentrations that are not at steady state, serum concentrations not obtained at the specific times needed to employ simpler methods, and unstable pharmacokinetic parameters.
  - When only a limited number of cyclosporine steady-state concentrations are available, Bayesian pharmacokinetic computer programs can be used to compute a complete patient pharmacokinetic profile that includes clearance, volume of distribution, and half life.

- Many Bayesian pharmacokinetic computer programs are available, and most should provide answers similar to the program used in the following examples. The program used to solve problems in this book is DrugCalc, written by Dr. Dennis Mungall and available at his Internet web site (www.clinpharmacologist.bigstep.com/consumersurvey.html).[45]

▶*Example 9*   LK is a 50-year-old, 75-kg (height 5'10") male renal transplant recipient who is receiving 400 mg of oral cyclosporine capsules every 12 hours. He has normal liver function (bilirubin = 0.7 mg/dl, albumin = 4.0 g/dl). His current steady-state cyclosporine blood concentration is 375 ng/ml. Compute a cyclosporine dose that will provide a steady-state concentration of 200 ng/ml.

1. *Enter patient demographic, drug dosing, and serum concentration/time data into a Bayesian pharmacokinetic computer program.*
2. *Compute pharmacokinetic parameters for the patient using the computer program.* The pharmacokinetic parameters computed by the program are a volume of distribution of 403 L, a half-life of 17.6 hours, and a clearance of 15.9 L/h.
3. *Compute dose required to achieve desired cyclosporine serum concentrations.* The one-compartment-model first-order absorption equations used by the program to compute doses indicate that a dose of 200 mg every 12 hours will produce a steady-state cyclosporine concentration of 210 µg/ml. Using the linear pharmacokinetics and pharmacokinetic parameter methods previously described in the chapter produced the same answer for this patient.

▶*Example 10*   FD is a 60-year-old, 85-kg (height 6'1") male liver transplant patient who is receiving 75 mg of intravenous cyclosporine every 12 hours. He has elevated liver function tests (bilirubin = 3.2 mg/dl, albumin = 2.5 g/dl). His current steady-state cyclosporine concentration is 215 ng/ml. Compute a cyclosporine dose that will provide a steady-state concentration of 350 ng/ml.

1. *Enter patient demographic, drug dosing, and serum concentration/time data into a Bayesian pharmacokinetic computer program.*
2. *Compute pharmacokinetic parameters for the patient using the computer program.* The pharmacokinetic parameters computed by the program are a volume of distribution of 403 L, a half-life of 13.8 hours, and a clearance of 20.3 L/h.
3. *Compute dose required to achieve desired cyclosporine serum concentrations.* The one-compartment-model first-order absorption equations used by the program to compute doses indicate that a dose of 125 mg every 12 hours will produce a steady-state cyclosporine concentration of 380 µg/ml. Using the linear pharmacokinetics and pharmacokinetic parameter methods previously described in the chapter produced the same answer for this patient.

▶*Example 11*   YT is a 25-year-old, 55-kg (height 5'2") female bone marrow transplant recipient who received 300 mg of oral cyclosporine capsules every 12 hours for two doses after transplant, but because her renal function decreased, her dose was empirically changed to 200 mg every 12 hours. She has normal liver function (bilirubin = 0.9 mg/dl, albumin = 3.9 g/dl).

TABLE 15-2 Dosing Strategies

Dosing approach/ philosophy	Initial dosing	Use of serum concentrations to alter doses
Pharmacokinetic parameters/ equations	Pharmacokinetic dosing method	Pharmacokinetic parameter method
Literature-based/ concept	Literature-based recommended dosing method	Linear pharmacokinetic method
Computerized	Bayesian computer program	Bayesian computer program

The cyclosporine blood concentration obtained 12 hours after her first dose of the lower dosage regimen was 280 ng/ml. Compute a cyclosporine dose that will provide a steady-state concentration of 250 ng/ml.

1. *Enter patient demographic, drug dosing, and serum concentration/time data into a Bayesian pharmacokinetic computer program.*
2. *Compute pharmacokinetic parameters for the patient using the computer program.* The pharmacokinetic parameters computed by the program are a volume of distribution of 401 L, a half-life of 35 hours, and a clearance of 8 L/h.
3. *Compute dose required to achieve desired cyclosporine serum concentrations.* The one-compartment-model first-order absorption equations used by the program to compute doses indicate that a dose of 100 mg every 12 hours will produce a steady-state cyclosporine concentration of 250 µg/ml.

DOSING STRATEGIES

• Initial dose and dosage adjustment techniques using serum concentrations can be used in any combination as long as the limitations of each method are observed.
• Some dosing schemes link together logically when considered according to their basic approaches or philosophies. Dosage strategies that follow similar pathways are given in Table 15-2.

REFERENCES

1. Johnson HJ, Heim-Duthoy KL. Renal transplantation. In: DiPiro JT, Talbert RL, Yee GC, Matzke GR, Wells BG, Posey LM, eds. Pharmacotherapy. 5th ed. New York: McGraw-Hill, 2002:843–66.
2. Lake KD, Aaronson KD. Cardiac transplantation. In: DiPiro JT, Talbert RL, Yee GC, Matzke GR, Wells BG, Posey LM, eds. Pharmacotherapy. 5th ed. New York: McGraw-Hill, 2002:321–36.
3. Maurer JR. Lung transplantation. In: Braunwald E, Fauci AS, Kasper DL, Hauser SL, Longo DL, Jameson JL, eds. Principles of internal medicine. 15th ed. New York: McGraw-Hill, 2001:1531–34.
4. Perkins JB, Yee GC. Bone marrow transplantation. In: DiPiro JT, Talbert RL, Yee GC, Matzke GR, Wells BG, Posey LM, eds. Pharmacotherapy. 5th ed. New York: McGraw-Hill, 2002:2425–44.

5. Stoffel JA, Somani AZ. Liver transplantation. In: DiPiro JT, Talbert RL, Yee GC, Matzke GR, Wells BG, Posey LM, eds. Pharmacotherapy. 5th ed. New York: McGraw-Hill, 2002:743–52.

6. Krensky AM, Strom TB, Bluestone JA. Immunomodulators—immunosuppressive agents and immunostimulants. In: Hardman JG, Limbird LE, Gilman AG, eds. The pharmacological basis of therapeutics. 10th ed. New York: McGraw-Hill, 2001: 1463–84.

7. Yee GC, Salomon DR. Cyclosporine. In: Evans WE, Schentag JJ, Jusko WJ, Relling MV, eds. Applied pharmacokinetics. 3rd ed. Vancouver, WA: Applied Therapeutics, 1992;28:1–40.

8. Min DI. Cyclosporine. In: Schumacher GE, ed. Therapeutic drug monitoring. 1st ed. Stamford, CT: Appleton & Lange, 1995:449–68.

9. Wacke R, Rohde B, Engel G, et al. Comparison of several approaches of therapeutic drug monitoring of cyclosporin A based on individual pharmacokinetics. Eur J Clin Pharmacol 2000;56:43–8.

10. Grevel J. Area-under-the-curve versus trough level monitoring of cyclosporine concentration: critical assessment of dosage adjustment practices and measurement of clinical outcome. Ther Drug Monit 1993;15(6):488–91.

11. Grant D, Kneteman N, Tchervenkov J, et al. Peak cyclosporine levels (C_{max}) correlate with freedom from liver graft rejection: results of a prospective, randomized comparison of neoral and sandimmune for liver transplantation (NOF-8). Transplantation 1999;67(8):1133–7.

12. Kronbach T, Fischer V, Meyer UA. Cyclosporine metabolism in human liver: identification of a cytochrome P-450III gene family as the major cyclosporine-metabolizing enzyme explains interactions of cyclosporine with other drugs. Clin Pharmacol Ther 1988;43(6):630–5.

13. Grevel J, Welsh MS, Kahan BD. Linear cyclosporine pharmacokinetics. Clin Pharmacol Ther 1988;43:175.

14. Lindholm A. Factors influencing the pharmacokinetics of cyclosporine in man. Ther Drug Monit 1991;13(6):465–77.

15. Fahr A. Cyclosporin clinical pharmacokinetics. Clin Pharmacokinet 1993;24(6): 472–95.

16. Neoral package insert. East Hanover, NJ: Novartis Pharmaceuticals, 1999.

17. Gupta SK, Manfro RC, Tomlanovich SJ, Gambertoglio JG, Garovoy MR, Benet LZ. Effect of food on the pharmacokinetics of cyclosporine in healthy subjects following oral and intravenous administration. J Clin Pharmacol 1990;30(7):643–53.

18. Naoumov NV, Tredger JM, Steward CM, et al. Cyclosporin A pharmacokinetics in liver transplant recipients in relation to biliary T-tube clamping and liver dysfunction. Gut 1989;30(3):391–6.

19. Tredger JM, Naoumov NV, Steward CM, et al. Influence of biliary T tube clamping on cyclosporine pharmacokinetics in liver transplant recipients. Transplant Proc 1988;20(2 suppl 2):512–5.

20. Burckart GJ, Starzl T, Williams L. Cyclosporine monitoring and pharmacokinetics in pediatric liver transplant patients. Transplant Proc 1985;17:1172.

21. Atkinson K, Britton K, Paull P. Detrimental effect of intestinal disease on absorption of orally administered cyclosporine. Transplant Proc 1983;15:2446.

22. Hansten PD, Horn JR. Drug interactions analysis and management. Vancouver, WA: Applied Therapeutics, 1999.

23. Wu CY, Benet LZ, Hebert MF, et al. Differentiation of absorption and first-pass gut and hepatic metabolism in humans: studies with cyclosporine. Clin Pharmacol Ther 1995;58(5):492–7.

24. Legg B, Rowland M. Cyclosporin: measurement of fraction unbound in plasma. J Pharm Pharmacol 1987;39(8):599–603.

25. Legg B, Gupta SK, Rowland M, Johnson RW, Solomon LR. Cyclosporin: pharmacokinetics and detailed studies of plasma and erythrocyte binding during intravenous and oral administration. Eur J Clin Pharmacol 1988;34(5):451–60.

26. Lemaire M, Tillement JP. Role of lipoproteins and erythrocytes in the in vitro binding and distribution of cyclosporin A in the blood. J Pharm Pharmacol 1982;34(11): 715–8.

27. Rosano TG. Effect of hematocrit on cyclosporine (cyclosporin A) in whole blood and plasma of renal-transplant patients. Clin Chem 1985;31(3):410–2.
28. Sgoutas D, MacMahon W, Love A, Jerkunica I. Interaction of cyclosporin A with human lipoproteins. J Pharm Pharmacol 1986;38(8):583–8.
29. Henricsson S. A new method for measuring the free fraction of cyclosporin in plasma by equilibrium dialysis. J Pharm Pharmacol 1987;39(5):384–5.
30. Ptachcinski RJ, Venkataramanan R, Burckart GJ. Clinical pharmacokinetics of cyclosporin. Clin Pharmacokinet 1986;11(2):107–32.
31. Flechner SM, Kolbeinsson MC, Lum B, Tam J, Moran T. The effect of obesity on cyclosporine pharmacokinetics in uremic patients. Transplant Proc 1989;21(1 pt 2): 1446–8.
32. Flechner SM, Kolbeinsson ME, Tam J, Lum B. The impact of body weight on cyclosporine pharmacokinetics in renal transplant recipients. Transplantation 1989;47(5):806–10.
33. Flechner SM, Haug M, Fisher RK, Modlin CS. Cyclosporine disposition and long-term renal function in a 500-pound kidney transplant recipient. Am J Kidney Dis 1998;32(4):E4.
34. Yee GC, McGuire TR, Gmur DJ, Lennon TP, Deeg HJ. Blood cyclosporine pharmacokinetics in patients undergoing marrow transplantation. Influence of age, obesity, and hematocrit. Transplantation 1988;46(3):399–402.
35. Yee GC, Lennon TP, Gmur DJ, Cheney CL, Oeser D, Deeg HJ. Effect of obesity on cyclosporine disposition. Transplantation 1988;45(3):649–51.
36. Swan SK, Bennett WM. Drug dosing guidelines in patients with renal failure. West J Med 1992;156(6):633–8.
37. Bennett WM. Guide to drug dosage in renal failure. Clin Pharmacokinet 1988; 15(5):326–54.
38. Follath F, Wenk M, Vozeh S, et al. Intravenous cyclosporine kinetics in renal failure. Clin Pharmacol Ther 1983;34(5):638–43.
39. Golper TA. Update on drug sieving coefficients and dosing adjustments during continuous renal replacement therapies. Contrib Nephrol 2001(132):349–53.
40. Golper TA, Marx MA. Drug dosing adjustments during continuous renal replacement therapies. Kidney Int Suppl 1998;66:S165–8.
41. Lindholm A, Henricsson S, Lind M, Dahlqvist R. Intraindividual variability in the relative systemic availability of cyclosporin after oral dosing. Eur J Clin Pharmacol 1988;34(5):461–4.
42. Anderson JE, Munday AS, Kelman AW, et al. Evaluation of a Bayesian approach to the pharmacokinetic interpretation of cyclosporin concentrations in renal allograft recipients. Ther Drug Monit 1994;16(2):160–5.
43. Kahan BD, Kramer WG, Williams C, Wideman CA. Application of Bayesian forecasting to predict appropriate cyclosporine dosing regimens for renal allograft recipients. Transplant Proc 1986;18(6 suppl 5):200–3.
44. Ruggeri A, Martinelli M. A program for the optimization of cyclosporine therapy using population kinetics modeling. Comput Methods Programs Biomed 2000; 61(1):61–9.
45. Wandell M, Mungall D. Computer assisted drug interpretation and drug regimen optimization. Am Assoc Clin Chem 1984;6:1–11.

16 | Tacrolimus (FK506)

Tacrolimus (also known as FK506) is a macrolide compound with immunosuppressant action that is used for the prevention of graft rejection in solid-organ transplant patients.[1-5] Currently, it is approved for use in liver and renal transplant patients.[1,5] It is also used in heart, heart–lung, and other solid-organ transplant recipients, and is under investigation for the treatment of graft-versus-host disease in bone marrow transplant patients.[2-4]

- The immunomodulating effects of tacrolimus are due to its ability to block the production of intraleukin-2 and other cytokines produced by T lymphocytes.[6] Tacrolimus binds to FK-binding protein (FKPB), an intracellular cytoplasmic protein found in T cells. The tacrolimus–FKPB complex interacts with calcineurin, inhibits the catalytic activity of calcineurin, and blocks the production of intermediaries involved with the expression of genes that regulate the production of cytokines.

THERAPEUTIC AND TOXIC CONCENTRATIONS

- The therapeutic range for tacrolimus used by most transplantation centers is 5–20 ng/ml in blood.[5,7,8] Although plasma tacrolimus concentrations have been measured and an equivalent therapeutic range in this matrix suggested (0.5–2 ng/ml), the two most widely used assays for the drug use blood samples.[7,8]

  - Because tacrolimus is bound extensively to erythrocytes, blood concentrations average about 15 times greater than concurrently measured serum or plasma concentrations.[7]
  - Two different assay systems are in widespread use. The enzyme-linked immunosorbent assay (ELISA; Pro-Trac®, IncStar) and microparticulate enzyme immunoassay (MEIA; IMx®, Abbott Diagnostics) incorporate the same monoclonal antibody. Using blood as the assay matrix, these two different assay systems produce similar results.[9-11]
  - For the purposes of the pharmacokinetic computations and problems presented in this book, tacrolimus concentrations in the blood determined with the ELISA or MEIA assay systems will be used.

- Because predose trough steady-state concentrations correlate well with steady-state area under the concentration/time curve measurements, tacrolimus trough concentrations are used in patient-monitoring situations.[7,12,13]
- Desired tacrolimus concentrations differ for the various types of organ transplants, change with time during the posttransplantation phase, and are determined by protocols specific to the transplantation service and institution.[1-5,7] Because of these factors, it is very important for clinicians to be aware of these situations, since acceptable tacrolimus concentrations under these various circumstances may be different from those given by the clinical laboratory or those suggested in this book.
- For patients receiving solid-organ transplants such as kidney, liver, heart, lung, or heart–lung transplants, the goal of tacrolimus therapy is to prevent acute or chronic rejection of the transplanted organ while minimizing drug side effects.[1-3,5,7]

- Because tacrolimus can cause nephrotoxicity, some centers delay tacrolimus therapy in renal transplant patients for a few days or until the kidney begins functioning, to avoid untoward effects on the newly transplanted organ. Also, desired tacrolimus concentrations in renal transplant patients are generally lower than for other transplant patients (typically 5–15 ng/ml versus 5–20 ng/ml using whole blood), to avoid toxicity in the new renal graft.
- For other solid-organ transplant patients, tacrolimus therapy may be started several hours before surgery. Intravenous tacrolimus may be given to these patients during the immediate postoperative phase.
- For long-term management of immunosuppression in solid-organ tissue transplant patients, tacrolimus doses are gradually tapered to the lowest concentration and dose possible over a 6–12-month time period as long as rejection episodes do not occur.
- Tacrolimus is being investigated as an immunosuppressant in bone marrow transplant recipients.[4] For patients receiving tacrolimus after a bone marrow transplant, the goal of therapy is to prevent graft-versus-host disease while avoiding adverse effects of immunosuppressant therapy.

  - If prophylaxis of acute graft-versus-host disease is successful, tacrolimus doses are tapered beginning on about posttransplant day 50, with the goal of drug discontinuation by about posttransplant day 180.
  - For allogeneic bone marrow transplant patients with HLA-mismatched or HLA-identical unrelated donors, the risk of acute graft-versus-host disease is higher, so tacrolimus therapy may be more prolonged for these patients.
  - Chronic graft-versus-host disease may occur after posttransplantation day 100, and tacrolimus is also being investigated as an agent to treat this type of immunological response.

- Neurotoxicity (coma, delirium, psychosis, encephalopathy, seizures, tremor, confusion, headaches, paresthesias, insomnia, nightmares, photophobia, anxiety), nephrotoxicity, hypertension, electrolyte imbalances (hyperkalemia, hypomagnesemia), glucose intolerance, gastrointestinal upset (diarrhea, nausea, vomiting, anorexia), hepatotoxicity, pruritus, alopecia, and leukocytosis are all typical adverse effects of tacrolimus treatment.[1–7]

  - Neurological side effects tend to be associated with high (≥25 ng/ml) tacrolimus blood concentrations and usually respond to dosage decreases.
  - Hypertension is a common side effect associated with tacrolimus therapy, and is treated with traditional antihypertensive drug therapy.
  - Nephrotoxicity is similar to that seen with cyclosporine, and is separated into acute and chronic varieties.

    - Acute nephrotoxicity is concentration- or dose-dependent and reverses with a dosage decrease.
    - Chronic nephrotoxicity is accompanied by kidney tissue damage, including interstitial fibrosis, nonspecific tubular vacuolization, and structural changes in arteries, arterioles, and proximal tubular epithelium.
    - Increased serum creatinine and blood urea nitrogen (BUN) values and hyperkalemia occur with tacrolimus-induced nephrotoxicity. The clinical features of tacrolimus nephrotoxicity and acute graft rejection in renal transplant patients are similar, so renal biopsies may be conducted to differentiate between these possibilities. Because biopsy findings are similar between tacrolimus-induced nephrotoxicity and chronic rejection of kidney transplants, this technique is less helpful in this situation.[1]

- Dosage decreases may be necessary to limit adverse drug effects associated with tacrolimus therapy.

CLINICAL MONITORING PARAMETERS

- Solid-organ transplant patients should be monitored for graft rejection consistent with the transplanted organ.[1–3,5]

  - For renal transplant patients, increased serum creatinine, azotemia, hypertension, edema, weight gain secondary to fluid retention, graft tenderness, fever, and malaise may be due to an acute rejection episode.[1]
  - Hypertension, proteinuria, a continuous decline in renal function (increases in serum creatinine and BUN levels), and uremia are indicative of chronic rejection in renal transplant patients.
  - For hepatic transplant patients, acute rejection signs and symptoms include fever, lethargy, graft tenderness, increased white blood cell count, change in bile color or amount, hyperbilirubinemia, and increased liver function tests.[5]
  - Chronic rejection in a liver transplant patient may be accompanied only by increased liver function tests and jaundice.
  - For heart transplant patients, acute rejection is accompanied by low-grade fever, malaise, heart failure (presence of S_3 heart sound), or atrial arrhythmia.[2]
  - Chronic rejection in heart transplant patients, also known as cardiac allograft vasculopathy, which is characterized by accelerated coronary artery atherosclerosis, may include the following symptoms: arrhythmias, decreased left ventricular function, heart failure, myocardial infarction, and sudden cardiac death.
  - For all solid-organ transplant patients, tissue biopsies may be taken from the transplanted tissue to confirm the diagnosis of organ rejection.[1–3,5]

- Bone marrow transplant patients should be monitored for the signs and symptoms associated with graft-versus-host disease.[4] These include a generalized maculopapular skin rash, diarrhea, abdominal pain, ileus, hyperbilirubinemia, and increased liver function tests (serum transaminases and alkaline phosphatase). Patients with severe chronic graft-versus-host disease may have involvement of the skin, liver, eyes, mouth, esophagus, or other organs similar to what might be seen with systemic autoimmune diseases.
- Typical adverse effects of tacrolimus treatment include neurotoxicity, nephrotoxicity, hypertension, hyperkalemia, hypomagnesemia, glucose intolerance, gastrointestinal upset, hepatotoxicity, pruritus, alopecia, and leukocytosis.[1–6] The management of these more common drug side effects are discussed in the previous section.
- Other adverse drug reactions to tacrolimus that occur less frequently include hyperlipidemia and thrombocytopenia.
- Because of the pivotal role that tacrolimus plays as an immunosuppressant in transplant patients, as well as the severity of its concentration- and dose-dependent side effects, tacrolimus concentrations should be measured in every patient receiving the drug.
- If a patient experiences signs or symptoms of organ rejection or graft-versus-host disease, tacrolimus concentration should be checked to ensure that levels have not fallen below the therapeutic range.
- If a patient encounters a possible clinical problem that could be an adverse drug effect of tacrolimus therapy, tacrolimus concentration should be measured to determine if levels are in the toxic range.

- During the immediate posttransplantation phase, tacrolimus concentrations are measured daily in most patients even though steady state may not yet have been achieved, in order to prevent acute rejection in solid-organ transplant patients or acute graft-versus-host disease in bone marrow transplant patients.

  - After discharge from the hospital, tacrolimus concentrations continue to be obtained at most clinic visits.
  - In patients receiving allogeneic bone marrow transplants from HLA-identical sibling donors, it is usually possible to decrease tacrolimus doses and concentrations about 2 months after the transplant and stop tacrolimus therapy altogether after about 6 months posttransplant if no or only mild acute rejection episodes have taken place.
  - In allogeneic bone marrow transplant patients with HLA-mismatched related or HLA-identical unrelated donors and all solid-organ transplant patients, chronic tacrolimus therapy is usually required. In these cases, tacrolimus doses and concentrations are decreased to the minimum required to prevent graft-versus-host reactions or rejection episodes in order to decrease drug adverse effects.
  - Because of a good correlation with the tacrolimus steady-state area under the concentration/time curve, predose steady-state trough tacrolimus concentration determinations are used to adjust drug doses.[7,12,13]

BASIC CLINICAL PHARMACOKINETIC PARAMETERS

- Tacrolimus is eliminated almost completely by hepatic metabolism (>99%). Hepatic metabolism is mainly via the CYP3A4 enzyme system, and the drug is a substrate for P-glycoprotein.[14–17]
- There are more than 15 identified tacrolimus metabolites.[7] None of these metabolites appears to have significant immunosuppressive effects in humans. Most of the metabolites are eliminated in the bile.[18]
- Less than 1% of a tacrolimus dose is recovered as unchanged drug in the urine.[19]
- There is a large amount of intrasubject variability in tacrolimus concentrations obtained on a day-to-day basis, even when the patient should be at steady state.[7] There are many reasons for this variability.

  - Tacrolimus has low water solubility, and its gastrointestinal absorption can be influenced by many variables. While oral absorption rate is generally fast for most patients (times to maximum concentration between 0.5 and 1 hour), some patients absorb tacrolimus very slowly, which yields a flat concentration/time profile.[12,19–21]
  - Absorption lag times of up to 2 hours have been reported in liver transplant patients.[12]
  - While the average oral bioavailability is 25%, there is a large amount of variation in this parameter among patients (4–89%).[7]

    - Renal transplant patients may have reduced oral bioavailability for tacrolimus. When tacrolimus is given with meals, especially meals with high fat content, oral bioavailability of tacrolimus decreases.[7] To avoid possible effects of food on tacrolimus bioavailability, the drug should be given at a constant time in relation to meals.
    - Oral tacrolimus should not be taken with grapefruit juice, since this vehicle inhibits CYP3A4 and/or P-glycoprotein in the gastrointestinal tract and markedly increases bioavailability.[22]

- After liver transplantation, bile production and flow may not begin immediately, or bile flow may be diverted from the gastrointestinal tract using a T-tube. Unlike cyclosporine, tacrolimus gastrointestinal absorption does not seem to be influenced by the presence or absence of bile.[19,23]
  - Other drug therapy can also increase or decrease the intestinal first-pass clearance of tacrolimus.[22]

- Tacrolimus is a drug with a low hepatic extraction ratio drug.[7] As a result, its hepatic clearance is influenced by unbound fraction in the blood (f_B) and intrinsic clearance (Cl'_{int}).

  - Tacrolimus binds primarily to erythrocytes, α_1-acid glycoprotein, and albumin.[24-27] The exact value for protein binding (72–99%) depends on the technique used and the matrix tested, and these factors have resulted in a large range of reported values for unbound fractions in the blood.[7]

    - Erythrocyte concentrations vary in transplant patients, especially those who have received bone marrow or kidney transplants. Concentrations of α_1-acid glycoprotein also vary greatly among patients.

  - Hepatic intrinsic clearance is different among individuals, and there is a large amount of variability in this value among individual liver transplant patients that changes according to the viability of the graft and time after transplantation surgery.
  - Other drug therapy can also increase or decrease the hepatic intrinsic clearance of tacrolimus.[22]

- Tacrolimus capsules are available in 0.5-, 1-, and 5-mg strengths.
- Tacrolimus injection for intravenous administration is available at a concentration of 5 mg/ml. Before administration, it should be diluted in normal saline or 5% dextrose, and the drug should be given as a continuous infusion.

  - Anaphylactic reactions have occurred with this dosage form, possibly due to the castor oil dilutant used to enhance dissolution of the drug.

- The initial dose of tacrolimus varies greatly among various transplant centers, with a range of 0.1–0.3 mg/kg/d for orally administered drug and 0.03–0.1 mg/kg/d for intravenously administered drug.[5,7]
- For patients with liver dysfunction, these doses may be reduced by 25–50%.[23,28,29]
- Recommended initial oral doses of tacrolimus are 0.2 mg/kg/d for adult kidney transplant patients, 0.10–0.15 mg/kg/d for adult liver transplant patients, and 0.15–0.2 mg/kg/d for pediatric hepatic transplant recipients. Oral tacrolimus is usually given in two divided daily doses given every 12 hours.

EFFECTS OF DISEASE STATES AND CONDITIONS ON TACROLIMUS PHARMACOKINETICS AND DOSING

- Transplantation type does not appear to have a substantial effect on tacrolimus pharmacokinetics.[7] The overall mean for all transplant groups is a clearance of 0.06 L/h/kg, a volume of distribution of 1 L/kg, and a half-life of 12 hours for adults.[7]
- In children (≤16 years old), average clearance and volume of distribution are higher (0.138 L/h/kg and 2.6 L/kg, respectively), but the mean half-life is about the same as for adults (12 hours).[7]

- These results, as with the other pharmacokinetic parameters discussed in this chapter, are based on an enzyme-linked immunosorbent assay (ELISA; Pro-Trac®, IncStar) or a microparticulate enzyme immunoassay (MEIA; IMx®, Abbott Diagnostics) assay conducted using whole blood samples. Concurrently measured plasma or serum concentrations are lower than whole blood concentrations.
- Because the drug is eliminated primarily by hepatic metabolism, average clearance is lower (0.04 L/h/kg) in adult patients with liver dysfunction.[23,28,29] Also, mean volume of distribution is larger (3 L/kg) and half-life is prolonged and variable (mean = 60 hours, range 28–141 hours) in this patient population.
- Immediately after liver transplantation, tacrolimus metabolism is depressed until the graft begins functioning in a stable manner.
- Patients with transient liver dysfunction, regardless of transplantation type, will have decreased tacrolimus clearance and increased half-life values.
- Renal failure does not change tacrolimus pharmacokinetics significantly, and tacrolimus dosage adjustments are not necessary for patients receiving hemodialysis or peritoneal dialysis.[30,31]

DRUG INTERACTIONS

- Drug interactions with tacrolimus fall into two basic categories.[22]
  - The first are agents known to cause nephrotoxicity when administered by themselves. The fear is that administration of a known nephrotoxin with tacrolimus will increase the incidence of renal damage over that observed when tacrolimus or the other agent is given separately.
    - Compounds in this category of drug interactions include aminoglycoside antibiotics, vancomycin, cotrimoxazole (trimethoprim-sulfamethoxazole), amphotericin B, and nonsteroidal anti-inflammatory drugs. Co-administration of tacrolimus with cyclosporine has resulted in augmented nephrotoxic side effects.
  - The second category of drug interactions involves inhibition or induction of tacrolimus metabolism.[22] Tacrolimus is metabolized by CYP3A4 and is a substrate for P-glycoprotein, so the potential for many pharmacokinetic drug interactions exists with agents that inhibit these pathways or are also cleared by these mechanisms.
    - Because both of these drug elimination systems also exist in the gastrointestinal tract, inhibition drug interactions may also enhance tacrolimus oral bioavailability by diminishing the intestinal and hepatic first-pass effects.
    - Drugs that may inhibit tacrolimus clearance include the calcium channel blockers (verapamil, diltiazem, nicardipine), azole antifungals (fluconazole, itraconazole, ketoconazole), macrolide antibiotics (erythromycin, clarithromycin, troleandomycin), antivirals (indinavir, nelfinavir, ritonavir, saquinavir), steroids (methylprednisolone, oral contraceptives, androgens), and psychotropic agents (fluvoxamine, nefazodone), as well as other compounds (cimetidine, grapefruit juice).
    - Inducing agents include other antibiotics (nafcillin, rifampin, rifabutin), anticonvulsants (phenytoin, carbamazepine, phenobarbital, primidone), barbiturates, aminoglutethimide, and troglitazone.
  - Because of the large number of potentially interacting agents, and the critical nature of the drugs involved in the treatment of transplant patients, complete

avoidance of drug interactions with tacrolimus is not possible. Thus, most drug interactions with tacrolimus are managed using appropriate tacrolimus dosage modification with tacrolimus concentration monitoring as a guide.
- If the drug is given with antacids, tacrolimus concentrations may decrease.[22] The mechanism of action of this drug interaction appears to be pH-mediated destruction of tacrolimus for sodium bicarbonate or magnesium oxide and physical adsorption of tacrolimus to the antacid for aluminum hydroxide gel.
- Gastrointestinal prokinetic agents (cisapride, metoclopramide) may increase tacrolimus concentrations by an unknown mechanism.
- Tacrolimus also has the potential to change the clearance of other drugs via competitive inhibition of CYP3A4 and/or P-glycoprotein.[22]

INITIAL DOSAGE DETERMINATION METHODS
- Several methods to initiate tacrolimus therapy are available.

  - The *pharmacokinetic dosing method* is the most flexible of the techniques. It allows individualized target serum concentrations to be chosen for a patient, and each pharmacokinetic parameter can be customized to reflect specific disease states and conditions present in the patient.
  - *Literature-based recommended dosing* is a very commonly used method to prescribe initial doses of tacrolimus. Doses are based on those that commonly produce steady-state concentrations near the lower end of the therapeutic range, although there is a wide variation in the actual concentrations for a specific patient.

Pharmacokinetic Dosing Method
- The goal of initial dosing of tacrolimus is to compute the best dose possible for the patient in order to prevent graft rejection or graft-versus-host disease given the set of disease states and conditions that influence tacrolimus pharmacokinetics, while avoiding adverse drug reactions. In order to do this, pharmacokinetic parameters for the patient are estimated using average parameters measured in other patients with similar disease state and condition profiles.

Clearance Estimate
- Tacrolimus is almost completely metabolized by the liver. Unfortunately, there is no good way to estimate the elimination characteristics of liver-metabolized drugs using an endogenous marker of liver function in the same fashion that serum creatinine and estimated creatinine clearance are used to estimate the elimination of agents that are eliminated renally.
- Therefore, a patient is categorized according to the disease states and conditions that are known to change tacrolimus clearance, and clearances previously measured in studies is used as an estimate of the current patient's clearance rate.

Selection of Appropriate Pharmacokinetic Model and Equations
- When tacrolimus given by intravenous infusion or orally, it follows a two-compartment model.

  - When oral therapy is chosen, the drug is often absorbed erratically, with variable absorption rates.

- Because of the complex absorption profile and the fact that the drug is usually administered twice daily, a simple pharmacokinetic equation that calculates the average tacrolimus steady-state concentration (Css in ng/ml = μg/L) is widely used and allows maintenance-dose computation:

$$Css = [F(D/\tau)]/Cl \quad \text{or} \quad D = (Css \cdot Cl \cdot \tau)/F$$

where F is the bioavailability fraction for the oral dosage form (F averages 0.25 or 25% for most patient populations), D is the dose of tacrolimus in mg, Cl is tacrolimus clearance in L/h, and τ is the dosage interval in hours.
- If the drug is to be given as a continuous intravenous infusion, the equivalent equation for that route of administration is

$$Css = k_0/Cl \quad \text{or} \quad k_0 = Css \cdot Cl$$

where k_0 is the infusion rate in mg/h.

Steady-State Concentration Selection

- The generally accepted therapeutic range for tacrolimus in the blood is 5–20 ng/ml.

  - More important than these general guidelines are the specific requirements for each graft type as defined by the transplant center where the surgery was conducted. Clinicians should become familiar with the tacrolimus protocols used at the various institutions at which they practice.
  - Although it is unlikely that steady state has been achieved, tacrolimus concentrations are usually obtained on a daily basis, even when dosage changes were made the previous day, due to the critical nature of the therapeutic effect provided by the drug.

▶ ***Example 1*** HO is a 50-year-old, 75-kg (height 5′10″) male renal transplant patient 2 days posttransplant surgery. The patient's liver function tests are normal. Suggest an initial oral tacrolimus dose designed to achieve a steady-state tacrolimus trough blood concentration of 15 ng/ml.

1. *Estimate clearance according to disease states and conditions present in the patient.* The mean tacrolimus clearance for adult patients is 0.06 L/h/kg. The tacrolimus blood clearance for this patient is expected to be

$$Cl = 0.06 \text{ L/h/kg} \cdot 75 \text{ kg} = 4.5 \text{ L/h}$$

2. *Compute dosage regimen.* A 12-hour dosage interval will be used for this patient. (*Note:* ng/ml = μg/L, and this concentration is substituted for Css in the calculations so that unit conversion is not required. Also, a conversion constant of 1000 μg/mg is used to change the dose amount to mg.) The dosage equation for oral tacrolimus is

$$D = (Css \cdot Cl \cdot \tau)/F = (15 \text{ μg/L} \cdot 4.5 \text{ L/h} \cdot 12 \text{ h})/(0.25 \cdot 1000 \text{ μg/mg})$$

$$= 3.2 \text{ mg, rounded to 3 mg every 12 h}$$

Tacrolimus concentrations should be obtained on a daily basis, with steady-state expected to occur in about 3 days (5 half-lives = 5 · 12 h = 60 h).

▶ ***Example 2*** Same patient as in Example 1, except compute an initial dose using intravenous tacrolimus.

1. *Estimate clearance according to disease states and conditions present in the patient.* The mean tacrolimus clearance for adult patients is 0.06 L/h/kg. The tacrolimus blood clearance for this patient is expected to be

$$Cl = 0.06 \text{ L/h/kg} \cdot 75 \text{ kg} = 4.5 \text{ L/h}$$

2. *Compute dosage regimen.* A continuous infusion will be used for this patient. (*Note:* ng/ml = μg/L, and this concentration is substituted for Css in the calculations so that unit conversion is not required. Also, a conversion constant of 1000 μg/mg is used to change the dose amount to mg.) The dosage equation for intravenous tacrolimus is

$$k_0 = Css \cdot Cl = (15 \text{ μg/L} \cdot 4.5 \text{ L/h})/(1000 \text{ μg/mg}) = 0.07 \text{ mg/h}$$

Tacrolimus concentrations should be obtained on a daily basis, with steady state expected to occur in about 3 days (5 half-lives = 5 · 12 h = 60 h).

Literature-Based Recommended Dosing

- Because of the large amount of variability in tacrolimus pharmacokinetics, even when concurrent disease states and conditions are identified, many clinicians believe that the use of standard tacrolimus doses for various situations is warranted.
- Most transplant centers use doses that are determined using a tacrolimus dosage protocol. The original computations of these doses were based on the pharmacokinetic dosing method described in the previous section, and the doses were subsequently modified based on clinical experience.

  - The expected tacrolimus steady-state concentration used to compute these doses depends on the type of transplanted tissue and the posttransplantation time line.

- Initial oral doses of 0.1–0.3 mg/kg/d are needed to achieve therapeutic tacrolimus steady-state concentrations.[5,7]
- Usual initial continuous infusion intravenous doses are 0.03–0.1 mg/kg/d.[5,7]
- For patients with liver dysfunction, these doses may be reduced by 25–50%.[23,28,29]
- To illustrate how this technique is used, the same patient examples utilized in the previous section will be repeated for this dosage approach for comparison purposes.

► *Example 3*   HO is a 50-year-old, 75-kg (height 5′10″) male renal transplant patient 2 days posttransplant surgery. The patient's liver function tests are normal. Suggest an initial oral tacrolimus dose designed to achieve a steady-state tacrolimus trough blood concentration within the therapeutic range.

1. *Choose tacrolimus dose based on disease states and conditions present in the patient and transplant type.* The tacrolimus oral dosage range for adult patients is 0.1–0.3 mg/kg/d. Because this is a renal transplant patient, a dose near the lower end of the range (0.1 mg/kg/d) will be used in order to avoid nephrotoxicity. The initial tacrolimus dose for this patient is 8 mg/d given as 4 mg every 12 hours:

$$Dose = 0.1 \text{ mg/kg/d} \cdot 75 \text{ kg}$$

$$= 7.5 \text{ mg/d, rounded to 8 mg/d or 4 mg every 12 h}$$

Tacrolimus concentrations should be obtained on a daily basis, with steady state expected to occur after 3 days (5 half-lives = 5 · 12 h = 60 h) of treatment.

▶ *Example 4*   Same patient as in Example 3, except compute an initial dose using intravenous tacrolimus.

1. *Choose tacrolimus dose based on disease states and conditions present in the patient and transplant type.* The tacrolimus intravenous dosage range for adult patients is 0.03–0.1 mg/kg/d. Because this is a renal transplant patient, a dose near the lower end of the range (0.03 mg/kg/d) will be used in order to avoid nephrotoxicity. The initial tacrolimus intravenous infusion dose for this patient is

$$\text{Dose} = (0.03 \text{ mg/kg/d} \cdot 75 \text{ kg})/(24 \text{ h/d}) = 0.09 \text{ mg/h}$$

Tacrolimus concentrations should be obtained on a daily basis, with steady state expected to occur after 3 days (5 half-lives = $5 \cdot 12$ h = 60 h) of treatment.

USE OF TACROLIMUS CONCENTRATIONS TO ALTER DOSES

- Because of the large amount of pharmacokinetic variability among patients, it is likely that doses computed using patient population characteristics will not always produce tacrolimus concentrations that are expected or desirable.
- Because of pharmacokinetic variability, the narrow therapeutic index of tacrolimus, and the severity of tacrolimus adverse side effects, measurement of tacrolimus concentrations is mandatory for patients, to ensure that therapeutic, nontoxic levels are present.
- In addition to tacrolimus concentrations, important patient parameters (transplanted organ function tests or biopsies, clinical signs and symptoms of graft rejection or graft-versus-host disease, potential tacrolimus side effects, etc.) should be followed to confirm that the patient is responding to treatment and not developing adverse drug reactions.
- When tacrolimus concentrations are measured in patients and a dosage change is necessary, clinicians should use the simplest, most straightforward method available to determine a dose that will provide safe and effective treatment.

  - In most cases a simple dosage ratio can be used to change tacrolimus doses, assuming the drug follows *linear pharmacokinetics.*
  - Sometimes it is useful to compute tacrolimus pharmacokinetic constants for a patient and base dosage adjustments on these. In this case it may be possible to calculate and use *pharmacokinetic parameters* to alter the tacrolimus dose.
  - Finally, computerized methods that incorporate expected population pharmacokinetic characteristics (*Bayesian pharmacokinetic computer programs*) can be used in difficult cases, when concentrations are obtained at suboptimal times or the patient was not at steady state when concentrations were measured.

Linear Pharmacokinetics Method

- Assuming that tacrolimus follows linear, dose-proportional pharmacokinetics,[32] steady-state concentrations change in proportion to dose according to the following equation:

$$D_{new}/Css_{new} = D_{old}/Css_{old} \quad \text{or} \quad D_{new} = (Css_{new}/Css_{old})D_{old}$$

where D is the dose, Css is the steady-state concentration, old indicates the dose that produced the steady-state concentration the patient is currently receiving, and new denotes the dose necessary to produce the desired steady-state concentration.

- The advantages of this method are that it is quick and simple. The main disadvantage is that steady-state concentrations are required.

▶ *Example 5* LK is a 50-year-old, 75-kg (height 5′10″) male renal transplant recipient who is receiving 5 mg of oral tacrolimus capsules every 12 hours. He has normal liver function. His current steady-state tacrolimus blood concentration is 24 ng/ml. Compute a tacrolimus dose that will provide a steady-state concentration of 15 ng/ml.

1. *Compute a new dose to achieve the desired concentration.* The patient can be expected to achieve steady-state conditions after the third day ($5t_{1/2} = 5 \cdot 12$ h = 60 h) of therapy. Using linear pharmacokinetics, the new dose to attain the desired concentration should be proportional to the old dose that produced the measured concentration (total daily dose = 5 mg/dose $\cdot$ 2 doses/d = 10 mg/d):

$$D_{new} = (Css_{new}/Css_{old})D_{old} = [(15 \text{ ng/ml})/(24 \text{ ng/ml})](10 \text{ mg/d})$$

$$= 6.3 \text{ mg/d, rounded to 6 mg/d}$$

The new suggested dose is 6 mg/d or 3 mg of tacrolimus capsules every 12 hours, to be started at the next scheduled dosing time.

A steady-state trough tacrolimus concentration should be measured after steady state is attained in 3–5 half-lives. Since the drug is expected to have a half-life of 12 hours, a tacrolimus steady-state concentration can be obtained at any time after the third day of dosing (5 half-lives = $5 \cdot 12$ h = 60 h). Tacrolimus concentrations should also be measured if the patient experiences signs or symptoms of graft rejection, or if the patient develops potential signs or symptoms of tacrolimus toxicity.

▶ *Example 6* FD is a 60-year-old, 85-kg (height 6′1″) male liver transplant patient who is receiving 0.15 mg/h of intravenous tacrolimus as a continuous infusion. The patient's current steady-state tacrolimus concentration is 9 ng/ml. Compute a tacrolimus dose that will provide a steady-state concentration of 15 ng/ml.

1. *Compute a new dose to achieve the desired concentration.* The patient can be expected to achieve steady-state conditions after the third day ($5t_{1/2} = 5 \cdot 12$ h = 60 h) of therapy. Using linear pharmacokinetics, the new dose to attain the desired concentration should be proportional to the old dose that produced the measured concentration:

$$D_{new} = (Css_{new}/Css_{old})D_{old} = [(15 \text{ ng/ml})/(9 \text{ ng/ml})](0.15 \text{ mg/h})$$

$$= 0.25 \text{ mg/h}$$

A tacrolimus concentration should be measured after steady state is attained in 3–5 half-lives. Since the drug is expected to have a half-life of 12 hours, a tacrolimus steady-state concentration can be obtained at any time after the third day of dosing (5 half-lives = $5 \cdot 12$ h = 60 h). Tacrolimus concentrations should also be measured if the patient experiences signs or symptoms of graft rejection, or if the patient develops potential signs or symptoms of tacrolimus toxicity.

Pharmacokinetic Parameter Method

- The pharmacokinetic parameter method of adjusting drug doses was among the first techniques available to change doses using drug concentrations. It allows the computation of an individual's own, unique pharmacokinetic constants and uses those to calculate a dose that achieves desired tacrolimus concentrations.

• The pharmacokinetic parameter method requires that steady state has been achieved and uses only a steady-state tacrolimus concentration.

  • Tacrolimus clearance can be measured using a single steady-state tacrolimus concentration and the following formula for orally administered drug:

$$Cl = [F(D/\tau)]/Css$$

  where Cl is tacrolimus clearance in L/h, F is the bioavailability factor for tacrolimus (F = 0.25), τ is the dosage interval in hours, and Css is the tacrolimus steady-state concentration in ng/ml, which equals μg/L.

  • If tacrolimus is administered intravenously, it is not necessary to take bioavailability into account:

$$Cl = k_0/Css$$

  where Cl is tacrolimus clearance in L/h, k_0 is the tacrolimus infusion rate in mg/h, and Css is the tacrolimus steady-state concentration in ng/ml, which also equals μg/L.

• Although this method does allow computation of tacrolimus clearance, it yields exactly the same tacrolimus dose as the use of linear pharmacokinetics. As a result, most clinicians prefer to calculate the new dose directly, using the simpler linear pharmacokinetics method.

• To demonstrate this point, the patient cases used to illustrate the linear pharmacokinetics method will be used as examples for the pharmacokinetic parameter method.

▶ **Example 7** LK is a 50-year-old, 75-kg (height 5′10″) male renal transplant recipient who is receiving 5 mg of oral tacrolimus capsules every 12 hours. He has normal liver function. His current steady-state tacrolimus blood concentration is 24 ng/ml. Compute a tacrolimus dose that will provide a steady-state concentration of 15 ng/ml.

1. *Compute pharmacokinetic parameters.* The patient can expected to achieve steady-state conditions after the third day ($5t_{1/2} = 5 \cdot 12$ h = 60 h) of therapy. Tacrolimus clearance can be computed using a steady-state tacrolimus concentration:

$$Cl = [F(D/\tau)]/Css = [0.25 \cdot (5 \text{ mg}/12 \text{ h}) \cdot 1000 \text{ } \mu\text{g/mg}]/(24 \text{ } \mu\text{g/L})$$
$$= 4.3 \text{ L/h}$$

  (*Note:* μg/L = ng/ml, and this concentration unit was substituted for Css in the calculations so that unit conversion was not required.)

2. *Compute tacrolimus dose.* Tacrolimus clearance is used to compute the new dose:

$$D = (Css \cdot Cl \cdot \tau)/F = [(15 \text{ } \mu\text{g/L}) \cdot (4.3 \text{ L/h}) \cdot 12 \text{ h}]/(0.25 \cdot 1000 \text{ } \mu\text{g/mg})$$
$$= 3.1 \text{ mg, rounded to 3 mg every 12 h}$$

  A steady-state trough tacrolimus concentration should be measured after steady state is attained in 3–5 half-lives. Since the drug is expected to have a half-life of 12 hours, a tacrolimus steady-state concentration can be obtained at any time after the third day of dosing (5 half-lives = 5 · 12 h = 60 h). Tacrolimus concentrations should also be measured if the patient experiences signs or symptoms of graft rejection, or if the patient develops potential signs or symptoms of tacrolimus toxicity.

► *Example 8*   FD is a 60-year-old, 85-kg (height 6'1″) male liver transplant patient who is receiving 0.15 mg/h of intravenous tacrolimus as a continuous infusion. His current steady-state tacrolimus concentration is 9 ng/ml. Compute a tacrolimus dose that will provide a steady-state concentration of 15 ng/ml.

1. *Compute pharmacokinetic parameters.* The patient can be expected to achieve steady-state conditions after the third day ($5t_{1/2}$ = 5 · 12 h = 60 h) of therapy. Tacrolimus clearance can be computed using a steady-state tacrolimus concentration:

$$Cl = k_0/Css = (0.15 \text{ mg/h} \cdot 1000 \text{ µg/mg})/(9 \text{ µg/L}) = 16.7 \text{ L/h}$$

   (*Note:* µg/L = ng/ml, and this concentration unit was substituted for Css in the calculations so that unit conversion was not required.)

2. *Compute tacrolimus dose.* Tacrolimus clearance is used to compute the new dose:

$$k_0 = Css \cdot Cl = (15 \text{ µg/L} \cdot 16.7 \text{ L/h})/1000 \text{ µg/mg} = 0.25 \text{ mg/h}$$

   A steady-state trough tacrolimus concentration should be measured after steady state is attained in 3–5 half-lives. Since the drug is expected to have a half-life of 12 hours, a tacrolimus steady-state concentration can be obtained at any time after the third day of dosing (5 half-lives = 5 · 12 h = 60 h). Tacrolimus concentrations should also be measured if the patient experiences signs or symptoms of graft rejection, or if the patient develops potential signs or symptoms of tacrolimus toxicity.

BAYESIAN PHARMACOKINETIC COMPUTER PROGRAMS

- Computer programs are available that can assist in the computation of pharmacokinetic parameters for patients. The most reliable computer programs use a nonlinear regression algorithm that incorporates components of Bayes' theorem.

- An advantage of this approach is that consistent dosage recommendations can be made when several different practitioners are involved in therapeutic drug monitoring programs. However, since simpler dosing methods work just as well for patients with stable pharmacokinetic parameters and steady-state drug concentrations, many clinicians reserve the use of computer programs for more difficult situations. Those situations include drug concentrations that are not at steady state, drug concentrations not obtained at the specific times needed to employ simpler methods, and unstable pharmacokinetic parameters.

  - When only a limited number of tacrolimus steady-state concentrations are available, Bayesian pharmacokinetic computer programs can be used to compute a complete patient pharmacokinetic profile that includes clearance, volume of distribution, and half-life.

  - Many Bayesian pharmacokinetic computer programs are available, and most should provide answers similar to the program used in the following examples. The program used to solve problems in this book is DrugCalc, written by Dr. Dennis Mungall and available at his Internet web site (www.clinpharmacologist.bigstep.com/consumersurvey.html).[33]

▶ *Example 9*   LK is a 50-year-old, 75-kg (height 5′10″) male renal transplant recipient who is receiving 5 mg of oral tacrolimus capsules every 12 hours. He has normal liver (bilirubin = 0.7 mg/dl, albumin = 4.0 g/dl). His current steady-state tacrolimus blood concentration is 24 ng/ml. Compute a tacrolimus dose that will provide a steady-state concentration of 15 ng/ml.

1. *Enter patient demographic, drug dosing, and concentration/time data into a Bayesian pharmacokinetic computer program.*
2. *Compute pharmacokinetic parameters for the patient using the computer program.* The pharmacokinetic parameters computed by the program are a volume of distribution of 76 L, a half-life of 15.8 hours, and a clearance of 3.3 L/h.
3. *Compute dose required to achieve desired tacrolimus concentrations.* The one-compartment-model first-order absorption equation used by the program to compute doses indicates that a dose of 2 mg every 12 hours will produce a steady-state tacrolimus concentration of 15 ng/ml. Using the linear pharmacokinetics and pharmacokinetic parameter methods previously described in the chapter produced a similar answer for this patient.

▶ *Example 10*   FD is a 60-year-old, 85-kg (height 6′1″) male liver transplant patient who is receiving 0.15 mg/h of intravenous tacrolimus as a continuous infusion. He has normal liver function tests (bilirubin = 1.1 mg/dl, albumin = 3.5 g/dl). His current steady-state tacrolimus concentration is 9 ng/ml. Compute a tacrolimus dose that will provide a steady-state concentration of 15 ng/ml.

1. *Enter patient demographic, drug dosing, and concentration/time data into a Bayesian pharmacokinetic computer program.*
2. *Compute pharmacokinetic parameters for the patient using the computer program.* The pharmacokinetic parameters computed by the program are a volume of distribution of 85 L, a half-life of 3.6 hours, and a clearance of 16.3 L/h.
3. *Compute dose required to achieve desired tacrolimus concentrations.* The one-compartment-model continuous infusion equation used by the program to compute doses indicates that a dose of 0.24 mg/h will produce a steady-state tacrolimus concentration of 15 ng/ml. Using the linear pharmacokinetics and pharmacokinetic parameter methods previously described in the chapter produced a similar answer for this patient.

▶ *Example 11*   YT is a 25-year-old, 55-kg (height 5′2″) female renal transplant recipient who received 4 mg of oral tacrolimus capsules every 12 hours for two doses after transplant, but because her renal function decreased, her dose was empirically changed to 2 mg every 12 hours. She has normal liver function (bilirubin = 0.9 mg/dl, albumin = 3.9 g/dl). The tacrolimus blood concentration obtained 12 hours after her first dose of the lower dosage regimen was 22 ng/ml. Compute a tacrolimus dose that will provide a steady-state concentration of 15 ng/ml.

1. *Enter patient demographic, drug dosing, and concentration/time data into a Bayesian pharmacokinetic computer program.*
2. *Compute pharmacokinetic parameters for the patient using the computer program.* The pharmacokinetic parameters computed by the program are a volume of distribution of 54 L, a half-life of 1.8 hours, and a clearance of 21 L/h.

TABLE 16-1 Dosing Strategies

Dosing approach/ philosophy	Initial dosing	Use of serum concentrations to alter doses
Pharmacokinetic parameter/ equations	Pharmacokinetic dosing method	Pharmacokinetic parameter method
Literature-based/ concept	Literature-based recommended dosing method	Linear pharmacokinetics method
Computerized	Bayesian computer program	Bayesian computer program

3. *Compute dose required to achieve desired tacrolimus concentrations.* The one-compartment-model first-order absorption equation used by the program to compute doses indicates that a dose of 1 mg every 12 hours will produce a steady-state tacrolimus concentration of 15 ng/ml.

DOSING STRATEGIES

• Initial dose and dosage adjustment techniques using serum concentrations can be used in any combination as long as the limitations of each method are observed.
• Some dosing schemes link together logically when considered according to their basic approaches or philosophies. Dosage strategies that follow similar pathways are given in Table 16-1.

REFERENCES

1. Johnson HJ, Heim-Duthoy KL. Renal transplantation. In: DiPiro JT, Talbert RL, Yee GC, Matzke GR, Wells BG, Posey LM, eds. Pharmacotherapy. 5th ed. New York: McGraw-Hill, 2002:843–66.
2. Lake KD, Aaronson KD. Cardiac transplantation. In: DiPiro JT, Talbert RL, Yee GC, Matzke GR, Wells BG, Posey LM, eds. Pharmacotherapy. 5th ed. New York: McGraw-Hill, 2002:321–36.
3. Maurer JR. Lung transplantation. In: Braunwald E, Fauci AS, Kasper DL, Hauser SL, Longo DL, Jameson JL, eds. Principles of internal medicine. 15th ed. New York: McGraw-Hill, 2001:1531–33.
4. Perkins JB, Yee GC. Bone marrow transplantation. In: DiPiro JT, Talbert RL, Yee GC, Matzke GR, Wells BG, Posey LM, eds. Pharmacotherapy. 5th ed. New York: McGraw-Hill, 2002:2425–44.
5. Stoffel JA, Somani AZ. Liver transplantation. In: DiPiro JT, Talbert RL, Yee GC, Matzke GR, Wells BG, Posey LM, eds. Pharmacotherapy. 5th ed. New York: McGraw-Hill, 2002:743–52.
6. Krensky AM, Strom TB, Bluestone JA. Immunomodulators: immunosuppressive agents, tolerogens, and immunostimulants. In: Hardman JG, Limbird LE, Gilman AG, eds. The pharmacological basis of therapeutics. 10th ed. New York: McGraw-Hill, 2001:1463–84.
7. Venkataramanan R, Swaminathan A, Prasad T, et al. Clinical pharmacokinetics of tacrolimus. Clin Pharmacokinet 1995;29(6):404–30.
8. Jusko WJ, Thomson AW, Fung J, et al. Consensus document: therapeutic monitoring of tacrolimus (FK-506). Ther Drug Monit 1995;17(6):606–14.

9. D'Ambrosio R, Girzaitis N, Jusko WJ. Multicenter comparison of tacrolimus (FK 506) whole blood concentrations as measured by the Abbott IMX analyzer and enzyme immunoassay with methylene chloride extraction. Ther Drug Monit 1994; 16(3):287–92.

10. Matsunami H, Tada A, Makuuchi M, Lynch SV, Strong RW. New technique for measuring tacrolimus concentrations in blood [letter]. Am J Hosp Pharm 1994; 51(1):123.

11. Winkler M, Christians U, Stoll K, Baumann J, Pichlmayr R. Comparison of different assays for the quantitation of FK 506 levels in blood or plasma. Ther Drug Monit 1994;16(3):281–6.

12. Jusko WJ, Piekoszewski W, Klintmalm GB, et al. Pharmacokinetics of tacrolimus in liver transplant patients. Clin Pharmacol Ther 1995;57(3):281–90.

13. Regazzi MB, Rinaldi M, Molinaro M, et al. Clinical pharmacokinetics of tacrolimus in heart transplant recipients. Ther Drug Monit 1999;21(1):2–7.

14. Floren LC, Bekersky I, Benet LZ, et al. Tacrolimus oral bioavailability doubles with coadministration of ketoconazole. Clin Pharmacol Ther 1997;62(1):41–9.

15. Hebert MF, Fisher RM, Marsh CL, Dressler D, Bekersky I. Effects of rifampin on tacrolimus pharmacokinetics in healthy volunteers. J Clin Pharmacol 1999;39(1): 91–6.

16. Sattler M, Guengerich FP, Yun CH, Christians U, Sewing KF. Cytochrome P-450 3A enzymes are responsible for biotransformation of FK506 and rapamycin in man and rat. Drug Metab Dispos 1992;20(5):753–61.

17. Karanam BV, Vincent SH, Newton DJ, Wang RW, Chiu SH. FK 506 metabolism in human liver microsomes: investigation of the involvement of cytochrome P450 isozymes other than CYP3A4 [published erratum appears in Drug Metab Dispos 1994 Nov–Dec;22(6):979]. Drug Metab Dispos 1994;22(5):811–4.

18. Iwasaki K, Shiraga T, Nagase K, Hirano K, Nozaki K, Noda K. Pharmacokinetic study of FK 506 in the rat. Transplant Proc 1991;23(6):2757–9.

19. Venkataramanan R, Jain A, Warty VS, et al. Pharmacokinetics of FK 506 in transplant patients. Transplant Proc 1991;23(6):2736–40.

20. Gruber SA, Hewitt JM, Sorenson AL, et al. Pharmacokinetics of FK506 after intravenous and oral administration in patients awaiting renal transplantation. J Clin Pharmacol 1994;34(8):859–64.

21. Venkataramanan R, Jain A, Warty VW, et al. Pharmacokinetics of FK 506 following oral administration: a comparison of FK 506 and cyclosporine. Transplant Proc 1991;23(1 pt 2):931–3.

22. Hansten PD, Horn JR. Drug interactions analysis and management. Vancouver, WA: Applied Therapeutics, 1999.

23. Jain AB, Venkataramanan R, Cadoff E, et al. Effect of hepatic dysfunction and T tube clamping on FK 506 pharmacokinetics and trough concentrations. Transplant Proc 1990;22(1):57–9.

24. Kobayashi M, Tamura K, Katayama N, et al. FK 506 assay past and present— characteristics of FK 506 ELISA. Transplant Proc 1991;23(6):2725–9.

25. Kay JE, Sampare-Kwateng E, Geraghty F, Morgan GY. Uptake of FK 506 by lymphocytes and erythrocytes. Transplant Proc 1991;23(6):2760–2.

26. Piekoszewski W, Jusko WJ. Plasma protein binding of tacrolimus in humans. J Pharm Sci 1993;82(3):340–1.

27. Nagase K, Iwasaki K, Nozaki K, Noda K. Distribution and protein binding of FK506, a potent immunosuppressive macrolide lactone, in human blood and its uptake by erythrocytes. J Pharm Pharmacol 1994;46(2):113–7.

28. Winkler M, Ringe B, Rodeck B, et al. The use of plasma levels for FK 506 dosing in liver-grafted patients. Transpl Int 1994;7(5):329–33.

29. Jain AB, Abu-Elmagd K, Abdallah H, et al. Pharmacokinetics of FK506 in liver transplant recipients after continuous intravenous infusion [see comments]. J Clin Pharmacol 1993;33(7):606–11.

30. Bennett WM. Guide to drug dosage in renal failure. Clin Pharmacokinet 1988; 15(5):326–54.

31. Swan SK, Bennett WM. Drug dosing guidelines in patients with renal failure. West J Med 1992;156(6):633–8.
32. Bekersky I, Dressler D, Mekki QA. Dose linearity after oral administration of tacrolimus 1-mg capsules at doses of 3, 7, and 10 mg. Clin Ther 1999;21(12): 2058–64.
33. Wandell M, Mungall D. Computer assisted drug interpretation and drug regimen optimization. Am Assoc Clin Chem 1984;6:1–11.

6 | OTHER DRUGS

17 | Lithium

Lithium is an alkali metal that is administered as a monovalent cation (Li$^+$) for the treatment of bipolar disorder. In the United States, orally administered carbonate and citrate salts of lithium are available. While lithium is still used as a primary treatment for bipolar disorders, its use as the primary agent is being challenged by valproic acid and carbamazepine for some subsets of the disease.[1]

- Although this drug has been used in psychiatric medicine since the 1940s, the mechanism of action of lithium is largely unknown. Among the current theories are competition with other cations at receptor and tissue sites, dopamine-receptor supersensitivity blockage, decreased stimulation of β-receptor-induced adenylate cyclase, and enhanced sensitivity to serotonin (5-HT), acetylcholine, and γ-aminobutyric acid (GABA).[1,2]

THERAPEUTIC AND TOXIC CONCENTRATIONS

- The general therapeutic range for lithium is 0.6–1.5 mmol/L. Because lithium is a monovalent cation, the therapeutic range expressed in mEq/L is identical to these values (i.e., 0.6–1.5 mEq/L).

  - Most clinicians apply different therapeutic concentration ranges depending on the clinical situation of the patient.[3]

    - For individuals with acute mania, a minimum lithium concentration of 0.8 mmol/L is usually recommended. The usual desired range for these individuals is 0.8–1 mmol/L. If patients with acute mania do not respond to these levels, it may be necessary to use lithium concentrations of 1– 1.2 mmol/L and in some instances concentrations as high as 1.2–1.5 mmol/L.
    - For long-term maintenance use, the usual desired range is 0.6–0.8 mmol/L. If patients do not respond to these levels during maintenance treatment, use of lithium concentrations of 0.9–1 mmol/L may be required, and in some cases concentrations as high as 1–1.2 mmol/L are necessary to gain an adequate outcome.

- These therapeutic ranges are based on steady-state lithium serum concentrations obtained 12 hours after a dose. The adoption of a standardized 12-hour postdose lithium concentration to assess dose and response has been paramount in establishing the therapeutic ranges for the agent.[4]

  - After oral administration, lithium concentrations follow a complex concentration/time curve that is best described using multicompartment models (Figure 17-1).[4–8] There is a great deal of variability among patients in the time needed for distribution between serum and tissues to occur, and under these conditions using a uniform time for the determination of steady-state serum concentrations is important.

- When lithium serum concentration monitoring is anticipated for an individual, the patient needs to understand that it is important to take the medication as instructed for 2–3 days before the blood sample is obtained, to have the blood sample withdrawn 12 ± 0.5 hours after the last dose, and to report any discrepancies in compliance and blood sampling time to the care provider.

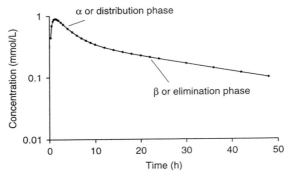

FIG. 17-1   Lithium ion serum concentration/time curve after a single 900-mg oral dose of lithium carbonate (24.4 mmol or mEq of lithium ion) rapid-release capsules. Maximum serum concentrations occur 2–3 hours after the dose is given. After the peak concentration is achieved, the distribution phase lasts for 6–10 hours, followed by the elimination phase. In patients with good renal function (creatinine clearance >80 ml/min), the average elimination half-life for lithium is 24 hours. Because of the long distribution phase, lithium serum concentrations used for dosage-adjustment purposes should be obtained no sooner than 12 hours after dosage administration.

- Short-term side effects observed when starting lithium or after a dosage increase include muscle weakness, lethargy, polydipsia, polyuria, nocturia, headache, impairment of memory or concentration, confusion, impaired fine-motor performance, and hand tremors.[1,2,9] Many of these adverse effects diminish with continued dosing of lithium.

  - Some intervention may be needed for the tremor, including a shorter dosage interval using the same total daily dose in order to decrease peak lithium concentrations, a decreased lithium dose, or concurrent treatment with a β-blocker.

- Long-term adverse effects of lithium therapy include a drug-induced diabetes insipidus, renal toxicity (glomerulosclerosis, renal tubular atrophy, interstitial nephritis, urinary casts), hypothyroidism with or without goiter formation, electrocardiographic abnormalities, leukocytosis, weight gain, and dermatological changes.[1,2,9]

  - At lithium serum concentrations near the upper end of the therapeutic range (1.2–1.5 mmol/L), the following adverse effects may be noted in patients: decreased memory and concentration, drowsiness, fine hand tremor, weakness, lack of coordination, nausea, diarrhea, vomiting, or fatigue.[1,2,9]
  - At concentrations just above the therapeutic range (1.5–3 mmol/L), confusion, giddiness, agitation, slurred speech, lethargy, blackouts, ataxia, nystagmus, blurred vision, tinnitus, vertigo, hyperreflexia, hypertonia, dysarthria, coarse hand tremors, and muscle fasciculations may occur in patients.
  - If concentrations exceed 3 mmol/L, severe toxicity occurs, with choreoathetosis, seizures, irreversible brain damage, arrhythmias, hypotension, respiratory and cardiovascular complications, stupor, coma, and death.

- At toxic lithium concentrations, lithium can cause a nonspecific decrease in glomerular filtration, which in turn decreases lithium clearance. The decrease in lithium clearance causes a further increase in the lithium serum concentration. This phenomenon can cause a viscous circle of decreased clearance leading to increased lithium serum concentration, which leads to additional decreases in lithium clearance, and so on.

  - Because of this problem and its severe toxic side effects, lithium concentrations above 3.5–4 mmol/L may require hemodialysis to remove the drug as quickly as possible.[1,9]

CLINICAL MONITORING PARAMETERS

- The signs and symptoms of bipolar disease include those of both depression and mania.[1]

  - *Depression:* Depressed affect, sad mood, decreased interest and pleasure in normal activities, decreased appetite and weight loss, insomnia or hypersomnia, psychomotor retardation or agitation, decreased energy or fatigue, feelings of worthlessness or guilt, impaired decision making and concentration, suicidal ideation or attempts.
  - *Mania:* Abnormal and persistently elevated mood, grandiosity, decreased need for sleep, pressure of speech, flight of ideas, distractible with poor attention span, increased activity or agitation, excessive involvement in high-risk activities.

- Generally, onset of action for lithium is 1–2 weeks, and a 4–6-week treatment period is required to assess complete therapeutic response to the drug.[1,9]
- Before initiating lithium therapy, patients should undergo a complete physical examination, and a general serum chemistry panel (including serum electrolytes and serum creatinine), complete blood cell count with differential, thyroid function tests, urinalysis (including osmolality and specific gravity), and urine toxicology screen for substances of abuse should be obtained.

  - For patients with renal dysfunction (measured 24-hour creatinine clearance) or baseline cardiac disease (electrocardiogram), additional testing is recommended.
  - Clinicians should consider ordering a pregnancy test for females of child-bearing age.

- Follow-up testing in the following areas should be conducted every 6–12 months: serum electrolytes, serum creatinine (measured 24-hour creatinine clearance in patients with renal dysfunction), thyroid function tests, complete blood cell count with differential. If urine output exceeds 3 L/d, a urinalysis with osmolality and specific gravity should also be measured.
- Lithium serum concentrations should be measured in every patient receiving the drug. As discussed previously, dosage schedules should be arranged so that serum samples for lithium measurement are obtained 12 ± 0.5 hours after a dose.[4]

  - Usually this requires administration of the drug every 12 hours for twice-daily dosing.
  - For three-times-a-day dosing, it is necessary to give the drug so that there is a 12-hour time period overnight. Examples of two common dosage schemes are 0900 H, 1500 H, and 2100 H or 0800 H, 1400 H, and 2000 H.

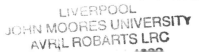

- Upon initiation of therapy, serum concentrations can be measured every 2–3 days for safety reasons in patients who are predisposed to lithium toxicity, even though steady state has not yet been achieved.
- Once the desired steady-state lithium concentration has been achieved, lithium concentrations should be rechecked every 1–2 weeks for approximately 2 months or until concentrations have stabilized.
- Because patients with acute mania can have increased lithium clearance, lithium concentrations should be remeasured in these patients once the manic episode is over and clearance returns to normal. Otherwise, lithium concentrations may accumulate to toxic levels due to the decrease in lithium clearance.
- During lithium maintenance therapy, steady-state lithium serum concentrations should be repeated every 3–6 months. This time period should be altered to every 6–12 months for patients whose mood is stable or every 1–2 months for patients with frequent mood alterations.
- If lithium dosage alterations are needed, or therapy with another drug known to interact with lithium is added, lithium serum concentrations should be measured within 1–2 weeks after the change.

BASIC CLINICAL PHARMACOKINETIC PARAMETERS

- Lithium is eliminated almost completely (>95%) unchanged in the urine.[8] The ion is filtered freely at the glomerulus, and subsequently 60–80% of the amount filtered is reabsorbed by the proximal tubule of the nephron.
- Lithium eliminated in saliva, sweat, and feces accounts for less than 5% of the administered dose.[9]
- On average, lithium clearance is approximately 20% of the patient's creatinine clearance.[9–11]
- Lithium is administered orally as carbonate or citrate salts.

  - Lithium carbonate capsules (150, 300, 600 mg) and tablets (rapid release, 300 mg; sustained release, 300, 450 mg) are available. There are 8.12 mmol (or 8.12 mEq) of lithium in 300 mg of lithium carbonate.
  - Lithium citrate syrup (8 mmol or mEq/5 ml) is another oral dosage form.

- Oral bioavailability is good for all lithium salts and dosage forms and equals 100%.[12,13]
- The peak lithium concentration occurs 15–30 minutes after a dose of lithium citrate syrup, 1–3 hours after a dose of rapid-release lithium carbonate tablets or capsules, and 4–8 hours after a dose of sustained-release lithium carbonate tablets.
- Lithium ion is not plasma protein-bound.
- The typical dose of lithium carbonate is 900–2400 mg/d in adult patients with normal renal function.

EFFECTS OF DISEASE STATES AND CONDITIONS ON LITHIUM PHARMACOKINETICS

- Adults with normal renal function (creatinine clearance >80 ml/min) have an average elimination half-life of 24 hours, volume of distribution of 0.9 L/kg, and clearance of 20 ml/min for lithium.[4–8]
- During an acute manic phase, lithium clearance can increase by as much as 50%, which produces a half-life that is about half the normal value.[14]

- In children 9–12 years of age, average elimination half-life is 18 hours, volume of distribution is 0.9 L/kg, and clearance is 40 ml/min for the ion.[15]
- Because glomerular filtration and creatinine clearance decrease with age, lithium clearance can be decreased in elderly patients, producing half-lives of up to 36 hours.[10,11]
- Because of the circadian rhythm of glomerular filtration, lithium clearance is about 30% higher during daytime hours.[16]

Renal Dysfunction

- Because lithium is eliminated almost exclusively by the kidney, renal dysfunction is the most important disease state that effects lithium pharmacokinetics. Lithium clearance rate decreases in proportion to creatinine clearance.
  - In adults, the lithium clearance/creatinine clearance ratio is 20%, but during a manic phase it increases to about 30%.[10,11,14]
  - The relationship between renal function and lithium clearance forms the basis for the initial dosage computations later in the chapter. Because of the decrease in clearance, the average lithium half-life is 40–50 hours in renal failure patients.

Sodium/Hydration

- The renal clearance of lithium for a patient is influenced by the state of sodium balance and fluid hydration in that individual.
  - Lithium is reabsorbed in the proximal tubule of the nephron via the same mechanisms used to maintain sodium balance.[4] When a patient is in negative sodium balance, the kidney increases sodium reabsorption as a compensatory maneuver and lithium reabsorption increases as a result.
  - The kidney also increases sodium reabsorption when a patient becomes dehydrated, and, again, lithium reabsorption increases.
  - In both cases, increased lithium reabsorption leads to decreased lithium clearance.
- Some common things that cause sodium depletion and/or dehydration include sodium-restricted diets for the treatment of other conditions; vomiting, diarrhea, or fever that might be due to viral or other illnesses; heavy or intense exercise; excessive sweating; use of saunas or hot tubs; and hot weather.
  - Overuse of coffee, tea, soft drinks, or other caffeine-containing liquids and ethanol should be avoided by patients taking lithium.
  - Patients should be advised to maintain adequate fluid intake at all times (2.5–3 L/d) and to increase fluid intake as needed.[1]

Acute Mania

- During periods of acute mania, lithium clearance can be increased by as much as 50%.[14]

Pregnancy/Lactation

- Lithium is generally not used during the first trimester of pregnancy because of possible teratogenic effects on the fetus.[1,9] Due to increased glomerular filtration, lithium clearance may be increased in pregnant women, especially during the third trimester. Lithium crosses the placenta, and human milk concentrations are 30–100% that of concurrent serum concentrations.[17]

Dialysis/Hemofiltration

- Lithium is removed from the body by hemodialysis, peritoneal dialysis, and arteriovenous hemodiafiltration, with clearance values of 30–50 ml/min, 13–15 ml/min, and 21 ml/min, respectively.[9,18,19] The sieving coefficient for lithium during hemofiltration is 0.90. Replacement doses of lithium during dialysis or hemofiltration should be determined using serum concentration monitoring.

DRUG INTERACTIONS

- Many diuretics have drug interactions with lithium.[20]

  - Thiazide diuretics cause sodium and water depletion, which leads to increased sodium reabsorption in the proximal tubule of the kidney as a compensatory mechanism. Since lithium is reabsorbed by the same mechanisms as sodium, lithium reabsorption increases and lithium clearance decreases by 40–50% during treatment with thiazide diuretics.
  - Other diuretics that work at the site of the distal tubule of the kidney may cause a similar interaction with lithium (chlorthalidone, metolazone).
  - Although there are case reports of loop diuretics causing a similar interaction, there are also reports of no drug interaction between lithium and these agents. Because of this, many clinicians favor the use of a loop diuretic, with careful monitoring of adverse effects and lithium serum concentrations, in patients taking lithium.
  - Amiloride has also been reported to have minimal effects on lithium clearance.

- Nonsteroidal anti-inflammatory agents (NSAIDs) also decrease lithium clearance and increase lithium concentrations. The probable mechanism is a NSAID-induced decrease in renal blood flow via inhibition of prostaglandins. Of these agents, sulindac and aspirin appear to have little or no drug interaction with lithium.
- Angiotensin-converting enzyme inhibitors (ACEIs) and angiotensin receptor blockers (ARBs) have been reported to inhibit the elimination of lithium by an undefined mechanism. Of the two classes of drugs, more documentation exists for the ACEIs, for which lithium serum concentrations have increased by as much as 200–300% from pretreatment levels.
- Some serotonin-specific reuptake inhibitors (SSRIs) have been reported to cause a serotonergic hyperarousal syndrome when taken in conjunction with lithium. Case reports of this problem are currently available for fluoxetine, sertraline, and fluvoxamine.

  - In addition to elevated lithium concentrations, patients have developed stiffness of arms and legs, course tremors, dizziness, ataxia, dysarthric speech, and seizures when taking these SSRI agents with lithium. Although there are also literature reports of these combinations used safely, caution should be exercised when concurrent treatment with SSRIs and lithium is indicated.

- Theophylline increases the lithium clearance/creatinine clearance ratio by as much as 58%, resulting in an average decrease of 21% in steady-state lithium concentrations.
- A rare, but severe, drug interaction between lithium and antipsychotic drugs has been reported in which patients are more susceptible to the development

of extrapyramidal symptoms or irreversible brain damage. Although there are reports of using antipsychotic agents and lithium together successfully, patients requiring this combination therapy should be closely monitored for adverse drug reactions.

INITIAL DOSAGE DETERMINATION METHODS

- Several methods to initiate lithium therapy are available.

  - The *pharmacokinetic dosing method* is the most flexible of the techniques. It allows individualized target serum concentrations to be chosen for a patient, and each pharmacokinetic parameter can be customized to reflect specific disease states and conditions present in the patient. However, it is computationally intensive.
  - *Literature-based recommended dosing* is a very commonly used method to prescribe initial doses of lithium. Doses are based on those that commonly produce steady-state concentrations near the lower end of the therapeutic range, although there is a wide variation in the actual concentrations for a specific patient.
  - *Test dose methods* use concentrations measured after one or more lithium test doses to rapidly individualize lithium therapy.

Pharmacokinetic Dosing Method

- The goal of initial dosing of lithium is to compute the best dose possible for the patient given the set of disease states and conditions that influence lithium pharmacokinetics and the type and severity of the bipolar disease. In order to do this, pharmacokinetic parameters for the patient are estimated using average parameters measured in other patients with similar disease state and condition profiles.

Clearance Estimate

- Lithium ion is eliminated almost totally unchanged in the urine, and there is a consistent relationship between lithium clearance and creatinine clearance, with a ratio of 20% between the two (lithium clearance/creatinine clearance).[9–11]

  - This relationship allows estimation of lithium clearance for a patient, which can be used to compute an initial dose of the drug. Mathematically, the equation for the straight line shown in Figure 17-2 is

$$Cl = 0.2(CrCl)$$

  where Cl is lithium clearance in ml/min and CrCl is creatinine clearance in ml/min.

- For dosing purposes, it is more useful to have lithium clearance expressed in L/d. The equation converted to these units is

$$Cl = 0.288(CrCl)$$

  where Cl is lithium clearance in L/d and CrCl is creatinine clearance in ml/min.
- For patients with acute mania, lithium clearance is increased by about 50%, and the corresponding equation for these individuals is

$$Cl = 0.432(CrCl)$$

  where Cl is lithium clearance in L/d and CrCl is creatinine clearance in ml/min.[14]

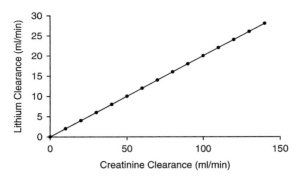

FIG. 17-2 The ratio between lithium clearance and creatinine clearance is 0.2 for patients requiring maintenance therapy with lithium. This relationship is used to estimate lithium clearance for patients requiring initial dosing with the drug.

Selection of Appropriate Pharmacokinetic Model and Equation

- When lithium is given orally, it follows a two-compartment model (Figure 17-1).[4-8]
- After the peak concentration is achieved, serum concentrations drop rapidly because of distribution of drug from blood to tissues (α or distribution phase). By 6–10 hours after administration of the drug, lithium concentrations decline more slowly, and the elimination rate constant for this segment of the concentration/time curve is the one that varies with renal function (β or elimination phase).
- While this model is the most correct from a strict pharmacokinetic viewpoint, it cannot easily be used clinically because of its mathematical complexity. During the elimination phase of the concentration/time curve, lithium serum concentrations drop very slowly due to the long elimination half-life (24 hours with normal renal function, up to 50 hours with end-stage renal disease).

  - As a result, a simple pharmacokinetic equation that computes the average lithium steady-state serum concentration (Css in mmol/L = mEq/L) is widely used and allows maintenance dosage calculation:

  $$Css = [F(D/\tau)]/Cl \qquad or \qquad D/\tau = (Css \cdot Cl)/F$$

  where F is the bioavailability fraction for the oral dosage form (F = 1 for oral lithium), D is the lithium dose in mmoles, τ is the dosage interval in days, and Cl is lithium clearance in L/d.
  - Because this equation computes lithium ion requirement and lithium carbonate doses are prescribed in mg, the ratio of lithium ion content to lithium carbonate salt (8.12 mmol Li$^+$/300 mg lithium carbonate) is used to convert the result from this equation into a lithium carbonate dose.

- Total daily amounts of lithium are usually given as near-equally divided doses twice or three times a day; single doses above 1200 mg/d of lithium carbonate are usually not given in order to avoid gastrointestinal upset.

Steady-State Concentration Selection

- Lithium serum concentrations are selected based on the presence or absence of acute mania and titrated to response.[3]

  - For individuals with acute mania, a minimum lithium concentration of 0.8 mmol/L is usually recommended. The usual desired range for these individuals is 0.8–1 mmol/L. If patients with acute mania do not respond to these levels, it may be necessary to use lithium concentrations of 1–1.2 mmol/L and in some instances concentrations as high as 1.2–1.5 mmol/L.
  - For long-term maintenance use, the usual desired range is 0.6–0.8 mmol/L. If patients do not respond to these levels during maintenance treatment, lithium concentrations of 0.9–1 mmol/L may be required, and in some cases concentrations as high as 1–1.2 mmol/L are necessary to gain an adequate outcome.

▶ ***Example 1***   MJ is a 50-year-old, 70-kg (height = 5′10″) male with bipolar disease. He is not currently experiencing an episode of acute mania. His serum creatinine is 0.9 mg/dl. Compute an oral lithium dose for this patient for maintenance therapy.

1. *Estimate creatinine clearance.* This patient has stable serum creatinine and is not obese. The Cockcroft-Gault equation can be used to estimate creatinine clearance:

$$CrCl_{est} = \frac{(140 - age)BW}{72 \cdot S_{Cr}} = \frac{(140 - 50\,y)70\,kg}{72 \cdot 0.9\,mg/dl}$$
$$CrCl_{est} = 97\,ml/min$$

2. *Estimate clearance.* The drug clearance/creatinine clearance relationship is used to estimate the lithium clearance for this patient:

$$Cl = 0.288(CrCl) = 0.288(97\,ml/min) = 27.9\,L/d$$

3. *Use the average steady-state concentration equation to compute a lithium maintenance dose.* For a patient requiring maintenance therapy for bipolar disease, the desired lithium concentration is 0.6–0.8 mmol/L. A serum concentration of 0.6 mmol/L will be chosen for this patient, and oral lithium carbonate will be used (F = 1, 8.12 mmol Li^+/300 mg of lithium carbonate).

$$D/\tau = (Css \cdot Cl)/F = (0.6\,mmol/L \cdot 27.9\,L/d)/1 = 16.7\,mmol/d$$
$$D/\tau = (300\,mg\,lithium\,carbonate/8.12\,mmol\,Li^+)16.7\,mmol/d$$
$$= 617\,mg/d,\,rounded\,to\,600\,mg/d$$

This dose would be given as 300 mg of lithium carbonate every 12 hours.

Upon initiation of therapy, serum concentrations can be measured every 2–3 days for safety reasons in patients who are predisposed to lithium toxicity, even though steady state has not yet been achieved. Once the desired steady-state lithium concentration has been achieved, lithium concentrations should be rechecked every 1–2 weeks for approximately 2 months or until concentrations have stabilized.

▶ *Example 2*   Same patient profile as in Example 1, but serum creatinine is 3.5 mg/dl, indicating renal impairment.

1. *Estimate creatinine clearance.* This patient has stable serum creatinine and is not obese. The Cockcroft-Gault equation can be used to estimate creatinine clearance:

$$CrCl_{est} = \frac{(140 - age)BW}{72 \cdot S_{Cr}} = \frac{(140 - 50\,y)70\text{ kg}}{72 \cdot 3.5\text{ mg/dl}}$$

$$CrCl_{est} = 25\text{ ml/min}$$

2. *Estimate clearance.* The drug clearance/creatinine clearance relationship is used to estimate the lithium clearance for this patient:

$$Cl = 0.288(CrCl) = 0.288(25\text{ ml/min}) = 7.2\text{ L/d}$$

3. *Use the average steady-state concentration equation to compute a lithium maintenance dose.* For a patient requiring maintenance therapy for bipolar disease, the desired lithium concentration is 0.6–0.8 mmol/L. A serum concentration of 0.6 mmol/L will be chosen for this patient, and oral lithium carbonate will be used (F = 1, 8.12 mmol Li^+/300 mg of lithium carbonate).

$$D/\tau = (Css \cdot Cl)/F = (0.6\text{ mmol/L} \cdot 7.2\text{ L/d})/1 = 4.3\text{ mmol/d}$$

$$D/\tau = (300\text{ mg lithium carbonate/8.12 mmol } Li^+)\,4.3\text{ mmol/d}$$

$$= 159\text{ mg/d, rounded to 150 mg/d}$$

This dose would be given as 150 mg of lithium carbonate daily.

Upon initiation of therapy, serum concentrations can be measured every 2–3 days for safety reasons in patients who are predisposed to lithium toxicity, even though steady state has not yet been achieved. Once the desired steady-state lithium concentration has been achieved, lithium concentrations should be rechecked every 1–2 weeks for approximately 2 months or until concentrations have stabilized.

▶ *Example 3*   Same patient profile as in Example 1, but serum creatinine is 0.9 mg/dl, and the patient is being treated for acute mania. Compute an oral lithium carbonate dose for this patient.

1. *Estimate creatinine clearance.* This patient has stable serum creatinine and is not obese. The Cockcroft-Gault equation can be used to estimate creatinine clearance:

$$CrCl_{est} = \frac{(140 - age)BW}{72 \cdot S_{Cr}} = \frac{(140 - 50\,y)70\text{ kg}}{72 \cdot 0.9\text{ mg/dl}}$$

$$CrCl_{est} = 97\text{ ml/min}$$

2. *Estimate clearance.* The drug clearance/creatinine clearance relationship is used to estimate the lithium clearance for this patient:

$$Cl = 0.432(CrCl) = 0.432(97\text{ ml/min}) = 41.9\text{ L/d}$$

3. *Use the average steady-state concentration equation to compute a lithium maintenance dose.* For a patient requiring therapy for the acute manic

phase of bipolar disease, the desired lithium concentration is 0.8 mmol/L. Oral lithium carbonate will be used (F = 1, 8.12 mmol Li^+/300 mg of lithium carbonate).

$$D/\tau = (Css \cdot Cl)/F = (0.8 \text{ mmol/L} \cdot 41.9 \text{ L/d})/1 = 33.5 \text{ mmol/d}$$

$$D/\tau = (300 \text{ mg lithium carbonate}/8.12 \text{ mmol } Li^+)33.5 \text{ mmol/d}$$

$$= 1238 \text{ mg/d, rounded to } 1200 \text{ mg/d}$$

This dose would be given as 600 mg of lithium carbonate every 12 hours.

Upon initiation of therapy, serum concentrations can be measured every 2–3 days for safety reasons in patients who are predisposed to lithium toxicity, even though steady state has not yet been achieved. Once the desired steady-state lithium concentration has been achieved, lithium concentrations should be rechecked every 1–2 weeks for approximately 2 months or until concentrations have stabilized. Because patients with acute mania can have increased lithium clearance, lithium concentrations should be remeasured in these patients once the manic episode is over and clearance returns to normal.

Literature-Based Recommended Dosing

- Because of the large amount of variability in lithium pharmacokinetics, even when concurrent disease states and conditions are identified, many clinicians believe that the use of standard lithium doses for various situations is warranted. The original computations of these doses was based on the pharmacokinetic dosing method described in the previous section, and the doses were subsequently modified based on clinical experience.

  - For the treatment of acute mania, initial doses are usually 900–1200 mg/d of lithium carbonate.[1,9]
  - If the drug is being used for bipolar disease prophylaxis, an initial dose of 600 mg/d lithium carbonate is recommended.[1,9]
  - In both cases, the total daily dose is given in 2–3 divided daily doses.
  - To avoid adverse side effects, lithium doses are slowly increased by 300–600 mg/d every 2–3 days according to clinical response and lithium serum concentrations.

- Renal dysfunction is the major condition that alters lithium pharmacokinetics and dosage.[21–24]

  - If creatinine clearance is 10–50 ml/min, the prescribed initial dose is 50–75% of that recommended for patients with normal renal function.
  - For creatinine clearance values below 10 ml/min, the prescribed dose should be 25–50% of the usual dose in patients with good renal function.

- Zetin and associates have developed a multiple-regression equation that computes lithium carbonate doses for patients based on hospitalization status, age, gender, and weight of the patient as well as the presence or absence of concurrent tricyclic use by the patient.[25,26] However, since renal function was not assessed as an independent parameter in their study population, this dosage method is not presented.

- To illustrate the similarities and differences between this method of initial dosage calculation and the pharmacokinetic dosing method, the same examples used in the previous section will be used.

▶ *Example 4*   MJ is a 50-year-old, 70-kg (height = 5′10″) male with bipolar disease. He is not currently experiencing an episode of acute mania. His serum creatinine is 0.9 mg/dl. Recommend an oral lithium dose for this patient for maintenance therapy.

1. *Estimate creatinine clearance.* This patient has stable serum creatinine and is not obese. The Cockcroft-Gault equation can be used to estimate creatinine clearance:

$$CrCl_{est} = \frac{(140 - age)BW}{72 \cdot S_{Cr}} = \frac{(140 - 50 \text{ y})70 \text{ kg}}{72 \cdot 0.9 \text{ mg/dl}}$$

$$CrCl_{est} = 97 \text{ ml/min}$$

2. *Choose a lithium dose based on disease states and conditions present in the patient.* The patient requires prophylactic lithium therapy for bipolar disease, and he has good renal function. A lithium carbonate dose of 600 mg/d, given as 300 mg every 12 hours, is recommended as the initial dose. The dosage rate will be increased 300–600 mg/d every 2–3 days as needed to provide adequate therapeutic effect, avoid adverse effects, and produce therapeutic lithium steady-state concentrations.

▶ *Example 5*   Same patient profile as in Example 4, but serum creatinine is 3.5 mg/dl indicating renal impairment.

1. *Estimate creatinine clearance.* This patient has stable serum creatinine and is not obese. The Cockcroft-Gault equation can be used to estimate creatinine clearance:

$$CrCl_{est} = \frac{(140 - age)BW}{72 \cdot S_{Cr}} = \frac{(140 - 50 \text{ y})70 \text{ kg}}{72 \cdot 3.5 \text{ mg/dl}}$$

$$CrCl_{est} = 25 \text{ ml/min}$$

2. *Choose a lithium dose based on disease states and conditions present in the patient.* The patient requires prophylactic lithium therapy for bipolar disease, and he has moderate renal function. With an estimated creatinine clearance of 25 ml/min, lithium carbonate doses should be 50–75% of the usual amount. A lithium carbonate dose of 300 mg/d, given as 150 mg every 12 hours, is recommended as the initial dose. The dosage rate will be increased 150–300 mg/d every 5–7 days as needed to provide adequate therapeutic effect, avoid adverse effects, and produce therapeutic lithium steady-state concentrations.

▶ *Example 6*   Same patient profile as in Example 4, but serum creatinine is 0.9 mg/dl, and the patient is being treated for the acute mania phase of bipolar disease. Compute an oral lithium carbonate dose for this patient.

1. *Estimate creatinine clearance.* This patient has stable serum creatinine and is not obese. The Cockcroft-Gault equation can be used to estimate creatinine clearance:

$$CrCl_{est} = \frac{(140 - age)BW}{72 \cdot S_{Cr}} = \frac{(140 - 50 \text{ y})70 \text{ kg}}{72 \cdot 0.9 \text{ mg/dl}}$$

$$CrCl_{est} = 97 \text{ ml/min}$$

2. *Choose a lithium dose based on disease states and conditions present in the patient.* The patient requires lithium therapy for acute mania, and he has good renal function. A lithium carbonate dose of 900 mg/d, given as 300 mg at 0800 H, 1400 H, and 2000 H, is recommended as the initial dose. The dosage rate will be increased 300–600 mg/d every 2–3 days as needed to provide adequate therapeutic effect, avoid adverse effects, and produce therapeutic lithium steady-state concentrations.

Test Dose Methods to Assess Initial Lithium Dosage Requirements

- Several methods to assess initial lithium dosage requirement using one or more lithium test doses and one or more lithium serum concentrations are available for clinical use. These methods can be used to rapidly individualize lithium maintenance doses to achieve desired steady-state concentrations.

Cooper Nomogram

- The Cooper nomogram for lithium maintenance dosage assessment requires the administration of a single test dose of 600 mg of lithium carbonate and a single lithium serum concentration measured 24 hours later.[27,28]
- The 24-hour lithium serum concentration is compared to a table that converts the observed concentration into the lithium carbonate dose required to produced a steady-state lithium concentration between 0.6 and 1.2 mmol/L (Table 17-1).

TABLE 17-1 Cooper Nomogram for Lithium Dosing[27,28]
Lithium carbonate dosage required to produce steady-state lithium serum concentrations between 0.6–1.2 mmol/L[a]

Lithium serum concentration 24 h after the test dose (mmol/L)	Lithium carbonate dosage requirement[b]
<0.05	1200 mg three times daily (3600 mg/d)[c]
0.05–0.09	900 mg three times daily (2700 mg/d)
0.10–0.14	600 mg three times daily (1800 mg/d)
0.15–0.19	300 mg four times daily (1200 mg/d)
0.20–0.23	300 mg three times daily (900 mg/d)
0.24–0.30	300 mg twice daily (600 mg/d)
>0.30	300 mg twice daily[d] (600 mg/d)

[a]Lithium dosage requirements should be reassessed with changes in clinical status (mania versus maintenance treatment), renal function, or other factors that alter lithium pharmacokinetics.
[b]Dosage schedule determined to provide minimum fluctuation in lithium serum concentration and maximum patient compliance. A change in dosage interval can be made by the prescribing clinician, but the total daily dose should remain the same.
[c]Use extreme caution. Patient appears to have an increased clearance and short half-life for lithium, which would require large lithium carbonate maintenance doses. However, this large of a maintenance dose requires careful patient monitoring for response and adverse side effects.
[d]Use extreme caution. Patient appears to have a reduced clearance and long half-life for lithium, and may accumulate steady-state lithium concentrations above the therapeutic range.

- The theoretical basis for this dosage approach lies in the relationship between the serum concentration of a drug obtained about 1 half-life after dosage and the elimination rate constant for the drug in a patient.
- This nomogram can also be expressed as an equation for the total daily lithium dosage requirement (D in mmol/d):

$$D = e^{(4.80-7.5C_{test})}$$

where C_{test} is the 24-hour postdose lithium concentration for a 600-mg lithium carbonate dose.[9]

- Perry and associates have suggested a similar nomogram that employs a larger test dose of 1200 mg of lithium carbonate.[29,30]

- An important requirement for these methods is an accurate lithium assay that can reproducibly measure the lithium concentrations that occur after a single dose of the drug. Additionally, at the time the lithium carbonate test dose is given, the lithium serum concentration in the patient must be zero.

▸ *Example 7*　　LK is a 47-year-old, 65-kg (height = 5′5″) female with bipolar disease. She is not currently experiencing an episode of acute mania. Her serum creatinine is 0.9 mg/dl. Compute an oral lithium dose for this patient during maintenance therapy using the Cooper nomogram.

1. *Administer a 600-mg lithium carbonate test dose and measure 24-hour postdose lithium concentration. Use the Cooper nomogram to recommend a lithium carbonate maintenance dose.* After the test dose was given, the 24-hour lithium concentration was 0.12 mmol/L. The recommended lithium carbonate dose maintenance dose is 600 mg three times daily. The doses will be given at 0900 H, 1500 H, and 2100 H to allow a 12-hour window after the evening dose so that lithium serum concentration measurements can be made.

   Upon initiation of therapy, serum concentrations can be measured every 2–3 days for safety reasons in patients who are predisposed to lithium toxicity, even though steady state has not yet been achieved. Once the desired steady-state lithium concentration has been achieved, lithium concentrations should be rechecked every 1–2 weeks for approximately 2 months or until concentrations have stabilized. Because patients with acute mania can have increased lithium clearance, lithium concentrations should be remeasured in these patients once the manic episode is over and clearance returns to normal.

Perry Method

- The Perry method conducts a small pharmacokinetic experiment in a patient after the administration of a lithium carbonate test dose.[31]

  - First, a test dose (600–1500 mg) of lithium carbonate is given to the patient. Then, lithium serum concentrations are measured 12 and 36 hours after the test dose was given.
  - The two lithium concentrations are used to compute the elimination rate constant for the individual:

$$k_e = (\ln C_{12\,h} - \ln C_{36\,h})/\Delta t$$

where k_e is the elimination rate constant in h^{-1} for lithium, $C_{12\,h}$ and $C_{36\,h}$ are the lithium concentrations in mmol/L (or mEq/L) at 12 and 36 hours, respectively, after the test dose was given, and Δt is the difference between times (24 hours) that the two serum concentrations were obtained.

- With knowledge of the elimination rate constant (k_e), the accumulation ratio (R) can be computed for any dosage interval:

$$R = 1/(1 - e^{-k_e \tau})$$

where τ is the dosage interval in hours. The accumulation ratio (R) is also equal to the ratio of the concentration at any time, t, after a single dose ($C_{SD,t}$ in mmol/L) and the steady-state concentration at that same time after the dose during multiple dosing (Css_t in mmol/L):

$$R = Css_t/C_{SD,t} \qquad \text{or} \qquad Css_t = R \cdot C_{SD,t}$$

- Once a steady-state concentration can be computed for a dosage regimen, linear pharmacokinetic principles can be used to compute the dose required to achieve a target lithium steady-state serum concentration:

$$D_{new} = (Css_{new}/Css_{old})D_{old}$$

where D is the dose, Css is the steady-state concentration, old indicates the dose that produced the steady-state concentration the patient is currently receiving, and new denotes the dose necessary to produce the desired steady-state concentration.

- As with the Cooper nomogram, the lithium serum concentration must be zero before the test dose is administered.

▶ **Example 8**   HG is a 32-year-old, 58-kg (height = 5′1″) female with bipolar disease. She is not currently experiencing an episode of acute mania. Her serum creatinine is 0.9 mg/dl. A single test dose of lithium (1200 mg) was given to the patient, and lithium concentrations were measured as 0.6 mmol/L and 0.3 mmol/L at 12 hours and 36 hours, respectively, after the drug was given. Compute an oral lithium dose for this patient which will produce a steady-state serum concentration of 0.8 mmol/L using the Perry method.

1. *Administer a lithium carbonate test dose and measure 12- and 36-hour postdose lithium concentrations. Compute the lithium elimination rate constant and accumulation ratio for the patient.* The lithium elimination rate constant is computed using the two serum concentrations:

$$k_e = (\ln C_{12\,h} - \ln C_{36\,h})/\Delta t$$
$$= [\ln(0.6\ \text{mmol/L}) - \ln(0.3\ \text{mmol/L})]/24\ h = 0.0289\ h^{-1}$$

The lithium accumulation ratio is computed using the elimination rate constant and desired lithium dosage interval of 12 hours:

$$R = 1/(1 - e^{-k_e \tau}) = 1/(1 - e^{-(0.0289\ h^{-1})(12\ h)}) = 3.4$$

2. *Compute the estimated lithium concentration at steady state for the test dose that was given. Use this relationship to compute the dosage regimen for the patient.* Using the lithium concentration at 12 hours, the steady-state lithium concentration for 1200 mg every 12 hours can be computed:

$$Css_t = R \cdot C_{SD,t} = 3.4 \cdot 0.6\ \text{mmol/L} = 2.0\ \text{mmol/L}$$

Linear pharmacokinetic principles can be used to compute the dose required to achieve the target lithium steady-state serum concentration:

$$D_{new} = [(0.8\ \text{mmol/L})/(2\ \text{mmol/L})](1200\ \text{mg}) = 480\ \text{mg}$$

This dose should be rounded to 450 mg of lithium carbonate every 12 hours.

Upon initiation of therapy, serum concentrations can be measured every 2–3 days for safety reasons in patients who are predisposed to lithium toxicity, even though steady state has not yet been achieved. Once the desired steady-state lithium concentration has been achieved, lithium concentrations should be rechecked every 1–2 weeks for approximately 2 months or until concentrations have stabilized. Because patients with acute mania can have increased lithium clearance, lithium concentrations should be remeasured in these patients once the manic episode is over and clearance returns to normal.

Repeated One-Point or Ritschel Method

- The method to individualize lithium dose proposed by Ritschel and associates utilizes another way to compute the elimination rate constant for a patient.[32,33]
- In this case, two equal lithium doses are administered apart from each other by the desired dosage interval (usually 12 hours). A single serum concentration is obtained before the second test dose is given and another is gathered after the second dose is given at a time equaling the anticipated dosage interval.
- These values are used to compute the elimination rate constant (k_e in h^{-1}) for the patient:

$$k_e = \frac{\ln[C_1/(C_2 - C_1)]}{\tau}$$

where C_1 is the lithium concentration in mmol/L obtained after the first test dose, C_2 is the lithium concentration in mmol/L obtained after the second test dose, and τ is the expected dosage interval in hours for lithium dosing and is also the postdose time at which the lithium concentrations were obtained.

- With knowledge of the elimination rate constant (k_e), the accumulation ratio (R) can be computed for the dosage interval:

$$R = 1/(1 - e^{-k_e \tau})$$

where τ is the dosage interval in hours.

- The accumulation ratio (R) is also equal to the ratio of the concentration at any time, t, after a single dose ($C_{SD,t}$ in mmol/L) and the steady-state concentration at that same time after the dose is administered as multiple doses (Css_t in mmol/L):

$$R = Css_t/C_{SD,t} \qquad \text{or} \qquad Css_t = R \cdot C_{SD,t}$$

- Once a steady-state concentration can be computed for a dosage regimen, linear pharmacokinetic principles can be used to compute the dose required to achieve a target lithium steady-state serum concentration:

$$D_{new} = (Css_{new}/Css_{old})D_{old}$$

where D is the dose, Css is the steady-state peak or trough concentration, old indicates the dose that produced the steady-state concentration the patient is currently receiving, and new denotes the dose necessary to produce the desired steady-state concentration.

- As with the Cooper and Perry methods, the lithium serum concentration must be zero before the test dose is administered.

▶ **Example 9** CB is a 27-year-old, 75-kg (height = 6′2″) male with bipolar disease. He is currently experiencing an episode of acute mania. His serum creatinine is 1.0 mg/dl. Two test doses of lithium (600 mg each, 12 hours apart) were given to the patient, and lithium concentrations were measured as 0.3 mmol/L and 0.5 mmol/L 12 hours after the first and second doses, respectively. Compute an oral lithium dose for this patient which will produce a steady-state serum concentration of 1.2 mmol/L using the Ritschel repeated one-point method.

1. *Administer lithium carbonate test doses and measure lithium concentrations. Compute the lithium elimination rate constant and accumulation ratio for the patient.* The lithium elimination rate constant is computed using the two serum concentrations:

$$k_e = \frac{\ln[C_1/(C_2 - C_1)]}{\tau} = \frac{\ln[(0.3 \text{ mmol/L})/(0.5 \text{ mmol/L} - 0.3 \text{ mmol/L})]}{12 \text{ h}}$$
$$= 0.0338 \text{ h}^{-1}$$

The lithium accumulation ratio is computed using the elimination rate constant and desired lithium dosage interval of 12 hours: $R = 1/(1 - e^{-k_e \tau}) = 1/(1 - e^{-(0.0338 \text{ h}^{-1})(12 \text{ h})}) = 3.0$

2. *Compute the estimated lithium concentration at steady state for the test dose that was given. Use this relationship to compute the dosage regimen for the patient.* Using the lithium concentration at 12 hours, the steady-state lithium concentration for 600 mg every 12 hours can be computed:

$$Css_t = R \cdot C_{SD,t} = 3.0 \cdot 0.3 \text{ mmol/L} = 0.9 \text{ mmol/L}$$

Linear pharmacokinetic principles can be used to compute the dose required to achieve the target lithium steady-state serum concentration:

$$D_{new} = [(1.2 \text{ mmol/L})/(0.9 \text{ mmol/L})](600 \text{ mg}) = 800 \text{ mg}$$

This dose is rounded to 900 mg of lithium carbonate every 12 hours.

Upon initiation of therapy, serum concentrations can be measured every 2–3 days for safety reasons in patients who are predisposed to lithium toxicity, even though steady state has not yet been achieved. Once the desired steady-state lithium concentration has been achieved, lithium concentrations should be rechecked every 1–2 weeks for approximately 2 months or until concentrations have stabilized. Because patients with acute mania can have increased lithium clearance, lithium concentrations should be remeasured in these patients once the manic episode is over and clearance returns to normal.

USE OF LITHIUM SERUM CONCENTRATIONS TO ALTER DOSAGES

- Because of pharmacokinetic variability among patients, it is likely that doses computed using patient population characteristics will not always produce lithium serum concentrations that are expected. Therefore, lithium serum concentrations are measured in all patients, to ensure that therapeutic, nontoxic levels are present.
- Important patient parameters should be followed to confirm that the patient is responding to treatment and not developing adverse drug reactions.
- When lithium serum concentrations are measured in patients and a dosage change is necessary, clinicians should use the simplest, most straightforward method available to determine a dose that will provide safe and effective treatment.

  - In most cases a simple dosage ratio can be used to change lithium doses, since this drug follows *linear pharmacokinetics*.
  - Computerized methods that incorporate expected population pharmacokinetic characteristics (*Bayesian pharmacokinetic computer programs*) can

be used in difficult cases, when renal function is changing, serum concentrations are obtained at suboptimal times, or the patient was not at steady state when serum concentrations were measured.

Linear Pharmacokinetics Method

- Because lithium follows linear, dose-proportional pharmacokinetics, steady-state serum concentrations change in proportion to dose according to the following equation:

$$D_{new}/Css_{new} = D_{old}/Css_{old} \quad \text{or} \quad D_{new} = (Css_{new}/Css_{old})D_{old}$$

where D is the dose, Css is the steady-state peak or trough concentration, old indicates the dose that produced the steady-state concentration the patient is currently receiving, and new denotes the dose necessary to produce the desired steady-state concentration.
- The main advantage of this method is that it is quick and simple.
- The principal disadvantage is that steady-state concentrations are required.

▶ ***Example 10*** YC is a 37-year-old, 55-kg (height = 5′1″) female with bipolar disease. She is currently not experiencing an episode of acute mania and she requires prophylactic treatment with lithium. Her serum creatinine is 0.6 mg/dl. The patient is receiving 900 mg of lithium carbonate at 0800 H, 1400 H, and 2000 H, and her 12-hour postdose steady-state lithium serum concentration is 1.1 mmol/L. Compute a new lithium dose to achieve a steady-state concentration of 0.6 mmol/L.

1. *Compute a new dose to achieve the desired serum concentration.* Using linear pharmacokinetics, the new dose to attain the desired concentration should be proportional to the old dose (2700 mg/d) that produced the measured concentration:

$$D_{new} = (Css_{new}/Css_{old})D_{old} = [(0.6 \text{ mmol/L})/(1.1 \text{ mmol/L})](2700 \text{ mg/d})$$

$$= 1473 \text{ mg/d, round to } 1500 \text{ mg/d}$$

The patient should be administered 600 mg of lithium carbonate at 0800 H and 2000 H, and 300 mg of lithium carbonate at 1400 H.

When lithium dosage alterations are needed, lithium serum concentrations should be measured within 1–2 weeks after the change. During lithium maintenance therapy, steady-state lithium serum concentrations should be repeated every 3–6 months. This time period should be altered to every 6–12 months for patients whose mood is stable or to every 1–2 months for patients with frequent mood alterations.

BAYESIAN PHARMACOKINETIC COMPUTER PROGRAMS

- Computer programs are available that can assist in the computation of pharmacokinetic parameters for patients.[14] The most reliable computer programs use a nonlinear regression algorithm that incorporates components of Bayes' theorem.
- An advantage of this approach is that consistent dosage recommendations can be made when several different practitioners are involved in therapeutic drug monitoring programs. However, since simpler dosing methods work just as well for patients with stable pharmacokinetic parameters and steady-state drug concentrations, many clinicians reserve the use of computer programs for more difficult situations.

- Those situations include serum concentrations that are not at steady state, serum concentrations not obtained at the specific times needed to employ simpler methods, and unstable pharmacokinetic parameters.
- When only a limited number of lithium steady-state concentrations are available, Bayesian pharmacokinetic computer programs can be used to compute a complete patient pharmacokinetic profile that includes clearance, volume of distribution, and half-life.

- Many Bayesian pharmacokinetic computer programs are available, and most should provide answers similar to the program used in the following examples. The program used to solve problems in this book is DrugCalc, written by Dr. Dennis Mungall and available at his Internet web site (www.clinpharmacologist.bigstep.com/consumersurvey.html).[34]
- For comparison purposes, three cases presented previously using other dosage determination methods are managed using a Bayesian pharmacokinetic computer program.

▶ *Example 11* YC is a 37-year-old, 55-kg (height = 5′1″) female with bipolar disease. She is currently not experiencing an episode of acute mania, and she requires prophylactic treatment with lithium. Her serum creatinine is 0.6 mg/dl. The patient is receiving 900 mg of lithium carbonate at 0800 H, 1400 H, and 2000 H, and her steady-state lithium serum concentration is 1.1 mmol/L. Compute a new lithium dose to achieve a steady-state concentration of 0.6 mmol/L.

1. *Enter patient demographic, drug dosing, and serum concentration/time data into a Bayesian pharmacokinetic computer program.* Lithium doses must be entered into DrugCalc as mmoles of lithium ion. Thus, 900 mg of lithium carbonate provides 24.4 mmol of lithium ion: 900 mg (8.12 mmol Li^+/300 mg lithium carbonate) = 24.4 mmol Li^+.
2. *Compute pharmacokinetic parameters for the patient using the computer program.* The pharmacokinetic parameters computed by the program are a volume of distribution of 38 L, a half-life of 17.9 hours, and a clearance of 1.48 L/h.
3. *Compute the dose required to achieve desired lithium serum concentrations.* The one-compartment first-order absorption equation used by the program to compute doses indicates that a dose of 13 mmol Li^+ every 12 hours will produce a steady-state concentration of 0.6 mmol/L. This dose is equivalent to 480 mg of lithium carbonate [13 mmol(300 mg lithium carbonate/8.12 mmol Li^+) = 480 mg lithium carbonate]. Rounding this dose to an amount available as an oral dosage form, 450 mg of lithium carbonate would be given every 12 hours.

▶ *Example 12* LK is a 47-year-old, 65-kg (height = 5′5″) female with bipolar disease. She is not currently experiencing an episode of acute mania. Her serum creatinine is 0.9 mg/dl. After a test dose of 600 mg of lithium carbonate was given, the 24-hour lithium concentration was 0.12 mmol/L. Compute an oral lithium dose for this patient for maintenance therapy that will achieve a steady-state concentration of 0.6 mmol/L.

1. *Enter patient demographic, drug dosing, and serum concentration/time data into a Bayesian pharmacokinetic computer program.* Lithium doses must be entered into DrugCalc as mmoles of lithium ion. Thus, 600 mg of lithium carbonate provides 16.2 mmol of lithium ion: 600 mg (8.12 mmol Li^+/300 mg lithium carbonate) = 16.2 mmol Li^+.

2. *Compute pharmacokinetic parameters for the patient using the computer program.* The pharmacokinetic parameters computed by the program are a volume of distribution of 77 L, a half-life of 38 hours, and a clearance of 1.42 L/h.

3. *Compute the dose required to achieve desired lithium serum concentrations.* The one-compartment first-order absorption equation used by the program to compute doses indicates that a dose of 10 mmol Li^+ every 8 hours will produce a steady-state concentration of 0.8 mmol/L. This dose is equivalent to 369 mg of lithium carbonate [10 mmol(300 mg lithium carbonate/8.12 mmol Li^+) = 369 mg lithium carbonate]. Rounding this dose to an amount available as an oral dosage form, 300 mg of lithium carbonate would be given three times daily, at 0800 H, 1400 H, and 2000 H, to provide a 12-hour window for serum concentration monitoring after the evening dose.

▶ *Example 13*   CB is a 27-year-old, 75-kg (height = 6′2″) male with bipolar disease. He is currently experiencing an episode of acute mania. His serum creatinine is 1.0 mg/dl. Two test doses of lithium (600 mg each) were given to the patient at 0800 H and 2000 H, and lithium concentrations were measured as 0.3 mmol/L and 0.5 mmol/L 12 hours after the first and second doses, respectively. Compute an oral lithium dose for this patient which will produce a steady-state serum concentration of 1.2 mmol/L.

1. *Enter patient demographic, drug dosing, and serum concentration/time data into a Bayesian pharmacokinetic computer program.* Lithium doses must be entered into DrugCalc as mmoles of lithium ion. Thus, 600 mg of lithium carbonate provides 16.2 mmol of lithium ion: 600 mg (8.12 mmol Li^+/300 mg lithium carbonate) = 16.2 mmol Li^+.

2. *Compute the pharmacokinetic parameters for the patient using the computer program.* The pharmacokinetic parameters computed by the program are a volume of distribution of 38 L, a half-life of 19.2 hours, and a clearance of 1.37 L/h.

3. *Compute the dose required to achieve desired lithium serum concentrations.* The one-compartment first-order absorption equation used by the program to compute doses indicates that a dose of 22 mmol Li^+ every 12 hours will produce a steady-state concentration of 1.2 mmol/L. This dose is equivalent to 813 mg of lithium carbonate [22 mmol(300 mg lithium carbonate/8.12 mmol Li^+) = 813 mg lithium carbonate]. Rounding this dose to an amount available as an oral dosage form, 900 mg of lithium carbonate would be given every 12 hours.

When lithium dosage alterations are needed, lithium serum concentrations should be measured within 1–2 weeks after the change. During lithium maintenance therapy, steady-state lithium serum concentrations should be repeated every 3–6 months. This time period should be altered to every 6–12 months for patients whose mood is stable or to every 1–2 months for patients with frequent mood alterations.

DOSING STRATEGIES

• Initial dose and dosage adjustment techniques using serum concentrations can be used in any combination as long as the limitations of each method are observed.

• Some dosing schemes link together logically when considered according to their basic approaches or philosophies. Dosage strategies that follow similar pathways are given in Table 17-2.

TABLE 17-2 Dosing Strategies

Dosing approach/ philosophy	Initial dosing	Use of serum concentrations to alter doses
Pharmacokinetic parameters/ equations	Pharmacokinetic dosing method	Linear pharmacokinetic method
Literature-based concepts	Literature-based recommended dosing method	Linear pharmacokinetics method
Test dose	Cooper nomogram or Perry method or Repeated one-point method	Linear pharmacokinetics method
Computerized	Bayesian computer program	Bayesian computer program

REFERENCES

1. Fankhauser MP. Bipolar disorder. In: DiPiro JT, Talbert RL, Yee GC, Matzke GR, Wells BG, Posey LM, eds. Pharmacotherapy. 5th ed. New York: McGraw-Hill, 2002:1265–88.
2. Baldessarini RJ, Tarazi FI. Drugs and the treatment of psychiatric disorders—depression and mania. In: Hardman JG, Limbird LE, Gilman AG, eds. The pharmacological basis of therapeutics. 10th ed. New York: McGraw-Hill, 2001: 485–520.
3. Weber SS, Saklad SR, Kastenholz KV. Bipolar affective disorders. In: Koda-Kimble M-A, Young LY, Kradjan WA, Guglielmo BJ, eds. Applied therapeutics. 5th ed. Vancouver, WA: Applied Therapeutics, 1992:58-1–17.
4. Amdisen A. Serum level monitoring and clinical pharmacokinetics of lithium. Clin Pharmacokinet 1977;2(2):73–92.
5. Thornhill DP, Field SP. Distribution of lithium elimination rates in a selected population of psychiatric patients. Eur J Clin Pharmacol 1982;21(4):351–4.
6. Nielsen-Kudsk F, Amdisen A. Analysis of the pharmacokinetics of lithium in man. Eur J Clin Pharmacol 1979;16:271–7.
7. Goodnick PJ, Meltzer HL, Fieve RR, Dunner DL. Differences in lithium kinetics between bipolar and unipolar patients. J Clin Psychopharmacol 1982;2(1):48–50.
8. Mason RW, McQueen EG, Keary PJ, James NM. Pharmacokinetics of lithium: elimination half-time, renal clearance and apparent volume of distribution in schizophrenia. Clin Pharmacokinet 1978;3(3):241–6.
9. Vertrees JE, Ereshefsky L. Lithium. In: Schumacher GE, ed. Therapeutic Drug Monitoring. 1st ed. Stamford, CT: Appleton & Lange, 1995:493–526.
10. Hardy BG, Shulman KI, Mackenzie SE, Kutcher SP, Silverberg JD. Pharmacokinetics of lithium in the elderly. J Clin Psychopharmacol 1987;7(3):153–8.
11. Chapron DJ, Cameron IR, White LB, Merrall P. Observations on lithium disposition in the elderly. J Am Geriatr Soc 1982;30(10):651–5.
12. Caldwell HC, Westlake WJ, Schriver RC, Bumbier EE. Steady-state lithium blood level fluctuations in man following administration of a lithium carbonate conventional and controlled-release dosage form. J Clin Pharmacol 1981;21(2):106–9.
13. Meinhold JM, Spunt AL, Trirath C. Bioavailability of lithium carbonate: in vivo comparison of two products. J Clin Pharmacol 1979;19(11-12):701–3.
14. Williams PJ, Browne JL, Patel RA. Bayesian forecasting of serum lithium concentrations. Comparison with traditional methods. Clin Pharmacokinet 1989;17(1):45–52.

15. Vitiello B, Behar D, Malone R, Delaney MA, Ryan PJ, Simpson GM. Pharmacokinetics of lithium carbonate in children. J Clin Psychopharmacol 1988;8(5): 355–9.
16. Lauritsen BJ, Mellerup ET, Plenge P, Rasmussen S, Vestergaard P, Schou M. Serum lithium concentrations around the clock with different treatment regimens and the diurnal variation of the renal lithium clearance. Acta Psychiatr Scand 1981; 64(4):314–9.
17. Schou M. Lithium treatment during pregnancy, delivery, and lactation: an update. J Clin Psychiatry 1990;51(10):410–3.
18. Pringuey D, Yzombard G, Charbit JJ, et al. Lithium kinetics during hemodialysis in a patient with lithium poisoning. Am J Psychiatry 1981;138(2):249–51.
19. Zetin M, Plon L, Vaziri N, Cramer M, Greco D. Lithium carbonate dose and serum level relationships in chronic hemodialysis patients. Am J Psychiatry 1981;138(10): 1387–8.
20. Hansten PD, Horn JR. Drug interactions analysis and management. Vancouver, WA: Applied Therapeutics, 1998.
21. Bennett WM, Aronoff GR, Morrison G, et al. Drug prescribing in renal failure: dosing guidelines for adults. Am J Kidney Dis 1983;3(3):155–93.
22. Swan SK, Bennett WM. Drug dosing guidelines in patients with renal failure. West J Med 1992;156(6):633–8.
23. Bennett WM, Muther RS, Parker RA, et al. Drug therapy in renal failure: dosing guidelines for adults. Part II: sedatives, hypnotics, and tranquilizers; cardiovascular, antihypertensive, and diuretic agents; miscellaneous agents. Ann Intern Med 1980;93(2):286–325.
24. Bennett WM, Muther RS, Parker RA, et al. Drug therapy in renal failure: dosing guidelines for adults. Part I: Antimicrobial agents, analgesics. Ann Intern Med 1980; 93(1):62–89.
25. Zetin M, Garber D, Cramer M. A simple mathematical model for predicting lithium dose requirement. J Clin Psychiatry 1983;44(4):144–5.
26. Zetin M, Garber D, De Antonio M, et al. Prediction of lithium dose: a mathematical alternative to the test-dose method. J Clin Psychiatry 1986;47(4):175–8.
27. Cooper TB, Bergner PE, Simpson GM. The 24-hour serum lithium level as a prognosticator of dosage requirements. Am J Psychiatry 1973;130(5):601–3.
28. Cooper TB, Simpson GM. The 24-hour lithium level as a prognosticator of dosage requirements: a 2-year follow-up study. Am J Psychiatry 1976;133(4):440–3.
29. Perry PJ, Prince RA, Alexander B, Dunner FJ. Prediction of lithium maintenance doses using a single point prediction protocol. J Clin Psychopharmacol 1983;3(1): 13–7.
30. Perry PJ, Alexander B, Prince RA, Dunner FJ. The utility of a single-point dosing protocol for predicting steady-state lithium levels. Br J Psychiatry 1986;148:401–5.
31. Perry PJ, Alexander B, Dunner FJ, Schoenwald RD, Pfohl B, Miller D. Pharmacokinetic protocol for predicting serum lithium levels. J Clin Psychopharmacol 1982;2(2):114–8.
32. Ritschel WA, Banarer M. Lithium dosage regimen design by the repeated one-point method. Arzneimittelforschung 1982;32(2):98–102.
33. Marr MA, Djuric PE, Ritschel WA, Garver DL. Prediction of lithium carbonate dosage in psychiatric inpatients using the repeated one-point method. Clin Pharm 1983;2(3):243–8.
34. Wandell M, Mungall D. Computer assisted drug interpretation and drug regimen optimization. Am Assoc Clin Chem 1984;6:1–11.

18 | Theophylline

Theophylline is a methylxanthine compound that is used for the treatment of asthma, chronic obstructive pulmonary disease (COPD; chronic bronchitis and emphysema), and premature apnea.

- The bronchodilatory response via smooth muscle relaxation in the lung to theophylline is postulated to occur due to several mechanisms.[1] Of these, the two predominant mechanisms of action are antagonism of adenosine receptors and inhibition of phosphodiesterases, which increases intracellular cyclic AMP. In addition to bronchodilation, theophylline increases diaphragmatic contractility, increases mucociliary clearance, and exerts some anti-inflammatory effects.
- Theophylline is a general central nervous system stimulant and specifically stimulates the medullary respiratory center.

THERAPEUTIC AND TOXIC CONCENTRATIONS

- The generally accepted therapeutic ranges for theophylline are 10–20 µg/ml for the treatment of asthma or chronic obstructive pulmonary disease, or 6–13 µg/ml for the treatment of premature apnea. Recent guidelines suggest that for initial treatment of pulmonary disease, clinical response to theophylline concentrations between 5 and 15 µg/ml should be assessed before higher concentrations are used.[2]

  - Many patients requiring chronic theophylline therapy will derive sufficient bronchodilatory response with a low likelihood of adverse effects at concentrations of 8–12 µg/ml. However, theophylline therapy must be individualized for each patient in order to achieve optimal responses and minimal side effects.

- At the upper end of the therapeutic range (>15 µg/ml), some patients will experience minor caffeine-like side effects due to theophylline treatment.[3] These adverse effects include nausea, vomiting, dyspepsia, insomnia, nervousness, and headache.
- Theophylline concentrations exceeding 20–30 µg/ml can cause various tachyarrhythmias including sinus tachycardia.
- At theophylline concentrations above 40 µg/ml, serious life-threatening adverse effects including ventricular arrhythmias (premature ventricular contractions, ventricular tachycardia or fibrillation) or seizures can occur.

  - Theophylline-induced seizures are an ominous sign, as they respond poorly to antiepileptic therapy and can result in postseizure neurological sequelae or death. Unfortunately, minor side effects do not always occur before severe, life-threatening adverse effects are manifested.
  - Seizures due to theophylline therapy have been reported to occur in patients at theophylline concentrations as low as 25 µg/ml.

- Because of the potential for serious adverse drug reactions, serum concentration monitoring is mandatory for patients receiving theophylline.

- Not all patients with "toxic" theophylline serum concentrations in the listed ranges will exhibit signs or symptoms of theophylline toxicity. Rather, theophylline concentrations in the ranges given increase the likelihood that an adverse effect will occur.

CLINICAL MONITORING PARAMETERS

- Measurement of pulmonary function tests is an important component of assessing response to bronchodilator therapy in patients with asthma or chronic obstructive pulmonary disease.[4,5] Forced expiratory volume over one second (FEV_1) should be measured on a regular basis for asthmatic patients, and peak-flow meter monitoring can be performed routinely by these individuals at home.

  - Other spirometric tests that are useful for patients with chronic obstructive pulmonary disease include vital capacity (VC), total lung capacity (TLC), forced vital capacity (FVC), and forced expiratory flow over the middle 50% of the expiratory curve ($FEF_{25\%-75\%}$ or $FEF_{50\%}$).

- Patients should also be monitored for clinical signs and symptoms of their disease states, including frequency and severity of the following events: dyspnea, coughing, wheezing, impairment of normal activity.
- During acute exacerbations or in severe cases of either pulmonary disease state, arterial blood gases may be determined and used as a monitoring parameter.
- When theophylline is used to treat premature infants with apnea, the frequency of apneic events are monitored as a measure of therapeutic effect.
- Theophylline serum concentration monitoring is mandatory in patients receiving the drug. If a patient is experiencing clinical signs or symptoms that could be due to a theophylline adverse effect, a theophylline serum concentration should be obtained to rule out drug-induced toxicity.

  - For dose-adjustment purposes, theophylline serum concentrations should be measured at steady state after the patient has received a consistent dosage regimen for 3–5 drug half-lives. Theophylline half-life varies from 3 to 5 hours in children and tobacco-smoking individuals to 50 hours or more in patients with severe heart or liver failure.

- If theophylline is given as a continuous intravenous infusion, it can take a considerable amount of time for some patients to achieve effective concentrations, so an intravenous loading dose is commonly administered to patients (Figure 18-1).

  - The ideal situation is to administer an intravenous loading dose that will achieve the desired concentration immediately, then start an intravenous continuous infusion that will maintain that concentration (Figure 18-1).

    - In order to attain this perfect situation, the theophylline volume of distribution (V in L) must be known to compute the loading dose (LD in mg): $LD = Css \cdot V$, where Css is the desired theophylline concentration in mg/L. However, this pharmacokinetic parameter is rarely, if ever, known for a patient, so a loading dose based on a population average volume of distribution is used to calculate the amount of theophylline needed.
    - Since the patient's own, unique volume of distribution will most likely be greater (resulting in too low a loading dose) or less (resulting in too large a loading dose) than the population average volume of distribution

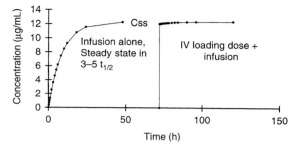

FIG. 18-1　When intravenous theophylline or aminophylline is administered to a patient as a continuous infusion, it will take 3–5 half-lives for serum theophylline concentrations to reach steady-state levels. As a result, maximal drug response will take time to achieve. To hasten the onset of drug action, loading doses are given to attain effective theophylline concentrations immediately.

used to compute the loading dose, the desired steady-state theophylline concentration will not be achieved.

- As a result, it will still take 3–5 half-lives for the patient to reach steady-state conditions while receiving a constant intravenous infusion rate (Figure 18-2). Thus, theophylline intravenous loading doses do not usually achieve steady-state serum concentrations immediately, but they should result in therapeutic concentrations and response sooner than simply starting an intravenous infusion alone.

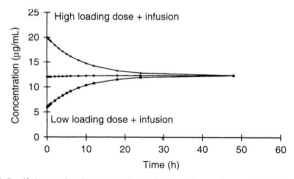

FIG. 18-2　If the patient's own, unique theophylline volume of distribution (V) is known, the exact loading dose (LD) of intravenous theophylline or aminophylline to immediately achieve steady-state theophylline concentrations (Css) can be calculated (LD = Css · V). However, the volume of distribution for the patient is rarely known when loading doses need to be administered, and for practical purposes, an average population volume of distribution for theophylline is used to estimate the parameter for the patient (V = 0.5 L/kg, use ideal body weight if > 30% overweight). Therefore, the computed loading dose will almost always be too large or too small to reach the desired steady-state theophylline concentration, and it will still take 3–5 half-lives to attain steady-state conditions.

- If oral theophylline-containing products are used to treat a patient, steady-state predose, or "trough," concentrations should be used to monitor therapy after the patient has received a stable dosage regimen for 3–5 half-lives.
- After an efficacious theophylline dosage regimen has been established for a patient, theophylline serum concentrations remain fairly stable in patients receiving long-term therapy. In these cases, theophylline dosage requirements and steady-state serum concentrations should be reassessed on a yearly basis.
- In patients with congestive heart failure or liver cirrhosis, theophylline dosage requirements can vary greatly according to the status of the patient.
- Acute viral diseases, especially in children, have been associated with theophylline adverse effects in patients previously stabilized on effective, nontoxic theophylline dosage regimens.[6,7]

BASIC CLINICAL PHARMACOKINETIC PARAMETERS

- Theophylline is eliminated primarily by hepatic metabolism (>90%). Hepatic metabolism is mainly via the CYP1A2 enzyme system, with a smaller amount metabolized by CYP2E1 and CYP3A.
- About 10% of a theophylline dose is recovered in the urine as unchanged drug.[8,9]
- Strictly speaking, theophylline follows nonlinear pharmacokinetics.[10–12] However, for the purposes of clinical drug dosing in patients, linear pharmacokinetic concepts and equations can be used effectively to compute doses and estimate serum concentrations.

  - Occasionally, theophylline serum concentrations increase in a patient more than expected after a dosage increase for an unidentifiable reason, and nonlinear pharmacokinetics may explain the observation.[10–12]

- Three different forms of theophylline are available. Aminophylline is the ethylenediamine salt of theophylline, and anhydrous aminophylline contains about 85% theophylline while aminophylline dihydrate contains about 80% theophylline. Oxtriphylline is the choline salt of theophylline and contains about 65% theophylline.

  - Theophylline and aminophylline are available for intravenous injection and oral use. Oxtriphylline is available only for oral use.
  - The oral bioavailability of all three theophylline-based drugs is very good and generally equals 100%. However, some older sustained-release oral dosage forms have been reported to exhibit incomplete bioavailability and loss of slow-release characteristics under certain circumstances due to their tablet or capsule design.

- Theophylline plasma protein binding is only 40%.[13,14]

EFFECTS OF DISEASE STATES AND CONDITIONS ON THEOPHYLLINE PHARMACOKINETICS AND DOSING

- Normal adults without the disease states and conditions discussed later in this section and with normal liver function have an average theophylline half-life of 8 hours (range 6–12 hours) and a volume of distribution of 0.5 L/kg (range 0.4–0.6 L/kg; Table 18-1).[15–17]

TABLE 18-1 Disease States and Conditions That Alter Theophylline Pharmacokinetics

Disease state/condition	Half-life (h)	Volume of distribution (L/kg)	Comment
Adult, normal liver function	8 (range 6–12 hours)	0.5 (range 0.4–0.6)	
Adult, tobacco or marijuana smoker	5	0.5	Tobacco and marijuana smoke induce CYP1A2 enzyme system and accelerate theophylline clearance.
Adult, hepatic disease (liver cirrhosis or acute hepatitis)	24	0.5	Theophylline is metabolized >90% by hepatic microsomal enzymes (primary, CYP1A2; secondary, CYP2E1, CYP3A), so loss of functional liver tissue decreases theophylline clearance. Pharmacokinetic parameters are highly variable in liver disease patients.
Adult, mild heart failure (NYHA CHF class I or II)	12	0.5	Decreased liver blood flow secondary to reduced cardiac output due to heart failure reduces theophylline clearance.
Adult, moderate–severe heart failure (NYHA CHF class III or IV) or cor pulmonale	24	0.5	Moderate–severe heart failure reduces cardiac output even more than mild heart failure, resulting in large and variable reductions in theophylline clearance. Cardiac status must be monitored closely in heart failure patients receiving theophylline, since theophylline clearance changes with acute changes in cardiac output.
Adult, obese (>30% over ideal body weight, IBW)	According to other disease states/conditions that affect theophylline pharmacokinetics	0.5 (IBW)	For patients who weigh more that 30% above IBW, theophylline doses should be based on ideal body weight.
Children, 1–9 y, normal cardiac and hepatic function	3.5	0.5	Children have increased theophylline clearance. Adult doses can be used when puberty is reached, taking into account disease states and conditions that alter theophylline pharmacokinetics.
Elderly, >65 y	12	0.5	Elderly individuals with concurrent disease states/conditions known to alter theophylline clearance should be dosed using those specific recommendations.

- Most disease states and conditions that change theophylline pharmacokinetics and dosage requirements alter clearance, but volume of distribution remains stable at ~0.5 L/kg in these situations.

Smoking

- Tobacco and marijuana smoke causes induction of hepatic CYP1A2, which accelerates the clearance of theophylline.[15–20] In patients who smoke these substances, the average theophylline half-life is 5 hours.

  - When patients stop smoking these compounds, theophylline clearance slowly approaches its baseline level for the patient over a 6–12-month period if the patient does not encounter "second-hand" smoke produced by other users.[21]
  - If the patient inhales a sufficient amount of second-hand smoke, theophylline clearance for the ex-smoker may remain in the fully induced state or at some intermediate induced state.[22]

Liver Dysfunction

- Patients with liver cirrhosis or acute hepatitis have reduced theophylline clearance, which results in a prolonged average theophylline half-life of 24 hours.[16,23–25] However, the effect of liver disease on theophylline pharmacokinetics is highly variable and difficult to predict accurately.

  - It is possible for a patient with liver disease to have relatively normal or grossly abnormal theophylline clearance and half-life.
  - An index of liver dysfunction can be gained by applying the Child-Pugh clinical classification system to the patient (Table 18-2). Child-Pugh scores are discussed more fully in Chapter 3 (Drug Dosing in Special Populations: Renal and Hepatic Disease, Dialysis, Heart Failure, Obesity, and Drug Interactions).

    - The Child-Pugh score consists of five laboratory tests or clinical symptoms: serum albumin, total bilirubin, prothrombin time, ascites, and hepatic encephalopathy. Each of these areas is given a score of 1 (normal) to 3 (severely abnormal; Table 18-2), and the scores for the five areas are summed.
    - The Child-Pugh score for a patient with normal liver function is 5, while the score for a patient with grossly abnormal serum albumin, total bilirubin, and prothrombin time values in addition to severe ascites and hepatic encephalopathy is 15.

TABLE 18-2 Child-Pugh Scores for Patients with Liver Disease[71]

Test/symptom	Score 1 point	Score 2 points	Score 3 points
Total bilirubin (mg/dl)	<2.0	2.0–3.0	>3.0
Serum albumin (g/dl)	>3.5	2.8–3.5	<2.8
Prothrombin time (seconds prolonged over control)	<4	4–6	>6
Ascites	Absent	Slight	Moderate
Hepatic Encephalopathy	None	Moderate	Severe

- A Child-Pugh score greater than 8 is grounds for a decrease in the initial daily drug dose for theophylline ($t_{1/2}$ = 24 hours). As in any patient, with or without liver dysfunction, initial doses are meant as starting points for dosage titration based on patient response and avoidance of adverse effects.
- Theophylline serum concentrations and the presence of adverse drug effects should be monitored frequently in patients with liver cirrhosis.

Heart Failure

- Heart failure causes reduced theophylline clearance because of decreased hepatic blood flow secondary to compromised cardiac output.[16,26–29] Venous stasis of blood within the liver may also contribute to the decrease in theophylline clearance found in heart failure patients.
- Patients with mild heart failure (New York Heart Association or NYHA class I or II, Table 18-3) have an average theophylline half-life of 12 hours (range 5–24 hours), while those with moderate to severe heart failure (NYHA class III or IV) or cor pulmonale have an average theophylline half-life of 24 hours (range 5–50 hours).
- The effect of heart failure on theophylline pharmacokinetics is highly variable and difficult to predict accurately. It is possible for a patient with heart failure to have relatively normal or grossly abnormal theophylline clearance and half-life.
- For heart failure patients, initial doses are meant as starting points for dosage titration based on patient response and avoidance of adverse effects.
- Theophylline serum concentrations and the presence of adverse drug effects should be monitored frequently in patients with heart failure.

Obesity

- Obese patients (>30% above ideal body weight or IBW) should have volume of distribution estimates based on ideal body weight.[30–33] Theophylline half-life

TABLE 18-3 New York Heart Association (NYHA) Functional Classification for Heart Failure[72]

NYHA heart failure class	Description
I	Patients with cardiac disease but without limitations of physical activity. Ordinary physical activity does not cause undue fatigue, dyspnea, or palpitation.
II	Patients with cardiac disease that results in slight limitations of physical activity. Ordinary physical activity results in fatigue, palpitation, dyspnea, or angina.
III	Patients with cardiac disease that results in marked limitations of physical activity. Although patients are comfortable at rest, less than ordinary activity will lead to symptoms.
IV	Patients with cardiac disease that results in an inability to carry on physical activity without discomfort. Symptoms of congestive heart failure are present even at rest. With any physical activity, increased discomfort is experienced.

should be based on the concurrent disease states and conditions present in the patient. If weight-based dosage recommendations (mg/kg/d or mg/kg/h) are to be used, ideal body weight should be used to compute doses for obese individuals.

Age

- Patient age has an effect on theophylline clearance and half-life.

  - Newborns have decreased theophylline clearance because hepatic drug-metabolizing enzymes are not yet fully developed at birth.

    - Premature neonates have average theophylline half-lives of 30 hours at 3–15 days after birth and 20 hours at 25–57 days after birth.[34–36]
    - Full-term infants have average theophylline half-lives of 25 hours at 1–2 days after birth, and 11 hours at 3–30 weeks after birth.[37–39]

  - Children between the ages of 1 and 9 years have accelerated theophylline clearance rates resulting in an average half-life of 3.5 hours (range 1.5–5 hours).[40–42] As children reach puberty, their theophylline clearance and half-life approach the values of an adult.
  - For elderly patients, over the age of 65, some studies indicate that theophylline clearance and half-life are the same as in younger adults, while other investigations have found that theophylline clearance is slower and half-life is longer (average half life = 12 hours, range 8–16 hours).[43–47]

    - A confounding factor found in theophylline pharmacokinetic studies conducted in older adults is the possible accidental inclusion of subjects who have subclinical or mild cases of the disease states associated with reduced theophylline clearance (heart failure, liver disease, etc). Thus, the pharmacokinetics of theophylline in elderly individuals is somewhat controversial.

Fever

- Febrile illnesses can temporarily decrease the clearance of theophylline and require an immediate dosage decrease to avoid toxicity.[6,7] The mechanism of this acute change in theophylline disposition is unclear, but probably involves decreased clearance due to the production of interleukins.
- Children seem to be at especially high risk of adverse reactions to theophylline because febrile illnesses are prevalent in this population and high theophylline doses (on a mg/kg/d basis) may be prescribed.

Hypothyroidism

- Hypothyroid patients have decreased basal metabolic rates, and require smaller theophylline doses until a euthyroid condition is established.[48]

Renal Dysfunction

- Because only a small amount of theophylline is eliminated unchanged in the urine (<10% of a dose), dosage adjustments are not necessary in patients with renal impairment.[8,9]

Dialysis and Hemoperfusion

- Theophylline is removed by hemodialysis, so, if possible, doses should be withheld until after the dialysis procedure is complete.[49–54] The hemoperfusion sieving coefficient for theophylline is 0.80, which indicates significant removal by these techniques.[55,56]

  - If a pulmonary exacerbation occurs due to decreased theophylline concentrations, individualized supplemental doses of theophylline may need to be given during or after the procedure is complete.

- Theophylline is not appreciably removed by peritoneal dialysis.[52]

DRUG INTERACTIONS

- Drug interactions with theophylline are common and occur with a variety of medications.[57]
- Serious inhibition drug interactions are those that decrease theophylline clearance more than 30%.

  - Clinicians should consider an arbitrary decrease in theophylline dose of 30–50% for patients receiving these agents until the actual degree of hepatic enzyme inhibition can be assessed using theophylline serum concentration monitoring. Patients should be actively monitored for the signs and symptoms of theophylline toxicity.
  - The magnitude of hepatic enzyme inhibition drug interactions is highly variable, so some patients may require even larger theophylline dosage decreases while others may exhibit no drug interaction at all.
  - Cimetidine given at higher doses (≥1000 mg/d) on a multiple daily dosage schedule decreases theophylline clearance by 30–50%. Other cimetidine doses (≤800 mg/d) given once or twice daily decrease theophylline clearance by 20% or less.[58,59]
  - Ciprofloxacin and enoxacin, both quinolone antibiotics, and troleandomycin, a macrolide antibiotic, also decrease theophylline clearance by 30–50%.
  - Estrogen and estrogen-containing oral contraceptives, propranolol, metoprolol, mexiletine, propafenone, pentoxifylline, ticlopidine, tacrine, thiabendazole, disulfiram, and fluvoxamine can also decrease theophylline clearance by this extent.

- Moderate-sized inhibition drug interactions are those that decrease theophylline clearance by 10–30%.

  - For this magnitude of drug interaction, many clinicians believe that a routine decrease in theophylline dose is unnecessary for patients with steady-state theophylline concentrations below 15 μg/ml, but should be considered on a case-by-case basis for those with concentrations above this level. Should a decrease be warranted in a patient, theophylline doses can be cut by 20% to avoid adverse effects.
  - Patients should be actively monitored for the signs and symptoms of theophylline toxicity.
  - The calcium channel blockers, verapamil and diltiazem, have been reported to cause decreases in theophylline clearance of 15–25%.
  - Clarithromycin and erythromycin, both macrolide antibiotics, and norfloxacin, a quinolone antibiotic, can also decrease theophylline clearance by this magnitude.

- At doses of 600 mg/d or above, allopurinol has been reported to decrease theophylline clearance by 25%.

- Theophylline elimination is also subject to induction of hepatic microsomal enzymes, which increases theophylline clearance. Because hepatic microsomal enzyme induction is quite variable in patients, some individuals may require theophylline dosage increases while others require no alteration in dosage requirements.

  - Hepatic microsomal enzyme induction takes time to occur, and maximal effects may not be seen before 2–4 weeks of treatment with enzyme inducers.
  - Patients treated with a drug that increases theophylline clearance need to be carefully monitored for the signs and symptoms of their respective disease state, and steady-state theophylline concentrations should be measured. Disease exacerbations may be due to decreased theophylline concentrations, and a dosage increase may be warranted in some patients.
  - Phenytoin, carbamazepine, phenobarbital, rifampin, and moricizine all increase theophylline clearance.

INITIAL DOSAGE DETERMINATION METHODS

- Several methods to initiate theophylline therapy are available.

  - The *pharmacokinetic dosing method* is the most flexible of the techniques. It allows individualized target serum concentrations to be chosen for a patient, and each pharmacokinetic parameter can be customized to reflect specific disease states and conditions present in the patient.
  - *Literature-based recommended dosing* is a very commonly used method to prescribe initial doses of theophylline. Doses are based on those that commonly produce steady-state concentrations near the lower end of the therapeutic range, although there is a wide variation in the actual concentrations for a specific patient.

Pharmacokinetic Dosing Method

- The goal of initial dosing of theophylline is to compute the best dose possible for the patient given the set of disease states and conditions that influence theophylline pharmacokinetics and the pulmonary disorder being treated. In order to do this, pharmacokinetic parameters for the patient are estimated using average parameters measured in other patients with similar disease state and condition profiles.

Half-Life and Elimination Rate Constant Estimate

- Theophylline is metabolized predominately by the liver. Unfortunately, there is no good way to estimate the elimination characteristics of liver-metabolized drugs using an endogenous marker of liver function in the same manner that serum creatinine and estimated creatinine clearance are used to estimate the elimination of agents that are eliminated renally.

  - As a result, a patient is categorized according to the disease states and conditions that are known to change theophylline half-life, and half-lives measured in previous studies are used as an estimate of the current patient's half-life.

- To produce the most conservative theophylline doses in patients with multiple concurrent disease states or conditions that affect theophylline pharmacokinetics, the disease state or condition with the longest half-life should be used to compute doses. This approach will avoid accidental overdosage has much as is currently possible.
- Once the correct half-life has been identified for the patient, it can be converted into the theophylline elimination rate constant (k) using the following equation:

$$k = 0.693/t_{1/2}$$

Volume of Distribution Estimate

- Theophylline volume of distribution is relatively stable in patients, regardless of the disease states and conditions that are present. Volume of distribution is assumed to be 0.5 L/kg for nonobese patients.
- For obese patients (>30% above ideal body weight), ideal body weight is used to compute theophylline volume of distribution.

Selection of Appropriate Pharmacokinetic Model and Equations

- When theophylline is given by continuous intravenous infusion or orally, the drug follows a one-compartment pharmacokinetic model (Figures 18-1, 18-3, and 18-4).
- When oral therapy is required, most clinicians utilize a sustained-release dosage form that has good bioavailability (F = 1), supplies a continuous release of theophylline into the gastrointestinal tract, and provides a smooth theophylline serum concentration/time curve that emulates an intravenous infusion after once- or twice-daily dosing.

- A simple pharmacokinetic equation that computes the average theophylline steady-state serum concentration (Css in μg/ml = mg/L) is widely used and

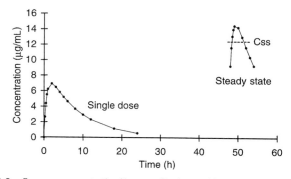

FIG. 18-3 Serum concentration/time profile for rapid-release theophylline or aminophylline oral dosage forms (given every 6 hours) after a single dose and at steady state. The curves shown are typical for an adult cigarette smoker receiving theophylline 300 mg. The steady-state serum concentration (Css) expected from an equivalent theophylline or aminophylline continuous infusion is shown by the dotted line in the steady-state concentrations.

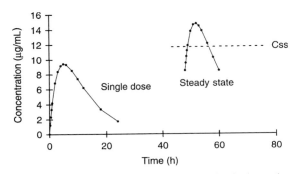

FIG. 18-4   Serum concentration/time profile for sustained-release theophylline or aminophylline oral dosage forms after (given every 12 hours) a single dose and at steady-state. The curves shown are typical for an adult cigarette smoker receiving 600 mg of theophylline. The steady-state serum concentration (Css) expected from an equivalent theophylline or aminophylline continuous infusion is shown by the dotted line in the steady-state concentrations.

allows maintenance dosage calculation:

$$\text{Css} = [\text{F} \cdot \text{S} \, (\text{D}/\tau)]/\text{Cl} \qquad \text{or} \qquad \text{D} = (\text{Css} \cdot \text{Cl} \cdot \tau)/(\text{F} \cdot \text{S})$$

where F is the bioavailability fraction for the oral dosage form (F = 1 for most oral theophylline sustained-release products), S is the fraction of the theophylline salt form that is active theophylline (S = 1 for theophylline, S = 0.80 for aminophylline dihydrate, S = 0.85 for S = 0.65 for oxtriphylline), D is the dose of theophylline salt in mg, and τ is the dosage interval in hours. Cl is theophylline clearance in L/h and is computed using estimates of theophylline elimination rate constant (k) and volume of distribution:

$$\text{Cl} = \text{kV}$$

• When intravenous therapy is required, a similar pharmacokinetic equation that computes the theophylline steady-state serum concentration (Css in μg/ml = mg/L) is widely used and allows dosage calculation for a continuous infusion:

$$\text{Css} = [\text{S} \cdot \text{k}_0]/\text{Cl} \qquad \text{or} \qquad \text{k}_0 = (\text{Css} \cdot \text{Cl})/\text{S}$$

where S is the fraction of the theophylline salt form that is active theophylline (S = 1 for theophylline, S = 0.80 for aminophylline dihydrate anhydrous aminophylline), and k_0 is the dose of theophylline salt in mg. Cl is theophylline clearance in L/h and is computed using estimates of theophylline elimination rate constant (k) and volume of distribution:

$$\text{Cl} = \text{kV}$$

• The equation used to calculate an intravenous loading dose (LD in mg) is based on a simple one-compartment model:

$$\text{LD} = (\text{Css} \cdot \text{V})/\text{S}$$

where Css is the desired theophylline steady-state concentration in μg/ml, which is equivalent to mg/L, V is the theophylline volume of distribution, and S is the fraction of the theophylline salt form that is active theophylline (S = 1 for theophylline, S = 0.80 for aminophylline dihydrate S = 0.85 for anhydrous aminophylline). Intravenous theophylline loading doses should be infusions over at least 20–30 minutes.

Steady-State Concentration Selection

- The generally accepted therapeutic ranges for theophylline are 10–20 μg/ml for the treatment of asthma or chronic obstructive pulmonary disease, or 6–13 μg/ml for the treatment of premature apnea.
- Recent guidelines suggest that for initial treatment of pulmonary disease, clinical response to theophylline concentrations between 5 and 15 μg/ml should be assessed before higher concentrations are used.[2]
- Many patients requiring chronic theophylline therapy will derive sufficient bronchodilatory response with a low likelihood of adverse effects at concentrations of 8–12 μg/ml.
- However, theophylline therapy much be individualized for each patient in order to achieve optimal responses and minimal side effects.

▶ ***Example 1*** LK is a 50-year-old, 75-kg (height 5′10″) male with chronic bronchitis who requires therapy with oral theophylline. He smokes 2 packs of cigarettes daily, and has normal liver and cardiac function. Suggest an initial theophylline dosage regimen designed to achieve a steady-state theophylline concentration of 8 μg/ml. (*Note:* μg/ml = mg/L, and this concentration unit is substitued for Css in the calculations so that unit conversion is not required.)

1. *Estimate half-life and elimination rate constant according to disease states and conditions present in the patient.* Cigarette smoke induces the enzyme systems responsible for theophylline metabolism, and the expected theophylline half-life ($t_{1/2}$) is 5 hours. The elimination rate constant is computed using the following formula:

$$k = 0.693/t_{1/2} = 0.693/5 \text{ h} = 0.139 \text{ h}^{-1}$$

2. *Estimate volume of distribution and clearance.* The patient is not obese, so the estimated theophylline volume of distribution is based on actual body weight:

$$V = 0.5 \text{ L/kg} \cdot 75 \text{ kg} = 38 \text{ L}$$

Estimated theophylline clearance is computed by taking the product of the volume of distribution and the elimination rate constant:

$$Cl = kV = 0.139 \text{ h}^{-1} \cdot 38 \text{ L} = 5.28 \text{ L/h}$$

3. *Compute dosage regimen.* Oral sustained-release theophylline tablets will be prescribed for this patient (F = 1, S = 1). Because the patient has rapid theophylline clearance and short drug half-life, the initial dosage interval (τ) will be set to 8 hours. (*Note:* μg/ml = mg/L, and this concentration unit is substitued for Css in the calculations so that unit conversion is not required.) The dosage equation for oral theophylline is

$$D = (Css \cdot Cl \cdot \tau)/(F \cdot S) = (8 \text{ mg/L} \cdot 5.28 \text{ L/h} \cdot 8 \text{ h})/(1 \cdot 1)$$
$$= 338 \text{ mg, rounded to } 300 \text{ every } 8 \text{ h}$$

A steady-state trough theophylline serum concentration should be measured after steady state is attained in 3–5 half-lives. Since the drug is expected to have a half-life of 5 hours, a theophylline steady-state concentration can be obtained at any time after the first day of dosing (5 half-lives = $5 \cdot 5$ h = 25 h). Theophylline serum concentrations should also be measured if the patient experiences an exacerbation of lung disease, or if the patient develops potential signs or symptoms of theophylline toxicity.

▶ *Example 2*   OI is a 60-year-old, 85-kg (height 6′1″) male with emphysema who requires therapy with oral theophylline. He has liver cirrhosis (Child-Pugh score = 11) and normal cardiac function. Suggest an initial theophylline dosage regimen designed to achieve a steady-state theophylline concentration of 10 μg/ml.

1. *Estimate half-life and elimination rate constant according to disease states and conditions present in the patient.* Patients with severe liver disease have highly variable theophylline pharmacokinetics and dosage requirements. Hepatic disease destroys liver parenchyma, where hepatic drug-metabolizing enzymes are found, and the expected theophylline half-life ($t_{1/2}$) is 24 hours. The elimination rate constant is computed using the following formula:

$$k = 0.693/t_{1/2} = 0.693/24 \text{ h} = 0.029 \text{ h}^{-1}$$

2. *Estimate volume of distribution and clearance.* The patient is not obese, so the estimated theophylline volume of distribution is based on actual body weight:

$$V = 0.5 \text{ L/kg} \cdot 85 \text{ kg} = 43 \text{ L}$$

Estimated theophylline clearance is computed by taking the product of the volume of distribution and the elimination rate constant:

$$Cl = kV = 0.029 \text{ h}^{-1} \cdot 43 \text{ L} = 1.25 \text{ L/h}$$

3. *Compute dosage regimen.* Oral sustained-release theophylline tablets will be prescribed for this patient (F = 1, S = 1). The initial dosage interval (τ) will be set to 12 hours. (*Note:* μg/ml = mg/L, and this concentration unit is substituted for Css in the calculations so that unit conversion is not required.) The dosage equation for oral theophylline is

$$D = (Css \cdot Cl \cdot \tau)/(F \cdot S) = (10 \text{ mg/L} \cdot 1.25 \text{ L/h} \cdot 12 \text{ h})/(1 \cdot 1)$$
$$= 150 \text{ mg every 12 h}$$

A steady-state trough theophylline serum concentration should be measured after steady state is attained in 3–5 half-lives. Since the drug is expected to have a half-life of 24 hours, a theophylline steady-state concentration can be obtained at any time after the fifth day of dosing (5 half-lives = $5 \cdot 24$ h = 120 h or 5 days). Theophylline serum concentrations should also be measured if the patient experiences an exacerbation of lung disease, or if the patient develops potential signs or symptoms of theophylline toxicity.

• To illustrate the differences and similarities between oral and intravenous theophylline dosage regimen design, the same cases will be used to compute intravenous theophylline loading doses and continuous infusions.

▶ *Example 3*   LK is a 50-year-old, 75-kg (height 5'10") male with chronic bronchitis who requires therapy with intravenous theophylline. He smokes 2 packs of
cigarettes daily, and has normal liver and cardiac function. Suggest an initial
intravenous aminophylline dosage regimen designed to achieve a steady-state
theophylline concentration of 8 µg/ml.

1. *Estimate half-life and elimination rate constant according to disease states
   and conditions present in the patient.* Cigarette smoke induces the enzyme
   systems responsible for theophylline metabolism, and the expected theophylline half-life ($t_{1/2}$) is 5 hours. The elimination rate constant is computed using the following formula:

$$k = 0.693/t_{1/2} = 0.693/5 \text{ h} = 0.139 \text{ h}^{-1}$$

2. *Estimate volume of distribution and clearance.* The patient is not obese, so
   the estimated theophylline volume of distribution is based on actual body
   weight:

$$V = 0.5 \text{ L/kg} \cdot 75 \text{ kg} = 38 \text{ L}$$

   Estimated theophylline clearance is computed by taking the product of
   the volume of distribution and the elimination rate constant:

$$Cl = kV = 0.139 \text{ h}^{-1} \cdot 38 \text{ L} = 5.28 \text{ L/h}$$

3. *Compute dosage regimen.* Theophylline will be administered as the
   aminophylline dihydrate salt form (S = 0.8). (*Note:* µg/ml = mg/L, and
   this concentration unit is substituted for Css in the calculations so that
   unit conversion is not required.) Therapy will be started by administering an intravenous loading dose (LD) of aminophylline to the patient:

$$LD = (Css \cdot V)/S = (8 \text{ mg/L} \cdot 38 \text{ L})/0.8$$
$$= 380 \text{ mg, rounded to } 400 \text{ mg IV over } 20\text{--}30 \text{ min}$$

   An aminophylline continuous intravenous infusion will be started immediately after the loading dose has been administered. (*Note:* µg/ml = mg/L,
   and this concentration unit is substituted for Css in the calculations so that
   unit conversion is not required.) The dosage equation for intravenous
   aminophylline is

$$k_0 = (Css \cdot Cl)/S = (8 \text{ mg/L} \cdot 5.28 \text{ L/h})/0.8$$
$$= 53 \text{ mg/h, rounded to } 55 \text{ mg/h}$$

   A steady-state theophylline serum concentration should be measured
   after steady state is attained in 3–5 half-lives. Since the drug is expected
   to have a half-life of 5 hours, a theophylline steady-state concentration
   can be obtained at any time after the first day of dosing (5 half-
   lives = 5 · 5 h = 25 h). Theophylline serum concentrations should also
   be measured if the patient experiences an exacerbation of lung disease, or if he develops potential signs or symptoms of theophylline
   toxicity.

▶ *Example 4*   OI is a 60-year-old, 85-kg (height 6'1") male with emphysema who requires therapy with intravenous aminophylline. He has liver
cirrhosis (Child-Pugh score = 11) and normal cardiac function. Suggest an
initial intravenous aminophylline dosage regimen designed to achieve a
steady-state theophylline concentration of 10 µg/ml.

1. *Estimate half-life and elimination rate constant according to disease states and conditions present in the patient.* Patients with severe liver disease have highly variable theophylline pharmacokinetics and dosage requirements. Hepatic disease destroys liver parenchyma, where hepatic drug-metabolizing enzymes are found, and the expected theophylline half-life $(t_{1/2})$ is 24 hours. The elimination rate constant is computed using the following formula:

$$k = 0.693/t_{1/2} = 0.693/24 \text{ h} = 0.029 \text{ h}^{-1}$$

2. *Estimate volume of distribution and clearance.* The patient is not obese, so the estimated theophylline volume of distribution is based on actual body weight:

$$V = 0.5 \text{ L/kg} \cdot 85 \text{ kg} = 43 \text{ L}$$

Estimated theophylline clearance is computed by taking the product of the volume of distribution and the elimination rate constant:

$$Cl = kV = 0.029 \text{ h}^{-1} \cdot 43 \text{ L} = 1.25 \text{ L/h}$$

3. *Compute dosage regimen.* Theophylline will be administered as the aminophylline dihydrate salt form $(S = 0.8)$. (*Note:* $\mu g/ml = mg/L$, and this concentration unit is substituted for Css in the calculations so that unit conversion is not required.) Therapy will be started by administering an intravenous loading dose of aminophylline to the patient:

$$LD = (Css \cdot V)/S = (10 \text{ mg/L} \cdot 43 \text{ L})/0.8$$
$$= 538 \text{ mg, rounded to 500 mg IV over 20–30 min}$$

An aminophylline continuous intravenous infusion will be started immediately after the loading dose has been administered. (*Note:* $\mu g/ml = mg/L$, and this concentration unit is substituted for Css in the calculations so that unit conversion is not required.) The dosage equation for intravenous aminophylline is

$$k_0 = (Css \cdot Cl)/S = (10 \text{ mg/L} \cdot 1.25 \text{ L/h})/0.8$$
$$= 16 \text{ mg/h, rounded to 15 mg/h}$$

A steady-state theophylline serum concentration should be measured after steady state is attained in 3–5 half-lives. Since the drug is expected to have a half-life of 24 hours, a theophylline steady-state concentration can be obtained at any time after the fifth day of dosing (5 half-lives = $5 \cdot 24$ h = 120 h or 5 days). Theophylline serum concentrations should also be measured if the patient experiences an exacerbation of lung disease, or if the patient develops potential signs or symptoms of theophylline toxicity.

Literature-Based Recommended Dosing

- Because of the large amount of variability in theophylline pharmacokinetics, even when concurrent disease states and conditions are identified, many clinicians believe that the use of standard theophylline doses for various situations is warranted.[16,60,61]
- The original computations of these doses were based on the pharmacokinetic dosing method described in the previous section, and the doses were

TABLE 18-4 Theophylline Dosage Rates for Patients with Various Disease States and Conditions[61]

Disease state/condition	Mean dose (mg/kg/h)
Children 1–9 y	0.8
Children 9–12 y or adult smokers	0.7
Adolescents 12–16 y	0.5
Adult nonsmokers	0.4
Elderly nonsmokers (>65 y)	0.3
Decompensated CHF, cor pulmonale, cirrhosis	0.2

subsequently modified based on clinical experience. In general, the expected theophylline steady-state serum concentration used to compute these doses was 10 μg/ml.

- Suggested theophylline maintenance doses stratified by disease states and conditions known to alter theophylline pharmacokinetics are given in Table 18-4.[61]

  - For obese individuals (>30% over ideal body weight), ideal body weight should be used to compute doses.[30–33]

- Because the doses are given in terms of theophylline, doses for other theophylline salt forms need to be adjusted accordingly (S = 0.8 for aminophylline dihydrate, S = 0.85 for anhydrous aminophylline, S = 0.65 for oxtriphylline).

- If theophylline is to be given orally, the dose given in Table 18-4 (in mg/kg/h) must be multiplied by the appropriate dosage interval for the dosage form being used:

$$D = (\text{theophylline dose} \cdot \text{Wt} \cdot \tau)/S$$

where Wt is patient weight, τ is the dosage interval, and S is the appropriate salt-form correction factor for aminophylline or oxtriphylline.

- If theophylline is to be given as a continuous intravenous infusion, the following equation is used to compute the infusion rate:

$$k_0 = (\text{theophylline dose} \cdot \text{Wt})/S$$

where Wt is patient weight and S is the appropriate salt-form correction factor for aminophylline.

- When more than one disease state or condition is present in a patient, choosing the lowest dose suggested by Table 18-4 will result in the safest, most conservative dosage recommendation.

- If an intravenous loading dose is necessary, 5 mg/kg of theophylline or 6 mg/kg of aminophylline is used; ideal body weight is used to compute loading doses for obese patients (>30% over ideal body weight).

- To illustrate the similarities and differences between this method of dosage calculation and the pharmacokinetic dosing method, the same examples used in the previous section will be used.

▶ *Example 1* LK is a 50-year-old, 75-kg (height 5′10″) male with chronic bronchitis who requires therapy with oral theophylline. He smokes 2 packs of cigarettes daily, and has normal liver and cardiac function. Suggest an initial theophylline dosage regimen for this patient.

1. *Choose theophylline dose based on disease states and conditions present in the patient.* A theophylline dose of 0.7 mg/kg/h is suggested by the table for an adult cigarette smoker.
2. *Compute dosage regimen.* Oral sustained-release theophylline tablets will be prescribed for this patient (F = 1, S = 1). Because the patient has rapid theophylline clearance and drug half-life, the initial dosage interval (τ) will be set to 8 hours:

$$D = (\text{theophylline dose} \cdot \text{Wt} \cdot \tau)/S = (0.7 \text{ mg/kg/h} \cdot 75 \text{ kg} \cdot 8 \text{ h})/1$$

$$= 420 \text{ mg, rounded to } 400 \text{ mg every } 8 \text{ h}$$

This dose is similar to that suggested by the pharmacokinetic dosing method of 300 mg every 8 hours.

A steady-state trough theophylline serum concentration should be measured after steady state is attained in 3–5 half-lives. Since the drug is expected to have a half-life of 5 hours, a theophylline steady-state concentration can be obtained at any time after the first day of dosing (5 half-lives = 5 $\cdot$ 5 h = 25 h). Theophylline serum concentrations should also be measured if the patient experiences an exacerbation of lung disease, or if the patient develops potential signs or symptoms of theophylline toxicity.

▶ *Example 2* OI is a 60-year-old, 85-kg (height 6′1″) male with emphysema who requires therapy with oral theophylline. He has liver cirrhosis (Child-Pugh score = 11) and normal cardiac function. Suggest an initial theophylline dosage regimen for this patient.

1. *Choose theophylline dose based on disease states and conditions present in the patient.* A theophylline dose of 0.2 mg/kg/h is suggested by the table for an adult with cirrhosis.
2. *Compute dosage regimen.* Oral sustained-release theophylline tablets will be prescribed for this patient (F = 1, S = 1). The initial dosage interval (τ) will be set to 12 hours:

$$D = (\text{theophylline dose} \cdot \text{Wt} \cdot \tau)/S = (0.2 \text{ mg/kg/h} \cdot 85 \text{ kg} \cdot 12 \text{ h})/1$$

$$= 204 \text{ mg, rounded to } 200 \text{ mg every } 12 \text{ h}$$

This dose is similar to that suggested by the pharmacokinetic dosing method of 150 mg every 12 hours.

A steady-state trough theophylline serum concentration should be measured after steady state is attained in 3–5 half-lives. Since the drug is expected to have a half-life of 24 hours, a theophylline steady-state concentration can be obtained at any time after the fifth day of dosing (5 half-lives = 5 $\cdot$ 24 h = 120 h or 5 days). Theophylline serum concentrations should also be measured if the patient experiences an exacerbation of lung disease, or if the patient develops potential signs or symptoms of theophylline toxicity.

• To illustrate the differences and similarities between oral and intravenous theophylline dosage regimen design, the same cases will be used to compute intravenous theophylline loading doses and continuous infusions.

▶ *Example 3* LK is a 50-year-old, 75-kg (height 5′10″) male with chronic bronchitis who requires therapy with intravenous theophylline. He smokes

2 packs of cigarettes daily, and has normal liver and cardiac function. Suggest an initial theophylline dosage regimen for this patient.

1. *Choose theophylline dose based on disease states and conditions present in the patient.* A theophylline dose of 0.7 mg/kg/h is suggested by the table for an adult smoker.

2. *Compute dosage regimen.* Theophylline will be administered as the intravenous drug $(S = 1)$:

$$k_0 = (\text{theophylline dose} \cdot \text{Wt})/S = (0.7 \text{ mg/kg/h} \cdot 75 \text{ kg})/1$$
$$= 53 \text{ mg/h, rounded to } 55 \text{ mg/h}$$

A loading dose of theophylline 5 mg/kg will also be prescribed for the patient:

$$LD = 5 \text{ mg/kg} \cdot 75 \text{ kg}$$
$$= 375 \text{ mg, rounded to } 400 \text{ mg of IV over } 20–30 \text{ min}$$

These doses are similar to those that were suggested by the pharmacokinetic dosing method.

A theophylline serum concentration should be measured after steady state is attained in 3–5 half-lives. Since the drug is expected to have a half-life of 5 hours, a theophylline steady-state concentration can be obtained at any time after the first day of dosing (5 half-lives = $5 \cdot 5$ h = 25 h). Theophylline serum concentrations should also be measured if the patient experiences an exacerbation of lung disease, or if the patient develops potential signs or symptoms of theophylline toxicity.

▶ *Example 4*   OI is a 60-year-old, 85-kg (height 6′1″) male with emphysema who requires therapy with intravenous theophylline. He has liver cirrhosis (Child-Pugh score = 11) and normal cardiac function. Suggest an initial intravenous aminophylline dosage regimen for this patient.

1. *Choose theophylline dose based on disease states and conditions present in the patient.* A theophylline dose of 0.2 mg/kg/h is suggested by the table for an adult with cirrhosis.

2. *Compute dosage regimen.* Theophylline will be administered as the aminophylline dihydrate salt form $(S = 0.8)$:

$$D = (\text{theophylline dose} \cdot \text{Wt})/S = (0.2 \text{ mg/kg/h} \cdot 85 \text{ kg})/0.8$$
$$= 21 \text{ mg/h, rounded to } 20 \text{ mg/h}$$

A loading dose of 6 mg/kg of aminophylline will also be prescribed for the patient:

$$LD = 6 \text{ mg/kg} \cdot 85 \text{ kg} = 510 \text{ mg, rounded to } 500 \text{ mg IV over } 20–30 \text{ min}$$

These doses are similar to those suggested by the pharmacokinetic dosing method of a 500-mg loading dose followed by a 15-mg/h continuous infusion.

A steady-state theophylline serum concentration should be measured after steady state is attained in 3–5 half-lives. Since the drug is expected to have a half-life of 24 hours, a theophylline steady-state concentration can be obtained at any time after the fifth day of dosing (5 half-lives = $5 \cdot 24$ h = 120 h or 5 days). Theophylline serum concentrations should also be measured if the patient experiences an exacerbation of lung disease, or if the patient develops potential signs or symptoms of theophylline toxicity.

USE OF THEOPHYLLINE SERUM CONCENTRATIONS TO ALTER DOSES

- Because of the large amount of pharmacokinetic variability among patients, it is likely that doses computed using patient population characteristics will not always produce theophylline serum concentrations that are expected or desirable.
- Because of pharmacokinetic variability, the narrow therapeutic index of theophylline, and the severity of theophylline adverse side effects, measurement of theophylline serum concentrations is mandatory for patients to ensure that therapeutic, nontoxic levels are present.
- In addition to theophylline serum concentrations, important patient parameters (pulmonary function tests, clinical signs and symptoms of the pulmonary disease state, potential theophylline side effects, etc.) should be followed to confirm that the patient is responding to treatment and not developing adverse drug reactions.
- When theophylline serum concentrations are measured in patients and a dosage change is necessary, clinicians should use the simplest, most straightforward method available to determine a dose that will provide safe and effective treatment.

  - In most cases, a simple dosage ratio can be used to change theophylline doses, assuming the drug follows *linear pharmacokinetics*.
    - Although it has been clearly demonstrated in research studies that theophylline follows nonlinear pharmacokinetics,[10–12] in the clinical setting most patients' steady-state serum concentrations change proportionally to theophylline dose below and within the therapeutic range, and assuming linear pharmacokinetics is adequate for dosage adjustments in most patients.

  - Sometimes it is useful to compute theophylline pharmacokinetic constants for a patient and base dosage adjustments on these. In these cases it may be possible to calculate and use *pharmacokinetic parameters* to alter the theophylline dose.
  - In some situations it may be necessary to compute theophylline clearance for the patient during a continuous infusion before steady-state conditions occur using the *Chiou method* and utilize this pharmacokinetic parameter to calculate the best drug dose.
  - Computerized methods that incorporate expected population pharmacokinetic characteristics (*Bayesian pharmacokinetic computer programs*) can be used in difficult cases, when serum concentrations are obtained at suboptimal times or the patient was not at steady state when serum concentrations were measured.

Linear Pharmacokinetics Method

- Because theophylline follows linear, dose-proportional pharmacokinetics in most patients with concentrations within and below the therapeutic range, steady-state serum concentrations change in proportion to dose according to the following equation:

$$D_{new}/Css_{new} = D_{old}/Css_{old} \quad \text{or} \quad D_{new} = (Css_{new}/Css_{old})D_{old}$$

where D is the dose, Css is the steady-state concentration, old indicates the dose that produced the steady-state concentration the patient is currently receiving,

and new denotes the dose necessary to produce the desired steady-state concentration.
- The advantages of this method are that it is quick and simple.
- The disadvantages are that steady-state concentrations are required, and the assumption of linear pharmacokinetics may not be valid in all patients.
  - When steady-state serum concentrations increase more than expected after a dosage increase or decrease less than expected after a dosage decrease, nonlinear theophylline pharmacokinetics is a possible explanation for the observation.
  - Therefore, suggested dosage increases greater than 75% using this method should be scrutinized by the prescribing clinician, and the risk versus benefit for the patient assessed before initiating large dosage increases (>75% over current dose).

▶ *Example 1*   LK is a 50-year-old, 75-kg (height 5′10″) male with chronic bronchitis who is receiving 300 mg of an oral sustained-release theophylline tablet every 8 hours. He smokes 2 packs of cigarettes daily, and has normal liver and cardiac function. His current steady-state theophylline concentration is 8 µg/ml. Compute a theophylline dose that will provide a steady-state concentration of 12 µg/ml.

1. *Compute new dose to achieve desired serum concentration.* The patient smokes tobacco-containing cigarettes and can be expected to achieve steady-state conditions after the first day ($5t_{1/2} = 5 \cdot 5$ h $= 25$ h) of therapy. Using linear pharmacokinetics, the new dose to attain the desired concentration should be proportional to the old dose that produced the measured concentration (total daily dose = 300 mg/dose $\cdot$ 3 doses/d = 900 mg/d):

$$D_{new} = (Css_{new}/Css_{old})D_{old}$$
$$= [(12 \text{ µg/ml})/(8 \text{ µg/ml})](900 \text{ mg/d}) = 1350 \text{ mg/d}$$

The new suggested dose is 1350 mg/d or 450 mg of sustained-release theophylline tablets every 8 hours, to be started at the next scheduled dosing time.

   A steady-state trough theophylline serum concentration should be measured after steady state is attained in 3–5 half-lives. Since the drug is expected to have a half-life of 5 hours, a theophylline steady-state concentration can be obtained at any time after the first day of dosing (5 half-lives = $5 \cdot 5$ h $= 25$ h). Theophylline serum concentrations should also be measured if the patient experiences an exacerbation of lung disease, or if the patient develops potential signs or symptoms of theophylline toxicity.

▶ *Example 2*   OI is a 60-year-old, 85-kg (height 6′1″) male with emphysema who is receiving 200 mg of an oral sustained-release theophylline tablet every 12 hours. He has liver cirrhosis (Child-Pugh score = 11) and normal cardiac function. His current steady-state theophylline concentration is 15 µg/ml, and he is experiencing some minor caffeine-type adverse effects (insomnia, jitteriness, nausea). Compute a theophylline dose that will provide a steady-state concentration of 10 µg/ml.

1. *Compute new dose to achieve desired serum concentration.* The patient has severe liver disease and can be expected to achieve steady-state conditions after 5 days ($5t_{1/2} = 5 \cdot 24$ h $= 120$ h or 5 d) of therapy. Using linear pharmacokinetics, the new dose to attain the desired concentration

should be proportional to the old dose that produced the measured concentration (total daily dose = 200 mg/dose $\cdot$ 2 doses/d = 400 mg/d):

$$D_{new} = (Css_{new}/Css_{old})D_{old}$$
$$= [(10 \ \mu g/ml)/(15 \ \mu g/ml)](400 \ mg/d) = 267 \ mg/d$$

The new suggested dose is 267 mg/d or 134 mg every 12 hours, rounded to 150 mg of sustained-release theophylline tablets every 12 hours, to be started after withholding 1–2 doses and until adverse effects have subsided.

A steady-state trough theophylline serum concentration should be measured after steady state is attained in 3–5 half-lives. Since the drug is expected to have a half-life of 24 hours, a theophylline steady-state concentration can be obtained at any time after the fifth day of dosing (5 half-lives = 5 $\cdot$ 24 h = 120 h or 5 days). Theophylline serum concentrations should also be measured if the patient experiences an exacerbation of lung disease, or if the patient develops potential signs or symptoms of theophylline toxicity.

• To illustrate the differences and similarities between oral and intravenous theophylline dosage regimen design, the same cases will be used to compute altered intravenous theophylline continuous infusions using steady-state serum concentrations.

▸ ***Example 3*** LK is a 50-year-old, 75-kg (height 5′10″) male with chronic bronchitis who is receiving an aminophylline constant intravenous infusion at a rate of 50 mg/h. He smokes 2 packs of cigarettes daily, and has normal liver and cardiac function. His current steady-state theophylline concentration is 8 μg/ml. Compute an aminophylline infusion rate that will provide a steady-state concentration of 12 μg/ml.

1. *Compute new dose to achieve desired serum concentration.* The patient smokes tobacco-containing cigarettes and can be expected to achieve steady-state conditions after the first day (5t$_{1/2}$ = 5 $\cdot$ 5 h = 25 h) of therapy. Using linear pharmacokinetics, the new infusion rate to attain the desired concentration should be proportional to the old infusion rate that produced the measured concentration:

$$D_{new} = (Css_{new}/Css_{old})D_{old}$$
$$= [(12 \ \mu g/ml)/(8 \ \mu g/ml)](50 \ mg/h) = 75 \ mg/h$$

The new suggested infusion rate is 75 mg/h of aminophylline.

A steady-state theophylline serum concentration should be measured after steady state is attained in 3–5 half-lives. Since the drug is expected to have a half-life of 5 hours, a theophylline steady-state concentration can be obtained at any time after the first day of dosing (5 half-lives = 5 $\cdot$ 5 h = 25 h). Theophylline serum concentrations should also be measured if the patient experiences an exacerbation of lung disease, or if the patient develops potential signs or symptoms of theophylline toxicity.

▸ ***Example 4*** OI is a 60-year-old, 85-kg (height 6′1″) male with emphysema who is receiving a 20-mg/h continuous infusion of theophylline. He has liver cirrhosis (Child-Pugh score = 11) and normal cardiac function. His current steady-state theophylline concentration is 15 μg/ml, and he is experiencing some minor caffeine-type adverse effects (insomnia, jitteriness, nausea). Compute a theophylline dose that will provide a steady-state concentration of 10 μg/ml.

1. *Compute new dose to achieve desired serum concentration.* The patient has severe liver disease and can be expected to achieve steady-state conditions after 5 days ($5t_{1/2} = 5 \cdot 24$ h = 120 h or 5 d) of therapy. Using linear pharmacokinetics, the new infusion rate to attain the desired concentration should be proportional to the old infusion rate that produced the measured concentration:

$$D_{new} = (Css_{new}/Css_{old})D_{old} = [(10 \text{ μg/ml})/(15 \text{ μg/ml})](20 \text{ mg/h})$$
$$= 13 \text{ mg/h, rounded to 15 mg/h}$$

The new suggested dose is 15 mg/h of theophylline as a continuous infusion. If necessary, the infusion can be stopped for 12–24 hours until the adverse effects of theophylline have subsided.

A steady-state trough theophylline serum concentration should be measured after steady state is attained in 3–5 half-lives. Since the drug is expected to have a half-life of 24 hours, a theophylline steady-state concentration can be obtained at any time after the fifth day of dosing (5 half-lives = $5 \cdot 24$ h = 120 h or 5 days). Theophylline serum concentrations should also be measured if the patient experiences an exacerbation of lung disease, or if the patient develops potential signs or symptoms of theophylline toxicity.

Pharmacokinetic Parameter Method

- The pharmacokinetic parameter method of adjusting drug doses was among the first techniques available to change doses using serum concentrations. It allows the computation of an individual's own, unique pharmacokinetic constants and uses those to calculate a dose that achieves desired theophylline concentrations.
- The pharmacokinetic parameter method requires that steady state has been achieved and uses only a steady-state theophylline concentration (Css).

  - During a continuous intravenous infusion, the following equation is used to compute theophylline clearance (Cl):

$$Cl = [S \cdot k_0]/Css$$

  where S is the fraction of the theophylline salt form that is active theophylline (S = 1 for theophylline, S = 0.80 for aminophylline dihydrate S = 0.85 for anhydrous aminophylline) and k_0 is the dose of theophylline salt in mg/h.
  - If the patient is receiving oral theophylline therapy, theophylline clearance (Cl) can be calculated using the following formula:

$$Cl = [F \cdot S(D/\tau)]/Css$$

  where F is the bioavailability fraction for the oral dosage form (F = 1 for most oral theophylline sustained-release products), S is the fraction of the theophylline salt form that is active theophylline (S = 1 for theophylline, S = 0.80 for aminophylline dihydrate, S = 0.85 for anhydrous aminophylline, S = 0.65 for oxtriphylline), D is the dose of theophylline salt in mg, Css is the steady-state theophylline concentration, and τ is the dosage interval in hours.

- Occasionally, theophylline serum concentrations are obtained before and after an intravenous loading dose. Assuming a one-compartment model, the volume of distribution (V) is calculated using the following equation:

$$V = (S \cdot D)/(C_{postdose} - C_{predose})$$

where S is the fraction of the theophylline salt form that is active theophylline (S = 1 for theophylline, S = 0.80 for aminophylline dihydrate, S = 0.85 for anhydrous aminophylline), D is the dose of theophylline salt in mg, $C_{postdose}$ is the post–loading dose concentration in mg/L, and $C_{predose}$ is the concentration before the loading dose was administered in mg/L (both concentrations should be obtained within 30–60 minutes of dosage administration).

- If the predose concentration was also a steady-state concentration, theophylline clearance can also be computed. If both clearance (Cl) and volume of distribution (V) have been measured using these techniques, the half-life $[t_{1/2} = (0.693 \cdot V)/Cl]$ and elimination rate constant $(k = 0.693/t_{1/2} = Cl/V)$ can be computed.

- The clearance, volume of distribution, elimination rate constant, and half-life measured using these techniques are the patient's own, unique theophylline pharmacokinetic constants and can be used in one-compartment-model equations to compute the required dose to achieve any desired serum concentration.

- Because this method also assumes linear pharmacokinetics, theophylline doses computed using the pharmacokinetic parameter method and the linear pharmacokinetic method should be identical.

▶ ***Example 1*** LK is a 50-year-old, 75-kg (height 5′10″) male with chronic bronchitis who is receiving 300 mg of an oral sustained-release theophylline tablet every 8 hours. He smokes 2 packs of cigarettes daily, and has normal liver and cardiac function. His current steady-state theophylline concentration is 8 μg/ml. Compute a theophylline dose that will provide a steady-state concentration of 12 μg/ml.

1. *Compute pharmacokinetic parameters.* The patient smokes tobacco-containing cigarettes and can be expected to achieve steady-state conditions after the first day $(5t_{1/2} = 5 \cdot 5 \text{ h} = 25 \text{ h})$ of therapy. Theophylline clearance can be computed using a steady-state theophylline concentration:

$$Cl = [F \cdot S(D/\tau)]/Css = [1 \cdot 1(300 \text{ mg/8 h})]/(8 \text{ mg/L}) = 4.69 \text{ L/h}$$

(*Note:* μg/ml = mg/L, and this concentration unit was substituted for Css in the calculation so that unit conversion was not required.)

2. *Compute theophylline dose.* Theophylline clearance is used to compute the new dose:

$$D = (Css \cdot Cl \cdot \tau)/(F \cdot S) = (12 \text{ mg/L} \cdot 4.69 \text{ L/h} \cdot 8 \text{ h})/(1 \cdot 1)$$
$$= 450 \text{ mg every 8 h}$$

The new theophylline dosage regimen should be instituted at the next dosage time.

A steady-state trough theophylline serum concentration should be measured after steady state is attained in 3–5 half-lives. Since the drug is expected to have a half-life of 5 hours, a theophylline steady-state concentration can be obtained at any time after the first day of dosing (5 half-lives = 5 · 5 h = 25 h). Theophylline serum concentrations should also be measured if the patient experiences an exacerbation of lung disease, or if the patient develops potential signs or symptoms of theophylline toxicity.

▶ *Example 2*   OI is a 60-year-old, 85-kg (height 6′1″) male with emphysema who is receiving 200 mg of an oral sustained-release theophylline tablet every 12 hours. He has liver cirrhosis (Child-Pugh score = 11) and normal cardiac function. His current steady-state theophylline concentration is 15 μg/ml, and he is experiencing some minor caffeine-type adverse effects (insomnia, jitteriness, nausea). Compute a theophylline dose that will provide a steady-state concentration of 10 μg/ml.

1. *Compute pharmacokinetic parameters.* The patient has severe liver disease and can be expected to achieve steady-state conditions after 5 days $(5t_{1/2} = 5 \cdot 24 \text{ h} = 120 \text{ h or } 5 \text{ d})$ of therapy. Theophylline clearance can be computed using a steady-state theophylline concentration:

$$Cl = [F \cdot S(D/\tau)]/Css = [1 \cdot 1(200 \text{ mg}/12 \text{ h})]/(15 \text{ mg/L}) = 1.11 \text{ L/h}$$

(*Note:* μg/ml = mg/L, and this concentration unit was substituted for Css in the calculation so that unit conversion was not required.)

2. *Compute theophylline dose.* Theophylline clearance is used to compute the new dose:

$$D = (Css \cdot Cl \cdot \tau)/(F \cdot S) = (10 \text{ mg/L} \cdot 1.11 \text{ L/h} \cdot 12 \text{ h})/(1 \cdot 1)$$
$$= 133 \text{ mg, rounded to } 150 \text{ mg every } 12 \text{ h}$$

The new theophylline dose should be started after withholding 1–2 doses until adverse effects have subsided.

A steady-state trough theophylline serum concentration should be measured after steady state is attained in 3–5 half-lives. Since the drug is expected to have a half-life of 24 hours, a theophylline steady-state concentration can be obtained at any time after the fifth day of dosing (5 half-lives = $5 \cdot 24 \text{ h} = 120 \text{ h or } 5 \text{ days}$). Theophylline serum concentrations should also be measured if the patient experiences an exacerbation of lung disease, or if the patient develops potential signs or symptoms of theophylline toxicity.

• To illustrate the differences and similarities between oral and intravenous theophylline dosage regimen design, the same cases will be used to compute altered intravenous theophylline continuous infusions using steady-state serum concentrations.

▶ *Example 3*   LK is a 50-year-old, 75-kg (height 5′10″) male with chronic bronchitis who is receiving an aminophylline constant intravenous infusion at a rate of 50 mg/h. He smokes 2 packs of cigarettes daily, and has normal liver and cardiac function. His current steady-state theophylline concentration is 8 μg/ml. Compute a aminophylline infusion rate that will provide a steady-state concentration of 12 μg/ml.

1. *Compute pharmacokinetic parameters.* The patient smokes tobacco-containing cigarettes and can be expected to achieve steady-state conditions after the first day $(5t_{1/2} = 5 \cdot 5 \text{ h} = 25 \text{ h})$ of therapy. Theophylline clearance can be computed using a steady-state theophylline concentration:

$$Cl = [S \cdot k_0]/Css = [0.8 \cdot 50 \text{ mg/h}]/(8 \text{ mg/L}) = 5 \text{ L/h}$$

(*Note:* μg/ml = mg/L, and this concentration unit was substituted for Css in the calculation so that unit conversion was not required.)

2. *Compute theophylline dose.* Theophylline clearance is used to compute the new aminophylline infusion rate:

$$k_0 = (Css \cdot Cl)/S = (12\ mg/L \cdot 5\ L/h)/(0.8) = 75\ mg/h$$

The new aminophylline infusion rate should be instituted immediately.

A steady-state theophylline serum concentration should be measured after steady state is attained in 3–5 half-lives. Since the drug is expected to have a half-life of 5 hours, a theophylline steady-state concentration can be obtained at any time after the first day of dosing (5 half-lives = $5 \cdot 5$ h = 25 h). Theophylline serum concentrations should also be measured if the patient experiences an exacerbation of lung disease, or if the patient develops potential signs or symptoms of theophylline toxicity.

▶ *Example 4* OI is a 60-year-old, 85-kg (height 6′1″) male with emphysema who is receiving a 20-mg/h continuous infusion of theophylline. He has liver cirrhosis (Child-Pugh score = 11) and normal cardiac function. His current steady-state theophylline concentration is 15 μg/ml, and he is experiencing some minor caffeine-type adverse effects (insomnia, jitteriness, nausea). Compute a theophylline dose that will provide a steady-state concentration of 10 μg/ml.

1. *Compute pharmacokinetic parameters.* The patient has severe liver disease and can be expected to achieve steady-state conditions after 5 days ($5t_{1/2} = 5 \cdot 24$ h = 120 h or 5 d) of therapy. Theophylline clearance can be computed using a steady-state theophylline concentration:

$$Cl = [S \cdot k_0]/Css = [1 \cdot 20\ mg/h]/(15\ mg/L) = 1.33\ L/h$$

(*Note:* μg/ml = mg/L, and this concentration unit was substituted for Css in the calculation so that unit conversion was not required.)

2. *Compute theophylline dose.* Theophylline clearance is used to compute the new theophylline infusion rate:

$$k_0 = (Css \cdot Cl)/S = (10\ mg/L \cdot 1.33\ L/h)/(1)$$
$$= 13\ mg/h, \text{ rounded to } 15\ mg/h$$

The new suggested theophylline dose is 15 mg/h of theophylline as a continuous infusion. If necessary, the infusion can be stopped for 12–24 hours until theophylline adverse effects have subsided.

A steady-state theophylline serum concentration should be measured after steady state is attained in 3–5 half-lives. Since the drug is expected to have a half-life of 24 hours, a theophylline steady-state concentration can be obtained at any time after the fifth day of dosing (5 half-lives = $5 \cdot 24$ h = 120 h or 5 days). Theophylline serum concentrations should also be measured if the patient experiences an exacerbation of lung disease, or if the patient develops potential signs or symptoms of theophylline toxicity.

▶ *Example 5* PP is a 59-year-old, 65-kg (height 5′8″) male with emphysema who is receiving an aminophylline constant intravenous infusion at a rate of 15 mg/h. He smokes 2 packs of cigarettes daily and has normal liver function. However, he also has heart failure (NYHA CHF class IV). His current steady-state theophylline concentration is 6 μg/ml. Compute a aminophylline infusion rate that will provide a steady-state concentration of 10 μg/ml. In addition, in an attempt to boost theophylline concentrations as soon as possible, an intravenous aminophylline bolus of 300 mg over 30 minutes was given before the infusion rate was increased. The patient's theophylline serum concentration after the additional bolus dose was 12 μg/ml.

1. *Compute pharmacokinetic parameters.* The patient has severe heart failure and can be expected to achieve steady-state conditions after 5 days ($5t_{1/2} = 5 \cdot 24$ h $= 120$ h or 5 d) of therapy. Theophylline clearance can be computed using a steady-state theophylline concentration:

$$Cl = [S \cdot k_0]/Css = [0.8 \cdot 15 \text{ mg/h}]/(6 \text{ mg/L}) = 2 \text{ L/h}$$

(*Note:* μg/ml = mg/L, and this concentration unit was substituted for Css in the calculation so that unit conversion was not required.)

Theophylline volume of distribution can be computed using the pre–bolus dose (Css = 6 μg/ml) and post–bolus dose concentrations:

$$V = (S \cdot D)/(C_{postdose} - C_{predose}) = (0.8 \cdot 300 \text{ mg})/(12 \text{ mg/L} - 6 \text{ mg/L})$$
$$= 40 \text{ L}$$

(*Note:* μg/ml = mg/L, and this concentration unit was substituted for Css in the calculation so that unit conversion was not required.)

Theophylline half-life ($t_{1/2}$) and elimination rate constant (k) can also be computed:

$$t_{1/2} = (0.693 \cdot V)/Cl = (0.693 \cdot 40 \text{ L})/(2 \text{ L/h}) = 14 \text{ h}$$
$$k = Cl/V = (2 \text{ L/h})/(40 \text{ L}) = 0.05 \text{ h}^{-1}$$

2. *Compute theophylline dose.* Theophylline clearance is used to compute the new aminophylline infusion rate:

$$k_0 = (Css \cdot Cl)/S = (10 \text{ mg/L} \cdot 2 \text{ L/h})/(0.8) = 25 \text{ mg/h}$$

The new aminophylline infusion rate should be instituted immediately after the additional loading dose is given.

A theophylline serum concentration should be measured after steady state is attained in 3–5 half-lives. Since the drug has a half-life of 14 hours, a theophylline steady-state concentration can be obtained after 3 days of continuous dosing (5 half-lives = $5 \cdot 14$ h = 70 h). Theophylline serum concentrations should also be measured if the patient experiences an exacerbation of lung disease, or if the patient develops potential signs or symptoms of theophylline toxicity.

CHIOU METHOD

- For some patients it is desirable to individualize theophylline infusion rates as rapidly as possible, before steady state is achieved. Examples of these cases include patients with heart failure or hepatic cirrhosis, who have variable theophylline pharmacokinetic parameters and long theophylline half-lives.
- Two theophylline serum concentrations obtained at least 4–6 hours apart during a continuous infusion can be used to compute theophylline clearance and dosing rates.[62–64]

- It is essential that the only way theophylline can be entering the patient's body is via the intravenous infusion. Thus, the last dose of sustained-release theophylline must have been administered no less than 12–16 hours before this technique is used, or some residual oral theophylline will still be absorbed from the gastrointestinal tract and cause computation errors.
- The following equation is used to compute theophylline clearance (Cl) using the two theophylline serum concentrations:

$$Cl = \frac{2 \cdot S \cdot k_0}{C_1 + C_2} + \frac{2V(C_1 - C_2)}{(C_1 + C_2)(t_2 - t_1)}$$

where S is the fraction of the theophylline salt form that is active theophylline (S = 1 for theophylline, S = 0.80 for aminophylline dihydrate, S = 0.85 for anhydrous aminophylline), k_0 is the infusion rate of the theophylline salt, V is theophylline volume of distribution (assumed to equal 0.5 L/kg; use ideal body weight for obese patients >30% overweight), C_1 and C_2 are the first and second theophylline serum concentrations, and t_1 and t_2 are the times at which C_1 and C_2 were obtained.
- Once theophylline clearance (Cl) is determined, it can be used to adjust the theophylline salt infusion rate (k_0) using the following relationship:

$$k_0 = (Css \cdot Cl)/S$$

where S is the fraction of the theophylline salt form that is active theophylline (S = 1 for theophylline, S = 0.80 for aminophylline dihydrate, S = 0.85 for anhydrous aminophylline).

▶ **Example 1** JB is a 50-year-old, 60-kg (5′7″) male with heart failure (NYHA CHF class III) who was started on a 50-mg/h aminophylline infusion after being administered an intravenous loading dose. His theophylline concentrations were 15.6 µg/ml at 1000 H and 18.3 µg/ml at 1400 H. What aminophylline infusion rate is needed to achieve Css = 15 µg/ml?

1. *Compute theophylline clearance and dose.*

$$Cl = \frac{2 \cdot S \cdot k_0}{C_1 + C_2} + \frac{2V(C_1 - C_2)}{(C_1 + C_2)(t_2 - t_1)}$$

$$Cl = \frac{2[0.8(50\,\text{mg/h})]}{15.6\,\text{mg/L} + 18.3\,\text{mg/L}} + \frac{2(0.5\,\text{L/kg} \cdot 60\,\text{kg})(15.6\,\text{mg/L} - 18.3\,\text{mg/L})}{(15.6\,\text{mg/L} + 18.3\,\text{mg/L})(4\,\text{h})}$$

$$= 1.17\,\text{L/h}$$

(*Note:* µg/ml = mg/L, and this concentration unit was substituted for concentrations so that unnecessary unit conversion was not required. Also, the time difference between t_2 and t_1 was determined and input directly into the equation.)

$$k_0 = (Css \cdot Cl)/S = (15\,\text{mg/L} \cdot 1.17\,\text{L/h})/0.8$$

$$= 22\,\text{mg/h, rounded to 20 mg/h of aminophylline}$$

▶ **Example 2** YU is a 64-year-old, 80-kg (5′9″) male with COPD who smokes $1\frac{1}{2}$ packs of cigarettes per day. He was started on a 40-mg/h theophylline infusion after being administered an intravenous loading dose at

0900 H. His theophylline concentrations were 11.6 µg/ml at 1000 H and 8.1 µg/ml at 1600 H. What theophylline infusion rate is needed to achieve Css = 10 µg/ml?

1. *Compute theophylline clearance and dose.*

$$Cl = \frac{2 \cdot S \cdot k_0}{C_1 + C_2} + \frac{2V(C_1 - C_2)}{(C_1 + C_2)(t_2 - t_1)}$$

$$Cl = \frac{2[1(40\,mg/hr)]}{11.6\,mg/L + 8.1\,mg/L} + \frac{2(0.5\,L/kg \cdot 80\,kg)(11.6\,mg/L - 8.1\,mg/L)}{(11.6\,mg/L + 8.1\,mg/L)(6\,h)}$$

$$= 6.43\,L/h$$

(*Note:* µg/ml = mg/L, and this concentration unit was substituted for concentrations so that unit conversion was not required. Also, the time difference between t_2 and t_1 was determined and input directly into the equation.)

$$k_0 = (Css \cdot Cl)/S = (10\,mg/L \cdot 6.43\,L/h)/1$$
$$= 64\,mg/h,\ rounded\ to\ 65\,mg/h\ of\ theophylline$$

BAYESIAN PHARMACOKINETIC COMPUTER PROGRAMS

• Computer programs are available that can assist in the computation of pharmacokinetic parameters for patients. The most reliable computer programs use a nonlinear regression algorithm that incorporates components of Bayes' theorem. Nonlinear regression is a statistical technique that uses an iterative process to compute the best pharmacokinetic parameters for a concentration/time data set.

  • An advantage of this approach is that consistent dosage recommendations can be made when several different practitioners are involved in therapeutic drug monitoring programs. However, since simpler dosing methods work just as well for patients with stable pharmacokinetic parameters and steady-state drug concentrations, many clinicians reserve the use of computer programs for more difficult situations. Those situations include serum concentrations that are not at steady state, serum concentrations not obtained at the specific times needed to employ simpler methods, and unstable pharmacokinetic parameters.
  • When only a limited number of theophylline steady-state concentrations are available, Bayesian pharmacokinetic computer programs can be used to compute a complete patient pharmacokinetic profile that includes clearance, volume of distribution, and half-life.

• Many Bayesian pharmacokinetic computer programs are available, and most should provide answers similar to the program used in the following examples. The program used to solve problems in this book is DrugCalc, written by Dr. Dennis Mungall and available at his Internet web site (www.clinpharmacologist.bigstep.com/consumersurvey.html).[65]

▶ ***Example 1*** LK is a 50-year-old, 75-kg (height 5'10″) male with chronic bronchitis who is receiving 300 mg of an oral sustained-release theophylline tablet every 8 hours. He smokes 2 packs of cigarettes daily, and has normal liver (bilirubin = 0.7 mg/dl, albumin = 4.0 g/dl) and cardiac function. His current steady-state theophylline concentration is 8 μg/ml. Compute a theophylline dose that will provide a steady-state concentration of 12 μg/ml.

1. *Enter patient demographic, drug dosing, and serum concentration/time data into a Bayesian pharmacokinetic computer program.*

2. *Compute pharmacokinetic parameters for the patient using the computer program.* The pharmacokinetic parameters computed by the program are a volume of distribution of 37 L, a half-life of 5.9 hours, and a clearance of 4.33 L/h.

3. *Compute dose required to achieve desired theophylline serum concentrations.* The one-compartment-model first-order absorption equations used by the program to compute doses indicate that a dose of 450 mg every 8 hours will produce a steady-state theophylline concentration of 12 μg/ml. Using the linear pharmacokinetics and pharmacokinetic parameter methods described previously in the chapter produced the same answer for this patient.

▶ ***Example 2***   HJ is a 62-year-old, 87-kg (height 6′1″) male with emphysema who was given a new prescription for 300 mg of an oral sustained-release theophylline tablet every 12 hours. He has liver cirrhosis (Child-Pugh score = 12, bilirubin = 3.2 mg/dl, albumin = 2.5 g/dl) and normal cardiac function. The theophylline concentration after the sixth dose was 15 μg/ml, and he is experiencing some minor caffeine-type adverse effects (insomnia, jitteriness, nausea). Compute a theophylline dose that will provide a steady-state concentration of 10 μg/ml.

1. *Enter patient demographic, drug dosing, and serum concentration/time data into a Bayesian pharmacokinetic computer program.* In this patient case, it is unlikely that the patient is at steady state, so the linear pharmacokinetics method cannot be used.

2. *Compute pharmacokinetic parameters for the patient using the computer program.* The pharmacokinetic parameters computed by the program are a volume of distribution of 38 L, a half-life of 19 hours, and a clearance of 1.41 L/h.

3. *Compute dose required to achieve desired theophylline serum concentrations.* The one-compartment first-order absorption equations used by the program to compute doses indicate that a dose of 200 mg every 12 hours will produce a steady-state concentration of 11 μg/ml.

▶ ***Example 3***   JB is a 50-year-old, 60-kg (5′7″) male with heart failure (NYHA CHF class III) who was started on a 50-mg/h aminophylline infusion after being administered an intravenous loading dose of 500 mg of aminophylline over 20 minutes at 0800 H. His theophylline concentrations were 15.6 μg/ml at 1000 H and 18.3 μg/ml at 1400 H. What aminophylline infusion rate is needed to achieve Css = 15 μg/ml?

1. *Enter patient demographic, drug dosing, and serum concentration/time data into a Bayesian pharmacokinetic computer program.* In this patient case, it is unlikely that the patient is at steady state, so the linear pharmacokinetics method cannot be used. DrugCalc requires doses to be entered in terms of theophylline, so aminophylline doses must be converted to theophylline doses for entry into the program (LD = 500 mg aminophylline · 0.8 = 400 mg theophylline, k_0 = 50 mg/h aminophylline · 0.8 = 40 mg/h theophylline).

2. *Compute pharmacokinetic parameters for the patient using the computer program.* The pharmacokinetic parameters computed by the program are

a volume of distribution of 29 L, a half-life of 21 hours, and clearance of 0.98 L/h.

3. *Compute dose required to achieve desired theophylline serum concentrations.* The one-compartment-model intravenous infusion equations used by the program to compute doses indicate that a dose of aminophylline 20 mg/h will produce a steady-state concentration of 16 μg/ml. Using the Chiou method previously described in the chapter produced a comparable answer for this patient (20 mg/h to produce a steady-state concentration of 15 μg/ml).

DOSING STRATEGIES

- Initial dose and dosage adjustment techniques using serum concentrations can be used in any combination as long as the limitations of each method are observed.
- Some dosing schemes link together logically when considered according to their basic approaches or philosophies. Dosage strategies that follow similar pathways are given in Table 18-5.

USE OF THEOPHYLLINE BOOSTER DOSES TO IMMEDIATELY INCREASE SERUM CONCENTRATIONS

- If a patient has a subtherapeutic theophylline serum concentration in an acute situation, it may be desirable to increase the theophylline concentration as quickly as possible. In this setting, it is not acceptable simply to increase the maintenance dose and wait 3–5 half-lives for therapeutic serum concentrations to be established in the patient.
- A rational way to increase the serum concentrations rapidly is to administer a booster dose of theophylline, a process also known as "reloading" the patient with theophylline, computed using pharmacokinetic techniques.
- A modified loading-dose equation is used to accomplish computation of the booster dose (BD) which takes into account the current theophylline concentration present in the patient:

$$BD = [(C_{desired} - C_{actual})V]/S$$

where $C_{desired}$ is the desired theophylline concentration, C_{actual} is the actual current theophylline concentration for the patient, S is the fraction of the

TABLE 18-5 Dosing Strategies

Dosing approach/ philosophy	Initial dosing	Use of serum concentrations to alter doses
Pharmacokinetic parameter/ equations	Pharmacokinetic dosing method	Pharmacokinetic parameter method or Chiou method (IV infusion before steady state)
Literature-based/ concept	Literature-based recommended dosing method	Linear pharmacokinetics method
Computerized	Bayesian computer program	Bayesian computer program

theophylline salt form that is active theophylline (S = 1 for theophylline, S = 0.80 for aminophylline dihydrate, S = 0.85 for anhydrous aminophylline), and V is the volume of distribution for theophylline.

- If the volume of distribution for theophylline is known for the patient, it can be used in the calculation. However, this value is not usually known and is assumed to equal the population average of 0.5 L/kg (ideal body weight used for patients >30% overweight).

- Concurrent with the administration of the booster dose, the maintenance dose of theophylline is usually increased. Clinicians need to recognize that the administration of a booster dose does not alter the time required to achieve steady-state conditions when a new theophylline dosage rate is prescribed.

  - It still requires 3–5 half-lives to attain steady state when the dosage rate is changed. However, usually the difference between the post–booster dose theophylline concentration and the ultimate steady-state concentration is reduced by giving the extra dose of drug.

▶ *Example 1*   BN is a 22-year-old, 50-kg (height 5′2″) female with asthma who is receiving therapy with intravenous theophylline. She does not smoke cigarettes and has normal liver and cardiac function. After receiving an initial loading dose of aminophylline (300 mg) and a maintenance infusion of aminophylline of 20 mg/h for 16 hours, her theophylline concentration is measured at 5.6 μg/ml and her pulmonary function tests are worsening. Compute a booster dose of aminophylline to achieve a theophylline concentration of 10 μg/ml.

1. *Estimate volume of distribution according to disease states and conditions present in the patient.* For theophylline, the population average volume of distribution is 0.5 L/kg, and this value is used to estimate the parameter for the patient. The patient is not obese, so her actual body weight will be used in the computation:

$$V = 0.5 \text{ L/kg} \cdot 50 \text{ kg} = 25 \text{ L}$$

2. *Compute booster dose.* The booster dose is computed using the following equation:

$$BD = [(C_{desired} - C_{actual})V]/S = [(10 \text{ mg/L} - 5.6 \text{ mg/L})25 \text{ L}]/0.8$$

$$= 138 \text{ mg, rounded to 150 mg IV of aminophylline infused over 20–30 min}$$

(*Note:* μg/ml = mg/L, and this concentration unit was substituted for Css in the calculations so that unit conversion was not required.) If the maintenance dose is increased, it will take an additional 3–5 estimated half-lives for new steady-state conditions to be achieved. Theophylline serum concentrations should be measured at this time.

CONVERSION OF THEOPHYLLINE DOSES FROM INTRAVENOUS TO ORAL ROUTE OF ADMINISTRATION

- Occasionally there is a need to convert a patient stabilized on theophylline therapy from the oral route of administration to an equivalent continuous infusion or vice versa.[66] In general, oral theophylline dosage forms, including most sustained-release tablets and capsules, have a bioavailability of 1.

- Assuming that equal theophylline serum concentrations are desired, this makes conversion between the intravenous and oral routes of administration simple, since equivalent doses of drug (corrected for theophylline salt form) are prescribed:

$$k_0 = D_{po}/(24 \text{ h/d} \cdot S_{iv}) \quad \text{or} \quad D_{po} = S_{iv} \cdot k_0 \cdot 24 \text{ h/d}$$

where k_0 is the equivalent intravenous infusion rate for the theophylline salt in mg/h, D_{po} is the equivalent dose of oral theophylline in mg/d, and S_{iv} is the fraction of the intravenously administered theophylline salt form that is active theophylline.

▶ **Example 1**   JH is currently receiving 600 mg of oral sustained-release theophylline every 12 hours. She is responding well to therapy, has no adverse drug effects, and has a steady-state theophylline concentration of 14.7 μg/ml. Suggest an equivalent dose of aminophylline to be given as an intravenous infusion for this patient.

1. *Calculate equivalent intravenous dose of aminophylline.* The patient is currently receiving 600 mg every 12 hours, or 1200 mg/d (600 mg/dose · 2 doses/d = 1200 mg/d) of theophylline. The equivalent intravenous aminophylline dose is

$$k_0 = D_{po}/(24 \text{ h/d} \cdot S_{iv}) = (1200 \text{ mg/d})/(24 \text{ h/d} \cdot 0.8)$$
$$= 62.5 \text{ mg/h, rounded to 65 mg/h IV continuous infusion}$$

▶ **Example 2**   LK is currently receiving a continuous infusion of amino-phylline at the rate of 40 mg/h. He is responding well to therapy, has no adverse drug effects, and has a steady-state theophylline concentration of 11.3 μg/ml. Suggest an equivalent dose of sustained-release oral theophylline for this patient.

1. *Calculate equivalent oral dose of theophylline.* The patient is currently receiving 40 mg/h of intravenous aminophylline as a constant infusion. The equivalent oral sustained-release theophylline dose is

$$D_{po} = S_{iv} \cdot k_0 \cdot 24 \text{ h/d} = 0.8 \cdot 40 \text{ mg/h} \cdot 24 \text{ h/d}$$
$$= 768 \text{ mg/d, rounded to 800 mg/d}$$

The patient should be prescribed 400 mg of sustained-release theophylline tablets orally every 12 hours.

REMOVAL OF THEOPHYLLINE BODY STORES IN MANAGEMENT OF THEOPHYLLINE OVERDOSE

- In addition to supportive care, treatment of seizures with anticonvulsant agents, and treatment of cardiac arrhythmias with antiarrhythmic agents, removal of theophylline from the body should be considered in cases of acute or chronic overdose.[60]

  - Extracorporeal methods to remove theophylline in emergency situations include hemodialysis[49–54] and charcoal hemoperfusion.[67,68]

    - Hemoperfusion is a technique similar to hemodialysis except the blood is passed through a column of activated charcoal instead of through an artificial kidney.

- Charcoal hemoperfusion is very effective in removing theophylline from the blood, with an extraction ratio across the column in excess of 90%, but theophylline serum concentrations can rebound 5–10 µg/ml upon discontinuation of the procedure as theophylline in the tissues comes into equilibrium with the blood.[67,68]
- Theophylline serum concentrations should be closely monitored when charcoal hemoperfusion is instituted.
- Other complications of charcoal hemoperfusion include hypotension, hypocalcemia, platelet consumption, and bleeding.

- Theophylline can also be removed from the body using oral doses of activated charcoal.[69,70] This method to reduce theophylline body stores is about as effective as hemodialysis removal.

- Activated charcoal physically adsorbs theophylline, rendering it nonabsorbable from the gastrointestinal tract.
- If the patient is vomiting, appropriate antiemetic therapy must be instituted so that the charcoal is retained in the stomach. Phenothiazine antiemetics should be avoided, as they may decrease the seizure threshold.
- In an acute theophylline overdose, oral activated charcoal (0.5 g/kg up to 20 g, repeated at least once in 1–2 hours) will bind theophylline that has not yet been absorbed and hold it in the gastrointestinal tract.
- Oral activated charcoal will also enhance the clearance of theophylline by binding theophylline secreted in gastrointestinal juices and eliminating the drug in the stool.
- When used in this fashion, oral activated charcoal (0.5 g/kg up to 20 g) is given every 2 hours. In both cases, a dose of oral sorbitol should be given to hasten the removal of charcoal-bound theophylline from the intestine.

- After acute and chronic theophylline overdoses, a single dose of oral activated charcoal is recommended if the theophylline serum concentration is 20–30 µg/ml.
- For theophylline serum concentrations >30 µg/ml, multiple doses of oral activated charcoal should be used.

- Patients should be monitored for signs and symptoms of theophylline toxicity and treated appropriately. Theophylline serum concentrations should be measured every 2–4 hours in order to guide further therapy.

REFERENCES

1. Undem BJ, Lichtenstein LM. Drugs used in the treatment of asthma. In: Hardman JG, Limbird LE, Gillman AG, eds. The pharmacologic basis of therapeutics. 10th ed. New York: McGraw-Hill, 2001:733–54.
2. Report NEP. Guidelines for the diagnosis and management of asthma—update on selected topics 2002. 2nd ed. Bethesda, MD: National Institutes of Health, 2002.
3. Weinberger M, Hendeles L. Drug therapy: theophylline in asthma. N Engl J Med 1996;334(21):1380–8.
4. Kelly HW, Sorkness CA. Asthma. In: DiPiro JT, Talbert RL, Yee GC, Matzke GR, Wells BG, Posey LM, eds. Pharmacotherapy. 5th ed. New York: McGraw-Hill, 2002:475–510.
5. Konzem SL, Stratton MA. Chronic obstructive lung disease. In: DiPiro JT, Talbert RL, Yee GC, Matzke GR, Wells BG, Posey LM, eds. Pharmacotherapy. 5th ed. New York: McGraw-Hill, 2002:511–30.
6. Chang KC, Bell TD, Lauer BA, Chai H. Altered theophylline pharmacokinetics during acute respiratory viral illness. Lancet 1978;1(8074):1132–3.

7. Koren G, Greenwald M. Decreased theophylline clearance causing toxicity in children during viral epidemics. J Asthma 1985;22(2):75–9.
8. Levy G, Koysooko R. Renal clearance of theophylline in man. J Clin Pharmacol 1976;16(7):329–32.
9. Bauer LA, Bauer SP, Blouin RA. The effect of acute and chronic renal failure on theophylline clearance. J Clin Pharmacol 1982;22(1):65–8.
10. Sarrazin E, Hendeles L, Weinberger M, Muir K, Riegelman S. Dose-dependent kinetics for theophylline: observations among ambulatory asthmatic children. J Pediatr 1980;97(5):825–8.
11. Weinberger M, Ginchansky E. Dose-dependent kinetics of theophylline disposition in asthmatic children. J Pediatr 1977;91(5):820–4.
12. Tang-Liu DD, Williams RL, Riegelman S. Nonlinear theophylline elimination. Clin Pharmacol Ther 1982;31(3):358–69.
13. Vallner JJ, Speir WA Jr, Kolbeck RC, Harrison GN, Bransome ED, Jr. Effect of pH on the binding of theophylline to serum proteins. Am Rev Respir Dis 1979;120(1):83–6.
14. Shaw LM, Fields L, Mayock R. Factors influencing theophylline serum protein binding. Clin Pharmacol Ther 1982;32(4):490–6.
15. Hunt SN, Jusko WJ, Yurchak AM. Effect of smoking on theophylline disposition. Clin Pharmacol Ther 1976;19(5 Pt 1):546–51.
16. Jusko WJ, Gardner MJ, Mangione A, Schentag JJ, Koup JR, Vance JW. Factors affecting theophylline clearances: age, tobacco, marijuana, cirrhosis, congestive heart failure, obesity, oral contraceptives, benzodiazepines, barbiturates, and ethanol. J Pharm Sci 1979;68(11):1358–66.
17. Jusko WJ, Schentag JJ, Clark JH, Gardner M, Yurchak AM. Enhanced biotransformation of theophylline in marihuana and tobacco smokers. Clin Pharmacol Ther 1978;24(4):405–10.
18. Jenne H, Nagasawa H, McHugh R, MacDonald F, Wyse E. Decreased theophylline half-life in cigarette smokers. Life Sci 1975;17(2):195–8.
19. Grygiel JJ, Birkett DJ. Cigarette smoking and theophylline clearance and metabolism. Clin Pharmacol Ther 1981;30(4):491–6.
20. Powell JR, Thiercelin JF, Vozeh S, Sansom L, Riegelman S. The influence of cigarette smoking and sex on theophylline disposition. Am Rev Respir Dis 1977;116(1):17–23.
21. Lee BL, Benowitz NL, Jacob Pd. Cigarette abstinence, nicotine gum, and theophylline disposition. Ann Intern Med 1987;106(4):553–5.
22. Matsunga SK, Plezia PM, Karol MD, Katz MD, Camilli AE, Benowitz NL. Effects of passive smoking on theophylline clearance. Clin Pharmacol Ther 1989;46(4):399–407.
23. Mangione A, Imhoff TE, Lee RV, Shum LY, Jusko WJ. Pharmacokinetics of theophylline in hepatic disease. Chest 1978;73(5):616–22.
24. Staib AH, Schuppan D, Lissner R, Zilly W, von Bomhard G, Richter E. Pharmacokinetics and metabolism of theophylline in patients with liver diseases. Int J Clin Pharmacol Ther Toxicol 1980;18(11):500–2.
25. Piafsky KM, Sitar DS, Rangno RE, Ogilvie RI. Theophylline disposition in patients with hepatic cirrhosis. N Engl J Med 1977;296(26):1495–7.
26. Piafsky KM, Sitar DS, Rangno RE, Ogilvie RI. Theophylline kinetics in acute pulmonary edema. Clin Pharmacol Ther 1977;21(3):310–6.
27. Vicuna N, McNay JL, Ludden TM, Schwertner H. Impaired theophylline clearance in patients with cor pulmonale. Br J Clin Pharmacol 1979;7(1):33–7.
28. Jenne JW, Chick TW, Miller BA, Strickland RD. Apparent theophylline half-life fluctuations during treatment of acute left ventricular failure. Am J Hosp Pharm 1977;34(4):408–9.
29. Powell JR, Vozeh S, Hopewell P, Costello J, Sheiner LB, Riegelman S. Theophylline disposition in acutely ill hospitalized patients. The effect of smoking, heart failure, severe airway obstruction, and pneumonia. Am Rev Respir Dis 1978; 118(2):229–38.
30. Gal P, Jusko WJ, Yurchak AM, Franklin BA. Theophylline disposition in obesity. Clin Pharmacol Ther 1978;23(4):438–44.

31. Blouin RA, Elgert JF, Bauer LA. Theophylline clearance: effect of marked obesity. Clin Pharmacol Ther 1980;28(5):619–23.
32. Slaughter RL, Lanc RA. Theophylline clearance in obese patients in relation to smoking and congestive heart failure. Drug Intell Clin Pharm 1983;17(4):274–6.
33. Rohrbaugh TM, Danish M, Ragni MC, Yaffe SJ. The effect of obesity on apparent volume of distribution of theophylline. Pediatr Pharmacol 1982;2(1):75–83.
34. Hilligoss DM, Jusko WJ, Koup JR, Giacoia G. Factors affecting theophylline pharmacokinetics in premature infants with apnea. Dev Pharmacol Ther 1980;1(1):6–15.
35. Giacoia G, Jusko WJ, Menke J, Koup JR. Theophylline pharmacokinetics in premature infants with apnea. J Pediatr 1976;89(5):829–32.
36. Aranda JV, Sitar DS, Parsons WD, Loughnan PM, Neims AH. Pharmacokinetic aspects of theophylline in premature newborns. N Engl J Med 1976;295(8):413–6.
37. Rosen JP, Danish M, Ragni MC, Saccar CL, Yaffe SJ, Lecks HI. Theophylline pharmacokinetics in the young infant. Pediatrics 1979;64(2):248–51.
38. Simons FE, Simons KJ. Pharmacokinetics of theophylline in infancy. J Clin Pharmacol 1978;18(10):472–6.
39. Nassif EG, Weinberger MM, Shannon D, et al. Theophylline disposition in infancy. J Pediatr 1981;98(1):158–61.
40. Zaske DE, Miller KW, Strem EL, Austrian S, Johnson PB. Oral aminophylline therapy. Increased dosage requirements in children. JAMA 1977;237(14):1453–5.
41. Loughnan PM, Sitar DS, Ogilvie RI, Eisen A, Fox Z, Neims AH. Pharmacokinetic analysis of the disposition of intravenous theophylline in young children. J Pediatr 1976;88(5):874–9.
42. Ginchansky E, Weinberger M. Relationship of theophylline clearance to oral dosage in children with chronic asthma. J Pediatr 1977;91(4):655–60.
43. Bauer LA, Blouin RA. Influence of age on theophylline clearance in patients with chronic obstructive pulmonary disease. Clin Pharmacokinet 1981;6(6):469–74.
44. Antal EJ, Kramer PA, Mercik SA, Chapron DJ, Lawson IR. Theophylline pharmacokinetics in advanced age. Br J Clin Pharmacol 1981;12(5):637–45.
45. Cusack B, Kelly JG, Lavan J, Noel J, O'Malley K. Theophylline kinetics in relation to age: the importance of smoking. Br J Clin Pharmacol 1980;10(2):109–14.
46. Crowley JJ, Cusack BJ, Jue SG, Koup JR, Park BK, Vestal RE. Aging and drug interactions. II. Effect of phenytoin and smoking on the oxidation of theophylline and cortisol in healthy men. J Pharmacol Exp Ther 1988;245(2):513–23.
47. Nielsen-Kudsk F, Magnussen I, Jakobsen P. Pharmacokinetics of theophylline in ten elderly patients. Acta Pharmacol Toxicol (Copenh) 1978;42(3):226–34.
48. Pokrajac M, Simic D, Varagic VM. Pharmacokinetics of theophylline in hyperthyroid and hypothyroid patients with chronic obstructive pulmonary disease. Eur J Clin Pharmacol 1987;33(5):483–6.
49. Blouin RA, Bauer LA, Bustrack JA, Record KE, Bivins BA. Theophylline hemodialysis clearance. Ther Drug Monit 1980;2(3):221–3.
50. Slaughter RL, Green L, Kohli R. Hemodialysis clearance of theophylline. Ther Drug Monit 1982;4(2):191–3.
51. Levy G, Gibson TP, Whitman W, Procknal J. Hemodialysis clearance of theophylline. JAMA 1977;237(14):1466–7.
52. Lee CS, Peterson JC, Marbury TC. Comparative pharmacokinetics of theophylline in peritoneal dialysis and hemodialysis. J Clin Pharmacol 1983;23(7):274–80.
53. Lee CS, Marbury TC, Perrin JH, Fuller TJ. Hemodialysis of theophylline in uremic patients. J Clin Pharmacol 1979;19(4):219–26.
54. Kradjan WA, Martin TR, Delaney CJ, Blair AD, Cutler RE. Effect of hemodialysis on the pharmacokinetics of theophylline in chronic renal failure. Nephron 1982;32(1):40–4.
55. Golper TA. Update on drug sieving coefficients and dosing adjustments during continuous renal replacement therapies. Contrib Nephrol 2001(132):349–53.
56. Golper TA, Marx MA. Drug dosing adjustments during continuous renal replacement therapies. Kidney Int Suppl 1998;66:S165–8.

57. Hansten PD, Horn JR. Drug interactions analysis and management. Vancouver, WA: Applied Therapeutics, 1999.

58. Loi CM, Parker BM, Cusack BJ, Vestal RE. Aging and drug interactions. III. Individual and combined effects of cimetidine and cimetidine and ciprofloxacin on theophylline metabolism in healthy male and female nonsmokers. J Pharmacol Exp Ther 1997;280(2):627–37.

59. Nix DE, Di Cicco RA, Miller AK, et al. The effect of low-dose cimetidine (200 mg twice daily) on the pharmacokinetics of theophylline. J Clin Pharmacol 1999;39(8):855–65.

60. Hendeles L, Jenkins J, Temple R. Revised FDA labeling guideline for theophylline oral dosage forms [see comments]. Pharmacotherapy 1995;15(4):409–27.

61. Edwards DJ, Zarowitz BJ, Slaughter RL. Theophylline. In: Evans WE, Schentag JJ, Jusko WJ, Relling MV, eds. Applied Pharmacokinetics. 3rd ed. Vancouver, WA: Applied Therapeutics, 1992.

62. Anderson G, Koup J, Slaughter R, Edwards WD, Resman B, Hook E. Evaluation of two methods for estimating theophylline clearance prior to achieving steady state. Ther Drug Monit 1981;3(4):325–32.

63. Chiou WL, Gadalla MA, Peng GW. Method for the rapid estimation of the total body drug clearance and adjustment of dosage regimens in patients during a constant-rate intravenous infusion. J Pharmacokinet Biopharm 1978;6(2):135–51.

64. Pancorbo S, Davies S, Raymond JL. Use of a pharmacokinetic method for establishing doses of aminophylline to treat acute bronchospasm. Am J Hosp Pharm 1981;38(6):851–6.

65. Wandell M, Mungall D. Computer assisted drug interpretation and drug regimen optimization. Am Assoc Clin Chem 1984;6:1–11.

66. Stein GE, Haughey DB, Ross RJ, Vakoutis J. Conversion from intravenous to oral dosing using sustained-release theophylline tablets. Ann Pharmacother 1982;16:772–4.

67. Ehlers SM, Zaske DE, Sawchuk RJ. Massive theophylline overdose. Rapid elimination by charcoal hemoperfusion. JAMA 1978;240(5):474–5.

68. Russo ME. Management of theophylline intoxication with charcoal-column hemoperfusion. N Engl J Med 1979;300(1):24–6.

69. Sintek C, Hendeles L, Weinberger M. Inhibition of theophylline absorption by activated charcoal. J Pediatr 1979;94(2):314–6.

70. Davis R, Ellsworth A, Justus RE, Bauer LA. Reversal of theophylline toxicity using oral activated charcoal. J Fam Pract 1985;20(1):73–4.

71. Pugh RN, Murray-Lyon IM, Dawson JL, Pietroni MC, Williams R. Transection of the oesophagus for bleeding oesophageal varices. Br J Surg 1973;60(8):646–9.

72. Johnson JA, Parker RB, Patterson JH. Heart failure. In: DiPiro JT, Talbert RL, Yee GC, Matzke GR, Wells BG, Posey LM, eds. Pharmacotherapy—a pathophysiologic approach. 5th ed. New York: McGraw-Hill, 2002:185–218.

Index

Page numbers followed by italic *f* or *t* denote figures or tables, respectively.